Nishkarsh Gupta • Rohini Dattatri
Vinod Kumar • Sushma Bhatnagar
Editors

Problem Based Learning Discussions in Onco-Anesthesia and Onco-Critical Care

Springer

Editors
Nishkarsh Gupta
Department of Onco-anaesthesia &
Palliative Medicine, Dr BRA IRCH
All India Institute of Medical Sciences
New Delhi, Delhi, India

Rohini Dattatri
Department of Anaesthesia
Kasturba Medical College
Manipal, Karnataka, India

Vinod Kumar
Department of Anaesthesiology
University of Minnesota Medical School
Minneapolis, MN, USA

Sushma Bhatnagar
Department of Onco-anesthesia &
Palliative Medicine, Dr BRA IRCH
All India Institute of Medical Sciences
New Delhi, Delhi, India

ISBN 978-981-99-6338-6 ISBN 978-981-99-6339-3 (eBook)
https://doi.org/10.1007/978-981-99-6339-3

This Springer imprint is published by the registered company Springer Nature Singapore Pte Ltd.
The registered company address is: 152 Beach Road, #21-01/04 Gateway East, Singapore 189721, Singapore

Foreword

It is a pleasure and honour to write a foreword for the book entitled *Problem Based Learning Discussions in Onco-Anaesthesia and Onco-Critical Care* edited by Nishkarsh Gupta, Rohini Dattatri, Vinod Kumar and Sushma Bhatnagar.

In my 30 years of professional experience in the field of academic surgical oncology, I always felt the need for a dedicated sub-specialty of onco-anaesthesia exclusively dealing with patients undergoing cancer surgery. Patients undergoing onco-surgery have unique challenges due to host and tumour interactions affecting multiple organ systems. Cancer-associated cachexia, sarcopenia, chemotherapy-associated systemic affects cancer-associated metabolic and immunological derangements can profoundly influence intraoperative and postoperative outcomes of cancer patients and can also affect survival outcomes. A significant number of cancer surgeries are complex, challenging, long duration and need to be done on priority basis. Knowledge, experience and skills of anaesthesiologists are extremely important in managing complex cancer surgeries which can influence outcomes. Difficult intubations for advanced head and neck cancers, one lung ventilation for thoracic surgical patients, perioperative management of patients undergoing complex surgical procedures like CRS and HIPEC, microvascular reconstruction, major hepato-pancreatico-biliary resections are few examples highlighting the need for dedicated onco-anaesthesia services. In addition, anaesthesiologist also plays an important role in pain management and critical care. The perioperative care should focus on early return to the intended oncological therapy (RIOT). Recent research has shown that oncological outcomes could be affected based on pharmacological agents used and type of anaesthesia. There is a need for collaborative research between onco-surgeons and onco-anaesthesia fraternity to explore the complex interactions of anaesthesia and surgery on cancer outcomes.

This book provides a comprehensive insight into various domains of onco-anaesthesia field including preoperative assessment, pre-habilitation, perioperative challenges specific to procedure, fluid management, anaesthetic techniques, perioperative pain management, post-operative complications and oncological emergencies. I strongly feel that this book will be of immense value to anaesthesiologists pursuing a career in onco-anaesthesia and also to general anaesthesiologists handling cancer cases.

The team of authors led by Prof. Sushma Bhatnagar are pioneers in this field, and I was fortunate to be professionally associated with them and witness the establishment and growth of a new medical specialty "Onco-Anaesthesia". I wish them all the success and sincerely hope that they will achieve their professional objectives through this book.

Department of Surgical Oncology
BRA-IRCH and NCI, AIIMS,
New Delhi, India

Svs Deo

Contents

About the Editors

Nishkarsh Gupta (MD, DNB, MNAMS, PGCCHM, Fellowship in Palliative Medicine) is working as a Professor in the department of Onco-Anaesthesiology and Palliative Medicine at DR BRA IRCH, All India Institute of Medical Sciences, New Delhi. He is alumnus of Maulana Azad Medical College and a gold medallist. He is assistant editor of *Indian journal of Anaesthesia*, Section Editor *Indian Journal of Palliative Care* and on editorial board panel of various journal. He is the chief editor of the first SA edition of *Clinical Anesthesia by Barash* and *Understanding Anesthesia Equipment by Dorsh and Dorsh*. He is also an editor of five more books. He has numerous national and international publications in various reputed journals (more than 200) and authored several book chapters. He received *MK Dey Award*-2022 by Indian College of Anesthesiologists at Chandigarh. He also received 'Best Researcher Award' in 2021 by ISA, Varanasi and 'Best Reviewer Award' in ISACON, Ahmedabad apart from several other awards in the past. He is an instructor of various skill-based training programmes and has been faculty in several national and international conferences. He is involved in many research projects funded by AIIMS and national agencies like ICMR.

Rohini Dattatri MD, DM (Onco-anaesthesia) is working as Assistant Professor in the department of anaesthesiology, KMC Manipal. She completed her MD (Anaesthesia) from Karnataka Institute of Medical Sciences, Hubli and DM (Onco-anaesthesia) from IRCH, AIIMS, New Delhi. She has an avid interest in research and has publications national and international journals. She has many chapters to her credit as an author and co-author. It includes clinical anaesthesia by Barash (South Asian edition), understanding anaesthesia equipment by Dorsh and Dorsh (South Asia edition), critical care—bench to bedside, onco-critical care—an evidence-based approach, a complete guide to onco-anaesthesia, critical care and cancer pain. She is a good orator and bagged prizes in ISACON Guwahati, ISACON Shillong and YUVA ISACON.

Vinod Kumar is Professor in the department of onco-anaesthesia and palliative medicine at Dr BRA IRCH, All India Institute of Medical Sciences (AIIMS), New Delhi, India. He received his training in anaesthesia from PGIMER, Chandigarh, India. Dr Kumar has a teaching experience of 12 years and guides MD (Palliative medicine) and DM (Onco-anaesthesiology) residents for research. He has many publications in peer-reviewed national and international journals to his credit and has edited book on onco-critical care by Springer. Dr. Kumar is a reviewer for various national and international journals. He is a member of national anaesthesia, airway and palliative care societies. He is an invited faculty for various national and international conferences.

Sushma Bhatnagar (MD-Anaesthesiology and MSc in Palliative Medicine from Cardiff University, UK) is Chief, Dr BRA IRCH and Head, National Cancer Institute (NCI)-Jhajjar and Professor and Head, Department of Onco-Anaesthesia and Palliative Medicine, Dr BRA IRCH, AIIMS, New Delhi. She has teaching and research experience more than 30 years. She can be described as a real catalyst driving innovation in the medical field by *working towards development of the field of Pain and Palliative Care in India and the developing world.* At AIIMS New Delhi, she developed a *protocol to make 'Pain free AIIMS' and formulated the 'End of Life Care Policy'* to manage pain and distressing symptoms in patients *with a motto of pain-free dignity of life till the end.* She has started two courses at AIIMS, New Delhi - *MD, Palliative Medicine* and *DM, Onco-Anaesthesia.* She is also the Chief Coordinator of Cancer Treatment Centre Programme jointly organized by Lien Collaborative, Singapore, Asia Pacific Hospice Network, Singapore and AIIMS, New Delhi. She is president of Indian Association of Palliative Care. She is editor of books *Textbook of Oncoanesthesiology* (Springer) and *Freedom from Pain* (IK International House Pvt. Ltd., New Delhi). She has been involved in many research projects funded by ICMR, DRDO, Ayush ministry, etc. She has more than 300 publications in national and international journals. She was the chairperson of clinical services of COVID task force at NCI, Jhajjar, AIIMS, New Delhi during COVID-19 pandemic. She is advisory Member of International Association for the Study of Pain (IASP) Press Editorial Board.

1 Carcinoma Buccal Mucosa with Trismus Posted for Hemimandibulectomy and Free Flap Reconstruction

Riniki Sarma, Nishkarsh Gupta, and Anju Gupta

1.1 Introduction

Head and neck cancer includes cancers originating from mouth, nose, sinuses, and throat. They account for nine million new cases and four million deaths annually. The male:female ratio ranges from 2:1 to 4:1. In India the male incidence rate is 20 per 100,000. Mouth and tongue cancer are common in Indian males [1]. Smoking has been implicated as one of the major risk factor associated with head and neck cancers. Apart from that, tobacco chewing for long duration is also associated with squamous cell carcinoma of head and neck [2]. Other risk factors include alcohol, human papilloma virus (especially HPV 16 and squamous cell carcinoma of larynx), occupational exposure with nickel, lead and wood workers, diet rich in salted cured fish, etc. [3]. Carcinoma buccal mucosa is a common oral cancer in India due to widespread use of tobacco products. Most patients present at a later stage when the tumour growth starts hindering quality of life [4]. Treatment of choice in patients with oral cancer is surgery [5]. Presence of oral tumours poses significant threat to airway management that ranges from difficult mouth opening, decreased range of neck movement, loss of anatomical margins, etc. Concomitant use of radiotherapy further may lead to trismus, difficult mask ventilation, and even front of neck access [6]. Thus a multi-disciplinary approach with discussion among the onco-surgeons, plastic surgeon and anaesthesiologists about the proper steps of airway management plan is necessary.

Q. Why Preoperative Assessment in Carcinoma Buccal Mucosa Patients Is Important? How Is It Different from Other Cancer Patients?

1.2 Preoperative Assessment

Apart from cancer, these patients also may have a number of comorbidities as mostly they are aged [7]. So, the plan of anaesthesia should also take the comorbid conditions (COPD, hypertension, diabetes, coronary artery disease, etc.) as well as the age of the patient into consideration. Optimisation of the comorbid conditions should be done before taking the patient for surgery. Carcinoma buccal mucosa may also lead to poor dietary intake in these patients. Hence, nutritional optimisation is of paramount importance. Considerations for previous chemotherapy and radiotherapy should be given. During primary pre-anaesthetic check-up, a thorough physical examination, routine investigations and airway examination should be done. The airway anatomy may change at the time the patient

R. Sarma
Department of Anesthesiology, Pain and Critical Care, JPNATC, AIIMS, New Delhi, New Delhi, India

N. Gupta
Department of Onco-Anesthesiology and Palliative Medicine, DRBRAIRCH, AIIMS, New Delhi, New Delhi, India

A. Gupta (✉)
Department of Anesthesiology, Pain Medicine and Critical Care, AIIMS, New Delhi, New Delhi, India

N. Gupta et al. (eds.), *Problem Based Learning Discussions in Onco-Anesthesia and Onco-Critical Care*, https://doi.org/10.1007/978-981-99-6339-3_1

is scheduled for surgery and so plan of airway management should be discussed. Counselling regarding smoking cessation is to be started from the day of primary PAC. The patient should be counselled regarding postoperative facial disfigurement. Most of the patients present with increased anxiety and nervousness due to the nature of surgery; premedication is to be advised accordingly. Elderly patients with impending compromise of the airway should be given titrated dose of sedative premedications.

1.2.1 Implications of RT CT

Chemotherapy or radiotherapy exposure as part of treatment management is to be elicited as it may alter anaesthesia management. Although surgery is the primary mode of treatment in carcinoma buccal mucosa, radiotherapy is used either as post-operative adjuvant treatment or as definitive treatment in advanced cases with or without chemotherapy. Chemotherapy can be neo-adjuvant, adjuvant or palliative. Radiation results in oedema of the tissues followed by fibrosis or necrosis of that area. There can be pain due to radiation-induced mucositis. Lose teeth or missing teeth, purulent discharge from tumour site or oro-cutaneous fistula may render mask ventilation and laryngoscopy difficult. Fibrosis resulting in trismus, limited mouth opening or restriction of neck movements makes laryngoscopy and intubation difficult. Post-radiation epiglottic and glottic oedema makes visualisation of vocal cords difficult. Osteoradionecrosis of the jaw is a fatal complication of high-dose radiotherapy seen in 0.4–50% of patients [8]. It can cause reduction in mandibular space and alteration of morphometric measurements leading to difficult airway [9]. Apart from this, radiotherapy is associated with restrictive cardiomyopathy due to myo- and endocardial fibrosis. This is often dose-dependent.

Chemotherapy is mostly given to enhance response to radiotherapy. Commonly used chemotherapy agents are cisplatin, flurouracil, carboplatin, paclitaxel, methotrexate, etc. Bone marrow suppression caused by paclitaxel, docetaxel and methotrexate can lead to thrombocytopenia and neutropenia. Pulmonary toxicity due to paclitaxel or carboplatin can result in noncardiogenic pulmonary oedema, chronic pneumonitis, fibrosis and hypersensitivity pneumonitis [10]. Patients may present with cough, dyspnoea, low-grade fever with bibasal crepitus on examination. Chest X-ray may show ground glass opacities or consolidation. Pulmonary function tests may show decreased diffusion capacity for CO_2, total lung capacity and forced vital capacity. Anthracyclines are associated with dysrhythmias, decreased cardiac contractility and cardiomyopathy. Busulfan results in endocardial fibrosis. Cyclophosphamide causes myocardial tissue injury and doxorubicin results in prolonged QT interval. Clinically, the patient will present with arrhythmias, chest pain, congestive cardiac failure and signs of pericarditis [11]. Methotrexate causes diarrhoea, oral mucositis electrolyte imbalance and weight loss. Drugs like cisplatin and doxetacel are associated with CNS (central nervous system) toxicity.

1.3 Preoperative Investigations

All routine blood tests along with chest X-ray and ECG should be asked prior to surgery. Electrolyte abnormalities may be present in patients with carcinoma buccal mucosa with poor nutritional status. Head and neck cancer is also associated with hypercalcemia [12]. Liver function tests are essential to find out the effect of chemotherapy as well as nutritional status (serum albumin). Radiological investigations have gained prominence in predicting difficult airway management although no single parameter exists. Lateral view of soft tissue of the neck in X-rays can predict difficult airway. CT scan of the airway is more precise than X-rays and can evaluate airway narrowing and deviation of trachea. CT bronchoscopy and virtual bronchoscopy can reconstruct images comparable to real bronchoscopy. MRI can locate tracheobronchial invasion or compression by tumours and assist in airway planning. 3D printing can be used for simulating the patient's airway. It is a comparatively new technology and has only been used for complex airway management cases. Ultrasound of the airway is the most explored radiological entity and can provide real-time assessment [13–15].

1.4 Preoperative Nutritional Optimisation

Patients with carcinoma buccal mucosa suffer from nutritional deficiency not only due to cancer per se but the location of tumour results in poor oral intake as well as painful swallowing. Heavy smoking and drinking further contributes to additional barrier to good nutrition. Unintentional weight loss of >5–10% over 6 months and BMI <20 kg/m^2 is defined as malnutrition in head and neck cancer patients [16, 17]. Subjective global assessment of nutrition and more recently Nutritional Risk Score 2002 (NRS 2002) are used as screening tools in carcinoma buccal mucosa patients. Dietary counselling focuses on maintaining appropriate nutritional intake in patients undergoing chemoradiotherapy. European Society for Parenteral and Enteral Nutrition (ESPEN) and the American Society for Parenteral and Enteral Nutrition (ASPEN) guidelines recommend that ambulating patients with cancer receive 1.2–2 g/kg/day of protein and 30–35 kcal/kg/day of energy daily [18, 19]. It was found that patients maintaining this dietary intake had a better quality of life without the need for additional nutritional intervention [20]. Carcinoma buccal mucosa patients with chronic malnutrition with swallowing impairment and inadequate oral intake may need feeding tube placement. Prophylactic gastrostomy although advocated in some centres is not of much benefit [21]. Also the principle of carbohydrate loading preoperatively is followed in patients with carcinoma buccal mucosa. ERAS guidelines recommend 800 mL of 12.5% carbohydrate drink on the night before surgery and 400 mL on the morning of procedure [22, 23].

Q. How Will You Proceed to Manage the Airway in Such Cases? What Will Be Your Strategy in Case of Trismus?

1.5 Intraoperative Management

1.5.1 The Shared Airway

Clear communication is required between the operating team and anaesthetists. Securing the airway and maintaining it is challenging in the light of abnormal anatomy due to tumour as well as surgical exploration of the area. The surgeon requires complete access to the airway, without any disruption by presence of bulky equipments. Hence the anaesthetist is away from the head end and accessing the airway during emergency may become problematic. In patients undergoing repeated surgery, the anatomy may be distorted requiring extensive redissection and longer duration of surgery. All major society guidelines for difficult airway management emphasise on the use of a preplanned strategy for managing the airway with closed communication between anaesthetists and surgeons [24–26]. Prior consent from the patient should always be taken. At the same time, patients should be explained about the chances of failure of the planned procedure (plan A) and the need to fall back to rescue options (plan B, plan C, etc.).

Awake fibreoptic intubation is the plan of choice for most anaesthesiologists as it ensures that airway is not lost totally. But the preparation of the airway is of vital importance for awake intubation. DAS awake tracheal intubation guidelines emphasise on the ideal sedation, topicalisation and oxygenation techniques before actually performing the procedure [27]. Nasotracheal intubation is done so as to keep the oral airway free for surgeons to explore. A flexometallic tube is preferred as there is less kinking and compression as compared to a PVC tube [28]. After the airway is secured a throat pack is inserted to prevent blood and tissue debris from entering into the larynx and trachea. This can be inserted either by anaesthetists or operating surgeons [29]. The anaesthesiologist should also be proficient in other airway management techniques including intubation through supraglottic device, transtracheal jet ventilation, etc. as well as front of neck access should the need arise.

Q: What Will Be the Airway Management Plan in the Above Case Scenario?

1.6 Trismus

Trismus in oral cancer patients is mostly due to treatment related to the cancer or the tumour growth itself that causes tonic contraction of the muscles of mastication resulting in mouth opening less than 3.5 cm [30]. Trismus is a common side effect of head and neck cancer treatment. 38–42%

of people with carcinoma head and neck suffer from trismus. This occurs due to radiation-induced fibrosis of temporomandibular joint or muscles of mastication. Surgical procedures in that area may also result in restricted mouth opening [31].

1.6.1 Airway Management in Trismus

Trismus results in a state of difficult airway management. On the basis of mouth opening, trismus can be graded into mild, moderate or severe [31]. In trismus with mild grade where mouth opening is a possibility following muscle relaxation, a check laryngoscopy before giving relaxant can be done. In moderate to severe grade trismus awake fibreoptic intubation can be planned. If the anaesthetists are proficient a blind nasal intubation can be tried. Surgeons should always be on standby to perform tracheostomy whenever any emergency arises and the airway becomes endangered [32].

1.7 Intraoperative Monitoring

Apart from ASA standard monitors, invasive arterial blood pressure monitoring may be required if the patient has associated comorbidities. Arterial cannulas are to be avoided in the arm where radial forearm flap is planned. Urinary catheterisation is required as the surgery is of prolonged duration.

Q: What Are the Other Anaesthetic Concerns in This Case Apart from Difficult Airway?

1.8 Position of the Patient

The patient is placed in a reverse Trendelenburg position to prevent venous congestion, reduce blood loss and clear surgical fields. However, there is a chance of venous air embolism with such position and a close observation on the end-tidal CO_2 should be kept [33]. The arms are tucked to the side of the patient and adequate padding should be done to prevent peripheral nerve injury. The venous access in the upper limbs may be difficult to the arms being tucked away and need for extension tubings.

1.9 Perioperative Management Including ERAS

The ERAS guidelines for head and neck cancer can be summarised in the following points [23, 34]:

Preoperative phase:

1. Patients are given a diary that consists of steps at various time points before and after surgery.
2. Preoperative psychological optimisation by meeting with clinical psychologists and patients who have undergone similar procedure.
3. Patients are encouraged for preoperative exercises and nutritional optimisation.
4. Carbohydrate preloading before surgery.
5. Avoid long-acting sedative premedication.

Intraoperative phase:

1. Standard anaesthesia protocol to be followed.
2. Cardiac output monitoring for goal-directed fluid therapy.
3. Rationalisation on the use of tracheostomy.
4. Prevention of hypothermia, adequate analgesia and antibiotic prophylaxis are to be given.

Postoperative phase:

1. Early extubation plan.
2. Early ambulation.
3. Adequate analgesia.
4. Early oral feeding to be established as soon as possible after extubation.

Q: When Is Free Flap Done in Carcinoma Buccal Mucosa? What Are Its Anaesthetic Concerns? How Will You Monitor Flap Patency in the Postoperative Period?

1.10 Anaesthetic Considerations in Free Flap

Free flap reconstruction is required in surgeries with extensive defects. Here a neurovascular pedicle is removed from the donor site and transplanted into a new location via microvascular anastomosis. This gives rise to a secondary defect which is then repaired. Various donor sites for taking flap includes the radial/ulnar forearm, lattismus dorsi, rectus abdominis, etc. Since this is a microvascular surgery there are chances of failure. Factors resulting in graft failure include inadequate surgical anastomosis, flap oedema due to excess fluids, mechanical compression, vasospasm, thrombosis, excess flap manipulation, generalised vasoconstriction due to hypothermia, hypovolemia, pain, etc. [35]. The prime concern here is to maintain adequate blood supply to the anastomosis. The use of TIVA was associated with less hemodynamic fluctuations [36]. Analgesic management of flap site with epidural or continuous drug infusion catheter can be done. Regional anaesthesia results in sympathetic blockade and vasodilation leading to better flap outcomes. If heparin is used during flap reconstruction, careful monitoring is to be done before epidural removal. Free flap reconstruction procedure warrants the use of invasive arterial line for hemodynamic monitoring. Analgesia, glucose levels, blood loss and urine output should be monitored to prevent flap failure. The transfusion trigger should be maintained at a haematocrit level of 25% to prevent increase rate of blood transfusion [37]. Vasoconstrictors like noradrenaline use have been found to be beneficial in maintaining blood flow to the flap; use of intravenous dexmedetoidine has been found to have similar effect [38, 39].

1.10.1 Postoperative Flap Monitoring

Flaps should be monitored for 24 h postoperatively for any kind of vasospasm, oedema and signs of necrosis. Re-exploration may be required if signs of ischemia emerge Use of dexamethasone and mannitol along with head elevation has been found to decrease graft oedema [40]. Various techniques of flap viability monitoring include from simple clinical examination (colour of flap site, capillary refill, temperature monitoring, etc.) to use of Doppler to check vascular flow. PO_2 monitoring of flap site can also be done [41, 42].

1.11 Venous Thromboembolism Prophylaxis

The incidence of deep vein thrombosis (DVT) ranges from 15 to 30% in patients undergoing surgery without any prophylaxis. But the presence of cancer increases the risk to 40–80% [43]. Patients of head and neck cancer undergoing free flap reconstruction require VTE prophylaxis as they are at moderate to high risk for the same [44]. Pharmacologic prophylaxis in the form of low molecular weight heparin is the prophylaxis of choice here. There may be an increased risk for bleeding with simultaneous use of antiplatelets, and individualisation of prophylaxis is always better [23, 45].

1.12 Tracheostomy

Tracheostomy is not done preoperatively unless emergency as it can interfere with delineation of tumour anatomy and resection. Intraoperative tracheostomy is often performed at the end of the surgical procedure if mandibular resection crosses midline with excision of both genial tubercles that cause tongue fall, extensive palatal resection or buccal mucosa resection requiring a flap [46]. During change from endotracheal tube to tracheostomy, ventilation should be done with 100% oxygen and suctioning of oral cavity and ETT to be done before removal. Sometimes a J-shaped laryngectomy tube may be inserted through the tracheostomy and sutured to chest wall. Correct position of tracheostomy should be ascertained with end-tidal CO_2 monitoring and auscultation. Although it is a safe procedure, tracheostomy may increase hospital stay [47]. Decannulation and closure of stoma is done later with respiratory and swallowing rehabilitation. In most cases, patients can be safely decannulated within 1 week of surgery [23].

1.13 Extubation

Extubation in patients undergoing hemimandibulectomy for buccal mucosa cancer depends on various factors like duration of surgery, dissection during surgery, degree of oedema, etc. The patients are mostly kept intubated overnight in the intensive care unit to let the oedema subside and extubation attempted on the next morning. The extubation process like intubation should also be planned immaculately. Guidelines pertaining to extubation of the difficult airway should be followed [48, 49]. All equipments arranged for intubation purpose should be kept for extubation as well.

1.14 Criteria for ICU Admission in the Postoperative Perio

1. Elective mechanical ventilation.
2. Extensive resection with free flap reconstruction.
3. Intraoperative hemodynamic instability.
4. Elderly patients with comorbidities requiring monitoring.

Q: How Will You Manage Pain in This Case? If the Patient Was Already Taking Opioids Preoperatively, What Will Be Your Analgesia Management Plan?

1.15 Analgesia Management

Preemptive analgesia as part of multi-modal analgesia reduces postoperative pain. NSAIDs play a key role in pain management as the cancer pain in buccal mucosa tumour is inflammatory in nature [23]. Opioids as well as other adjuvants should be used together to decrease the cumulative dose of a single agent. Paracetamol should be given round the clock. Celecoxib can be added as it was found to have minimal effect on flap blood flow [50]. Use of COX-1 inhibitors has been found to be associated with surgical bleeding and should be individualised [51]. Use of patient-controlled analgesia (PCA) pumps with morphine or fentanyl has been found to be beneficial in the postoperative period [52]. Patients with severe cancer-related pain who are on opioids preoperatively with or without adjuvant therapy are difficult to treat in the perioperative period. It is imperative that these patients receive their usual dose of opioids before surgery and additional opioids can be administered intra- and postoperatively. Adequate adjuvants should be added in the postoperative period. Patients are to be monitored for signs of opioid withdrawal (hypertension, tachycardia, diaphoresis). According to FDA, an opioid-tolerant patient is one who receives: 60 mg/day oral morphine or transdermal fentanyl 25 mcg/h or oxycodone, hydromorphone, oxymorphone orally 30 mg/day, 8 mg/day. 25 mg/day respectively or any equianalgesic dose of other opioids for a period of at least 7 days. Patients who are opioid tolerant will require more opioid doses than opioid naïve patients [53]. The administration of opioids should be carefully titrated so as to decrease its side effects like respiratory depression, sedation, etc. while at the same time achieving its goal of adequate analgesia. Substituting a different opioid when one opioid is unable to provide adequate analgesia even with increase doses is called opioid rotation. This is mainly done in patients with opioid tolerance. Here, the new opioid is initially started at one-half to two-thirds equianalgesic dose and observed for side effects. Substituting a long acting opioid with a short acting one may result in precipitation of withdrawal symptoms [53, 54].

References

1. Global Cancer Observatory [Internet]. Cancer (IARC) TIA for R on. https://gco.iarc.fr/. Accessed 21 Jul 2022.
2. Argiris A, Karamouzis MV, Raben D, Ferris RL. Head and neck cancer. Lancet. 2008;371(9625):1695–709.
3. Moore SR, Johnson NW, Pierce AM, Wilson DF. The epidemiology of mouth cancer: a review of global incidence. Oral Dis. 2000;6(2):65–74.
4. Singhania V, Jayade BV, Anehosur V, Gopalkrishnan K, Kumar N. Carcinoma of buccal mucosa: a site specific clinical audit. Indian J Cancer. 2015;52(4):605.
5. Chi AC, Day TA, Neville BW. Oral cavity and oropharyngeal squamous cell carcinoma—an update. CA Cancer J Clin. 2015;65(5):401–21.

6. Sonowal DSJ. Anaesthetic considerations for head and neck cancers in patients undergoing reconstructive free flap surgeries—a review of 55 patients. Clin Med. 2020;7(2):8.
7. Tandon P, Dadhich A, Saluja H, Bawane S, Sachdeva S. The prevalence of squamous cell carcinoma in different sites of oral cavity at our Rural Health Care Centre in Loni, Maharashtra—a retrospective 10-year study. Contemp Oncol (Pozn). 2017;21(2):178–83.
8. Perrier M, Moeller P. Osteoradionecrosis. A review of the literature. Schweiz Monatsschr Zahnmed. 1994;104(3):271–7.
9. Balakrishnan M, Kuriakose R, Koshy RC. Radiation induced changes in the airway—anaesthetic implications. S Afr J Anaesth Analg. 2004;10(2):19–21.
10. Groenewold MD, Olthof CG, Bosch DJ. Anaesthesia after neoadjuvant chemotherapy, immunotherapy or radiotherapy. BJA Educ. 2022;22(1):12–9.
11. Pai VB, Nahata MC. Cardiotoxicity of chemotherapeutic agents: incidence, treatment and prevention. Drug Saf. 2000;22(4):263–302.
12. Liston SL. Hypercalcemia and head and neck cancer: bony metastases from tongue cancer. Arch Otolaryngol. 1978;104(10):597–600.
13. Jain K, Gupta N, Yadav M, Thulkar S, Bhatnagar S. Radiological evaluation of airway—what an anaesthesiologist needs to know! Indian J Anaesth. 2019;63(4):257–64.
14. Bhaskar SB. Newer airway assessment techniques: a view on their utility. Indian J Anaesth. 2017;61(10):779–81.
15. Kanaya N, Kawana S, Watanabe H, Niiyama Y, Niiya T, Nakayama M, et al. The utility of three-dimensional computed tomography in unanticipated difficult endotracheal intubation. Anesth Analg. 2000;91(3):752–4.
16. van den Berg MGA, Rasmussen-Conrad EL, van Nispen L, van Binsbergen JJ, Merkx MAW. A prospective study on malnutrition and quality of life in patients with head and neck cancer. Oral Oncol. 2008;44(9):830–7.
17. Nesemeier R, Dunlap N, McClave SA, Tennant P. Evidence-based support for nutrition therapy in head and neck cancer. Curr Surg Rep. 2017;5(8):18.
18. Arends J, Bachmann P, Baracos V, Barthelemy N, Bertz H, Bozzetti F, et al. ESPEN guidelines on nutrition in cancer patients. Clin Nutr. 2017;36(1):11–48.
19. August DA, Huhmann MB, American Society for Parenteral and Enteral Nutrition. A.S.P.E.N. clinical guidelines: nutrition support therapy during adult anticancer treatment and in hematopoietic cell transplantation. JPEN J Parenter Enteral Nutr. 2009;33(5):472–500. https://doi.org/10.1177/0148607109341804.
20. Roussel LM, Micault E, Peyronnet D, Blanchard D, Guarnieri S, Choussy O, et al. Intensive nutritional care for patients treated with radiotherapy in head and neck cancer: a randomized study and meta-analysis. Eur Arch Otorrinolaringol. 2017;274(2):977–87.
21. Ames JA, Karnell LH, Gupta AK, Coleman TC, Karnell MP, Van Daele DJ, et al. Outcomes after the use of gastrostomy tubes in patients whose head and neck cancer was managed with radiation therapy. Head Neck. 2011;33(5):638–44.
22. Lassen K, Soop M, Nygren J, Cox PBW, Hendry PO, Spies C, et al. Consensus review of optimal perioperative care in colorectal surgery: Enhanced Recovery After Surgery (ERAS) Group recommendations. Arch Surg. 2009;144(10):961–9.
23. Dort JC, Farwell DG, Findlay M, Huber GF, Kerr P, Shea-Budgell MA, et al. Optimal perioperative care in major head and neck cancer surgery with free flap reconstruction: a consensus review and recommendations from the enhanced recovery after surgery society. JAMA Otolaryngol Head Neck Surg. 2017;143(3):292–303.
24. Apfelbaum JL, Hagberg CA, Connis RT, Abdelmalak BB, Agarkar M, Dutton RP, et al. 2022 American Society of Anesthesiologists practice guidelines for management of the difficult airway*. Anesthesiology. 2022;136(1):31–81.
25. Myatra SN, Shah A, Kundra P, Patwa A, Ramkumar V, Divatia JV, et al. All India Difficult Airway Association 2016 guidelines for the management of unanticipated difficult tracheal intubation in adults. Indian J Anaesth. 2016;60(12):885–98.
26. Difficult Airway Society. DAS guidelines for management of unanticipated difficult intubation in adults 2015. https://das.uk.com/guidelines/das_intubation_guidelines. Accessed 6 Aug 2022.
27. Ahmad I, El-Boghdadly K, Bhagrath R, Hodzovic I, McNarry AF, Mir F, et al. Difficult Airway Society guidelines for awake tracheal intubation (ATI) in adults. Anaesthesia. 2020;75(4):509–28.
28. Garcha P, Sreevastava D, Singh S. Flexometallic endotracheal tube and nasal intubation. Med J Armed Forces India. 2000;56(1):88.
29. Gupta A, Sarma R, Gupta N, Kumar R. Current practices and beliefs regarding the use of oropharyngeal throat pack in India: a nationwide survey. Indian J Anaesth. 2021;65(3):241–7.
30. Agarwal P, Shiva Kumar HR, Rai KK. Trismus in oral cancer patients undergoing surgery and radiotherapy. J Oral Biol Craniofac Res. 2016;6(Suppl 1):S9–13.
31. Santiago-Rosado LM, Lewison CS. Trismus. In: StatPearls. Treasure Island (FL): StatPearls Publishing; 2022. http://www.ncbi.nlm.nih.gov/books/NBK493203/.
32. Kapre V. Anesthesia for surgery of trismus due to OSMF. In: Kapre M, Kothe S, editors. Surgery of trismus in oral submucous fibrosis. Singapore: Springer Singapore; 2018. p. 11–6. https://doi.org/10.1007/978-981-10-4892-0_3.
33. Türe H, Harput MV, Bekiroğlu N, Keskin Ö, Köner Ö, Türe U. Effect of the degree of head elevation on the incidence and severity of venous air embolism in cranial neurosurgical procedures with patients in the semisitting position. J Neurosurg. 2018;128(5):1560–9.
34. Coyle MJ, Main B, Hughes C, Craven R, Alexander R, Porter G, et al. Enhanced recovery after surgery

(ERAS) for head and neck oncology patients. Clin Otolaryngol. 2016;41(2):118–26.
35. Goswami U, Jain A. Anaesthetic implications of free-flap microvascular surgery for head and neck malignancies—a relook. J Anaesthesiol Clin Pharmacol. 2021;37(4):499–504.
36. Chang YT, Wu CC, Tang TY, Lu CT, Lai CS, Shen CH. Differences between total intravenous anesthesia and inhalation anesthesia in free flap surgery of head and neck cancer. PLoS One. 2016;11(2):e0147713.
37. Rossmiller SR, Cannady SB, Ghanem TA, Wax MK. Transfusion criteria in free flap surgery. Otolaryngol Head Neck Surg. 2010;142(3):359–64.
38. Monroe MM, Cannady SB, Ghanem TA, Swide CE, Wax MK. Safety of vasopressor use in head and neck microvascular reconstruction: a prospective observational study. Otolaryngol Head Neck Surg. 2011;144(6):877–82.
39. Yang X, Li Z, Gao C, Liu R. Effect of dexmedetomidine on preventing agitation and delirium after microvascular free flap surgery: a randomized, double-blind, control study. J Oral Maxillofac Surg. 2015;73(6):1065–72.
40. Offodile AC, Aherrera A, Wenger J, Rajab TK, Guo L. Impact of increasing operative time on the incidence of early failure and complications following free tissue transfer? A risk factor analysis of 2008 patients from the ACS-NSQIP database. Microsurgery. 2017;37(1):12–20.
41. Abdel-Galil K, Mitchell D. Postoperative monitoring of microsurgical free tissue transfers for head and neck reconstruction: a systematic review of current techniques—part I. Non-invasive techniques. Br J Oral Maxillofac Surg. 2009;47(5):351–5.
42. Abdel-Galil K, Mitchell D. Postoperative monitoring of microsurgical free-tissue transfers for head and neck reconstruction: a systematic review of current techniques—part II. Invasive techniques. Br J Oral Maxillofac Surg. 2009;47(6):438–42.
43. Agnelli G. Prevention of venous thromboembolism in surgical patients. Circulation. 2004;110(24 Suppl 1):IV4–12.
44. Shuman AG, Hu HM, Pannucci CJ, Jackson CR, Bradford CR, Bahl V. Stratifying the risk of venous thromboembolism in otolaryngology. Otolaryngol Head Neck Surg. 2012;146(5):719–24.
45. Bahl V, Shuman AG, Hu HM, Jackson CR, Pannucci CJ, Alaniz C, et al. Chemoprophylaxis for venous thromboembolism in otolaryngology. JAMA Otolaryngol Head Neck Surg. 2014;140(11):999–1005.
46. Chaukar D, Dandekar M. Surgical resection of cancer of the buccal mucosa. Open Access Atlas Otolarygngol Head Neck Oper Surg Cape Town UCT Librariespp. 33:1–21.
47. Moore MG, Bhrany AD, Francis DO, Yueh B, Futran ND. Use of nasotracheal intubation in patients receiving oral cavity free flap reconstruction. Head Neck. 2010;32(8):1056–61.
48. Kundra P, Garg R, Patwa A, Ahmed SM, Ramkumar V, Shah A, et al. All India Difficult Airway Association 2016 guidelines for the management of anticipated difficult extubation. Indian J Anaesth. 2016;60(12):915–21.
49. Difficult Airway Society Extubation Guidelines Group, Popat M, Mitchell V, Dravid R, Patel A, Swampillai C, Higgs A. Difficult Airway Society Guidelines for the management of tracheal extubation. Anaesthesia. 2012;67(3):318–40.
50. Wax MK, Reh DD, Levack MM. Effect of celecoxib on fasciocutaneous flap survival and revascularization. Arch Facial Plast Surg. 2007;9(2):120–4.
51. Stammschulte T, Brune K, Brack A, Augenstein H, Arends G, Gundert-Remy U. Unexpected hemorrhage complications in association with celecoxib. Spontaneously reported case series after perioperative pain treatment in gynecological operations. Anaesthesist. 2014;63(12):958–60.
52. Jellish WS, Leonetti JP, Sawicki K, Anderson D, Origitano TC. Morphine/ondansetron PCA for postoperative pain, nausea, and vomiting after skull base surgery. Otolaryngol Head Neck Surg. 2006;135(2):175–81.
53. Mehta V, Langford RM. Acute pain management for opioid dependent patients. Anaesthesia. 2006;61(3):269–76.
54. Texas AA PharmD, BCPS Assistant Professor Ambulatory Care Division Department of Pharmacy Practice Texas Tech University Health Sciences Center School of Pharmacy Clinical Pharmacy Specialist VA North Texas Health Care System—Dallas Dallas, Texas Nakia Duncan, PharmD, BCGP, BCPS Assistant Professor—Geriatrics Division Department of Pharmacy Practice Texas Tech University Health Sciences Center School of Pharmacy Palliative Care Clinical Pharmacy Specialist UT Southwestern Medical Center Dallas. Acute Pain Management in Patients With Opioid Tolerance [Internet]. https://www.uspharmacist.com/article/acute-pain-management-in-patients-with-opioid-tolerance. Accessed 7 Aug 2022.

2 Anaesthesia and Perioperative Concerns in Total Laryngectomy

Saurabh Vig, Ankit Sharma, and Swati Bhan

2.1 Case Vignette

A 54-year-old male presented to ENT OPD with chief complaints of hoarseness and foreign body sensation in the throat for 3 months. Initial laryngoscopic examination revealed a lesion with an irregular surface on his right vocal cord. Head and neck CT revealed that the lesion had invaded the anterior commissure of the larynx and the glottis through the length. The patient had no other significant medical or surgical history. He was an ex-smoker (20 pack-years, reformed for 3 months), and a social drinker. Whole-body PET-CT showed no sign of metastasis. The patient was referred to Head and Neck Oncology and posted for total laryngectomy.

2.1.1 Define Total Laryngectomy? Contrast It with Other Partial Surgical Modalities

Total laryngectomy is defined as the en-bloc removal of laryngeal structures (i.e. hyoid, epiglottis and some amount of upper trachea) and creation of a permanent tracheostome. A part of or total thyroid gland may be removed as a part of this procedure which may require postoperative thyroxine replacement [1]. Other surgical

S. Vig
Department of Onco-Anaesthesia and Palliative Medicine, National Cancer Institute, AIIMS, New Delhi, New Delhi, India

A. Sharma
Department of Onco-Anaesthesia and Palliative Medicine, BRAIRCH, AIIMS, New Delhi, New Delhi, India

S. Bhan (✉)
Department of Anaesthesia and Critical Care, VMMC and Safdarjung Hospital, New Delhi, India

N. Gupta et al. (eds.), *Problem Based Learning Discussions in Onco-Anesthesia and Onco-Critical Care*, https://doi.org/10.1007/978-981-99-6339-3_2

modalities available which preserve some part of larynx are:

- Cordectomy—Surgical removal of vocal cords.
- Hemi/partial laryngectomy—Only on half of larynx removed, voice is usually preserved in this surgery.
- Supraglottic laryngectomy—Removal of larynx above the glottis only, voice is preserved in this surgery.
- Transoral laser microsurgery—It is a minimally invasive endoscopic approach involving the use of suspension laryngoscopy with an operating microscope, a tissue-cutting laser, and microsurgical instruments to resect the laryngeal tumour. In contrast to partial laryngectomy, the cartilage framework of the larynx is preserved, thus reducing the need for tracheostomy allowing more rapid return of postoperative swallowing, and shorter hospital stays. The oncological results with this surgery are comparable with open partial laryngectomy.

2.1.2 What Are the Quality of Life Affecting Concerns in a Patient Planned for 'Total Laryngectomy'?

Laryngectomy impacts the life of a patient in a big way. Altered body image after surgery, inability to speak naturally for the rest of life, learning and training oneself with a new method of communication for the rest of life, and breathing through the neck are some of the main concerns which may plague the mind of a patient and the caregivers having negative impact on quality of life [2, 3].

Plan of rehabilitation discussed at the time of planning the surgery with multidisciplinary team involving a voice therapist, and nursing team specializing in care of a neck breather may help to alleviate these concerns and lead to better patient outcome and satisfaction.

2.1.3 What Is the Incidence of Laryngeal Cancer in India and Worldwide? What Are the Main Risk Factors Associated with This Malignancy?

Laryngeal cancer is the seventh most common malignancy among males in India and the ninth most common in males worldwide. It is more common in males and accounts for 3–6% of all cancers in males and 0.2–1% of all cancers in females in India. Common risk factors associated are tobacco use and alcohol consumption. The 5-year survival rate after treatment is around 28% [4].

2.1.4 Describe the TNM Staging for Ca Larynx

The 'T' staging ranges from T1 to T4b and consists of various sized and local spread of the lesion in supraglottic, glottic and subglottic areas. Underlying basis of classifying growths from T1, i.e. limited local site involvement to increasing in size and spreading to nearby structures in and outside larynx. T2 being invasion of adjacent structures, T3 being growths involving vocal cords, para glottic space and leading to cord fixation and T4 being invasion through the thyroid or cricoid cartilages into the prevertebral space, encasement of carotid artery and nearby mediastinal structures.

For lymph nodal spread description ranges from N0 to N3b where N0 means no lymph nodal spread, N1 being single ipsilateral lymph node which measures less than 3 cm, a single node on ipsilateral side of mass between 3–6 cm comes under N2a, and multiple ipsilateral nodes 3–6 cm are N2b, N2c is bilateral or contralateral nodes all less than 6 cm and any node more than 6 cm or any extranodal regional metastasis comes under N3a and N3b respectively.

2.1.5 How Do You Evaluate and Prehabilitate These Patients?

- A thorough preoperative assessment that includes relevant history and investigations should be done.
- Most of these patients are smokers, so cardiovascular and respiratory diseases are common. Symptoms like unstable angina, history of recent stenting, major cardiac conditions like heart failure on medication, or a valvular heart disease would warrant for a cardiologist opinion for risk stratification and perioperative management.
- Evaluating for exercise tolerance is an essential part of pre-anaesthetic check-up. Cardiopulmonary exercise testing (CPET) is a useful aid in risk-stratifying patients. But in patients with critical airway stenosis due to the laryngeal pathology, CPET can precipitate airway obstruction and hence, contra-indicated.
- Some of these patients could have received preoperative radiotherapy. It is essential to assess airway for potential difficulties in management. The attending anaesthesiologist should also be aware of the airway-related changes due to radiotherapy. Radiotherapy can result in oral mucositis, oral thrush, and oro-cutaneous fistulae which leads to friable mucosa and increased bleeding. It causes fibrosis of temporo-mandibular joint and floor of mouth, glossomegaly, tongue oedema (decreased tongue movement), risk of caries, increased mobility and loss of teeth, osteoradionecrosis and pathological fracture of mandible, micrognathia, altered neck consistency which becomes hard, woody and indurated leading to difficult mask ventilation and laryngoscopy. It also causes laryngeal oedema leading to difficult visualization of larynx and tracheal intubation. Acute or chronic baroreflex dysfunction, hypothyroidism can also occur following head and neck radiotherapy. Tissue Fibrosis due to radiation involves tissue atrophy and contractures (such as trismus), and cannot be relaxed with neuromuscular blocking agents (NMBAs).
- Few patients might have received concurrent chemoradiation with agents such as cisplatin, carboplatin, docetaxel, and cituxumab. They should be evaluated for the presence of renal toxicity, hypomagnesemia, neurological toxicity and haematological toxicity.
- Head and neck cancer patients could be on opioids for pain management. A perioperative opioid management plan is needed for optimal pain management.
- Nutritional assessment is an important part of evaluation and prehabilitation. Nutrition counselling and dietary advice, tube nutrition, parenteral nutrition, and nutritional supplements are some of the measures that can be used to combat malnutrition. A caloric intake of 25–30 kcal/kg/day together with 1.2–1.5 g protein/kg/day which could be increased to 2 g/kg/day in severe catabolism is recommended.
- Medical optimization which includes cessation of smoking and alcohol intake, weight optimization, correction of anaemia, blood glucose optimization, and optimization of co-morbidities should be started 4–6 weeks prior to surgery.
- Aerobic and resistance exercises help to improve the functional capacity of the patients.
- Psychological interventions such as deep breathing, meditation and hypnosis reduce anxiety and motivate patients to comply with medical and nutritional interventions.
- Scoring systems such as ACS-NSQIP, SORT, POSSSUM, APACHE 2 and Charlson index can be used in predicting morbidity although none of these has been validated for use in laryngectomy.

2.1.6 What Are the Toxicities Associated with Chemotherapeutic Agents Used in Ca Larynx?

Major toxicities of chemotherapy on various organ systems are listed in Table 2.1; toxicity profile of agents specifically used in head and neck malignancies are summarized in Table 2.2.

Table 2.1 Chemo-toxicities

Toxicity	Manifestations
Myelosuppression	Neutropenia, thrombocytopenia, anaemia, microangiopathic haemolytic anaemia (carboplatin)
Cardiotoxicity	• Brady and tachyarrhythmias, conduction disorders, myocardialIschaemia, may be seen with concomitant cisplatin therapy • Peripheral oedema due to fluid retention (docetaxel)
GI	Diarrhoea, mucositis, vomiting
CNS	Encephalopathy, ototoxicity, vestibulopathy, cognitive impairment, GB syndrome (rare), reversible posterior leukoencephalopathy syndrome
PNS	Paresthesias, dysesthesias of the hands, feet. Cold-induced pharyngolaryngeal dysesthesias; and muscle cramps. Distal axonal neuropathy without motor involvement
Pulmonary	Pneumonitis, interstitial pneumonia, eosinophilic pneumonia, diffuse alveolar damage, etc.
Electrolyte abnormalities	Hypokalaemia, hypomagnesemia
Dermatotoxicity	Infusion reactions, alopecia

Table 2.2 Toxicities associated with different chemotherapeutic agents

Chemotherapy agent	M	GI	C	CNS	PNS	R	E	H	D	HS	P	N
Cisplatin	+	–	–	++	+++	++	+	–	+		+	++
Carboplatin	+	+	–		+++	+				++		
Docetaxel	+	++		+							+	
Cetuximab	++		+		++	+	+	+	++	+		
5 FU	+	+	++	+					+			

M myelosuppression, *C* cardiotoxicity, *CNS* central nervous system, *R* renal toxicity, *E* electrolyte abnormalities, *H* hepatotoxicity, *D* dermatologic toxicity, *PN* peripheral nervous system, *GI* gastrointestinal, *HS* hypersensitivity reactions, *P* pulmonary toxicity, *N* nausea and vomiting

2.1.7 What Can Be the Airway-Related Concerns in a Patient of Ca Larynx Posted for Total Laryngectomy? [5–7]

The current surgical management protocols favour organ-preserving strategy and total laryngectomy is mainly done in advanced lesions (T4 on TNM staging). Also, preoperative tracheostomy is generally avoided as it is associated with poorer wound healing and higher rate of cancer recurrence in the tracheostomy stoma. Thus, the anaesthetist should be well versed in intubating a case of laryngeal cancer as the glottic aperture may be compromised with poor/restricted view on laryngoscopy. In addition to keeping in mind the difficult airway management guidelines [5–7] the following are the specific points of concern when anaesthetizing and securing airway in a carcinoma larynx for total laryngectomy:

A. Preoperative signs of airway obstruction.
B. Specific concerns in a patient with a history of radiotherapy to the larynx.
C. Estimating size of laryngeal aperture using preoperative radiological scans.
D. Choice of tracheostomy tube.
E. Planning and predicting difficult front of neck access for emergency airway management.

Each of the points of difficulty should be approached with a primary plan and an emergency plan B in mind.

A. Preoperative signs of airway obstruction—preoperative visit should specifically focus on eliciting signs and symptoms of airway obstruction. Points in history pointing to an airway obstruction are dysphagia, voice change, breathlessness, or orthopnoea. In a patient reporting breathing difficulty in supine position, the most comfortable position while sleeping should be noted and pre-oxygenation and anaesthetic induction should be done in this position. Narrowing of laryngeal aperture leading to obstruction of airway can also give rise to situations of difficult bag and mask ventilation as the overlying growth may be floppy and obstruct the airway completely once muscle relaxant has been given. High-flow nasal oxygen and THRIVE is helpful especially in patients with stridor.

B. Specific concerns due to radiotherapy of larynx—a patient previously treated with an organ-preserving approach with radiotherapy to the larynx will invariably be a difficult airway. Radiotherapy can produce an array of changes in the airway ranging from inflammation, oedema to fibrosis and narrowing of the laryngeal inlet with distortion of anatomy. In severe cases, radiotherapy-induced changes can lead to an entity called as '*Frozen Larynx*' which is defined as a fixed immobile larynx with cord palsies and dysphagia. Such an airway is particularly difficult to manage and every case of preoperative radiotherapy should be treated as an anticipated difficult airway.

C. Estimating laryngeal aperture size and specific endotracheal tubes for laryngectomy—

   A secure airway (inside the trachea and with a seal cuff) is necessary during laryngectomy to protect the pulmonary tree and alveoli from blood and secretions trickling down. A cuffed endotracheal tube also prevents leakage of anaesthetic gas or oxygen. Since the surgical field and the airway is a shared space between the anaesthetist and the surgeon the endotracheal tube may interfere with the surgical field and hence impede the dissection of the larynx and the neck. Thus, care should be taken to place an appropriately sized and carefully secure it keeping in mind the chances of dislodgment or kink during surgery.

   The size of the endotracheal tube can be predicted based on direct visualization techniques such as Indirect laryngoscopy (to see 'chink' between vocal cords) and nasendoscopy, which may also help to visualize any possible narrowing beyond the vocal cords. However, these techniques have a drawback of not providing an objective value for the size of the endotracheal tube, and may not predict any further narrowing beyond the vocal cords or any significant narrowing beyond which an endoscope may not advance.

   Computerized tomography (CT) and magnetic resonance imaging are available preoperatively for many surgical patients. The axial images can show narrow points of the airway—the thinner the slices the more accurate the details (Image 2.1). The sagittal and/or coronal

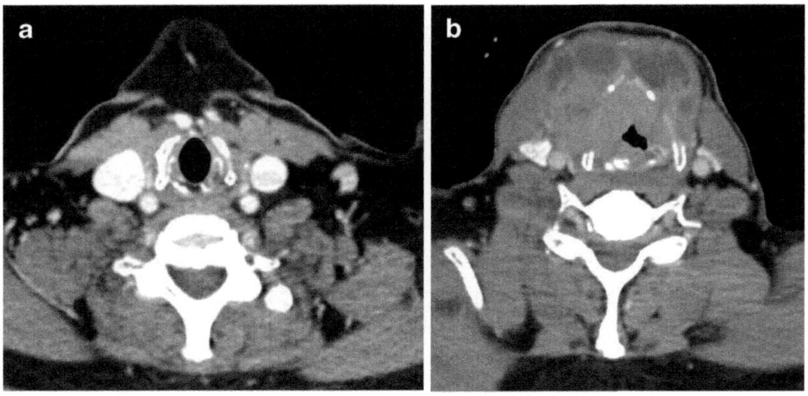

Image 2.1 (**a**) Axial section CT image at level of thyroid cartilage showing normal airway, (**b**) axial section at same level showing growth and reduced glottic aperture, minimal diameter at axial view used to calculate endotracheal tube size (minimum diameter on axial cut corresponds to maximum external diameter of the MLS/small sized flexometallic tube that can pass through the aperture. (*Image source—authors own personal image database, all patient details concealed)

cuts can estimate the length of such narrow segments. Using the scale available on these 'slices', we can objectively measure the largest diameter at the narrowest site, which will be the maximum permissible outer diameter of the endotracheal tube planned for the patient. 3D reconstruction of airway is now possible using CT images which may provide a virtual layout with accurate diameters, but it is a relatively new entity which may possibly be time-consuming and is resource-dependent.

Based on the predicted/measured narrowest diameter, the smallest endotracheal tube (ETT) capable of supporting ventilation should be used, and care should be taken to avoid laryngeal tissue injury if oral intubation is attempted.

Normal PVC single-lumen endotracheal tubes may be used, although microlaryngeal surgery (MLS) tubes (Image 2.1) have an advantage of having length equivalent to an adult 8 size endotracheal tube but available in small paediatric sized (size 4, 5 and 6—internal diameter 4, 5 and 6 mm and outer diameter 5.6, 6.9 and 8.2 mm respectively with each having same length of 368 mm) for the expected narrow glottic chink and to ensure maximal surgical exposure for the surgeon. These tubes have a special high-volume low-pressure cuff (resting cuff diameter of 25, 27 and 27 mm for size 4, 5 and 6 MLS tube respectively—Image 2.2) to ensure adequate seal of a small paediatric-sized tube in an adult trachea. Their main drawback are the high airway pressures generated during positive pressure ventilation which can lead to lung injury like bullae rupture especially in COPD patients. If appropriate small small-sized flexometallic tubes can also be used to intubate as they are easier to direct away from the external surgical field after fixation with no chances of kinking. Other special tubes available for laryngeal surgeries are—the laryngectomy J-shaped tube or the 'Montando tube'.

D. Device selection for laryngoscopy and role of awake fibreoptic bronchoscopy for intubation—the most useful device for optimal glottic view and the general first choice among airway devices as per international guidelines is a video laryngoscope. Awake fibreoptic is generally considered as the go to technique in any case of predicted difficult airway as the chances of airway loss are minimal, however in cases of laryngeal and growths with narrowed laryngeal inlet the diameter of the patent laryngeal aperture might just be equal to the diameter of the fibreoptic bronchoscope. Such a case leads to a dangerous situation described as *'Cork in the Bottle' phenomenon.* In this situation the laryngeal aperture is completely blocked by the fibreoptic and airway is lost, thus awake fibreoptic may be useful in supraglottic growths causing airway obstruc-

Image 2.2 Size 4 and 6 MLS tubes—note the high volume low pressure cuffs, Length equivalent to adult size 8 ETT (details in text)

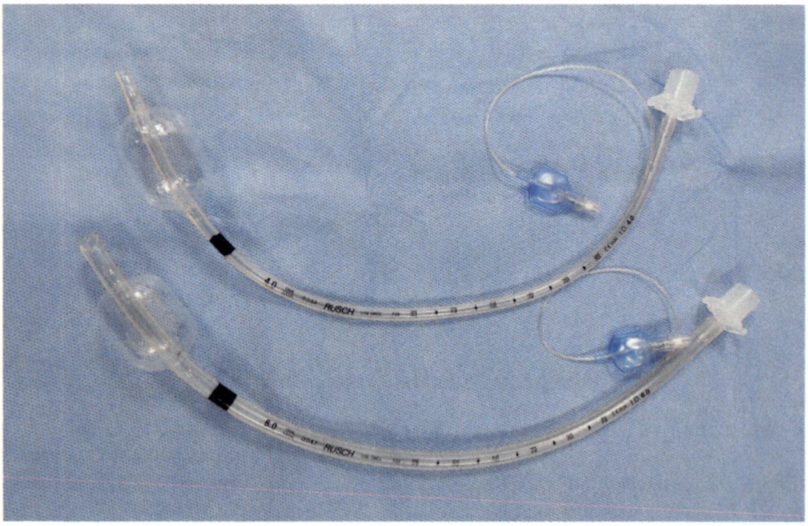

tion but not in glottic growths or laryngeal aperture narrowing.

E. Planning and predicting difficult front of neck access—tumours with subglottic or subcricoid extension, preoperative radiotherapy to the neck which may have altered anatomy due to tissue oedema and fibrosis may pose a challenge in front of neck access (FONA) for emergency tracheostomy or cricothyroidotomy. In such cases clear communication with the surgical team should be done regarding the site and approach for a surgical airway access if required.

F. Five questions would help in formulating the airway management strategy
   - How will I pre-oxygenate?
   - Is bag and mask ventilation possible or difficult?
   - Is it possible to get a good view of glottis?
   - Is intubation difficult?
   - Is FONA possible?

   Aintree Difficult Airway Management website is a good option for individual airway planning.

2.1.8 Specific Intraoperative Concerns?

Most specific intraoperative concern is the shared airway space between the anaesthetist and the surgeon. This poses the danger of kinking or displacement of the endotracheal tube during the surgery. In the process of surgical dissection and removal of larynx, the surgeon may require the endotracheal tube to be pulled up away from the surgical field. Periods of apnoea may occur during resection and when the tracheal stoma is created and a flexometallic tube is passed through the stoma for ventilation after removing the endotracheal tube.

2.1.9 Role of Enhanced Recovery After Surgery (ERAS) Protocols in Laryngectomy Cases?

There haven't been dedicated guidelines published for ERAS in laryngectomy. Protocols for perioperative management of free flap surgeries are available in the literature [8]. Since the concerns other than flap management and viability, such as those of major debulking, shared airway and proximity to important vascular structures are similar for any major head and neck surgery, many recommendations can be find application in laryngectomy surgery as well.

Importantly, comprehensive preoperative nutritional assessment, with a special focus on dysphagia and risk for refeeding syndrome is of paramount importance.

A standard enteral nutrition formula should be considered in patients requiring preoperative and/or postoperative nutrition support. There is no concrete evidence regarding immunonutrition. Preoperative fasting should be minimized. Clear fluids should be permitted for up to 2 h and solids for up to 6 h prior to anaesthesia and preoperative CHO treatment may be offered. Postoperatively, tube feeding should be initiated within 24 h. Nutrition interventions should be developed in consultation with the multidisciplinary team and individualized according to nutritional status and surgical procedure.

Cancer and major surgery confer risk of venous thromboembolism (VTE). Mechanical prophylaxis is recommended, and pharmacological prophylaxis against VTE should be individualized based on risks and benefit. Perioperative antibiotics in clean-contaminated cases should be given within 1 h of surgery and continued for 24 h.

Postoperative nausea and/or vomiting prophylaxis should include multiple drugs (combination of corticosteroid and antiemetic) should be considered. Long-acting anxiolytics and opioids should be avoided. The anaesthetic protocol should target preventing awareness while minimizing adverse effects and allowing rapid recovery. Normothermia should be maintained intraoperatively. Goal-directed perioperative fluid management, avoiding over and under hydration, is beneficial. Routine intensive care unit admission to facilitate an immediate postoperative period of deep sedation and artificial respiration is not necessary. Low-risk patients with uncomplicated surgery may be treated safely after recovery from anaesthesia in a high-dependency unit or specialist ward, provided adequate skilled nursing and medical coverage is provided. Opioid-sparing, multimodal analgesia, utilizing NSAIDs, COX inhibitors, and paracetamol, are preferred for such patients. Patient-controlled analgesia can be considered. No concrete evidence or recommendation is available regarding the utility of nerve blocks.

Early postoperative mobilization (preferably within the first 24 h of surgery) is recommended for faster recovery. Urinary catheters should be removed as soon as the patient is able to void, ideally less than 24 h after completion of surgery. Decannulation after tracheostomy and stoma closure (surgical) is recommended. Pulmonary physical therapy should be initiated as early as possible after head and neck reconstructions to avoid pulmonary complications.

2.1.10 Main Postoperative Concerns After Total Laryngectomy?

Main postoperative concerns in the immediate postoperative period (24–48 h) are analgesia, sedation, ventilation and feeding. Usually after total laryngectomy there is no or minimal need for prolonged deep sedation and mechanical ventilation. Efforts must be made to ensure early weaning off from sedation and ventilation to T-piece so the other components of the ERAS pathway like early mobilization, pulmonary physical therapy, removal of indwelling catheters and initiation of feeds can be done as per protocol. Feeding is usually done via nasogastric tube inserted at the time of surgery; however, early resumption of oral feeding after total laryngectomy also finds a mention in the literature [9].

2.1.11 What Are the Available Options for Postoperative Voice Rehabilitation After Laryngectomy and a Permanent Tracheostome? List Out Complications of Such Voice Prosthetic Devices

There are three elements of a functional speech production system—a power source, a sound source, and a sound modifier. In a normal laryngeal speaker, lung air is the power source, the larynx is the sound source, and the vocal tract (i.e., pharynx, oral cavity) functions as the sound modifier. If larynx is removed, the sound source is removed from the equation and hence the power source (lungs) lose their connection with the sound modifier [10, 11].

A tracheo oesophageal puncture (TEP), training in oesophageal speech or inserting a voice prosthetic device (valve/electronic) may be used to restore speech after laryngectomy [12].

- TEP is a surgically created fistula at the back of the tracheal stoma, which creates an opening between the trachea and the oesophagus. It can be done as part of laryngectomy surgery, or as a separate minor procedure after the surgery (a gap of at least 8 weeks). A small tube/catheter or a one-way valve (voice prosthesis) is inserted into the fistula to keep it patent. Once the area has healed, the catheter can be removed, and valve can be fit. If catheter is not inserted, NG tube needs to remain in-situ and feeding done via the same.
- The voice prosthesis is a valve that allows the patient to make sounds by pushing air from the lungs through the valve and up into the oral cavity. The patient has to cover/plug the stoma temporarily so that the air goes

through the valve and does not leak out of the stoma. Using voice prosthesis requires practice, and a speech therapist may help in adjustment to the same. As the pharyngeal muscles get used to it, it becomes easier with passage of time.

- Alternatively, hands-free valves may be used which automatically close the stoma when speaking valve is in use, e.g. Blom-Singer valve, Provox valve, Groningen valve. Blom-Singer and a few Provox valve varieties are external valves and have to be taken out and manually cleaned. Cleaning can be done by the patient after due training. If the valve gets blocked, air can't pass through it easily and the patient won't be able to speak. Groningen and some types of Provox valves are internal valves. They are left in place until they need changing (about every 6 months or if leaking, whichever is earlier). Only a specially trained therapist, doctor or nurse can and must change such a valve.

2.2 Complications of Speech Valves

Pharyngeal muscle spasms may go into spasm because of speech valve. A speech therapist can train the patient to loosen the muscles or botox injections may help. Inflammation and swelling around the valve are other common complications and are due to tissue reaction and/or acid reflux.

- Oesophageal speech is another method where the patient moves air down into the oesophagus which becomes the power source. Forceful swallowing of air is done into the oesophagus and then the air is pushed through the muscles of pharynx, and resultant vibrations can be learnt to be converted to speech by moving mouth and lips.

Advantage of oesophageal speech is no extra apparatus needed, while disadvantage is the limitation to short sentences as patients are unable to produce continuous speech, which requires large quantities of air to be moved into the oesophagus.

Oesophageal speech might also be a better option than an electrolarynx if you think you might have a problem holding something to your throat every time you need to speak.

- Another option is an electronic larynx (electrolarynx) which is a battery-operated machine that produces sound to create a voice. It is usually held against the neck or in the corner of the mouth where it can generate sound which can be modulated by tongue and lips into words. Electrolarynx is useful in patients with any medical contraindication to Voice Prosthesis, and/or too weak for oesophageal sound training. The speech has a mechanical timber which may not be acceptable to some, and it requires plenty of practice and training.

2.2.1 How Do You Manage a Post-laryngectomy Patient Posted for Other Surgical Procedures?

(A) Intubating and securing airway in a patient with partially removed larynx—Presence of tracheal stoma indicates that the whole larynx has been removed. However, absence of stoma is suggestive of partial laryngectomy, and it is important to know this prior to intubation. Partial laryngectomy may be in the form of:
  (a) Vertical partial laryngectomy—here half of the larynx has been excised in the vertical plane, the epiglottis is still present but the larynx appears narrowed.
  (b) Supracricoid laryngectomy here laryngeal structures are excised superior to the level of the cricoid, resulting in a more narrowed and rounded appearance of larynx.

- Tracheal intubation is possible following both of these procedures using a smaller tube size and using videolaryngoscope can aid in visualization of the laryngeal inlet position.

(B) **Management of Laryngectomy Stoma (Post Total Laryngectomy)**

- In these patients, it is important to remember that there is absence of any communication between the mouth and trachea.
- Preoxygenation is to be performed over the laryngeal stoma.
- Ventilation can be performed by placing a paediatric facemask over the stoma site, placing an inflated laryngeal mask airway or the end of a catheter mount over the stoma. Then, laryngectomy tube (J tube) or reinforced tracheal tube can be inserted through the stoma. A cuffed tracheostomy tube can also be placed.
- The main concerns include appropriate mode of delivery of oxygen and management of a 'neck breather' in an environment where they are not normally cared for.

2.2.2 What Are the Complications of Laryngectomy?

Acute complications include postoperative pain, bleeding, dysphagia or odynophagia, and postoperative infections. Chronic complications are tracheopharyngeal and laryngocutaneous fistulas, tracheostomy or feeding tube dependence, long-term fibrosis, dysphagia, and psychosocial distress. Complications of neck dissection include bleeding, raised intracranial pressure due to ligation of internal jugular vein, nerve palsies affecting marginal mandibular branch of the facial nerve (resulting in lower-lip weakness), the hypoglossal nerve (causing loss of movement of the ipsilateral tongue), or the accessory nerve (resulting in stiffening and weakness of shoulder movements). Paralysis of hemidiaphragm can occur due to phrenic nerve damage. Thoracic duct can be damaged leading to chyle leak which is recognized by the presence of a milky fluid in the surgical drains.

References

1. Ceachir O, Hainarosie R, Zainea V. Total laryngectomy—past, present, future. Maedica (Bucur). 2014;9(2):210–6. PMID: 25705281; PMCID: PMC4296768.
2. Perry A, Casey E, Cotton S. Quality of life after total laryngectomy: functioning, psychological well-being and self-efficacy. Int J Lang Commun Disord. 2015;50(4):467–75. https://doi.org/10.1111/1460-6984.12148. Epub 2015 Feb 19.
3. Woodard TD, Oplatek A, Petruzzelli GJ. Life after total laryngectomy: a measure of long-term survival, function, and quality of life. Arch Otolaryngol Head Neck Surg. 2007;133(6):526–32. https://doi.org/10.1001/archotol.133.6.526.
4. Mathur P, Sathishkumar K, Chaturvedi M, Das P, Sudarshan KL, Santhappan S. Cancer statistics, 2020: report from national cancer registry programme, India. JCO Glob Oncol. 2020;6:1063–75.
5. Patel SG, Lydiatt WM, Glastonbury CM, et al. Larynx. In: Amin MB, editor. AJCC cancer staging manual. 8th ed. New York: Springer; 2017.
6. Stephens M, Montgomery J, Urquhart CS. Management of elective laryngectomy. BJA Educ. 2017;17:306.
7. Sinha R, Trikha A, Subramanian R. Microlaryngeal endotracheal tube for lung isolation in pediatric patient with significant tracheal narrowing. Saudi J Anaesth. 2017;11(4):490–3. https://doi.org/10.4103/1658-354X.215427. PMID: 29033734; PMCID: PMC5637430.
8. Dawson P, Rosewane F, Wells D. The Montando laryngectomy tube. Can J Anaesth. 1989;36:486–7.
9. Dort JC, Farwell DG, Findlay M, Huber GF, Kerr P, Shea-Budgell MA, Simon C, Uppington J, Zygun D, Ljungqvist O, Harris J. Optimal perioperative care in major head and neck cancer surgery with free flap reconstruction: a consensus review and recommendations from the enhanced recovery after surgery society. JAMA Otolaryngol Head Neck Surg. 2017;143(3):292–303.
10. Süslü N, Hoşal AŞ. Early oral feeding after total laryngectomy: outcome of 602 patients in one cancer center. Auris Nasus Larynx. 2016;43(5):546–50.
11. Lorenz KJ. Rehabilitation after total laryngectomy—a tribute to the pioneers of voice restoration in the last two centuries. Front Med (Lausanne). 2017;4:81. https://doi.org/10.3389/fmed.2017.00081. PMID: 28695120; PMCID: PMC5483444.
12. https://www.cancerresearchuk.org/about-cancer/laryngeal-cancer/living-with/speaking-after-laryngectomy/voice-prosthesis.

3 Carcinoma Trachea for Tracheal Resection and Anastomosis

Namrata Ranganath, C. S. Sumitha, and Kavitha Lakshman

3.1 Case

A 60-year-old male patient with diagnosis of primary tracheal tumor was posted for emergency tracheal resection and reconstruction. The patient had history of cough, hemoptysis, breathlessness on lying down with audible stridor, diabetic, and hypertensive on treatment. Airway imaging showed tracheal narrowing.

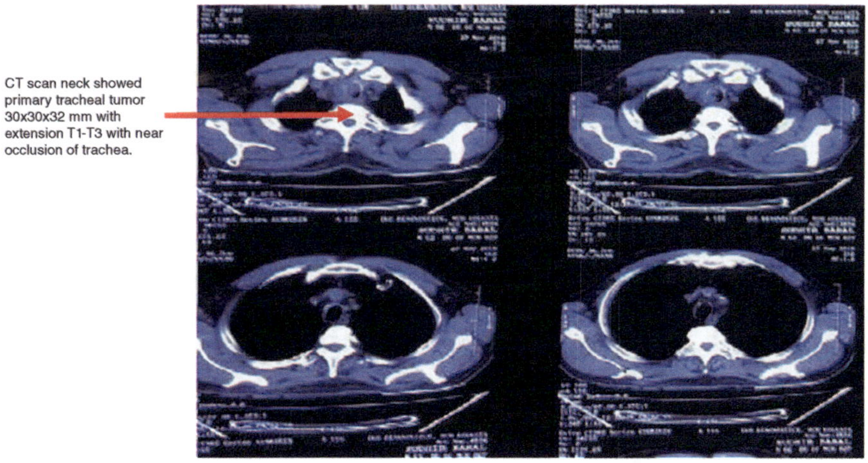

N. Ranganath (✉) · C. S. Sumitha · K. Lakshman
Kidwai Memorial Institute of Oncology,
Bangalore, India

N. Gupta et al. (eds.), *Problem Based Learning Discussions in Onco-Anesthesia and Onco-Critical Care*, https://doi.org/10.1007/978-981-99-6339-3_3

1. **What are the common tracheal tumors** [1]**?**
   (a) Primary tracheal tumors [rare-0.01% of malignancies]
   (b) Secondary tracheal tumors [more common]
   (c) Metastatic and locally invasive tumors [thyroid, lung, esophagus, breast, or other distant organs]

3.2 Preoperative Evaluation

3.2.1 Clinical Evaluation

2. **How does the patient clinically present?**
   (a) Nonspecific symptoms such as cough or dyspnea on exertion may be the first symptoms to appear. Symptoms may be ascribed to other conditions such as asthma, chronic obstructive pulmonary disease (COPD), and pneumonia which may delay the diagnosis.
   (b) Hemoptysis.
   (c) Dysphagia.
   (d) Hoarseness.
   (e) Recurrent infections [2]
3. **How critical a narrowing of trachea should happen for patients to show the symptoms at rest?**
   A normal tracheal anatomy
   (a) Extent: Lower edge of cricoid cartilage in neck to division into main stem bronchi.
   (b) Length: 10–13 cm.
   (c) Internal diameter: 2.3 cm laterally and 1.8 cm anteroposteriorly.
   A 50% reduction in the tracheal lumen (8 mm or less) will cause symptoms such as stridor, dyspnea on exertion. Any further reduction in diameter (5–6 mm or less) will cause these symptoms to appear even at rest [3]. The other determinants of the symptoms and their severity are:
   (a) The exact etiology of obstruction.
   (b) The rate of progression of the obstruction.
   (c) Location of the obstruction—a fixed airway narrowing at larynx and upper trachea manifests as inspiratory obstruction whereas lower airway obstructions manifest as expiratory symptoms, e.g., dynamic collapse.
4. **What will be the focus of our examination of the patient?**
   Detailed examination of the patient should be done as follows:
   (a) The ability of the patient to extend and flex the neck.
   (b) Ability to lie supine.
   (c) The pattern of breathing.
   (d) Presence of any stridor.
   (e) Amount of exercise tolerated without dyspnea.
   (f) Any respiratory infection.

3.3 Investigations

5. **What will be our focus when asking for investigations for tracheal tumor patient?**
   (a) Degree of lumen stenosis
   (b) Length of tracheal damage
   (c) Distance from vocal cord to upper end of lesion
   (d) Distance from lower end of lesion to carina
6. **What specific investigations should be asked for?**
   (a) X-ray—AP and lateral neck X-ray
   PA and lateral view chest X-rays
   (b) CT scan
   (c) Virtual endoscopy
   (d) PET scan
   (e) PFT: flow volume loops
   (f) Bronchoscopy

7. **How important are pulmonary function test?**

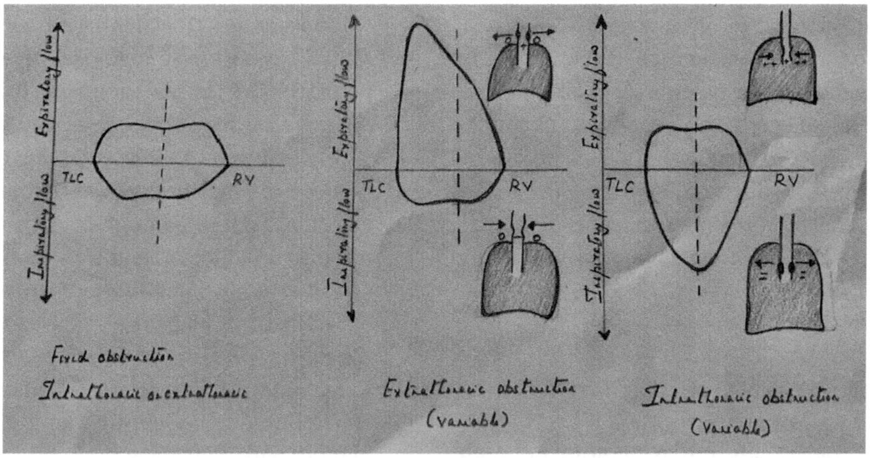

Appearance of flow volume loops can help distinguish between fixed (inspiratory or expiratory) versus dynamic (intrathoracic or extrathoracic) obstruction, depending on the pattern of flow.

8. **What is the role of flexible bronchoscopy prior to surgery in these patients?**

   Surgeon usually inspects the glottis and trachea via a flexible bronchoscope. Defines preoperatively the current anatomy [length and diameter of tracheal narrowing by direct vision] and pathology. It is confirmed that the planned surgical procedure is appropriate, and rules out the presence of a new acute process that could be improved with therapy [3, 4].

9. **What is the role of rigid bronchoscopy?**

   As airway is often tenuous, the rigid bronchoscopy is the preferred technique, so that airway can be established through bronchoscope if necessary. Bronchoscopy is usually performed prior to resection [4]. A careful endoscopic evaluation is done to assess parameters like

   (a) Location and extent of lesion to be resected.
   (b) The health and function of vocal cords.
   (c) Any areas of inflammation of trachea, including signs of aspiration.
   (d) Any areas of tracheomalacia.

3.4 Surgical Considerations

10. **What are the surgical considerations?**

    Tracheal lesions in the upper third of the trachea are amenable to repair via a cervical incision. Middle third tracheal lesions are commonly approached via a cervical incision with extension down onto the sternum (sternal split). Distal tracheal lesions usually require a right thoracotomy through the fourth or the fifth interspace. Long tracheal lesions involving the carina may be approached via a full sternotomy.

11. **What are contraindications for surgery?**

    Absolute contraindications:

    (a) Severe pulmonary disease
    (b) Ventilator dependence
    (c) Steroid dependence
    (d) Airway infection
    (e) Inability to cooperate with pulmonary toilet

    Relative contraindications:

    (a) Previous radiotherapy to neck or mediastinum
    (b) Invasive tumors
    (c) Long complex lesion [5]

12. **Why there is bigger role of communication between surgeon and anesthesiologists in such types of surgery?**

    A detailed preoperative discussion with the surgeon about planning airway management and an emergency plan in the event of a failed airway. Along with this, discussion on surgical steps, fire risk owing to the use of electrocautery, and requirements regarding critical portions of the shared airway should be carried out.

3.5 Intraoperative

13. **What airway equipment should be available for a major airway surgery?**
    (a) Endotracheal tubes (various sizes, reinforced and microlaryngeal tubes)
    (b) Laryngeal mask airways
    (c) Laryngoscopes [direct and video]
    (d) Circuit with gas sampling line
    (e) Bronchoscopes [fiberoptic, rigid]
    (f) Jet ventilator
    (g) Means of pressurized air delivery
    (h) Extracorporeal circuit with perfusionist on standby (for high-risk patients) [1]
14. **What monitors are required intraoperatively? Is an arterial line always indicated for tracheal resection?**

    In addition to the standard American Society of Anesthesiologists monitoring, an anesthesia depth monitor, train of four monitor, urinary catheter, and CVP optional.

    An arterial line may be useful in case of jet ventilation and hilar releases to monitor the partial pressure of arterial CO_2 ($PaCO_2$), in the absence of reliable end-tidal CO_2 pressure ($ETCO_2$) monitoring and to monitor hemodynamic changes [5].
15. **What are the different methods of anesthetic management for tracheal surgery?**
    (a) Conventional approach
    (b) Breathing nonintubated
    (c) Jet ventilation
    (d) Extracorporeal life support [6]
16. **What are the advantages and disadvantages of different modes of ventilation?**

Anesthetic management	Patient characteristics	Advantages	Disadvantages
Conventional approach General anesthesia Endotracheal intubation and distal/cross-field intubation Mechanical ventilation	Most common technique by default Contraindication to regional anesthesia	Secure airway and control of oxygenation/ventilation Protection from secretions and easy to suction fluid and blood from lower airway Easy to perform an astomotic leak test	Surgical exposure compromised by ETT Possible complications of intubation and mechanical ventilation (airway injury, disruption of friable tissue) Extubation might disrupt anastomosis Difficult to visualize vocal cord function
Spontaneous ventilation (nonintubated) mild to moderate sedation Regional, neuraxial, or local Native or laryngeal mask airway	Ideally suited for limited extent, benign disease Small incisions planned experienced team patients who can tolerate up to 3 h surgery Good cardiopulmonary function ASA class 1 or 2 BMI <25 kg/m^2No local anesthetic allergy	Ideal surgical exposure airway construction more anatomic Avoids complications of intubation (airway injury and disruption of friable tissue) Nonintubated trachea is more flexible—facilitates surgical re-approximation Decreased postoperative complications with residual opioids, anesthetics, and paralytics—early recovery Allows for checking vocal cords in the OR	Hypoxemia/hypercarbia difficult monitoring of ventilation Inadequate pain control increased risk of regional block complications and local anesthetic toxicity technically challenging for surgeon Risk of aspiration precise titration of anesthetics to prevent apnea or coughing Not possible in sicker patients and/or with extensive lesions

Anesthetic management	Patient characteristics	Advantages	Disadvantages
Jet ventilation (general anesthesia) High- or low-frequency jet ventilation	Rapid rescue technique Augmentation of other airway techniques Poor surgical visualization	Uninterrupted access for anastomosis of the whole circumference of trachea	Barotrauma and the mucosal damage Entrainment of blood and debris from surgical field in distal airway Lack of monitoring of $EtCO_2$, inspired oxygen, and anesthetic gas concentration
Extracorporeal life support VV-ECMO, VA-ECMO, or CPB	Any anesthesia and any airway (including no airway) Cases with near-total obstruction Patients with extensive tumor infiltration hemodynamically unstable patients	It is the ultimate rescue technique Provides best surgical exposure Provides reliable control of gas exchange Hemodynamic support	Coagulopathy hemodilution vascular injury

17. **After we have secured the airway, what is the course of anesthesia during tracheal resection in high- and mid-tracheal surgery?**
    (a) Induction and intubation—a critical period
    (b) Dissection—a period of relative calm during which excision of lesion is done
    (c) Open airway—a critical period in which anastomosis is being constructed and airway is intubated across the field
    (d) Closure
    (e) Emergence and extubation—a critical period during which the reconstructed, potentially edematous airway is extubated [5]
18. **What is distal tracheal intubation/cross-field intubation in conventional anesthetic management of upper and mid tracheal lesion?**

This technique of lung ventilation is, by far, the most frequently used. In its simplest form, the trachea is intubated above the lesion. Once the trachea is opened, the ETT is simply pushed across the gap and positioned by the surgeon in the distal trachea. Following tracheal intubation with the ETT above or sometimes through the lesion, the lungs are ventilated using IPPV. Once the trachea is transected by the surgeon, the proximal ETT is pulled back, but kept in the trachea, and a new and sterile ETT is inserted by the surgeon, through the surgical field, into the distal trachea. Sterile tubings are then attached to this distal ETT and passed to the anesthesiologist so that IPPV can be resumed. Once the segment of diseased trachea is excised, end-to-end anastomosis is carried out [2, 6].

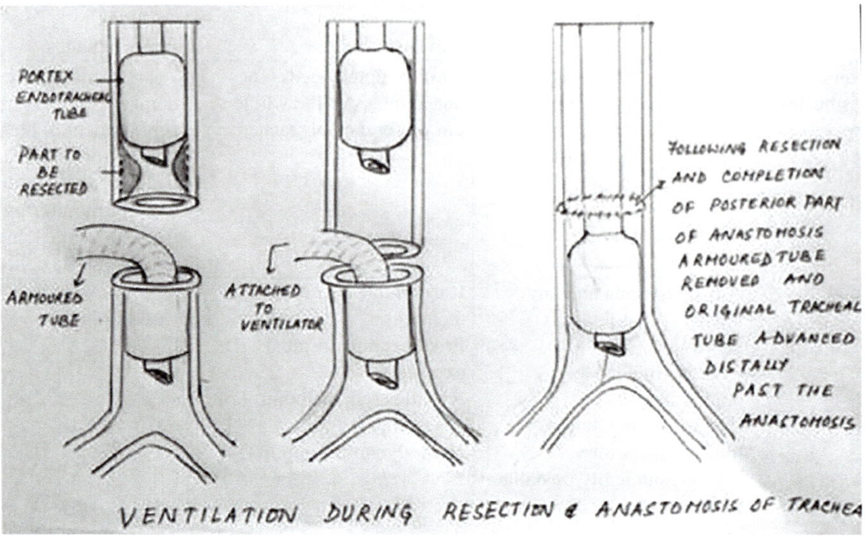

19. **For the surgeon to have a better vision while doing posterior anastomosis of trachea, what technique is used?**

Once the segment of diseased trachea is excised, end-to-end anastomosis is carried out. For this stage of operation, short intermittent apneic periods are permitted during which the distal ETT is removed from the trachea for suturing. There is no defined "optimal" apneic time. Patients should be receiving 100% O_2 to ensure an oxygen-rich FRC, and vital signs should be observed closely. The ventilation is resumed after a maximum of 3 min even if the saturation still reads above 98% or earlier if the saturation level decreases. Between the apneic periods, the lungs are manually hyperventilated with 100% O_2 to maintain a $PEtCO_2$ between a normal range of 30 and 35 mmHg. During this "hyperventilation-apnea" period, the surgeon starts by putting sutures on each end of the trachea without tying them, and then reapproximates the ends and ties the sutures on the posterior membrane. The neck is flexed during this part of surgery [2, 3, 6].

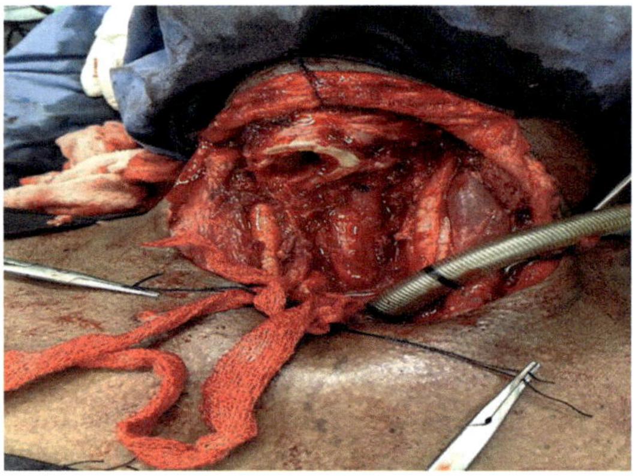

20. **When the surgeon asks to pull back our oral endotracheal tube, how can we avoid accidental extubation? At the end of the case, if the surgeon asks us to insert a larger endotracheal tube. How would we accomplish this?**

Once all the sutures are in place and the posterior membrane is securely anastomosed, the distal ETT is removed, and the proximal ETT is advanced beyond the anastomosis, either in the distal trachea or the mainstem bronchus. The surgeon then ties the remaining sutures. There are ways to secure the proximal ETT for readvancement in case of accidental extubation (the head is inaccessible to the anesthesiologist in most cases). Before pulling back the proximal ETT, a suture or surgical tape passed through the Murphy's eye can be secured on the surgical drapes, or a sterile flexible and long bougie can be passed retrogradely through the ETT and secured on one end by anesthesiologist and on the other end by the surgeon [2, 5, 7].

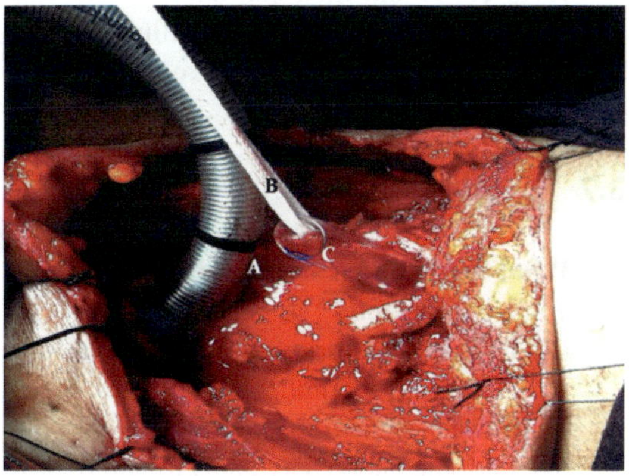

A—Flexometallic tube, B—Surgical tape, C—Endotracheal tube

21. **At the end of the procedure what measures are taken by the surgeon to check the patency of suture line?**

    On completion of the tracheal anastomosis, an "anastomosis leak test" is carried out by subjecting the airway to 20–30 cm of positive airway pressure for about 10 s with the anastomosed trachea submerged in saline [2, 6].

22. **What are the anesthesia concerns for low tracheal and carinal lesions?**

    Lower tracheal and carinal resection requires some modification of the technique the distal tube is advanced into left main stem bronchus below the lesion. The resected trachea and the right main stem bronchus are anastomosed, the orotracheal tube is advanced through the suture line and one lung ventilation to the right side is accomplished while left main stem bronchus is anastomosed to the side of the trachea. Endotracheal tube is then withdrawn above both suture lines until extubation. Intermittent apnea technique is used similar to high tracheal lesions. Independent distal cannulation of both bronchi has been described, and a variety of endotracheal tubes of different sizes should be available for distal cannulation and if required two anesthesia machines [2, 5, 6, 8].

23. **What is the role of chin stitch and how long can it be maintained?**

    An immobilizing guardian stitch, a suture is placed to connect the patient's chin to his or her chest, it is placed to maintain neck flexion in a neutral position and to prevent tension on the fresh anastomosis, goal is to prevent hyperextension not to force hyperflexion [8].

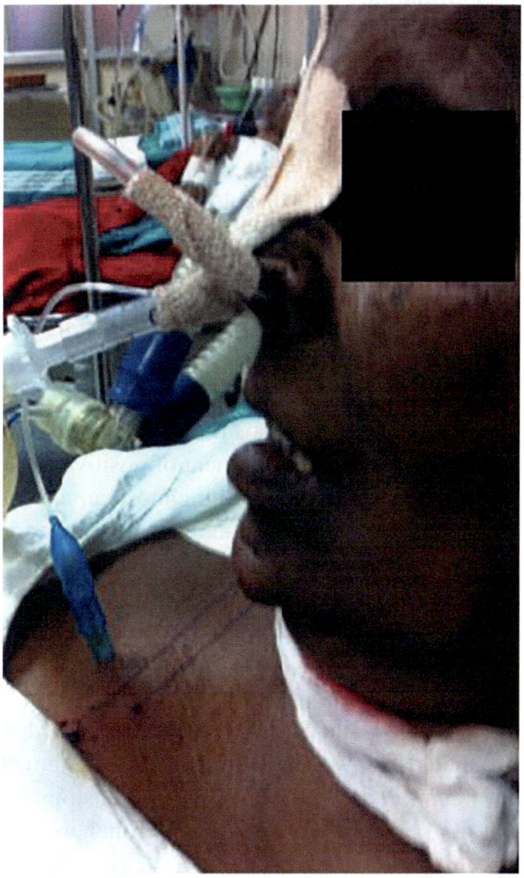

3.6 Extubation

24. **Should we extubate these patients?**

    It's a high-risk extubation in laryngotracheal surgery owing to the pathologies involved and the surgery performed. We should try to extubate as it is the primary goal in tracheal resection patients to relieve cuff pressure on the tracheal mucosa.

    Prior to extubation a check bronchoscopy for tracheobronchial suctioning inspection of anastomoses is desirable. Once extubation criteria are achieved patient is extubated in an awake state where airway patency is assured.

    Another option is to extubate the spontaneously breathing anesthetized patient and place a laryngeal mask, the aim is to avoid bucking and coughing.

25. **In what situations should we delay extubation?**

    In a minority of patients (expect vocal cord swelling due to proximal tracheal manipulation and rigid bronchoscopy), extubation may be deemed inadvisable and the decision thereafter is limited to extended intubation or a tracheostomy. The alternative is an advanced extubation technique, such as laryngeal mask airway exchange, or an airway rescue device left in place (e.g., airway exchange catheter, cricothyroid cannula). If we need to ventilate them it may include use of continuous positive airway pressure (CPAP) or bilevel positive airway pressure (BiPAP) with establishment of positive pressure limits. It is critical to choose an appropriately safe postoperative room for observation of the airway and a clear strategy for airway rescue [3].

26. **If we need to re-intubate, how we should do? Are there any issues with direct laryngoscopy?**

    If the patient needs to be reintubated it should be by a small ETT tube to minimize trauma and placement above the anastomotic site should be confirmed by bronchoscope. Flexible bronchoscope intubation can be performed safely while maintaining a neutral to slightly flexed position, thus allowing for precise ETT positioning and bronchial lavage and to provide diagnostic information for potential causes of postoperative failure. Direct laryngoscopy will require extension and cause strain on the suture line [8].

27. **How would we exclude recurrent laryngeal nerve damage postextubation?**

    The easiest way is to assess phonation/visualize by fiberoptic bronchoscopy of the vocal cords and then can address any concerns regarding vocal cord swelling or injury to the recurrent laryngeal nerve [8].

3.7 Postoperative

28. **What are the special concerns in the postoperative period?**
    (a) ICU care in the postoperative period to detect any complication of the anastomosed trachea.
    (b) Periodic blood gas analysis along with clinical monitoring.
    (c) Patients propped up at around 45° with head flexed with the help of guardian sutures. Comprehensive ancillary care comprising of humidified oxygen supplementation, nebulization, physiotherapy, and antitussive use.
    (d) A slow diet advancement strategy and gentle pulmonary toileting to prevent aspiration [6].

29. **What measures would you take for pain management?**

    Effective pain management is essential to prevent agitated patients.
    (a) Cervical incisions are managed well with systemic analgesics.
    (b) Thoracotomies require epidural analgesia (PCEA).
    (c) Multimodal analgesia helps prevent delirious patient and respiratory depression [6].

30. **What are the complications associated with this procedure?**

    Surgical

    (a) Dehiscence of anastomosis.
    (b) Recurrent laryngeal nerve dysfunction.
    (c) Hemorrhage.
    (d) Air leak.
    (e) Tracheoesophageal fistula.

    Nonsurgical complications

    (a) The residual effect of drugs (analgesics, neuromuscular blockers).
    (b) Atelectasis (due to secretions).
    (c) Respiratory failure.
    (d) Pneumonia.
    (e) Pulmonary embolism.
    (f) Deep vein thrombosis.
    (g) Myocardial infarction.
    (h) Tetraplegia [9].

31. **What is the role of regional anesthesia?**

    Literature describes four regional anesthesia techniques [10] for conducting tracheal resection and anastomosis, which have been tried since 2010. However, these techniques need further evaluation before they can be adopted as the sole technique. Cervical epidural catheters, cervical plexus block, local infiltration, thoracic epidural have been used to provide analgesia in these cases.

References

1. Smeltz AM, Bhatia M, Arora H, et al. Anesthesia for resection and reconstruction of the trachea and Carina. J Cardiothorac Vasc Anesth. 2020;34:1902.
2. Pinsonneault C, Fortier J, Donati F, et al. Tracheal resection and reconstruction. Can J Anaesth. 1999;46:439–55.
3. Al-Bazzaz F, Grillo H, Kazemi H. Response to exercise in upper airway obstruction. Am Rev Respir Dis. 1975;111(5):631–40.
4. Shapshay SM, Valdez TA. Bronchoscopic management of benign stenosis. Chest Surg Clin N Am. 2001;11:749–68.
5. Sandberg W. Anesthesia and airway management for tracheal resection and reconstruction. Int Anesthesiol Clin. 2000;38:55–75.
6. Marwaha A, Kumar A, Sharma S, Sood J. Anaesthesia for tracheal resection and anastomosis. J Anaesthesiol Clin Pharmacol. 2022;38:48–57.
7. Blasberg JD, Wright CD. Surgical considerations in tracheal and carinal resection. Semin Cardiothorac Vasc Anesth. 2012;16:190–5.
8. Hobai IA, Chhangani SV, Alfille PH. Anesthesia for tracheal resection and reconstruction. Anesthesiol Clin. 2012;30:709–30.
9. Auchincloss HG, Wright CD. Complications after tracheal resection and reconstruction: prevention and treatment. J Thorac Dis. 2016;8:S160–7.
10. Macchiarini P, Rovira I, Ferrarello S. Awake upper airway surgery. Ann Thorac Surg. 2010;89:387–90.

Anterior Mediastinal Mass for Mediastinoscopy and Proceed

4

Kiran Mahendru, Nishkarsh Gupta, and Anju Gupta

4.1 Case Scenario

A 25-year-old woman presented with history of cough and progressively increasing dyspnea in supine position for the last 2 months. Chest X-ray revealed a large mediastinal mass filling approximately two-thirds of the chest. The above finding was confirmed using CT scan with compression of the mid to distal trachea and 50% decrease in the cross-sectional area in the narrowest part. She has been referred to the anesthesia department for pre-anesthetic checkup for mediastinoscopy and proceed.

4.2 Introduction

Mediastinal masses are a diverse group of benign and malignant tumors [1]. They range from slow-growing, small, asymptomatic tumors to large aggressive symptomatic masses. Though they are uncommon, with advances in medicine they are increasingly being recognized and present to the anesthesiologist for both diagnostic and therapeutic procedures. They are a challenge to the anesthesiologist especially anterior mediastinal masses as they have the propensity to cause airway and vascular compression which is exacerbated under general anesthesia leading to increased risk of perioperative morbidity and mortality. Therefore, careful preoperative assessment with emphasis on the relation of the mediastinal mass to the surrounding vital structures and appropriate preparation for the worst is the key to successful management.

4.3 Describe Anatomy of Mediastinum?

The mediastinum is made up of four compartments namely superior, anterior, middle, and posterior. A line passing from the sternal angle anteriorly to the lower border of T4 vertebrae divides the mediastinum into superior and inferior compartments. The anterior, middle, and posterior are the three parts of inferior mediastinum.

The boundaries of the mediastinum are formed by the following structures [2]:

Superior	Thoracic inlet
Inferior	Diaphragm
Lateral	Mediastinal pleura
Anterior	Sternum
Posterior	Vertebral column

The extent of the anterior mediastinum is from the posterior surface of the sternum to anterior

K. Mahendru · A. Gupta
Department of Anesthesiology, Pain Medicine and Critical Care, AIIMS, New Delhi, New Delhi, India

N. Gupta (✉)
Department of Onco-Anesthesiology and Palliative Medicine, DRBRAIRCH, AIIMS, New Delhi, New Delhi, India

N. Gupta et al. (eds.), *Problem Based Learning Discussions in Onco-Anesthesia and Onco-Critical Care*, https://doi.org/10.1007/978-981-99-6339-3_4

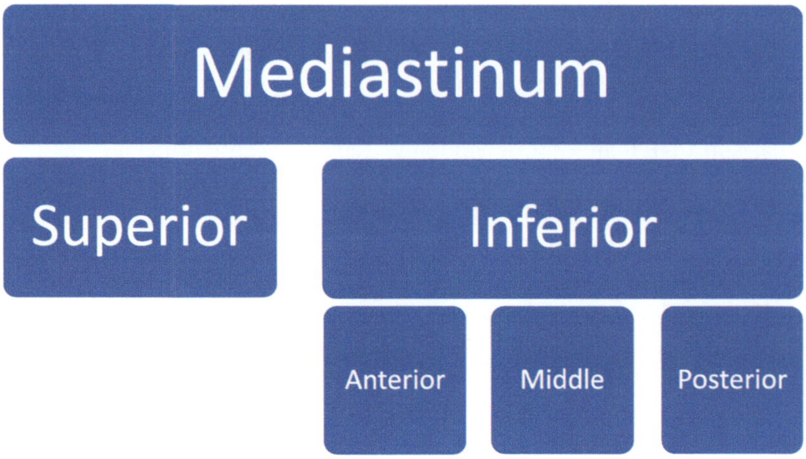

surface of pericardium and great vessels. The middle mediastinum is bounded anteriorly and posteriorly by the pericardium. The posterior mediastinum lies between posterior pericardium and anterior longitudinal ligament [3].

The contents of the mediastinum as per the compartments are as follows:

Superior mediastinum	Thymus Trachea Esophagus Arteries: aortic arch, brachiocephalic trunk, left common carotid artery, left subclavian artery Veins: superior vena cava, brachiocephalic veins, arch of azygous Thoracic duct
Anterior mediastinum	Thymus Trachea Esophagus Large arteries and veins Thoracic duct Sympathetic trunk Lymph nodes Ectopic thyroid and parathyroid tissue
Middle mediastinum	Heart and pericardium Great vessels Vagus Phrenic nerve
Posterior mediastinum	Thoracic spinal ganglion Sympathetic chain Intercostal nerves

4.4 What is Differential Diagnosis of a Mediastinal Mass?

The differential diagnosis for a mediastinal mass based on its location is as follows [4, 5]:

Superior mediastinum	Retrosternal thyroid
	Thymoma
Anterior mediastinum	Thymoma
	Thymic cyst
	Thymic hyperplasia
	Thymic carcinoma
	Lymphoma
	Germ cell tumor—teratoma/dermoid cyst/seminoma/nonseminoma
	Intrathoracic thyroid
	Parathyroid adenoma
	Hemangioma
	Lipoma/liposarcoma
	Fibroma/fibrosarcoma
	Foramen of morgagni hernia
Middle mediastinum	Pericardial cyst
	Bronchogenic cyst
	Lymphadenopathy—lymphoma/sarcoid/metastatic lung tumor
	Enteric cysts
	Esophageal tumor
	Vascular masses
Posterior mediastinum	Neurogenic tumors—neurofibroma/neurosarcoma/neuroblastoma/ganglioneuroma/gaglioneuroblastoma/neurilemmoma/chemodectoma/pheochromocytoma
	Spine lesions
	Hiatal hernia
	Meningoceles

Most commonly the masses are located in the anterior mediastinum. The masses more frequently seen in adult patients are thymoma, lymphoma, and germ cell tumors whereas lymphoma, neuroblastoma, and PNET are more commonly seen in the pediatric age group [6].

4.5 How do Patients with Mediastinal Mass Present Clinically?

The clinical presentation of a patient with mediastinal mass varies with the size, site, and nature of the lesion. The most notorious ones are the anterior mediastinal masses because of the risk of tracheobronchial and vascular compression. The presentation can vary from asymptomatic patients with incidental discovery of the mass to a patient with severe symptoms caused by tracheobronchial obstruction, superior vena cava syndrome, right heart compression, and pulmonary vascular compression. The patients can also have associated systemic symptoms of thyroid disorder, myasthenia gravis [7], caused by the disease processes associated with common mediastinal masses. The use of preoperative chemotherapy and radiotherapy can have various implications for the conduct of anesthesia.

4.6 Enumerate the Signs and Symptoms of Mediastanal Compression?

4.6.1 Tarcheobrpnchial Compresison

The patient may present with a history of nonspecific cough, chest discomfort, dyspnea, orthopnea, hoarseness, and noisy breathing. The signs include tachypnea, decreased breath sounds, ronchi, and stridor. The signs and symptoms can vary with positional changes, with increasing severity most commonly seen in supine position. The patient becomes comfortable in a specific position which is associated with least compression of the tracheobronchial tree. However, the severity of symptoms may not correlate with the degree of obstruction of the airway specially in pediatric patients. A child who is asymptomatic may develop airway obstruction post induction of anesthesia [8]. Children also tend to develop symptoms earlier as compared to adults because of the decreased caliber of the trachea, with symptoms developing with even a small decrease in tracheal diameter.

4.6.2 Vascular Compression

The signs and symptoms caused by vascular compression may mimic those caused by airway obstruction. The obstruction of the superior vena cava may lead to dyspnea, headache, visual disturbances, and altered mentation caused by the decreased venous return from the upper thorax. The patient develops edema of the face, neck, and arms. Development of collaterals occurs in the upper part of the body. The compression of the heart caused by the anterior mediastinal mass may lead to dyspnea of cardiac origin, syncope, arrhythmia, and murmur.

The grading of the signs and symptoms is as per the severity in supine position. A patient can be asymptomatic, have mild symptoms where the patient is comfortable in supine position with mild symptoms of compression, moderate symptoms where a patient can lie supine for only a short duration of time because of the manifestation of compressive symptoms, and severe where the patient cannot lie supine at all [9].

4.7 Enumerate Major Anesthetic Concernds in this Patient?

The major concerns for an anesthesiologist evaluating a patient with mediastinal mass is the risk of airway compromise and hemodynamic instability caused by the tracheobronchial and cardiovascular compression.

The major concerns are as follows:

- Mass effect on the tracheobronchial structures with risk of airway obstruction post induction of anesthesia
- Mass effect on the cardiovascular structures like superior vena cava, right heart, pulmonary artery with risk of cardiovascular collapse

- Positional changes associated with exacerbation of symptoms in supine position as compared to sitting or lateral
- Increased risk of loss of airway control after administration of neuromuscular blocking agents
- Effect of positive pressure ventilation leading to decreased venous return combined with the vasodilatory effect of the anesthetic agents can have synergistic effects in causing cardiovascular collapse
- Loss of airway patency during the surgical procedure as a result of injuries inflicted during resection
- Risk of blood loss due to hemorrhage caused by injury to the vascular structures and heart

4.7.1 Preoperative Evaluation and Investigations

The preoperative evaluation will include detailed history and clinical examination pertaining to the signs and symptoms associated with the compression of the vital structures. The main aim is to assess the size and relationship of the mass and extent of compression of the airway and cardiovascular structures. The signs and symptoms pertaining to the mass should be elicited in the history. It should focus on both the local symptoms caused by the mass like chest pain, dyspnea, dysphagia, syncope, hoarseness, cough, stridor, hemoptysis, and the systemic symptoms due to paraneoplastic syndromes like myasthenia gravis. The degree of severity of the symptoms and the exacerbating and relieving factors should be noted. The most important point in the history and examination is the positional changes which tend to alleviate the symptoms of the patient.

Apart from the routine preoperative investigations special emphasis is needed on the radiological studies, pulmonary function tests, flow volume loops, and transthoracic echocardiography.

- **Radiological imaging**: It helps to define the location, size, and relation of mass to surrounding structures. Reviewing the images can help anesthesiologist decide the plan of anesthetic management. Chest X-ray is a screening modality and CT scans provide the accurate assessment of the tumor [10]. MR imaging though not commonly used can be done in patients with contrast allergy or neurogenic lesions.

  It will give us the details of the compressive effects. A reduction of more than 50% of the cross-sectional area of the trachea is associated with more chances of airway-related morbidity. The extent of obstruction usually correlates with the symptomatology and also helps to predict the risk of complete airway obstruction post induction of anesthesia [11]. Detection of pericardial effusion on CT scan can be a warning for increased risk of perioperative complications and thus will require further cardiac evaluation [12].
- **Pulmonary function tests (PFT)**: Though it is an investigation done in preoperative evaluation of mediastinal tumors, their ability to identify degree of airway obstruction and hence changing the anesthetic management is questionable [13].
- **Flow volume loops**: They help to differentiate between intrathoracic and extrathoracic obstruction [14]. The patient with intrathoracic airway obstruction will present with reduced expiratory airflow and a patient with extrathoracic airway obstruction will have an inspiratory plateau [15].
- **Transthoracic echocardiography (TTE)**: It should be considered in patients with suspicion of compression or invasion of the cardiovascular structures as deciphered by either signs and symptoms or CT scan imaging. In case pericardial effusion is identified in CT scan, further evaluation using TTE is must [15].

Combining two investigations in a patient with mediastinal mass can help assess the risk of airway complications and hence decide the plan of anesthetic management. These are the peak expiratory flow rate (PEFR) and tracheal area [16].

Shamberger risk assessment box [16]

	Tracheal area <50%	Tracheal area >50%
PEFR >50%	Moderate risk	Low risk
PEFR <50%	High risk	Moderate risk

The patients in low-risk group can receive general anesthesia using neuromuscular blocking agents without any complications. In moderate risk category it is important to maintain spontaneous ventilation to avoid airway collapse. Whereas, in high-risk group it is wise to avoid GA, use local anesthesia for biopsy and consider pretreatment with chemotherapy and steroids.

4.7.2 Discuss Anesthetic Management in this Patient

The anesthetic management will depend on the type of surgical procedure which may be diagnostic or therapeutic. Diagnostic procedures are done to procure tissue for histological diagnosis which can be safely conducted under local anesthesia or regional techniques like intercostal nerve block, paravertebral block, or epidural. Position-related exacerbation of symptoms should be considered during these procedures and sedatives should be used cautiously to prevent airway compromise.

Patients undergoing therapeutic procedures will require general anesthesia. Routine standard American Society of Anesthesiology (ASA) monitoring is done along with invasive blood pressure monitoring preinduction because of the risk of sudden cardiovascular collapse following induction. Transesophageal echocardiography can be considered in patients with risk of cardiovascular compression. It is important to establish a good intravenous access with due consideration to secure a central venous catheter depending on a case-to-case basis. In a patient with SVC syndrome IV access should be secured in the lower limbs [17].

4.7.2.1 Induction and Intubation

The three methods to conduct anesthesia and secure airway in a patient undergoing mediastinal mass excision are:

1. Awake fiberoptic intubation
2. Inhalational induction
3. Routine intravenous induction

The method used needs to be individualized based on patient characteristics, site, and extent of tracheobronchial compression.

In a patient with large mediastinal mass causing significant or distal tracheobronchial obstruction, awake fiberoptic intubation will be the method of choice. The advantages of this technique are that it will allow the assessment of the level and degree of obstruction which can be useful later in case of respiratory compromise intraoperatively, will help maintain spontaneous respiration and hence is the most reversible technique out of all [18, 19]. All these factors make it the safest technique.

The use of inhalational technique for induction can precipitate airway obstruction [20]. Partial airway obstruction during inhalational anesthesia can generate negative pressures to such an extent that it can lead on to complete airway collapse.

In asymptomatic patients with radiological findings suggestive of no airway or cardiovascular compression, routine intravenous induction can be performed. It is important to be cautious while using this technique in asymptomatic pediatric patients as airway obstruction has been reported in such cases [8, 21].

Consideration must be given to the most appropriate position for conduct of anesthesia to prevent the risk of airway obstruction post induction. The positions used can be lateral, semierect, or sitting based on the patient's history [8, 22].

Intubation must be done distal to the level of tracheobronchial obstruction. Therefore, in some cases, endobronchial intubation may be required. Endobronchial tubes, microlaryngeal tubes, equipment for jet ventilation, and rigid bronchoscopes must be available in the operation theatre.

Cardiopulmonary bypass is considered as the technique in patients with uncertainty regarding the ability to ventilate like obstruction of distal third trachea, both mainstem bronchi or carina or extensive compression of the right heart or pulmonary artery with expected cardiopulmonary compromise post induction.

4.7.2.2 Ventilation

Maintenance of spontaneous ventilation is savior in management of these cases especially if the ability to intubate distal to the level of airway obstruction is uncertain. Short-acting muscle relaxants should only be administered if the ability to ventilate and secure an airway is certain. Once the patient is intubated distal to the level of obstruction, the tolerance of positive pressure ventilation is checked. If well tolerated patient is ventilated with positive pressure with or without the use of muscle relaxants. In case of any doubt related to the ability to ventilate or intubate distal to obstruction spontaneous ventilation is maintained with occasional assistance.

4.8 Enumerate Special Consoderations for Mediastinoscopy

Indications for doing mediastinoscopy are staging of lung cancer and to obtain biopsy for histological diagnosis. The two commonly used techniques are:

1. Cervical mediastinoscopy: done from beneath the manubrium sterni and requires general anesthesia. More commonly done procedure.
2. Anterior mediastinoscopy: done from second left intercostal space to inspect lower mediastinum and can be done under local anesthesia [23]. Less commonly done.

The following are the major considerations while conducting anesthesia for mediastinoscopy:

- Done under general anesthesia, therefore preoperative evaluation should be done as per mediastinal mass
- There is a risk of life-threatening major hemorrhage due to the proximity of the mediastinoscope to the major blood vessels like innominate artery and azygous vein
- Compression of the innominate artery can lead to cerebrovascular events and right upper limb ischemia. Therefore, it is important to monitor pulse oximeter and right arterial waveform to look for any compression
- Compression of the trachea can occur leading to respiratory compromise. It is therefore important to monitor peak airway pressures
- Compression of aorta causing reflex bradycardia
- Risk of injury to recurrent laryngeal nerve
- Risk of pneumothorax
- Air embolism

The patient is usually extubated on table and shifted to recovery. Postoperative chest X-ray is done to rule out pneumothorax.

4.9 Enumerate Complictaions in the Postoperative Period

The two major complications anticipated in these patients are respiratory and cardiovascular collapse.

4.9.1 Respiratory Collapse

In case of respiratory collapse during the intraoperative period

1. The first step will be to increase the inspired concentration of oxygen to 100%.
2. This should be followed by the application of continuous positive airway pressure (CPAP) which can help splint open the airways and restore the functional residual capacity [24].
3. Repositioning the patient to either lateral or prone [25] can help relieve the obstruction caused by the mass.
4. Use of intermittent positive ventilation with positive end-expiratory pressure can be considered.
5. Passing the tracheal tube past the site of obstruction can help restore oxygenation and ventilation. This may require using one lung ventilation.
6. Finally, a rigid bronchoscope will be the rescue device to be used in situation of crisis to be inserted beyond the point of obstruction to maintain oxygenation.

4.9.2 Cardiovascular Collapse

In case of cardiovascular collapse in the intraoperative period

1. First-line therapy will be the use of fluid boluses
2. This should be followed by reducing the depth of anesthesia
3. Repositioning of the patient to prevent compression of the cardiovascular structures
4. The last resort is to perform sternotomy and list the mass from the thoracic structures

The respiratory and cardiovascular complications are interrelated. Therefore, it is important to consider both in case of deteriorating condition of the patient. Extracorporeal membrane oxygenation or cardiopulmonary bypass should be preemptively kept ready in high-risk patients with increased chances of such complications.

4.9.3 Emergence and Recovery

The recovery can be complicated by risk of airway obstruction after diagnostic procedures, glottic edema, and postoperative stridor due to prolonged procedures or SVC syndrome. For enhancing the recovery post anesthesia short-acting anesthetic agents should be used and the patient should be extubated only fully awake, is obeying commands and the muscle strength is completely recovered. The patient should be monitored closely post extubation for airway and cardiovascular complications.

4.9.4 Postoperative Care

The appropriate level of care in the postoperative period will depend on the nature of the procedure and the intraoperative course. For a patient who has undergone a diagnostic procedure under anesthesia, there is a risk of airway complications postoperatively because of presence of the mass effect. Therefore, increased level of care is required in such cases. Whereas, for a patient who has undergone the surgical procedure involving the excision of the mediastinal mass, the compression effects have been alleviated. The patient can be extubated if fully awake with return of the protective airway reflexes and hemodynamically stable. Postoperative complications like bleeding, atelectasis, lung infection, and airway edema can happen and need close monitoring. The intensive care unit should be notified regarding the procedure so that appropriate management can be done as per need in case of perioperative complications. Postoperative mechanical ventilation may be required in patients with long complicated procedures associated with blood loss, fluid shifts, and hemodynamic instability.

Postoperative pain management is provided using multimodal analgesia depending on the invasiveness of the procedure. Intravenous agents like paracetamol, non-steroidal anti-inflammatory drugs, opioids infusion or patient-controlled analgesia (PCA), and regional techniques in the form of thoracic epidural and paravertebral infusions of local anesthetics will provide adequate analgesia and reduce the risk of postoperative pulmonary complications. They will also help in early ambulation thus enhancing the recovery in the postoperative period. Other techniques that can also be used include intercostal nerve blocks, use of intrathecal opioids, and use of intrapleural analgesia.

References

1. Yoneda KY, Louie S, Shelton DK. Mediastinal tumors. Curr Opin Pulm Med. 2001;7:226–33.
2. Pokorny WJ. Mediastinal tumors. In: Holder TM, Ashcraft KW, editors. Pediatric surgery. 2nd ed. Philadelphia: WB Saunders; 1993. p. 218–27.
3. Warren WH. Chapter 122: Anatomy of the mediastinum with special reference to surgical access. In: Pearson's thoracic and esophageal surgery. 3rd ed. Elsevier; 2009. p. 1472.
4. Slinger P, Karsli C. Management of the patient with a large anterior mediastinal mass: recurring myths. Curr Opin Anaesthesiol. 2007;20:1.
5. Rath L, Gullahorn G, Connolly N, et al. Anterior mediastinal mass biopsy and resection: anesthetic techniques and perioperative concerns. Semin Cardiothorac Vasc Anesth. 2012;16:235.
6. Dubashi B, Cyriac S, Tenali SG. Clinicopathological analysis and outcome of primary mediastinal malignancies—a report of 91 cases from a single institute. Ann Thorac Med. 2009;4:140–2.

7. Congedo E, Aceto P, Cardone A, Petrucci R, Dottarelli A, De Cosmo G. Perioperative management of thymectomy. Ann Ital Chir. 2007;78(5):367–70.
8. Bray RJ, Fernandes FJ. Mediastinal tumour causing airway obstruction in anaesthetized children. Anaesthesia. 1982;37:571–5.
9. Frawley G, Low J, Brown TCK. Anaesthesia for an anterior mediastinal mass with ketamine and midazolam infusion. Anaesth Intensive Care. 1995;23:610–2.
10. Graeber GM, Shriver CD, Albus RA, Burton NA, Collins GJ, Lough FC, et al. The use of computed tomography in the evaluation of mediastinal masses. J Thorac Cardiovasc Surg. 1986;91:662–6.
11. Azizkhan RG, Dudgeon DL, Buck JR, Colombani PM, et al. Life threatening airway obstruction as a complication to the management of mediastinal masses in children. J Pediatr Surg. 1985;20:816–22.
12. Mandell GA, Lantieri R, Goodman LR. Tracheobronchial compression in Hodgkin's lymphoma in children. Am J Radiol. 1982;139:1167–70.
13. Hnatiuk OW, Corcoran PC, Sierra A. Spirometry in surgery for anterior mediastinal masses. Chest. 2001;120:1152–6.
14. Prakash UB, Abel MD, Hubmayer RD. Mediastinal mass and tracheal obstruction during general anesthesia. Mayo Clin Proc. 1988;63:1004–11.
15. Neuman GG, Weingarten AE, Abramowitz RM, Kushins LG, Abramson AL, Ladner W. The anesthetic management of the patient with an anterior mediastinal mass. Anesthesiology. 1984;60:144–7.
16. Shamberger RC, Holzman RS, Griscom NT, et al. CT quantitation o tracheal cross-sectional area as a guide to the surgical and anesthetic management of children with anterior mediastinal masses. J Pediatr Surg. 1991;26:138–42.
17. Northrip DN, Bohman BK, Tsueda K. Total airway occlusion and SVC syndrome in a child with an anterior mediastinal tumor. Anesth Analg. 1986;65:1079–82.
18. Goh MH, Liu XY, Goh YS. Anterior mediastinal masses: an anaesthetic challenge. Anaesthesia. 1999;54:670–82.
19. Narang S, Harte BH, Body SC. Anesthesia for patients with a mediastinal mass. Anesthesiol Clin N Am. 2001;19:559–79.
20. Mackie AM, Watson CB. Anaesthesia and mediastinal masses. Anaesthesia. 1984;39:899–903.
21. Shamberger RC. Preanesthetic evaluation of children with anterior mediastinal masses. Semin Pediatr Surg. 1999;8:61–8.
22. O'Leary HT, Tracey JA. Mediastinal tumours causing airway obstruction: a case in an adult. Anaesthesia. 1983;38:67.
23. Rendina EA, Venuta F, De Giacomo T, Ciccone AM, Moretti MS, Ibrahim M, et al. Biopsy of anterior mediastinal masses under local anesthesia. Ann Thorac Surg. 2002;74:1720–2.
24. Hammer GB. Anaesthetic management for the child with a mediastinal mass. Paediatr Anaesth. 2004;14:95–7.
25. Latham GJ, Greenberg RS. Anesthetic considerations for the pediatric oncology patient—part 2. Pediatr Anesth. 2010;20:396–420.

5 Anesthetic Considerations for a Patient with Carcinoma Lung Scheduled for Lobectomy or Pneumonectomy

Umesh Goneppanavar and Jasvinder Kaur

5.1 Case Scenario

A 72-year-old gentleman, chronic smoker for the past 30 years has presented with history of blood-streaked sputum, cough, right-sided chest pain in the last 1 month. His current height and weight are 166 cm and 62 kg. He doesn't have any other associated co-morbidities. On investigation, he was found to be having a non-small cell carcinoma in the right lower lobe region. The thoracic surgeon has discussed with the patient regarding a plan for right lower lobectomy/right pneumonectomy.

5.2 Enumerate the Risk Factors, Major Types of Lung Malignancies, and Their Common Manifestations Along with Their Prognosis?

The manifestations vary based on organ system involvement, extent of involvement, spread of the malignancy, degree of shunt, existing co-morbidities, etc. Detection by clinical evaluation, radiology, and flexible bronchoscopy. Common presenting complaints include persistent cough, recurrent lung infections, hemoptysis, wheezing, weight loss, fatigue, and chest pain. Paraneoplastic syndromes, nerve entrapment leading to Horner's syndrome, and vena caval compression may also be the presenting features.

Small cell lung cancers (SCLC) have poor prognosis as they usually would have metastasized significantly by the time of diagnosis and hence are mostly suited for non-surgical management.

Non-small cell lung cancers (NSCLC) have relatively better prognosis (fortunately, they account for nearly 80% of lung malignancies) and often surgical management can be an option +/− subsequent radiotherapy and chemotherapy [1]. Lung tumors have been reclassified by the WHO in 2015, with subtypes which were earlier clubbed as NSCLC being segregated into separate groups based on cytology, as specimens nowadays are more frequently obtained during bronchoscopic sampling rather than at surgical resection. This also has bearing on treatment as specific tumor subtypes express receptors which serve as targets for immunotherapeutic agents [2].

U. Goneppanavar (✉) · J. Kaur
Department of Neuroanaesthesia, DIMHANS, Dharwad, Dharwad, India

N. Gupta et al. (eds.), *Problem Based Learning Discussions in Onco-Anesthesia and Onco-Critical Care*, https://doi.org/10.1007/978-981-99-6339-3_5

5.3 Enumerate the Advantages and Disadvantages of Different Surgical Options Available

These are detailed in Table 5.1 [3].

Table 5.1 Different lung cancer resection procedures

Procedures	Details
Lobectomy	Lobectomy with mediastinal lymph node dissection with open thoracotomy
VATS lobectomy	Lobectomy performed under thoracoscopy
Sleeve lobectomy	For centrally located tumors of the lung: Affected lobe along with its bronchial component removed along with reimplantation of remaining bronchial component and parenchyma
Segmentectomy and wedge resection	Segment of the lung to be removed along with removal of its related pulmonary artery, vein, and bronchus
Pneumonectomy	Removal of the entire lung by leaving a bronchial stump

5.4 What Different Evaluations Are Required for this Patient Apart from Routine Assessment?

Lung malignancy contributes to bulk of lung resections currently and most of these surgeries will be semi-urgent in nature. Therefore, this small preoperative time window should be used for determining patient fitness as well as detecting and optimizing (a) co-morbidities, (b) cardiopulmonary status, and (c) factors that may contribute to acute lung injury (ALI) postoperatively. The surgical procedure may be through a large incision (open approach) or through small ports (thoracoscopy) performed manually or with robotic assistance. Accordingly, anesthesiologists should plan management options for anesthesia and postoperative management including pain relief.

The 3-legged stool for preoperative evaluation of lung has been developed to identify the suitability of patients for proposed lung resection surgery. It involves assessment of the mechanical and parenchymal functioning of the lungs along with the overall cardiopulmonary reserves (Tables 5.2 and 5.3) [1, 4]. Minute ventilation to carbon diox-

Table 5.2 The 3-legged stool for assessment for fitness before lung resection surgery

3-legged stool to assess for fitness before lung surgery	Mechanical function (ability to deliver oxygen/air till alveoli)	Parenchymal function (ability to transfer oxygen across alveolo-pulmonary barrier)	Cardiopulmonary reserve (ability to deliver oxygen to tissues and meet their demands at different physical activities)
Parameters	ppo FEV1 Spirometry FEV1 FVC FEV1/FVC	Arterial blood gas (ABG) Diffusing capacity for carbon monoxide in lungs (DLCO)	Maximal oxygen consumption (VOmax) Six min walk test (cost-effective and equally reliable as Vomax)
Most valuable and reliable method to assess	Predicted postoperative FEV1% (ppo FEV1) = preoperative FEV1 × (1 − % of functional lung tissue removed/100)	Corrected DLCO = preoperative DLCO × (1 − % of functional lung tissue removed/100)	Vomax Six min walk test = number of meters walked in 6 min/30 (is approximately equal to Vomax)
Other predictors	FEV1/FVC for differentiating obstructive and restrictive components Plethysmography	Room air ABG: PO_2 <60 mmHg and/or PCO_2 >45 mmHg	Predicted Vomax <60% Anerobic threshold <11 mL/kg/min >4% drop in SpO_2 on >2 staircase climb Stair climbing <54 steps (<3 flights of stairs)

Table 5.3 Management plan for lung resections based on the risk assessment

ppoFEV1 or ppo DLCO	>40%	30-40%	20-30%	<20%
Consider the lowest of the two to make reliable predictions about outcomes	Safe, expected to do well	Grey zone, consider co-morbidities and limiting the resection	Enhanced risk, consider only for minimally invasive surgery To be performed in dedicated centres with experienced teams	Very high mortality risk Contra-indication for surgery
Extubation plan	Can be extubated in the operating room if the intraoperative period was uneventful, for patients warm, stable and comfortable	Individualize as per patient status, co-morbidities and anticipated future course Some can be extubated in the theatre, some require extubation following a period of ventilation/observation	Postoperative mechanical ventilation and subsequent decision in ICU	
Preoperative VOmax	> 20 mL/kg/min	15-20 mL/kg/min	15-20 mL/kg/min	<15 mL/kg/min

Prediction of risk during lung resection surgery (green zone is fit, grey zone is acceptable with risk, amber zone is to be performed in dedicated centers with significant backup and morbidity/mortality, red zone is contra-indication for lung resection procedures

ide output slope (VE/VCO$_2$ slope) also called the ventilatory efficiency curve is derived through cardiopulmonary exercise testing [5]. Values >35 indicate high risk of mortality following lung resection. Inability to climb 3 floors (12.16 m) by stairs within 37.5 s has been found to correlate with increased complications following thoracic surgery [6].

5.5 Determining the Actual Contribution of the Segments to Current Overall Functioning of the Lungs

Important aspect here is to know whether the resectable segment is contributing to functioning of the lungs or not (Fig. 5.1). Functionally contributing units when resected will affect the postoperative functioning whereas the already diseased segments that may not contribute functionally in the preoperative period itself may not affect the postoperative outcomes even when they are resected.

Imaging of the lungs and its vasculature: V/Q radionuclide scan, pulmonary quantitative CT scan, or 3D dynamic perfusion MRI with V/Q scan being the gold standard.

Split lung function tests: endobronchial intubation with normal ETT or DLT or bronchial blocker to other side than the one to be resected (one lung ventilation to check if the patient will be fine with the lung to remain after pneumonectomy) or occlusion of intended operative side pulmonary trunk.

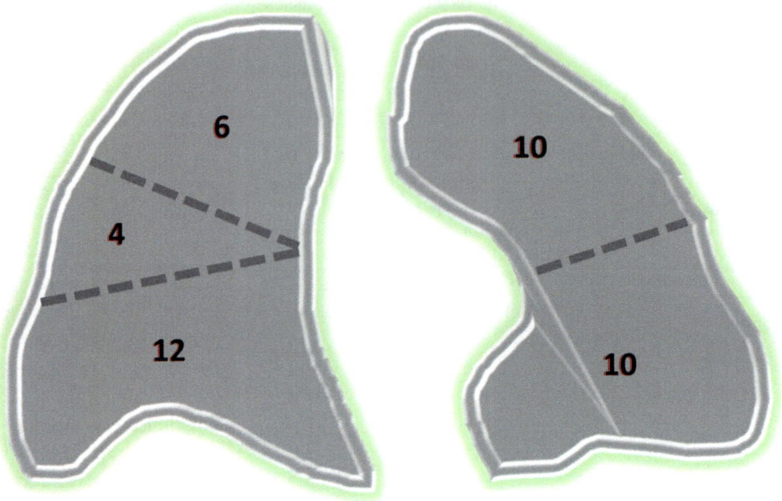

Fig. 5.1 The distribution of subsegments in each lobe of the lung for computing ppoFEV1. Example for computing the ppoFEV1 in a patient with 70% FEV1 scheduled to undergo right upper lobectomy: for right upper lobectomy which has 6 segments out of the maximum 42 segments, the equation will be: PPO FEV1 = 70% (1 − [6 × 100/42]/100) = 70% (1 − [100/7]/100) = 70% (1 − [14.3/100]) = 70% (1–0.143) = 70% (0.857) = ~60%

Apart from this, pre-existent lung disease in both lungs or in the lung to be preserved postoperatively will affect the outcomes. Also, the effects of lung malignancy should be considered from four different perspectives, i.e., their mass effects on surrounding tissues, their metabolic effects (including endocrinal manifestations), and metastatic effects. In addition, preoperative chemotherapy or radiotherapy effects should also be considered [1, 4, 7].

5.6 Other Risk Factors

Cardiac problems (myocardial ischemia, arrhythmias, and heart failure) constitute the second most frequently encountered complications following lung resection (intermediate-risk surgery for myocardial ischemia, peaks usually by 48–72 h postoperatively). Those with poor cardiopulmonary reserves require stress ECHO or technetium thallium scan. If perfusion scan is defective, require cardiac catheterization [1, 4].

Chronic smoking, current smoking, advanced age, impaired renal function, and extent of metastasis will affect outcomes.

5.7 What Aspects of Airway Evaluation Are Relevant to Management of These Patients?

Apart from routinely known predictors for poor glottic view on laryngoscopy, history of irradiation to neck and hard neck tissues on palpation should be considered. In addition, predictors for difficult lung isolation such as distortion, narrowing, invasion, or disruption of the tracheobronchial tree should be evaluated. Tracheostomy presents challenges in lung isolation. Since airway below the oropharynx is invisible to naked eye evaluation, radiological evaluation with X-ray chest and neck, ultrasound, CT, and MRI may be required for better understanding. Check flexible bronchoscopy will also provide useful information regarding the nature of airway pathology [1, 4, 7].

Assessment for the size and side of DLT and appropriate flexible bronchoscope are detailed in Table 5.4 [1, 4, 7, 8].

Table 5.4 Determination size of DLT with corresponding internal diameter and maximum flexible bronchoscope that can be inserted

Height of the patient	Tracheal diameter (measured at suprasternal notch level in CXR)	Size of the DLT	DLT lumen ID	Maximum allowable outer diameter of flexible bronchoscope
Males >170 cm	>18 mm	41 F	~5.5 mm	3.5–4.2 mm
Males <170 cm	16–18 mm	39 F	~5.0 mm	3.5–4.2 mm
Males <160 cm Females >160 cm	15–16 mm	≤37 F 37 F	~4.5 mm	3.5–4.2 mm
Females <160 cm	14–16 mm	35 F	~4.3–4.5 mm	3.5 mm
Adolescents Children		32 F 28 F (L) 26 F (L)	~3.5 mm ~3.5 mm ~3.0 mm	2.2 mm
Indications for right DLT	Left pneumonectomy, left lung transplantation, left sleeve dissection, anticipated difficult left mainstem bronchial intubation Except for these indications where right DLT is required, left DLT should be chosen as default option			

Indications for right DLT are also provided here

5.8 What Are the Various Optimization Options Available for this Patient?

Refer to Table 5.5 [1].

Table 5.5 Preoperative optimization measures prior to lung resection surgery

Risk factors	Interventions
Smoking	Cessation: >12 h reduces carboxyhemoglobin levels >4 weeks decreases pulmonary complications >8 weeks improves wound healing
Bronchospasm	Bronchodilators, sputum and infection control, hydration of airway, steroids, physiotherapy
Pulmonary infection	Antibiotics, sputum control, lung recruitment
Malnutrition	Appropriate nutrition
Cardiac	Coronary artery disease: depending upon stent/bypass or type of stent and anticoagulants, follow guidelines to space the thoracic surgery appropriately. Stable patients 4–6 weeks post MI can be planned for surgery Withhold ACE inhibitors and angiotensin receptor blockers inhibitors 24 h prior to surgery. Routine institution of beta-blockers is not encouraged due to enhanced stroke risk Patients previously on beta-blockers should continue them. Stable cardiac patients can proceed to surgery
Renal	Avoid ACE inhibitor, angiotensin receptor blocker, hydroxyethyl starch in the immediate preoperative period Improve serum albumin levels and control diabetes mellitus

5.9 Why Is One Lung Ventilation (Lung Isolation) Required? Briefly Describe the Various Available Lung Isolation Techniques. Present the Intricacies of Choosing an Appropriate Lung Isolation Device for a Given Patient

Lung isolation is required to mainly facilitate the surgery as still, spacious surgical field is helpful to the surgeon. Various lung isolation techniques available are deliberate endobronchial intubation with a conventional single lumen endotracheal tube, double lumen tubes, and bronchial blockers. Since the last two options are more sophisticated and yield much better patient outcomes, the advantages and disadvantages of these two techniques are given in Table 5.6. A DLT is suitable for most cases except when a right-sided DLT is to be chosen or where insertion of DLT is either difficult or not feasible (e.g., critically ill patients) or patient has tracheostomy that the bronchial blockers can be considered [4, 7, 8].

Table 5.6 Pros and Cons of different lung isolation devices

	DLT	Bronchial blockers, uninvent tubes
Advantages	Larger ID, less airway resistance, better suctioning	Difficult airway, critically ill, tracheostomized
	Better lung protection from soiling	Selective lobar blockade possible
	Easy switch between two lung and one lung ventilation	Nasal intubation can be used
Disadvantages	Difficulty choosing correct size	Frequent dislodgements, loss of seal
	Difficulty insertion and positioning	Inclusion in the stapling line
	Trauma	Longer time to collapse the lung
Advantages of one device serve as disadvantage of the other and vice versa		
Bronchial blockers are inflatable devices that are passed alongside or through a single-lumen endotracheal tube to selectively occlude a bronchial orifice		

5.10 Discuss the Anatomy of the Tracheobronchial Tree Relevant to One Lung Ventilation with Specific Emphasis on the Margin of Safety

The anatomy relevant is detailed in Fig. 5.2 [1, 4, 7]. Margin of safety is the length of the tracheobronchial tree between the most distal and the proximal acceptable positions for a DLT. The margin of safety for right and left bronchi are <10 mm and 15–20 mm respectively. The margin of safety is decreased in female gender and right main bronchus.

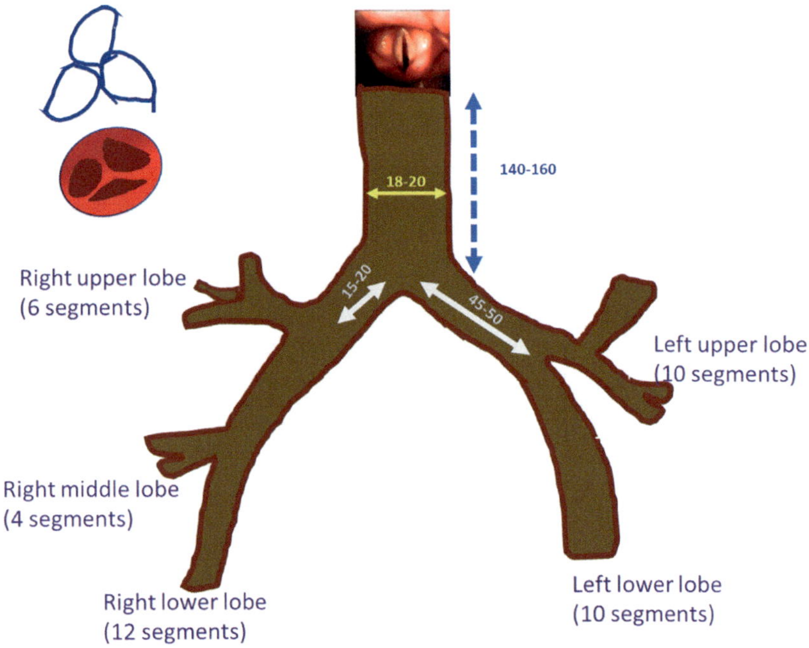

Fig. 5.2 Typical anatomy of the tracheobronchial tree. Characteristic *table fan* with three wings like appearance of right upper lobe bronchus on flexible bronchoscopy

5.11 Discuss the Relevance of Hypoxic Pulmonary Vasoconstriction (HPV) in These Patients. Detail the Influence of Anesthetic Agents on the HPV Response

Hypoxic pulmonary vasoconstriction (HPV) is a protective locally mediated vasomotor reflex response around the alveoli where in response to alveolar hypoxia, surrounding pulmonary vasculature constricts to redistribute the blood to better-ventilated areas thus improving ventilation-perfusion distribution. The characteristics of HPV response are that it responds most to alveolar hypoxia and not to appreciable degree to hypoxemia (reduced PaO_2). It is locally mediated, hence not abolished by vagotomy and is present in transplanted lung also. The response is biphasic in nature—early, develops over 10–15 min and late, develops over 4 h. Once triggered, continues to persist and subsides completely only hours after restoration of alveolar oxygen levels. Though it is beneficial when local hypoxia is present, generalized hypoxia (e.g., high altitudes) can precipitate pulmonary edema as HPV can be triggered all over the lungs. During anesthesia, relative HPV response between the non-dependent and the dependent lungs determines the degree of hypoxemia. Greater HPV response in non-dependent lung is desirable while HPV response in the dependent lung results in desaturation requiring changes in the anesthetic and ventilatory management.

Role of anesthetic agents and ventilatory management in HPV response: Most volatile anesthetics can influence the HPV response in a dose-dependent fashion. However, at <1 MAC levels, they have very little influence. Most IV induction agents do not affect the HPV response. But since VAs in clinical concentrations do not really disturb the HPV response much, it can be safely assumed that opting for TIVA over VA-based maintenance has no definite advantage. Regional anesthesia, especially epidural analgesia also doesn't appear to have any significant influence over the HPV response [9].

5.12 What Preoperative Investigations and Premedication Are Required for this Patient?

Apart from routine investigations, airway and cardiopulmonary-specific investigations are discussed under suitable headings already. Decision on administration of sedatives, analgesics, antacids, or proton pump inhibitors should be individualized to the patient, antisialogogue administration can be considered prior to flexible bronchoscopy [1].

5.13 Outline the Overall Flow of the Patient Scheduled for Thoracic Surgery

Patient enters operating room → Monitoring → nerve block → CVC, IBP (can also be done after induction) → Induction → Confirm lung isolation is accurate → Foley's, NG, etc., additional invasive monitors → position, confirm again accurate lung isolation → once lung isolation is achieved, appropriate ventilatory settings individualized to patient → mildly restrictive fluid therapy, mainly with isotonic crystalloids, blood 1:1 → end of surgery, consider extubating on table if appropriate → postoperative monitoring and management for ERAS, complications, extubation.

5.14 Discuss the Various Intraoperative Monitoring Options and Preparations Required During the Management of this Patient?

Presented in Table 5.7 [1, 4, 7, 8].

Table 5.7 Anesthetic preparations inside the operating room for patients scheduled to undergo lung resection surgery

Some of the essential requirements for immediate perioperative management during lung resection surgery
Monitors: Non-invasive: ECG (5 lead): left thoracotomy—V5 lead placed close to V1 location because V5 area will be used for incision, NIBP, SpO_2, $ETCO_2$, NMJ, depth of anesthesia, temperature, blood loss, NICO Invasive: IBP in dependent limb, CVP/PAWP, CO, spirometry, etc.
Airway cart
Medication cart
Lung isolation devices and flexible bronchoscope
CPAP delivery device for non-dependent lung
Warming devices
Equipment for positioning the patient
Mechanical DVT prophylaxis devices
Analgesia delivery devices: USG, PNS, epidural or paravertebral block kit; kit for peripheral nerve blocks (intercostal, serratus anterior plane or erector spinae block, etc.)
Other analgesic techniques: TENS, intrapleural catheter for LA infusion, TCA, cognitive therapy for relaxation/distraction, analgesics such as opioids/ketamine/NSAIDs, etc.

5.15 Describe the Technique of Left-Sided Double Lumen Tube Insertion and the Methods to Confirm Its Ideal Location

After induction of anesthesia and ensuring dense neuromuscular blockade (train of four 0), an optimal view of the glottis should be obtained on laryngoscopy. Then the DLT should be inserted with concavity of the bronchial part facing anteriorly till the bronchial cuff passes through the vocal cords. At this juncture, the DLT should be gently rotated toward the intended bronchus side while simultaneously the DLT is advanced till gentle resistance is felt or approximate estimated depth (usually about 29 cm at incisors in adults) is reached. Turning the patient head to the opposite side by an assistant while the intubator is rotating the DLT toward intended bronchus helps in directing the bronchial lumen toward the intended bronchus. Alternately, once the bronchial cuff has passed beyond the vocal cords, flexible bronchoscope can be passed via the bronchial lumen to advance the DLT toward intended bronchus under vision or bronchoscope is first advanced into the intended bronchus followed by railroading the bronchial lumen [4, 7, 8, 10].

5.16 Confirmation of Ideal Positioning of the DLT

Auscultation method—steps to be followed and possible scenarios are outlined in Table 5.8.

Flexible bronchoscope method—This is the ideal technique to ensure that the DLT is positioned in the intended bronchus in such a way that the bronchial cuff is not herniating at the carina and bronchial tube tip is not obstructing the upper lobar bronchial openings [4, 7, 8, 10].

Table 5.8 Sequence for auscultatory method of confirming correct placement of left DLT

	Right	Left	
Inflate tracheal cuff and ventilate	Heard Not heard Not heard	Heard Not heard Heard	Tracheal intubation Esophageal intubation Too far in (withdraw)
Inflate both cuffs and ventilate	Heard Heard	Heard Heard	Fair position or too far outside (push down)
Both cuffs inflated, right lumen clamped	Heard Not heard Heard	Heard Heard Not heard	Too far outside (push down) Reasonable position Accidental right endobronchial intubation (withdraw and re-insert)
Both cuffs inflated, left lumen clamped	Not heard Not heard	Not heard Heard	Too far outside or too far inside (L or R) Reasonable position
Only tracheal cuff inflated, left lumen clamped	Heard Not heard Heard	Heard Heard Not heard	Too far outside (push down) Too far inside left (withdraw) Too far inside right (withdraw and redirect)

When a DLT is inserted, it may be located in an acceptable position, might be too far down with both bronchial and tracheal openings inside either left or right mainstem bronchus or it may be too far outside with both tracheal and bronchial openings within the trachea

5.17 Describe the Technique of Insertion and Confirmation of Ideal Location of Bronchial Blockers

After confirming tracheal intubation with appropriate size single lumen endotracheal tube, the bronchial blocker can be placed under flexible bronchoscope guidance to intended bronchus or bronchiole as desired and the cuff inflated. Some of the bronchial blockers have wire loop through which the flexible bronchoscope can be inserted and the wire loop is subsequently tightened such that with bronchoscope tip advancement, the bronchial blocker will also move and once the tip of the bronchoscope is in desired position, the loop is loosened to let free the bronchial blocker and the cuff of the blocker inflated after withdrawing the bronchoscope [4, 7, 8, 10].

5.18 Discuss the Anesthetic Drug Choices for Induction and Maintenance of Anesthesia

Choice of drugs depends upon the patient condition, co-morbidities and their ability to influence the HPV. These are covered in other sections [1, 3, 4].

5.19 Enumerate the Main Precautions to be Taken While Positioning the Patient in Lateral Decubitus Position

These are detailed in Table 5.9 [11].

Table 5.9 Measures to be taken to prevent neurovascular injuries for patients to be positioned in lateral decubitus position for lung resection surgery

Preventive measures for lateral decubitus positioning related neurovascular injuries and equipment care
Adequate and proper padding of dependent eye, ear, and dependent limbs
Adequate padding for dependent axilla to prevent kinking of neurovascular bundle of dependent upper limb
Appropriate padding and positioning of the non-dependent upper limb to prevent kinking of neurovascular bundle
Padding between dependent and non-dependent legs
Ensure cervical and thoracic spine are in line and not acutely bent
Foley's catheter free from compression
ETT, lung isolation devices, monitoring lines, vascular access to be carefully positioned to prevent drag/dislodgement
Warming blankets, fluid warmers in situ
Mechanical DVT prophylaxis device applied

5.20 Discuss the Alterations in Ventilation and Perfusion Related to Lateral Decubitus Position, When Thorax Is Intact and When Open, with Patient Spontaneously Breathing and Paralyzed

These are detailed in Table 5.10 [4, 7, 8, 12, 13].

Table 5.10 V/Q differences in lateral decubitus position with patient breathing spontaneously or paralyzed and with thoracic wall intact or open

	Ventilation	Perfusion
Lateral decubitus, closed thorax, spontaneous breathing	Non-dependent lung: decrease Dependent lung: increase (spontaneous diaphragmatic activity) V/Q: Good	Non-dependent lung: Decrease Dependent lung: Increase (gravity) V/Q: Good
Lateral decubitus, open thorax, spontaneous breathing	Paradoxical breathing Pendelluft Mediastinal shift	
Lateral decubitus, closed or open thorax, paralyzed	Non-dependent lung: increase Dependent lung: decrease (weight of abdominal contents) V/Q: more dead space in non-dependent lung	Non-dependent lung: decrease Dependent lung: increase (gravity) V/Q: more shunt in dependent lung
Lateral decubitus, open thorax, paralyzed, OLV	Non-dependent lung: decreased (absent) Dependent lung: increased V/Q: atelectatic non-dependent lung	Non-dependent lung: decreased (HPV) Dependent lung: increased V/Q: relatively well matched

5.21 Enumerate the Various Options for Intraoperative and Postoperative Analgesia

These are detailed in Table 5.7 [4, 14, 15].

5.22 Discuss the Ventilatory Strategy for the Management of OLV

This is detailed in Table 5.11 [13].

Table 5.11 Mechanical ventilatory settings for OLV

Mechanical ventilation adjustments for OLV	
Mode of ventilation	PCV = VCV
Tidal volume	4–6 mL/kg Bronchospasm/severe hypoxia: 6–8 mL/kg with lower RR
RR	12–16/min Hypercapnia—increase along with increase in tidal volume
Minute ventilation	Targeted to modest permissive hypercapnia <70 mmHg; pH >7.25
FIO_2	Attempt to maintain around 0.4–0.5, higher FIO_2 can be detrimental (limited use during troubleshooting is acceptable)
I:E	**Bronchospasm normal lung restrictive lung** 1:3–4 1:2 1:1
Airway pressures	Peak <35 cmH_2O; plateau <25 cmH_2O
PEEP	**Bronchospasm normal lung restrictive lung** <5 cmH_2O: 5–10 cmH_2O: >10 cmH_2O
Recruitment maneuvers	Occasionally applied to dependent lung to improve V/Q

5.23 Detail Your Plan for Intraoperative Hypoxemia Management

Regarding which patient is likely to desaturate more during OLV intraoperatively, a simple understanding of the disease process will help. If the lung to be resected is healthy and or if the lung to be preserved is diseased, more problems can be anticipated. Conversely, if the lung to be resected is significantly diseased with pre-existent collapse and the lung that would remain is mostly healthy, then very minimal problems can be anticipated with maintaining saturation intra or postoperatively. Acceptable SpO_2 during OLV is 90–95%. Remember extremes of dependent lung volumes affect V/Q adversely—large volumes contribute to dead space and shunting of blood so also are small volumes as they contribute to increased shunt. Therefore, both upward and downward titration of PEEP should be considered to optimize V/Q to the dependent lung. Plan for intraoperative desaturation management is outlined in Table 5.12 [3, 4, 7, 13].

Table 5.12 Principles of management of hypoxemia/desaturation during OLV

	Management options for desaturation during OLV	
Modest hypoxia	FIO_2	Increase FIO_2 to achieve acceptable SpO_2 till other options work. Attempt to decrease FIO_2 to 0.4–0.5 as early as possible with acceptable SpO_2
	Confirm lung isolation	Confirm correct positioning of the lung isolation device
	Suction	Clear secretions with good suctioning directly or under flexible bronchoscopy guidance
	Communicate	Inform the surgeon regarding possibility of initiating both lung ventilation. Surgeon may reduce the traction or reducing the force on great vessels to improve saturation
	Non-dependent lung	Provide CPAP so that some oxygen is delivered. Alternatively, HFJV or passive oxygen insufflation can be done. Not an option for VATS procedures—instead, consider placing flexible bronchoscope tip in bronchus distal to the operative field in the non-dependent lung and deliver oxygen passively through suction port to that part of lung
	Dependent lung	Recruitment maneuver Titrate PEEP (incremental increase or decrease) as necessary to achieve better V/Q
	Oxygen delivery	Optimize cardiac output, blood pressure, and hemoglobin levels
	Anesthesia technique	Consider switching to TIVA from VA based technique Decrease or stop local anesthetic infusions if contributing to low BP
Severe hypoxia	Ventilation strategy	Initiate two lung ventilation with FIO_2 titrated to achieve acceptable SpO_2. Confirm correct position of the lung isolation device. Recruitment maneuver to both lungs
	Improve V/Q	Systemic vasopressor (phenylephrine) to increase HPV response in the non-dependent lung. Inhaled NO delivery to the dependent lung to optimize V/Q
	Surgeon	Partial or complete clamping of the pulmonary trunk to the operative lung (optimizes V/Q but can trigger right ventricular strain)
	Last resort	Extracorporeal membrane oxygenation or cardiopulmonary bypass

5.24 Discuss the Essential Principles in Fluid Management in These Patients

These are detailed in Table 5.13 [4, 12–15].

Table 5.13 Principles of fluid therapy during lung resection surgery

Principles of fluid therapy during lung resection surgery	
Preoperatively	Clear fluids can be allowed up to 2 h prior to surgery
Perioperative IV fluid of choice	Isotonic crystalloids (combination of or alternate use of Ringer's lactate and normal saline)
Maintenance IV fluid rate	1.5–2 mL/kg/h
Target	Normovolemia, restrictive fluid therapy, avoid excess positive fluid balance
GA/RA/medication induced hypotension	Judiciously use inotropes and vasopressors
Colloids	Avoid as far as possible Use selectively for rapid blood loss only in patients with normal renal function and absence of sepsis
Blood	1:1 ratio

5.25 Enumerate the High-Risk Factors for the Development of Post-procedure Acute Lung Injury

Preoperative factors: advanced age, female gender, lung injury, pulmonary infections, restrictive lung disease, alcohol abuse, poor lung function, chemotherapy.

Perioperative factors: Pneumonectomy, large and complex resections, blood and blood product administration, liberal tidal volume ventilation and or fluid therapy, prolonged duration of OLV (>90 min).

The team should concentrate on optimizing the preoperative factors and avoiding as much of the perioperative factors as possible to minimize the possibility of development of ALI [16].

5.26 Outline the Salient Points for On Table Extubation of Patients Following Various Types of Lung Resection Surgery

5.26.1 Enumerate the Essential Principles for Postoperative Care of These Patients

Extubation plan is detailed in Table 5.3. Good pulmonary toilet, adequate analgesia, encourage coughing and sputum clearance, early ambulation, bronchodilator therapy, antibiotics, and chest drain care are common to management of all postoperative patients. Prevention and management of postoperative complications, bronchoscopy and physiotherapy for lung expansion, appropriate oxygen therapy and invasive/non-invasive mechanical ventilation, and application of CPAP form core strategies for postoperative management [4, 12, 14–16].

5.26.2 Briefly Discuss the Immediate Life-Threatening Postoperative Problems and Discuss the Troubleshooting for the Same

Detailed in Table 5.14 [17].

5.26.3 Briefly Discuss the Differences Between Open Thoracotomy, VATS, and NIVATS with Respect to Anesthetic Techniques and Concerns

Detailed in Table 5.15 [4, 12, 14, 15].

5.26.4 Discuss the Principles of Enhanced Recovery After Thoracic Surgery

The main purpose of ERAS protocols is to fast-track the patients through the postoperative period. It requires concerted team efforts involving patient with attenders and the multidisciplinary teams involved with patient care.

Detailed in Table 5.16 [4, 18].

Table 5.14 Immediate life-threatening complications following lung resection and their management principles

	Tracheobronchial rupture	Cardiac herniation	Tension pneumothorax
Etiology	Surgery Lung isolation devices Excessive positive pressure ventilation	Pericardial disruption during or subsequent to pneumonectomy	Excessive positive pressure ventilation Absence of or malfunctioning of or clamping of in situ chest drain post surgery
Clinical features	Hemoptysis, desaturation Crepitus Mediastinal emphysema, pneumothoraces Respiratory distress Hemodynamic collapse	Unresolving tachycardia and hypotension Left herniation—myocardial ischemia, arrhythmias Right herniation—superior vena caval obstruction	Hypotension, tachycardia, desaturation
Modalities to diagnose	CXR USG CT	CXR ECHO	USG CXR
Immediate management	Preserve spontaneous ventilation SGA and flexible bronchoscopy to evaluate location and extent of injury Place tracheal tube tip below the injury under direct bronchoscopic vision Consider: ECMO, cardiopulmonary bypass in severe cases	DO NOT PLACE SURGICAL SIDE IN DEPENDENT POSITION Avoid/stop negative pressure from chest drain suction	Needle thoracostomy Chest tube insertion

Table 5.15 Anesthesia management principles for different surgical options for lung resection

	Open thoracotomy	VATS	NIVATS
Airway control	Anesthetized and paralyzed	Anesthetized and paralyzed or anesthetized and spontaneously breathing or under regional with patient sedated/awake	Under regional with patient awake/sedated
Breathing	Controlled	Controlled or spontaneous	Spontaneous
Cognitive dysfunction	Higher incidence	Lower incidence if mainly regional-based technique used	Lower incidence
Desaturation episodes	Higher incidence, longer duration	Lower incidence with spontaneous breathing	Lower incidence
Early discharge	+	+++	++++
Frequent complications	Ventilator-induced lung injury Mechanical airway injury	Spontaneously breathing: no VILI or mechanical airway injury Hypercapnia, cough Conversion to GA may be needed	Cough, pain, patient discomfort, hypercapnia Conversion to GA may be needed
			THRIVE can be used to improve oxygenation

Transnasal humidified rapid-insufflation ventilatory exchange (THRIVE) at around 20 L/min can be administered for improving oxygenation during NIVATS without risking expansion of the collapsed lung

Table 5.16 ERAS for lung resection

Preoperative	Intraoperative	Postoperative
Improving patient lifestyle (e.g., cessation of smoking, improving nutrition) Educating patient and caregiver Optimizing cardiopulmonary status and other co-morbidities Antibiotic and thromboprophylaxis Individualized management plan with coordinated team interactions	Least invasive surgical approach suitable for patient condition Lung protective ventilatory strategies Avoiding excessive oxygen use Restrictive fluid therapy Choice of drugs to facilitate on table extubation or early postoperative extubation	Early extubation, spontaneous breathing Early oral intake Early ambulation Early removal of indwelling catheters including chest drains Restrictive fluid therapy Respiratory therapy
Minimizing the duration of perioperative fasting Lung recruitment therapy Minimizing/avoiding colloid therapy and transfusion of blood and blood products Optimal multimodal analgesia centered around thoracic epidural analgesia		

5.27 What Are the Specific Considerations for the Patient with Post-pneumonectomy Status If Scheduled to Undergo (a) Another Lung Resection Surgery in the Future (b) to Undergo Incidental Surgery in the Future

Post-pneumonectomy itself is a condition of extreme pulmonary compromise. Following this, the patient may have disease in the remaining lung and or the surgical procedure itself may compromise the lung function further such as requirement for head low position or surgeries requiring lateral decubitus with the non-operated thorax in dependent position or laparoscopy surgery, etc. The pulmonary function would depend upon various factors such as age, time since, and the extent of compensation following pneumonectomy. Moreover, right pneumonectomy carries more morbidity and mortality compared to left pneumonectomy status. Therefore, anesthesiologist should carefully evaluate the effort tolerance, breath-holding capacity, lung functions, room air saturation, and blood gas evaluation to understand and optimize the lung function prior to any incidental surgery [19].

Success of additional lung resection surgery in a patient with post-pneumonectomy status depends essentially on careful choice of oncological and functional assessment of the patient and carrying out appropriate surgical procedure with due anesthetic considerations. PET CT lung should be performed to evaluate the extent and spread of the tumor within thorax along with radiology of brain to rule out metastasis. Only patients with ppoFEV1 and DLCO >40%, VOmax >10 mL/kg/min without evidence of serious pulmonary hypertension and right ventricular failure are suitable. Success of surgery requires absolute co-ordination between anesthesiologist and surgeon at every stage as there is no option of collapsing the only remaining lung though selective lobar bronchial isolation may be possible in few cases. HFJV is another option. Both teams have to mutually find suitable option for facilitating surgery with lung protective ventilatory strategy or with VATS or NIVATS where feasible. Where serious issues with pulmonary gas exchange are likely intraoperatively due to remaining lung condition, ECMO or cardiopulmonary bypass can be considered [20].

References

1. Slinger P, Darling G. Preanesthetic assessment for thoracic surgery. In: Slinger P, editor. Principles and practice of anesthesia for thoracic surgery. 2nd ed. Cham: Springer Nature; 2019. p. 13–42.
2. Travis WD, et al. The 2015 World Health Organization classification of lung tumors. J Thorac Oncol. 2015;10:1243–60.
3. Andrew Ochroch E, Wright GM, Riedel BJCJ. Anesthesia for open pulmonary resection: a systems approach. In: Slinger P, editor. Principles and

practice of anesthesia for thoracic surgery. 2nd ed. Cham: Springer Nature; 2019. p. 389–412.
4. Ankeny D, Chitilian H, Bao X. Anesthetic management for pulmonary resection current concepts and improving safety of anesthesia. Thorac Surg Clin. 2021;31:509–17.
5. Brunelli A, Belardinelli R, Pompili C, Xiumé F, Refai M, Salati M, Sabbatini A. Minute ventilation-to-carbon dioxide output (VE/VCO_2) slope is the strongest predictor of respiratory complications and death after pulmonary resection. Ann Thorac Surg. 2012;93(6):1802–6. https://doi.org/10.1016/j.athoracsur.2012.03.022.
6. Salati M, Brunelli A. Risk stratification in lung resection. Curr Surg Rep. 2016;4(11):37.
7. Marasigan BL. Separation of the two lungs: double-lumen tubes, endobronchial blockers, and endobronchial single-lumen tubes. In: Benumof and Hagberg's airway management. Philadelphia: Elsevier Saunders; 2013. p. 549–68.
8. Campos J. Lung isolation. In: Slinger P, editor. Principles and practice of anesthesia for thoracic surgery. 2nd ed. Cham: Springer Nature; 2019. p. 283–310.
9. Michael Jaeger J, Titus BJ, Blank RS. Essential anatomy and physiology of the respiratory system and the pulmonary circulation. In: Slinger P, editor. Principles and practice of anesthesia for thoracic surgery. 2nd ed. Cham: Springer Nature; 2019. p. 65–92.
10. Campos J. Fiberoptic bronchoscopy for positioning double-lumen tubes and bronchial blockers. In: Slinger P, editor. Principles and practice of anesthesia for thoracic surgery. 2nd ed. Cham: Springer Nature; 2019. p. 311–22.
11. Reimer C, Slinger P. Intraoperative patient positioning and neurological injuries. In: Slinger P, editor. Principles and practice of anesthesia for thoracic surgery. 2nd ed. Cham: Springer Nature; 2019. p. 337–42.
12. Schisler T, Lohser J. Clinical management of one-lung ventilation. In: Slinger P, editor. Principles and practice of anesthesia for thoracic surgery. 2nd ed. Cham: Springer Nature; 2019. p. 107–30.
13. Macpherson JA. Intraoperative ventilation strategies for thoracic surgery. In: Slinger P, editor. Principles and practice of anesthesia for thoracic surgery. 2nd ed. Cham: Springer Nature; 2019. p. 375–88.
14. Cohen E, Slinger P. Anesthesia for video-assisted thoracoscopic surgery (VATS). In: Principles and practice of anesthesia for thoracic surgery. Springer; 2019.
15. Slinger P. Anesthesia for non-intubated thoracic surgery. In: Slinger P, editor. Principles and practice of anesthesia for thoracic surgery. 2nd ed. Cham: Springer Nature; 2019. p. 425–8.
16. Slinger P. Perioperative lung injury. In: Slinger P, editor. Principles and practice of anesthesia for thoracic surgery. 2nd ed. Cham: Springer Nature; 2019. p. 181–96.
17. Tsai J, Moon T, Vachhani S, Lasala J, Norman PH, Purugganan R. Anesthesia for thoracic surgical procedures. In: Tsai J, et al., editors. Principles and practice of cardiothoracic surgery. IntechOpen; 2013. https://doi.org/10.5772/56104.
18. Dinic VD, Stojanovic MD, Markovic D, Cvetanovic V, Vukovic AZ, Jankovic RJ. Enhanced recovery in thoracic surgery: a review. Front Med. 2018;5:14. https://doi.org/10.3389/fmed.2018.00014.
19. Kumar S, Uppalapati V, Shukla R, et al. Anesthetic considerations for elective laparoscopic cholecystectomy in a patient with previous pneumonectomy. Cureus. 2022;14(2):e22176. https://doi.org/10.7759/cureus.22176.
20. Van Slambrouck J, Ceulemans LJ. Lung resection after pneumonectomy: is it worth the risk? Shanghai Chest. 2021;5:22. https://doi.org/10.21037/shc-20-75.

Malignant Melanoma Foot for Isolated Limb Perfusion

6

Raghav Gupta and Nishkarsh Gupta

6.1 Case

A 40-year-old male weighing 75 kg was diagnosed with hyperthermic isolated limb perfusion using melphalan due to recurrent malignant melanoma of the lower right leg with in-transit metastases. He had previously received adjuvant immunotherapy with Nivolumab and endured two large local excisions. The patient currently takes a 75 mcg levothyroxine tablet and reports a history of hypothyroidism.

6.2 What Is Malignant Melanoma (MM) and What Is the Incidence of the Disease?

One type of skin cancer that arises from melanocytes, or pigment-producing cells of the epidermis, is malignant melanoma. Although the frequency is only 4%, it is the most deadly form of skin cancer, accounting for 79% of all skin cancer-related deaths [1, 2].

R. Gupta · N. Gupta (✉)
Department of Onco-Anaesthesiology and Palliative Medicine, DRBRAIRCH, AIIMS, New Delhi, India

6.3 What Are the Risk Factors for Malignant Melanoma?

- Exposure to UV radiation (intermittent exposure to sunlight with subsequent sunburns increases the risk) in fair skinned individuals [3].
- Light skin pigmentation.
- Prominent freckling [4].
- Familial melanoma.

Because persons from higher socioeconomic strata had more free time and could spend longer vacations in warm, sunny weather with increased sun exposure, malignant melanoma has historically been referred to as "rich man's disease" [5].

Malignant melanoma incidence is equal both sex. It tends to develop commonly in white women on the extremities and in men on trunk, head, and neck region. If malignant melanoma is confined to a limb, 75% cases are found on lower limbs [6].

6.4 How Is the Diagnosis of Malignant Melanoma Done?

- Physical examination—Large size (>6 mm), asymmetry, various colors or hues, and erratic borders. Satellite lesions developing, bleeding, ulceration, and itching are further warn-

N. Gupta et al. (eds.), *Problem Based Learning Discussions in Onco-Anesthesia and Onco-Critical Care*, https://doi.org/10.1007/978-981-99-6339-3_6

ing indicators. Using the ABCD technique, one should regularly examine oneself: Diameter, Color, Border, and Asymmetry [7, 8].
- Dermatoscopy.
- Histological examination.

6.5 What Is the TNM Staging of Malignant Melanoma?

- Stage I—Local disease with primary lesion.
- Stage II—Primary tumor site, in addition to the presence of satellite tumors 3 cm from the primary lesion.
- Stage III—Metastasis to regional lymph nodes draining the tumor area.
- Stage IV—Distant metastasis [1].

6.6 What Are the Treatment Strategies Available for Malignant Melanoma?

- Chemotherapy.
- Biological therapy utilizing immunomodulators.
- Radiation therapy.
- Amputation, selective lymph node dissection, sentinel node mapping, surgical excision, and hyperthermic isolated limb perfusion (HILP).

The TNM staging at the time of diagnosis, the patient's age, the incidence of recurrence, and the types of prior therapy utilized all have a role in the management of malignant melanoma [3].

6.7 What Are the Indications for HILP for Treatment of MM?

- Therapeutic ILP for loco-regionally advanced malignant melanoma, including local recurrence of MM, satellitosis, and in-transit metastases [9].
- Locally advanced soft tissue sarcoma not suitable for surgical resection.
- Adjunct to local excision of a high-risk primary, or recurrent MM.

6.8 Briefly Describe the HILP in Brief

In the 1950s, the technique was initially described. Using 40–42 ° C oxygenated blood, an extracorporeal administration of a high-dose chemotherapy drug is administered intraarterially to the afflicted limb as part of the normal limp perfusion regimen. Leaks between the systemic and limb circulations are determined once isolated limb bypass is initiated. Chemotherapy is administered intraarterially and circulated at a high temperature for 60 min after the vascular isolation is complete. Following the completion of the perfusion, the limb is cleaned with 3–5 L of crystalloid solution and the perfusate is sent to a trash bag. The limb is infused with 0.5–2.5 L of low molecular weight dextran once the effluent is nearly clean. After that, perfusion is stopped, vascular repair is carried out, and any further scheduled [10, 11]. The response rates are high and ranges from 40% to 85%.

6.9 How Is HILP Different from Cardiopulmonary Bypass and What Precautions Are to Be Taken?

HILP uses both the limb and body circulatory systems, in contrast to cardiopulmonary bypass. Because the degree of systemic toxicity is determined by the extent of leakage between systems, the circulations must continue to be segregated. Leaks are directional and can go either way; blood can flow from body to limb or from limb to body, which is commonly referred to as a "systemic leak." If there is a considerable leakage of the chemotherapy-enriched perfusate from the limb into the systemic circulation, systemic toxicity occurs. Similarly, if a significant amount of systemic blood enters the limb, the patient's hemodynamic stability is compromised.

6.10 What Are the Special Anesthesia Preparations Required During the Preoperative Period?

In addition to routine pre-anesthesia examinations and investigations (complete blood counts with hemoglobin and hematocrit values, coagulation tests, and liver function tests), patients who are hospitalized for heart failure and premature lung injury (HILP) may receive subcutaneous heparin (5000 IU, eighth hourly) and oral aspirin (300 mg) as thromboembolism prevention measures. In order to keep the limb to be perfused warm, aluminum foil space blankets can also be put around it [12]. Patients with cardiovascular disease need to be thoroughly evaluated.

6.11 Describe the Intraoperative Anesthesia Management

- One or two additional large-bore intravenous cannulas (14G or 16G) must be inserted as access for volume replacement in addition to the relatively small peripheral intravenous cannula (20G or 18G) used for induction.
- Using propofol (1-2 mg/kg body weight; BW), fentanyl (0.5–1 mcg/kg BW), and rocuronium (0.6 mg/kg BW) for neuromuscular blockade, anesthesia can be induced following pre-medication with midazolam. Urinary catheter, nasogastric tube, arterial line, and central venous line insertion are required following orotracheal intubation.
- Vital signs, ECG, pulse oximetry, CVP, arterial pressures, urine output, end-tidal CO_2, nasopharyngeal temperature, cardiac output, blood loss, and given fluids and blood products are all required for patient monitoring. For every patient, three to five units of packed red blood cells (RBC) must be prepared. At certain points during the process, there may be a drop in the mean blood pressure and shock index (heart rate/systolic blood pressure).
- Low-flow inhalational anesthetics with a FiO_2 of 0.5 to 1.0 are required to maintain anesthesia. Neuromuscular blockers should not be administered again if necessary for surgical nerve monitoring. To control pressure differences and stop communication between the various "circuits," phenylephrine can be injected into the isolated limb or into the systemic circulation. Standard drugs, such as vasopressors, must also be readily available on the anesthetic emergency cart [13].
- Blood/fluid warmer and heated mattress must be used to conserve body heat. In addition, heat and moisture (HME) exchanger must be used to reduce heat loss from respiratory tract.

6.12 Describe the Operative and Perfusion Technique

The ipsilateral limb and the operation site (groin or axilla) need to be cleaned and sterilely wrapped once anesthesia is induced. It is necessary to perform a radical lymph node dissection. The patient has to receive 3 mg/kg of heparin after the relevant blood arteries have been exposed [13].

It is necessary to place large bore cannulae into the proper vein and artery. The cannulae must then be linked to an extracorporeal circuit that includes a heat exchanger, a membrane oxygenator, and a roller pump. Heparin (50 mg) and sodium bicarbonate (50 mmol) must be added to 1200 mL of Hartmann's solution and 2 units packed cells, which prime the extracorporeal circuit on a regular basis. Warming the perfusate to 40 °C, 3–4 1/min carbogen (02 95%; CO_2 5%) is added to oxygenate it. Melphalan must be given as a single bolus into the oxygenator reservoir and the limb must be warmed to 38 ± 0.5 °C after total isolation of the limb is accomplished by the use of a tourniquet.

It is necessary to modify perfusion flow rates to achieve flows of 0.7–1.5 1/min (about 90–180 mL/min/I tissue perfused) in order to prevent the limb venous pressure from rising above baseline levels by more than 15 mmHg before ILP starts. Warming the perfusate to 41 °C over 35–50 min is required to gradually raise the limb temperatures to 40 ± 0.5 °C after being held at 38 °C for 10 min.

The amount of melphalan leakage into the systemic circulation can be retrospectively assessed by taking blood samples from the perfusate and the systemic circulation at regular intervals while melphalan is being perfused. Using radiolabeled tracers, systemic leakage can also be continuously monitored. After HILP with melphalan is finished, any leftover melphalan in the limb needs to be cleaned out by quickly infusing 2 L of Hartmann's solution into the reservoir, running it through the roller pump, and discarding the venous effluent. After that, the tourniquet needs to be loosened, the limb has to be revascularized, blood vessels need to be fixed, and vascular cannulae removed. To completely reverse previous heparinization, protonate is first given as a test dose (0.2–0.5 mg) and subsequently at a dose of 0.5–1 mg/100 units of heparin.

6.13 What Are the Intraoperative Blood Testing Strategies?

In the intraoperative period after incision, during pre-cannulation phase, during perfusion every 30 min, after washout and after decannulation following blood testing should be done [14].

A. Arterial blood gas (ABG) analysis with values of hemoglobin and hematocrit.

B. Activated clotting time (ACT) analysis.

6.14 What Is the Dose of Melphalan to Be Given Intraarterially During the Procedure?

13 mg of Melphalan per liter of limb volume for the upper extremities (by water replacement method) and 10 mg per liter of limb volume for the lower extremities. Even in cases when the computed volume is larger, the maximum dosage is restricted to 120 mg [13].

6.15 What Are the Possible Side Effects Because of Usage of Melphalan?

- Nausea, vomiting, allergic reaction, and cardiorespiratory arrest.
- The hematopoietic system can get affected due to unavoidable leak leading to neutropenia.
- Regional limb toxicity is seen. Mild erythema or edema (Grade I-II) is seen in most cases. Higher grade toxicity requiring fasciotomy (for compartment syndrome) or amputation (for tissue loss) has been reported to occur in up to 1-2% of patients undergoing HILP [15, 16].

6.16 Should Regional Anesthesia in the Form of Central Neuraxial Block Be Used During the Intraoperative Phase?

Given the patient's systemic heparinization, localized anesthetic—such as epidural or spinal anesthesia—should not be considered; instead, general anesthesia should be used [14].

6.17 Why Core Body Temperature Monitoring Is Essential During the Surgery?

Monitoring core temperature is necessary to sustain normothermia, which will support the isolated limb's hyperthermic perfusion. Furthermore, when the perfusate is heated to 41 °C, a rise in core temperature would suggest a leak into the systemic circulation [17].

6.18 What Is the Importance of Close Monitoring of Limb Venous Pressure?

A partial obstruction of venous drainage is most likely the cause of a limb venous pressure increase that is more than 15 mmHg above baseline. This can lead to increased bleeding at the surgical site and leakage of the cytotoxic agent into the systemic circulation from the extracorporeal circuit [12].

6.19 Which Are the Different Leak Assessment Techniques and What Are the Qualities of a Good Leak Assessment Test?

Fluorescein dye, radiolabeled tracers, dye dilution, plasma melphalan levels, and exhaled desflurane levels are some of the methods used today for leak assessment. Changes in temperature, reservoir level, ACTs, and hematocrit are other secondary leak indicators. The method should be simple to use, measurable, repeatable, real-time, and economically viable. Sadly, none of these qualities can be found in a single technique [18].

6.20 Mention the Other Drugs Which Can Be Used Apart from Melphalan?

Melphalan can be taken either on its own or at smaller doses in combination with other medications. Among these are TNF-α, Interferon-γ, Actinomycin D, Cisplatin, Doxorubicin, Soxurubicin, and Thiotepa. A second-generation alkylating agent is called thiotepa. Instead of being an alkylating agent, cisplatin (platinol) is a platinum-containing chemical that is mostly utilized to treat solid tumors and their metastases. Less often used antibiotic that interacts with DNA is actinomycin D. Physician preference dictates whether to employ more than one agent. Usually, patients undergoing the surgery a second or third time will receive a combination of medications rather than just melphalan [10]. Table 6.1 provides the dosage of drugs used in ILP and HILP.

Table 6.1 Drugs used for ILP

S.I	Drug	Dosage
1.	Melphalan	Upper limb—13 mg/L Lower limb—10 mg/L
2.	Cisplatin	20 mg/L
3.	Actinomycin D	50-100mcg/L (commonly 75mcg/l)
4.	Doxorubicin	10-18 mg/L
5.	Soxorubicin	8.5 mg/L
6.	TNF-α	Upper limb—1-3 mg Lower limb—1-4 mg
7.	Interferon γ	0.2 mg

6.21 What Are the Important Considerations in the Postoperative Phase?

At the end of the surgery, ABG with hemoglobin values have to be measured again with ACT analysis to see whether action of heparin given is reversed or not. Also, complete blood count, liver function tests, ABG, and INR should be repeated. It is needed to be careful about blood, urine, and other body fluids secretions. The washout from the extremity, the pump filling, and the circuit must be put into cytostatic waste cans [13, 14]. Vigilance for occurrence of local and systemic complications is essential. Elevation of the operated extremity is recommended to reduce edema as well as to help in better assessment of the limb. Daily assessment of serum creatine kinase levels helps in early detection of muscle toxicity and prophylactic administration of systemic steroids if it is >1000 mg/l. Monitoring for the development of compartment syndrome for at least 24 h post-procedure is recommended. Early detection is essential as it requires fasciotomy.

6.22 Which Groups of Patients Are Considered High Risk and Not Eligible for the Procedure?

Patients at high risk who are not eligible for the operation include those who have peripheral neuropathy, lymphedema, severe peripheral vascular disease (PVD), or are pregnant. Individuals who are older and fit the requirements for the surgery do not have a higher risk of problems than younger individuals. The likelihood of additional disease variables, such as PVD, diabetes, severe heart disease, previous MI, and a longer smoking history, is more concerning in these patients than their age [6].

6.23 What Are the Other Oncological Cases Where the Use of Isolated Hyperthermia Perfusions Is Being Considered Apart from Malignant Melanoma?

Treatment for pulmonary metastases and limb-related osteogenic sarcomas has been established. In order to treat tumors that have spread from colon carcinoma, melanoma, metastatic sarcoma, renal cell carcinoma, and adenoid cystic carcinoma, it entails administering chemotherapy isolated to one or both lungs. Like HILP, it aims to deliver a targeted dose of chemotherapy with minimal systemic toxicity [19, 20].

6.24 What Are the Differences between HILP and ILI (Isolated Limb Infusion)?

Characteristics [21]	HILP	ILI
Vascular access	Open surgery	Percutaneous
Arterial catheter size	1-12 Fr	6-8 Fr
Venous catheter size	16–18 Fr	6-8 Fr
Perfusion time	60-90 min	30 min
Prefusion pressure	Systemic pressure	Low pressure
Flow rate	250-1200 mL/min	60-120 mL/min
Drugs used	Melphalan with or without TNF-alpha	Melphalan with or without actinomycin D
Dose of melphalan	10-13 mg/L limb volume	7.5-10 mg/L limb volume
Leakage risk	High	Low
pH	Normal	Acidotic
Oxygenation	High	Low
Temperature	40	37-39

6.25 What Are the Postoperative Complications of HILP and ILP?

Postoperative complications can be classified as local and systemic. Weiberdink et al. described 5 grades of local complications. Table 6.2 describes the grades of local toxicity. Grade 1 and 2 toxicity with an incidence of 32-100% have been reported in the majority of studies while grade 3 is seen in 1-19% [23–25]. Grade 4 complication (compartmental syndrome) requiring fasciotomy and grade 5 with extensive tissue loss and necrosis that requires amputation is seen in 1-2% patients [25]. Pain and local discomfort are seen in 25-40% patients and generally resolve in 2-3 weeks [22]. Compartmental syndrome is other dangerous complication that requires close monitoring of intra-compartmental pressure for at least 24 h post-procedure.

Systemic complications include

- Neurotoxicity—manifests as stabbing pain and paresthesia, Onset is 2-3 weeks after the procedures and resolves in few months. It is reported in 25-40% patients.
- Vascular complications—less common. Thrombosis at arteriotomy site has been reported in 2.5% cases and DVT in 10% cases. DVT can occur despite heparinization during the procedure due to the thrombogenic potential of tumor, use of cytotoxic agents, surgical trauma, edema, and decreased mobility.
- Systemic Inflammatory Response Syndrome may occur due to TNF-α that manifests as fever, increased cardiac output, decrease in

Table 6.2 —Weiberdink classification of post-ILP toxicity [22]

Grade	Description
Grade 1	Absence of subjective or objective evidence of reaction
Grade 2	Mild edema/and or erythema
Grade 3	Considerable edema/and or erythema with some blisters, slight alteration in mobility
Grade 4	Extensive epidermolysis with damage to deep tissues leading to functional disability as well as compartment syndrome
Grade 5	Severe reaction that might require amputation

systemic vascular resistance, increased cardiac index, coagulopathy, thrombocytopenia, hepatic failure requiring fluid resuscitation, and use of ionotropic agents. The severity depends on the dose and intensity of leakage into systemic circulation. Higher levels can be associated with multi-organ failure.

These complications occur due to leak from the perfusion circuit during the procedure.

6.26 Who all Must Be the Part of Multidisciplinary Team Management in a Case of HILP?

An experienced team of anesthesiologists, surgeons, perfusionists, anesthesia technicians, and nursing personnel, as well as careful monitoring and care during the whole perioperative phase, are necessary for the management of HILP.

References

1. American Committee on Cancer. AJCC cancer staging manual. Malignant melanoma of the skin. Philadelphia: Lippencott-Raven; 1997. p. 163–70.
2. Miller DL, Weinstock MA. Nonmelanoma skin cancer in the United States: incidence. J Am Acad Dermatol. 1994;30:774.
3. Langely RGB, Barnhill RL, Mihm MG, et al. Neoplasms: cutaneous melanoma. In: Eisen AZ, Wolff K, editors. Clinical dermatology. Freedberg IM. New York: McGraw-Hill; 1999. p. 1080–116.
4. Rhodes AR, et al. Risk factors for cutaneous melanoma: a practical method for recognizing predisposed individuals. JAMA. 1987;258:3146.
5. Elwood JM. Melanoma and sun exposure. Semin Oncol. 1996;23:650.
6. Ariyan S, Poo WJ. Safety and efficacy of isolated perfusion of extremities for recurrent tumor in elderly patients. Surgery. 1998;123:335–43.
7. Koh HK, et al. Evaluation of the American Academy of Dermatology's national skin cancer early detection and screening program. J Am Acad Dermatol. 1996;34:971–8.
8. Friedman RJ, Rigel SD, Kopf AW. Early detection of malignant melanoma: the role of physician examination and self-examination of the skin. CA Cancer J Clin. 1985;35:140–51.
9. Hohenberger P, Kettelhack C. Clinical management and current research in isolated limb perfusion for sarcoma and melanoma. Oncology. 1998;5:89–102.
10. Krementz ET, Sutherland CM, Muchmore JH. Isolated hyperthermia chemotherapy perfusion for limb melanoma. Surg Clin North Am. 1996;76:1313–30.
11. Klaase JM, Kroon BB, van Geel AN, et al. Prognostic factors for tumor response and limb recurrence free interval in patients with advanced melanoma of the limbs treated with regional isolated perfusion with melphalan. Surgery. 1994;115:39–44.
12. Kam PC, Thompson JF. Anaesthetic experience with isolated limb perfusion with melphalan for melanoma. Perfusion. 1996;11(5):395–9.
13. Ruschulte H, Shi S, Tseng WW, et al. Anesthesia management of patients undergoing hyperthermic isolated limb perfusion with melphalan for melanoma treatment: an analysis of 17 cases. BMC Anesthesiol. 2013;13(1):15.
14. Gupta R, Yadav HP, Gupta N, Deo SVS, Bhatnagar S. Multidisciplinary perioperative Management of Hyperthermic-Isolated Limb Perfusion for malignant melanoma: a case report. Indian J Surg Oncol. 2021;12(Suppl 2):371–3.
15. Vrouenraets BC, Eggermont AM, Hart AA, Klaase JM, van Geel AN, Nieweg OE. Regional toxicity after isolated limb perfusion with melphalan and tumour necrosis factor- alpha versus toxicity after melphalan alone. Eur J Surg Oncol. 2001;27:390–5.
16. Kettelhack C, Hohenberger P, Schulze G, Kilpert B, Schlag PM. Induction of systemic serum procalcitonin and cardiocirculatory reactions after isolated limb perfusion with recombinant human tumor necrosis factor-alpha and melphalan. Crit Care Med. 2000;28:1040–6.
17. Goldberg ME, Rosenblum HM, Seltzer JL, Rosato FE. Isolated regional perfusion: anaesthetic technique, monitoring and blood replacement. Can Anaesth Soc J. 1984;31:552–8.
18. Schaadt J, Crowley R, Miller D, Kavanah M. Isolated limb perfusion: a literature review. J Extra Corpor Technol. 2002;34(2):130–43.

19. Weksler B, Burt M. Isolated lung perfusion with antineoplastic agents for pulmonary metastases. Chest Surg Clin North Am. 1998;8:157–82.
20. Vaglini M, Bacci G, Baldini M. Limb salvage in osteogenic sarcoma of extremities a new therapeutic approach associated infusion and hyperthermic antiblastic perfusion. J Extra-Corp Technol. 1987;19:338–47.
21. Bagge RO, Carlson P, Razzazian R, Hansson C, Hjärpe A, Mattsson J, Katsarelias D. Minimally invasive isolated limb perfusion—technical details and initial outcome of a new treatment method for limb malignancies. Int J Hyperth. 2018;35(1):667–73.
22. Lejeune FJ, Deloof T, Ewalenko P, et al. Objective regression of unexcised melanoma in-transit metastases after hyperthermic isolation perfusion of the limbs with melphalan. Recent Result Cancer Res. 1983;86:268–76.
23. Pace M, Gattai R, Matteini M, Macera Mascitelli E, Bechi P. Toxicity and morbility after isolated lower limb perfusion in 242 chemo-hyperthermal treatments for cutaneous melanoma. The experience of the Tuscan re-ference Centre. J Exp Clin cancer res. 2008;27(1):67. 37. 26. Vrouenraets BC, Eggermont AM, Hart AA, et al. regional toxicity after isolated limb perfusion with melphalan and tumour necrosis factor-alpha versus toxicity after melphalan alone. Eur J Surg Oncol. 2001;27(4):390–5.
24. Beasley GM, Caudle A, Petersen RP, et al. A multi-institutional expe-rience of isolated limb infusion: defining response and toxicity in the US. J Am Coll Surg. 2009;208(5):706–15.
25. Klausner JM, Lev-Chelouche D, Meller I, Inbar M, Gutman M. Isolated Limb Perfusion in the Treatment of Advanced Soft-tissue Sarcomas. In: Malawer MM, Sugarbaker PH, editors. Musculoskeletal cancer surgery: treatment of sarcomas and allied diseases. 1st ed. Dordrecht: Springer Netherlands; 2001. p. 75–84.

7 Anesthetic Considerations for a Patient with Carcinoma Esophagus Scheduled for Ivor-Lewis Esophagectomy

Seema Mishra, Swagata Biswas, and Sandeep Bhoriwal

7.1 Case Scenario

A 62 year old male patient, known case of diabetes mellitus and hypertension, presents with chief complaints of difficulty in swallowing (solid>liquid), weight loss and loss of appetite for last 4 months. Patient has been diagnosed as a case of adenocarcinoma of lower third of esophagus. He has completed neoadjuvant chemoradiation 8 weeks back. He has been posted for Ivor Lewis Esophagectomy.

7.2 Introduction: Overview of Esophageal Carcinoma

7.2.1 Classify the Esophageal Neoplasms Based on Their Histological Characteristics

Three types of esophageal carcinomas have been recognized based on their histological characteristics [1, 2]:

(a) Epithelial tumors: 95% of the esophageal tumors are squamous cell carcinomas (SCC) and adenocarcinomas (ADC). Other types of esophageal carcinoma are adenoid cystic, adenosquamous, mucoepidermoid, verrucous, spindle cell carcinoma, and undifferentiated carcinoma.
(b) Mesenchymal tumors:
  - Benign: Granular cell tumor, hemangioma, leiomyoma, lipoma (benign).
  - Malignant: These include melanoma, synovial sarcoma, Kaposi sarcoma, gastrointestinal stromal tumor (GIST), leiomyosarcoma, and rhabdomyosarcoma.
(c) Others: These include lymphomas and neuroendocrine tumors.

7.2.2 Is There Any Difference in the Histological Types of Ca Esophagus Between Developing and Developed Countries? How Does It Differ Between Upper and Lower Esophagus?

In developing countries and the middle 1/third of the esophagus, SCC is the most commonly reported type of Ca esophagus, while in developed nations and the lower 1/third of the esophagus, adenocarcinoma has been reported more frequently [3].

S. Mishra (✉) · S. Biswas
Department of Onco-Anaesthesia and Palliative Medicine, Dr BRA, IRCH, AIIMS, New Delhi, India

S. Bhoriwal
Department of Surgical Oncology, Dr BRA, IRCH, AIIMS, New Delhi, India

N. Gupta et al. (eds.), *Problem Based Learning Discussions in Onco-Anesthesia and Onco-Critical Care*, https://doi.org/10.1007/978-981-99-6339-3_7

7.2.3 What Are the Risk Factors for Developing Ca Esophagus?

Two types of risk factors can contribute to the development of the Ca esophagus [3].

(a) Non-modifiable risk factors:
  - Increased age is a risk factor for developing adenocarcinoma.
  - Male gender (2–3 times more common in males than female).
  - Race: Caucasians have a higher risk of developing adenocarcinoma, whereas SCC is found more in sub-Saharan Africans.

(b) Modifiable risk factors:
  - Dietary habits: Pickled vegetables, preserved fish, and intake of hot beverages lead to an increased risk of developing SCC; whereas decreased consumption of fresh fruits and vegetables increases the risk of developing ADC.
  - Obesity: Adenocarcinoma is 16 times more common in people with a BMI > 30.
  - Socioeconomic status: SCC has a common occurrence in developing countries, whereas ADC has been found more frequently in developed nations.
  - Addiction: Alcohol consumption increases the risk of SCC, whereas smoking has been attributed to both ADC and SCC.
  - Associated diseases:
    - Squamous cell carcinoma: Achalasia cardia, caustic injury, nutritional deficiency, non-epidermolytic palmoplantar keratoderma, HPV infection, Head and neck cancer, thoracic radiation.
    - Adenocarcinoma: Hiatus hernia, scleroderma, Barrett's esophagus, gastroesophageal reflux disease (GERD), and thoracic radiation.

7.2.4 What Are the Common Presenting Symptoms of Carcinoma Esophagus?

- Progressive dysphagia.
- Halitosis.
- Odynophagia.
- Vomiting.
- Unintentional weight loss, cachexia.
- Dehydration.
- Anemia.
- Chest pain.
- Aspiration pneumonitis.
- Features of surrounding or distant organ involvement, e.g. recurrent laryngeal nerve infiltration leading to hoarseness of voice, development of stridor as a result of tracheal involvement, choking and cyanosis due to tracheoesophageal fistula formation.

7.2.5 What Are the Most Common Sites of Metastases in the Ca Esophagus? What Is the Median Survival/5-Year Survival Rate for Carcinoma Esophagus?

As the esophageal wall lacks serosal covering, the cancer tends to spread early, most commonly via lymphatic (70%), rest (25–30%) via the hematogenous route. The liver, pleura, lung, renal, bone, and adrenal gland are the commonest metastases sites.

The cancer stage at the time of initial diagnosis determines the 5-year survival rate in esophageal cancers. It is around 46% in early disease, decreases to 26% in case of regional spread further decreases to 5% in diseases with metastases [4].

7.2.6 Describe the Eighth AJCC Staging of Carcinoma Esophagus and Their Clinical Implications?

Separate classification for clinical (cTNM), pathologic (pTNM), and post-neoadjuvant (ypTNM) stage groups have been described by the American Joint Committee on Cancer (AJCC) staging [5] of epithelial cancers of the esophagus in its eighth edition.

Clinical categories (cTNM) are obtained by imaging studies and minimal histology. It has a role in deciding the treatment protocols. It includes details about the tumor size (T), nodal spread (N), and distant metastases (M).

Pathological staging involves the histological examination of the resected specimen of esophagectomy along with grading (G) and tumor length (L). It is a more precise tool for prognostication and survival than clinical staging, though decision-making for postoperative adjuvant therapies using pTNM is still not recommended.

Postneoadjuvant (ypTNM) staging was introduced in the eighth edition for pathological staging in patients who had received preoperative neoadjuvant therapies. This facilitated specific prognostication and identification of poor response to neoadjuvant therapy in the histological specimen. Details of these parameters and staging are described below (Tables 7.1, 7.2, 7.3 and 7.4).

Table 7.1 Criteria for defining categories for staging [5]

Categories	Criteria
T category TX T0 Tis T1 T1a[a] T1b[a] T2 T3 T4 T4a[a] T4b[a]	Tumor cannot be assessed No evidence of primary tumor High-grade dysplasia, defined as malignant cells confined by the basement membrane Tumor invades the lamina propria, muscularis mucosae, or submucosa Tumor invades the lamina propria or muscularis mucosae Tumor invades the submucosa Tumor invades the muscularis propria Tumor invades adventitia Tumor invades adjacent structures Tumor invades the pleura, pericardium, azygos vein, diaphragm, or peritoneum Tumor invades other adjacent structures, such as aorta, vertebral body, or trachea
N category NX N0 N1 N2 N3	Regional lymph nodes cannot be assessed No regional lymph node metastasis Metastasis in 1–2 regional lymph nodes Metastasis in 3–6 regional lymph nodes Metastasis in 7 or more regional lymph nodes
M category M0 M1	No distant metastasis Distant metastasis
Adenocarcinoma	
G category GX G1 G2 G3[b]	Differentiation cannot be assessed Well differentiated. >95% of tumor is composed of well-formed glands Moderately differentiated. 50–95% of tumor shows gland formation Poorly differentiated. Tumors composed of nest and sheets of cells with <50% of tumor demonstrating glandular formation
Squamous cell carcinoma	
G category GX G1 G2 G3[c]	Differentiation cannot be assessed Well-differentiated. Prominent keratinization with pearl formation and a minor component of non-keratinizing basal-like cells. Tumor cells are arranged in sheets, and mitotic counts are low Moderately differentiated. Variable histologic features, ranging from parakeratotic to poorly keratinizing lesions. Generally, pearl formation is absent Poorly differentiated. Consists predominantly of basal-like cells forming large and small nests with frequent central necrosis. The nests consist of sheets or pavement-like arrangements of tumor cells, and occasionally are punctuated by small numbers of parakeratotic or keratinizing cells

(continued)

Table 7.1 (continued)

Categories	Criteria
Squamous cell carcinoma L category[d]	
LX	Location unknown
Upper	Cervical esophagus to lower border of azygos vein
Middle	Lower border of azygos vein to lower border of inferior pulmonary vein
Lower	Lower border of inferior pulmonary vein to stomach, including esophagogastric junction

[a]Subcategories
[b]If further testing of "undifferentiated" cancers reveals a glandular component, categorize as adenocarcinoma G3
[c]If further testing of "undifferentiated" cancers reveals a squamous cell component, or if after further testing they remain undifferentiated, categorize as squamous cell carcinoma G3
[d]Location is defined by epicenter of esophageal tumor

Table 7.2 Clinical staging (cTNM) [5]

cStage group	cT	cN	cM
Squamous cell carcinoma			
0	Tis	N0	M0
I	T1	N0–1	M0
II	T2	N0–1	M0
	T3	N0	M0
III	T3	N1	M0
	T1–3	N2	M0
IVA	T4	N0–2	M0
	T1–4	N3	M0
IVB	T1–4	N0–3	M1
Adenocarcinoma			
0	Tis	N0	M0
I	T1	N0	M0
IIA	T1	N1	M0
IIB	T2	N0	M0
III	T2	N1	M0
	T3–4a	N0–1	M0
IVA	T1–4a	N2	M0
	T4b	N0–2	M0
	T1–4	N3	M0
IVB	T1–4	N0–3	M1

Table 7.3 Pathological (pTNM) staging [5]

pStage group	pT	pN	pM	pGrade	pLocation
Squamous cell carcinoma					
0	Tis	N0	M0	N/A	Any
IA	T1a	N0	M0	G1,X	Any
IB	T1b	N0	M0	G1, X	Any
	T1	N0	M0	G2–3	Any
	T2	N0	M0	G1	Any
IIA	T2	N0	M0	G2–3, X	Any
	T3	N0	M0	Any	Lower
	T3	N0	M0	G1	Upper/middle
IIB	T3	N0	M0	G2–3	Upper/middle
	T3	N0	M0	X	Any
	T3	N0	M0	Any	X
	T1	N1	M0	Any	Any

Table 7.3 (continued)

pStage group	pT	pN	pM	pGrade	pLocation
IIIA	T1	N2	M0	Any	Any
	T2	N1	M0	Any	Any
IIIB	T4a	N0–1	M0	Any	Any
	T3	N1	M0	Any	Any
	T2–3	N2	M0	Any	Any
IVA	T4a	N2	M0	Any	Any
	T4b	N0–2	M0	Any	Any
	T1–4	N3	M0	Any	Any
IVB	T1–4	N0–3	M1	Any	Any
Adenocarcinoma					
0	Tis	N0	M0	N/A	
IA	T1a	N0	M0	G1, X	
IB	T1a	N0	M0	G2	
	T1b	N0	M0	G1–2, X	
IC	T1	N0	M0	G3	
	T2	N0	M0	G1–2	
IIA	T2	N0	M0	G3, X	
IIB	T1	N1	M0	Any	
	T3 N0	M0	Any		
IIIA	T1	N2	M0	Any	
	T2	N1	M0	Any	
IIIB	T4a	N0–1	M0	Any	
	T3	N1	M0	Any	
	T2–3	N2	M0	Any	
IVA	T4a	N2	M0	Any	
	T4b	N0–2	M0	Any	
	T1–4	N3	M0	Any	
	T1–4	N0–3	M1	Any	

N/A not applicable, *X* not defined

Table 7.4 Postneoadjuvant therapy (ypTNM) staging [5]

ypStage group	ypT	ypN	ypM
I	T0–2	N0	M0
II	T3	N0	M0
IIIA	T0–2	N1	M0
IIIB	T4a	N0	M0
	T3	N1–2	M0
	T0–3	N2	M0
IVA	T4a	N1–2,X	M0
	T4b	N0–2	M0
	T1–4	N3	M0
IVB	T1–4	N0–3	M1

7.2.7 What Are the Staging Investigations for Carcinoma Esophagus?

Staging of the disease is done using Multi-modal imaging. These include endoscopic ultrasound(EUS) or oesophagogastroduodenoscopy, bronchoscopy for upper lesions or suspected tracheoesophageal fistula, positron-emission tomography (PET)/CT and CECT. In addition, liver function tests, metabolic parameters and pulmonary function tests (optional) should also be done [6, 7].

7.2.8 What Are the Treatment Options Available for Carcinoma Esophagus?

Ca esophagus patients present with an advanced disease in nearly 51% of the cases. Management of esophageal carcinoma is a multimodal approach using either or a combination of three therapies: chemotherapy, radiotherapy, and surgery [3, 8]. The decision-making process for treatment should consider the location of tumor, clinical staging, comorbidities of the patient, and functional status. For patients with operable tumor surgery is preceded by neoadjuvant therapies as it improves 5-year survival benefit (CROSS trial) [9].

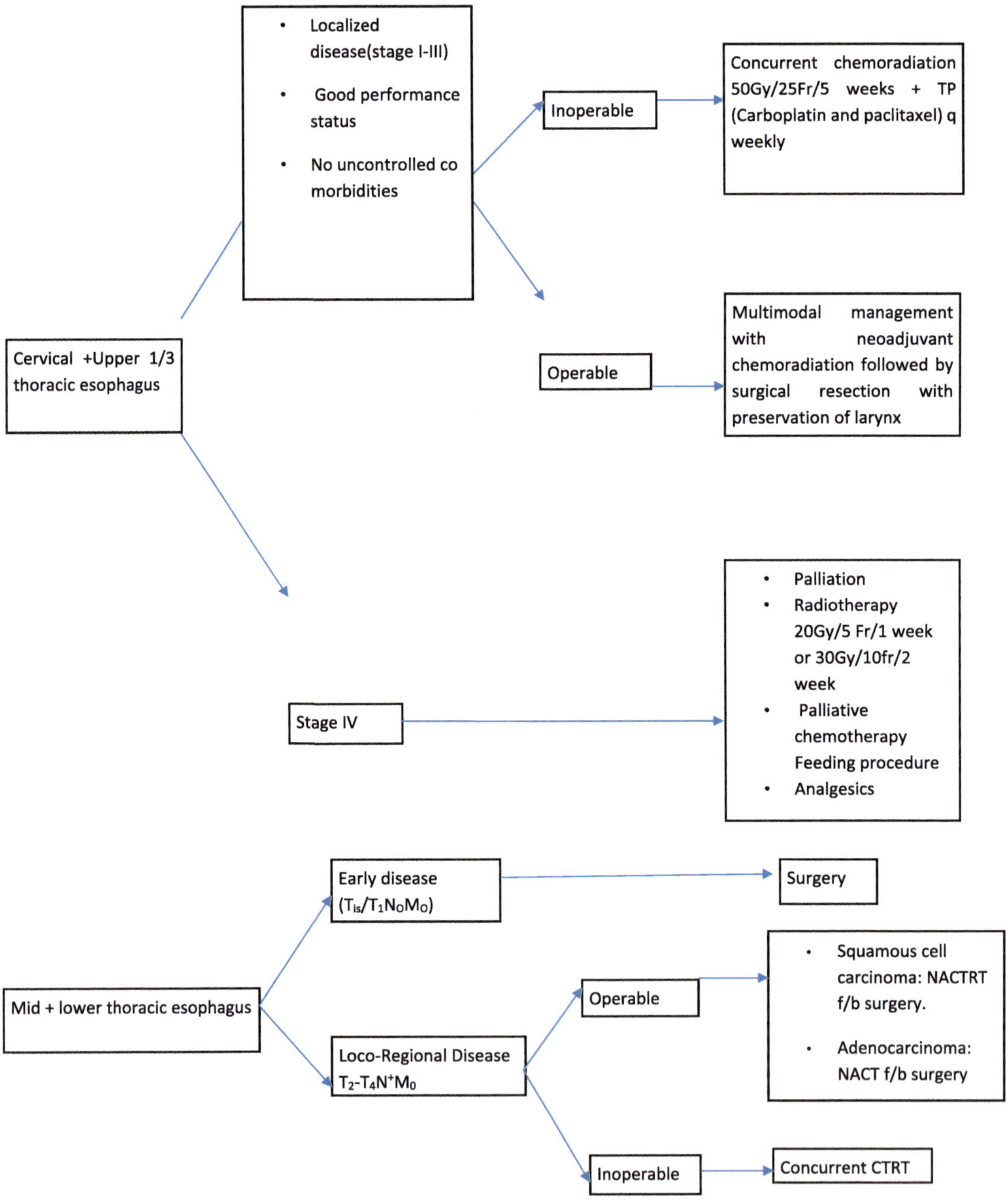

7.3 Preoperative Evaluation and Management

7.3.1 How Do You Evaluate These Patients in the PAC Clinic?

The medical history should include the following details:

(a) Age: It has been seen that in patients undergoing an esophagectomy, age does not have a major influence on the postoperative course, recurrent disease, or survival [10]. Hence, those with an advanced age should not be denied radical resection merely based on age. Rather, due attention to frailty and comorbid conditions is to be paid to these elderly patients.
(b) Race.
(c) Sex: M:F = 3:1 [3].
(d) H/O risk factors (e.g., heartburn, acid reflux, palmar keratosis, dietary habit, smoking, alcohol).
(e) H/O neoadjuvant therapies: drug details, dosages, duration since the last dose, any signs of toxicity.
(f) Any symptoms of surrounding structure involvement: hoarseness, coughing, choking with cyanosis, stridor, etc.
(g) Detailed history of comorbidities.

Physical Examination: Apart from routine general, systemic, and airway examinations, the following *details* should be noted:

(a) IV access: often difficult due to frailty and previous chemotherapies.
(b) Skin changes (frail, tylosis, palmar keratosis).
(c) Weight, height, BMI, skinfold thickness.

7.3.2 What Are the Systemic Toxicities of Preoperative Chemotherapies in a Patient with Carcinoma Esophagus?

Preoperative chemotherapy regimens for esophageal carcinoma vary in different institutions. Age, comorbidities, and physical status of patient are also deciding factors for choosing an appropriate regimen. The common regimens used are as follows [8, 11]:

- Carboplatin and paclitaxel.
- Oxaliplatin and Capecitabine/5 FU.
- Cisplatin and Irinotecan.
- Paclitaxel and 5-FU/Capecitabine.
- Epirubicin, Cisplatin, and 5-FU (ECF regimen).
- Docetaxel, Cisplatin, and 5-Fu (DCF regimen).

The toxicities of commonly used drugs are described below:

- Cisplatin:
  - *Ototoxicity:* It causes irreversible ototoxicity and thus should be used cautiously with other ototoxic drugs [12].
  - *Neurotoxicity:* Neurotoxicity occurs with a cumulative dose >300 mg/m^2 [13]. It presents with peripheral neuropathy and may present with tingling, burning sensation, and paresthesia. It also can precipitate seizures and autonomic dysfunction which must be evaluated and managed preoperatively [14–16].
  - *Nephrotoxicity:* It causes mostly reversible nephrotoxicity, but rarely can cause irreversible nephrotoxicity requiring dialysis [17]. It mostly causes proximal tubular damage. Predisposing factors for the development of nephrotoxicity are: age > 60 years, higher doses, baseline GFR <75 mL/min, daily dosing, cumulative dose, and low albumin. Adequate hydration, slow infusion of the drug over 24 h, and pretreatment with amifostine can prevent toxicity [18].
  - *Pancytopenia and mild bone marrow suppression.*
  - *Highly emetogenic*: at a dose >50 mg/m^2.
  - *Hypomagnesaemia.*
- Oxaliplatin, Carboplatin: Moderate emetogenicity, dose-related thrombocytopenia, hypersensitivity reactions, peripheral neuropathy.

- Paclitaxel: Dose-limiting myelosuppression (maximum effect by eighth to tenth day), cardiotoxicity (arrhythmias, heart block), hypersensitivity reaction, mucositis, peripheral neuropathy, and transient hyperbilirubinemia [19].
- 5-FU: Myelosuppression, oral mucositis, diarrhea, nausea and vomiting, hand-foot syndrome, peripheral neuropathy, cardiotoxicity (2–5%, coronary vasospasm, myocardial infraction, and cardiomyopathy) [20, 21].
- Capecitabine [22, 23]: Hand-foot syndrome, low emetogenic potential. If it is used with 5-FU, it can cause enhanced toxicity and death in elderly.

7.3.3 What Are the Toxicities of Thoracic Radiation in Carcinoma Esophagus?

Preoperative radiation is used in esophageal carcinoma along with chemotherapies in squamous cell carcinoma. These are the following side effects which have implications for perioperative anesthetic management:

- *Pulmonary toxicity: Thoracic irradiation can affect the lungs in the form of* radiation-induced lung injury (RILI) which is a serious complication [24]. Immediately after the radiation (hours to days) acute inflammatory asymptomatic phase starts followed by a latent and symptomatic acute exudative phase (12 weeks to 6 months) [25]. A final and fibrotic phase sets in after months to >1 year [25]. Several factors are associated with the development of RILI, e.g., > 13.5 Gy mean dose to the lung, the volume of normal lung receiving a radiation of 20 Gy or more(V20) > 30%, concomitant chemoradiation [25]. Patients may present after 3 weeks to 1 year with complaints of shortness of breath, non-productive cough and wheezing. CxR and HRCT reveal patchy opacities in the initial phase to fibrosis in the later phase [25]. PFTs reveal a restricted pattern, decreased DLCO and SPO_2. Initially, RILI is managed with prednisolone [25], pentoxyphylline [26], and enalapril [27, 28]. If there is poor response, it may require immunosuppression with azathioprine or cyclosporine [29]. Long-term chest physiotherapy, nebulization with bronchodilators, mucolytic and pneumococcal vaccination should be used for these patients.
- *Cardiac toxicity:* Radiation-induced cardiac diseases can occur after thoracic *radiation* for esophageal cancer, especially if the tumor is located at the middle and distal one-third [30, 31]. Involvement of pericardium and myocardium leads to development of acute pericarditis, constrictive pericarditis, pericardial effusion and acute myocarditis, cardiomyopathy respectively [32]. Pericardial effusion was reported to be most common (48%) form of cardiotoxicity after esophageal radiation and mostly develop within 2 years of treatment [33]. Inferior left ventricular ischemia is seen in patients with distal esophageal cancer who have received radiotherapy [34]. Even an asymptomatic patient may reveal diastolic dysfunction on a preoperative echocardiogram. The involvement of the conduction system is not so common with ECG showing nonspecific ST-T changes, low voltage complexes, and right bundle branch block (RBBB) [35]. These patients need regular follow-up for the rest of their lives as complete heart block can occur at various time intervals following radiation therapy [36]. Hence these patients should be followed up for life.
- *Radiation-induced dysphagia:* It is late sequelae (35–65%) of radiation occurring due to soft tissue fibrosis. It leads to preoperative poor oral intake and severe malnutrition, increases risk of aspiration due to impaired swallowing reflex [37].
- *Airway changes* [38, 39]: Early changes after radiation include ulceration in the oral and GI mucosa which increases the risk of bleeding during airway instrumentations. Radiation-induced edema of the airway leads to difficult laryngoscopy and difficult intubation. In the late stage, temporomandibular joint fibrosis sets in and leads to development of radiation-induced trismus, which may *progress* up to

9 months and makes airway management challenging. Radiation-induced osteonecrosis causing difficult mask ventilation is rare with thoracic radiation but may occur in case of tumor of upper esophagus.

- *Skin changes*: It can range from erythema, desquamation, ulceration to contraction and fibrosis.

7.3.4 What Is the Ideal Time to Schedule a Patient for Surgery Who Has Received Neoadjuvant Therapies?

An adequate time after neoadjuvant therapies should be allowed for the physiological systems to recover from the toxicities of neoadjuvant therapies. This benefit should be balanced with the risk of metastasis and recurrence while deciding the ideal interval period. ERAS guidelines *recommend* the optimum interval for surgery as 3–6 weeks after chemotherapy completion and 6–10 weeks following radiotherapy [40].

7.3.5 What Are the Preoperative Investigations Needed for This Patient?

- Blood tests: CBC, LFT, KFT, serum electrolytes, PT/INR, ABG at room air.
- Chest X-ray: Look for pulmonary pathologies, signs and severity of aspiration pneumonitis, radiation toxicities.
- PFT: May reveal obstructive lung disease (smoker, COPD) or restrictive lung disease (radiation pneumonitis, aspiration pneumonitis).
- ECG.
- 2D Echocardiography: It should be considered in elderly patients having various comorbidities or patients receiving preoperative chemoradiation [41, 42].
- Review the preoperative CECT & UGIE to know the exact location of the tumor.
- Cardiopulmonary exercise testing (CPET). Risk stratification in patients posted for esophagectomy can be done using CPET. It is an important preoperative tool for risk stratification of patients posted for esophagectomy. Patients can be categorized as low risk ($VO_2 > 20$ mL/kg/min), moderate risk (VO_2 15–20 mL/kg/min), and high risk ($VO_2 < 15$ mL/kg/min) based on CPET derivatives [43].

7.3.6 What Are the Preoperative Procedure-Specific Risk Stratification Tools for Patients Posted for Esophagectomy?

Preoperative risk stratification is an essential preoperative concern for prognostication of patients. Apart from general preoperative risk stratification tools (e.g., ASA classification, ECOG-PS, etc.) Reeh M et al. described the *PER (Preoperative Esophagectomy Risk) Score* for esophagectomy patients [44]. The short-term outcome of patients who underwent esophagectomy can be predicted with reasonable accuracy with PER score. The risk of morbidity and mortality is significantly increased in PER 2 and PER 3 compared to PER 1 patients. In addition, disease-free survival ($P < 0.001$) and overall survival ($P < 0.001$) were found to be lower in patients with a higher PER score (Table 7.5).

Cardiopulmonary exercise testing (CPET)—The risk stratification of these patients in the preoperative period can be done using CPET [45, 46]. Peak VO_2 and anaerobic threshold reduce following chemotherapy which improves with time and can be enhanced by prehabilitation. An increased risk of perioperative complications occurs with a peak $VO_2 < 800$ mL min − 1 m − 2 and anaerobic threshold (AT) <11 mL/kg/min correlates with increasing the perioperative risk [40]. Another parameter of CPET that can predict the long-term survival is an increased ventilatory equivalent of CO_2 (VE/VCO_2) [47].

Table 7.5 PER (Preoperative Esophagectomy Risk) Score [44]

Organ system	Tools	Values	Points	PER score	PER score risk group
Cardiovascular	RCRI	• 0 • 1 • 2 • ≥3	0 1 2 3	• <4 (no impaired organ system) • 4 (impairment of one organ system) • >4 (impairment of at least 2 organ systems)	• 1 (low, PER score < 4) • 2 (intermedi-ate, PER score 4) • 3 (high, PER Score > 4)
Pulmonary	Lung function test	• VC and FEV1 > 80% or VC > 80 and FEV1 > 60% to <80% or VC > 60% to <80% and FEV1 > 80%	1		
		• VC and FEV1 > 60% to <80% or VC > 80% and FEV1 < 60% or VC < 60% and FEV1 > 80%	2		
		• VC and FEV1 < 60% or VC > 60% to <80% and FEV1 < 60% or VC < 60% and FEV1 > 60% to <80%	3		
Hepato-renal	MELD score	–≤8 >8	1 2		

FEV1% forced expiratory volume in 1 s, *MELD* model of end-stage liver disease, *RCRI* revised cardiac risk index, *VC* vital capacity

7.3.7 How Will You Optimize the Patient with Carcinoma Esophagus Before Surgery?

Preoperative optimization involves a multidisciplinary approach for evaluation and problem-specific interventions. The major interventions are:

- Detailed evaluation and management of comorbidities.
- Preoperative counseling and informed consent taking from patient and caregivers decreases preoperative anxiety and enhances the compliance to treatment.
- Correction of anemia.
- Cessation of alcohol and smoking at least for 4 weeks before the surgery.
- Nutritional assessment and intervention: As per the ERAS guideline, the patients can be divided into three categories for risk of preoperative malnutrition [40] based on their oral intake, BMI, and unintentional weight loss (Table 7.6). Moderate to high-risk patients must consume 25–30 Kcal/Kg/day with a protein of 1–1.5 gm/kg/day [48]. Oral nutrition is preferred among enteral routes, whereas tube feeding may be considered if oral feeding is not feasible. The inability to meet at least 60% of the target energy consumption through the enteral route requires parenteral nutrition to be started. The role of immunonutrition has not been yet established and hence its use in the preoperative period is not beneficial.
- Physical exercise: Targeted, individualized exercise training in preoperative period improves the physiological reserve and decreases postoperative morbidities [49]. Every patient should undergo aerobic resistance training at least for 4–6 weeks before surgery [50–52]. A daily exercise schedule for 45–50 min (warm up: 5 min, aerobic exercise: 20 min, resistance training: 20 min, cool down: 5 min) is usually recommended. A CPET-guided exercise training program can also be used to evaluate recovery from systemic toxicities of neoadjuvant therapies [53].
- Pulmonary prehabilitation: Deep breathing exercises, incentive spirometry, deep diaphragmatic breathing, and inspiratory muscle training should be continued in the perioperative period [54]. A home-based prehabilitation program enhances compliance of the patients [55]. Some recent trials have also shown feasibility of tele-prehabilitation program for esophagectomy patients [56, 57].

Table 7.6 Nutritional risk stratification [40]

Nutritional risk categories	Diagnostic criteria	Intervention
Low nutritional risk	• Able to meet normal caloric intake with minimal loss of weight	Dietary advice
Moderate nutritional risk	• Presence of anorexia/dysphagia with 5–9% weight loss which is unintended	Protein and energy supplements
High nutritional risk	• Presence of severe dysphagia with BMI < 18 kg/m2 or weight loss>10% that is unintended	Requires enteral support often with Ryle's tube feeding to meet the target caloric requirements

7.3.8 What Will Be Your Preoperative Fasting Guidelines and Advice for Bowel Preparation for This Patient?

Prolonged fasting is avoided in the preoperative period to decrease the risk of postoperative nausea vomiting, insulin resistance, stress response, and postoperative morbidities and improve patient comfort. Intake of solids can be continued for 6 h before surgery while clear liquids can be continued 2 h before surgery. Carbohydrate drinks should also be allowed 2 h before the surgery [58], though it is cautioned in patients who have significant dysphagia or other symptoms suggestive of obstruction [40]. In patients undergoing esophagectomy with gastric reconstruction, routine bowel preparation is not recommended [40].

7.4 Intraoperative Management

7.4.1 Discuss the Premedication, Monitoring, and Anesthesia Plan for These Patients

Premedication: ERAS recommends to use short-acting sedatives and anxiolytics especially in elderly patients due to the increased risk of upper airway obstruction and postoperative cognitive dysfunction with the use of long-acting sedatives [40]. In patients with a high risk for PONV, a multimodal strategy is recommended.

Monitoring: Apart from ASA standard monitors (e.g., 5 lead ECG, SPO_2, NIBP, Temperature, etc. O_2) some additional monitors should be used in esophagectomy. As most of the patients are elderly, they need care full titration of anesthetic agents. Thus, BIS for monitoring depth of anesthesia, end-tidal concentration of anesthetic agents and neuromuscular monitoring for precise use of muscle relaxants should be done intraoperatively. Goal-directed fluid therapy must be used. Non-invasive cardiac output monitoring can be used in elderly patients with multiple comorbidities although its exact role is not established in low tidal volume lung protective ventilation [59] and one- lung ventilation with open thorax [60].

Anesthesia Plan: Anesthetic agents may have an impact on the recurrence of cancers. Volatile anesthetics may cause suppression of NK cell activity [61–63], whereas propofol-based total intravenous anesthesia may prevent cancer recurrence by directly suppressing the tumor cells [61, 62], inhibition of HIF-1, inhibiting matrix metalloproteinase [64], and activating CD4+ cells. A retrospective cohort study of 992 patients who underwent elective esophagectomy found the beneficial effects of propofol-based TIVA on overall and recurrence-free survival [65]. But overall the quality of evidence is poor and more prospective studies are needed to conclude. Thus, the use of volatile anesthesia and TIVA remains univocal for use in esophagectomy surgeries. The lung-protective effect of sevoflurane during one-lung ventilation due to its immuno-modulatory effects has been reported in a few studies [66, 67]. It causes a significantly lower level of inflammatory markers in bronchoalveolar fluids, but their clinical impact in reducing incidence of pulmonary complications is still doubtful [67]. A recent review has concluded that sevoflurane may have a better lung protective function, whereas propofol maintains better oxygenation during OLV due to decrease in pulmonary shunt fraction [68].

Regional anesthesia is another popular anesthetic technique which suppresses surgical stress response and may reduce cancer recurrence [69, 70]. Local anesthetics have anti-proliferative, pro-apoptotic, and anti-inflammatory effects [71]. TIVA along with epidural anesthesia reduces the surgical stress response [72]. Epidural analgesia provides good postoperative pain control. An increase in shunt fraction during OLV has been described with the use of thoracic epidural infusion [73, 74], though this occurs in higher dosages of local anesthetics only [75].

7.4.2 Enumerate the Different Surgical Techniques Available and Discuss the Pros and Cons for Individual Techniques

(a) Open esophagectomy.

There are 3 surgical approaches of open esophagectomy:

- Trans hiatal esophagectomy [76]:
  - Abdominal and cervical incision.
  - No thoracotomy.
  - It involves blunt dissection of the thoracic esophagus through the mediastinum.
  - This is followed by anastomosis in the cervical region (no risk of mediastinitis).
  - Risk of hemodynamic instability, mediastinal structures including major vessels and recurrent laryngeal nerve injury.
  - Chance of inadequate nodal clearance.

(b) Ivor Lewis esophagectomy [77]:

- Good for exposure of mid to upper esophageal lesions.
- Laparotomy and right thoracotomy with mediastinal anastomosis.

(c) McKeown/3 field esophagectomy [78]:

- This involves right thoracotomy, together with *abdominal* and cervical incision followed by anastomosis in the cervical region.
- No *risk* of mediastinitis.

(d) *Minimally invasive esophagectomy* [79]:

- It includes mobilization of esophagus by thoracoscope *(VATS assisted)* and mediastinal lymph nodes dissection along with laparoscopic mobilization of stomach. This is followed by a cervical or mediastinal anastomosis of the esophagus and gastric conduit.
- It causes less blood loss, less postoperative complications, early functional recovery, and less postoperative pain without compromising oncological outcome [80].
- It is a *long*-duration surgery done in prone position. It also requires a longer learning curve for surgeons.
- It is *associated* with complications of extraperitoneal CO_2, e.g., Capnothorax, capnomediastinum, surgical emphysema, etc. [81].
- *A robotic-assisted minimally invasive esophagectomy (RAMIE)*—It has lower rate of pulmonary complications, better range of motion, and vision of the field [82]. However, the disadvantages include difficulty in accessing the patient, difficulty in managing a displaced DLT or bronchial blocker, and nerve plexus injury [83].

7.4.3 Discuss the Concerns Associated with Surgical Techniques Contributing to Early Recovery in Esophagectomy Patients?

Modifications of surgical techniques are often very useful for an early recovery for patients as they cause less tissue damage, less postoperative pain, and early ambulation. ERAS recommends the following modifications [40] in the surgical technique of esophagectomy for an early and improved postoperative recovery:

- A recovery period of 3–6 weeks following the last session of chemotherapy and 6–10 weeks following the last radiotherapy session is required before surgery.
- Minimally invasive approaches are found to be equally effective as open approaches. But it causes less blood loss, less postoperative pulmonary complications, better pain control, and an early recovery.

- Though stomach, jejunum, and colon are equally suitable conduits for reconstruction, stomach is the preferred one for its rich vascularity.
- Two-field lymphadenectomy is recommended for mid and lower esophagus, whereas three-field lymphadenectomy is reserved for squamous cell carcinoma of upper one-third of esophagus. Three-field lymphadenectomy has better yield of lymph nodes but has a greater risk of recurrent laryngeal nerve damage and is done only in patients with good functional status and early stage of disease.

7.4.4 What Are the Concerns during Anesthesia Induction and Maintenance in These Surgeries?

Plan of anesthetic induction in these patients depends on multiple factors, e.g., cardiopulmonary status, hemodynamic stability, risk of aspiration, and mediastinal effect if any. Rapid sequence induction is preferred in these patients due to the presence of partial or complete esophageal obstruction and the high risk of aspiration. The stomach should be decompressed along with the esophageal conduit. To achieve this, a nasogastric tube must be placed after induction if it is not already placed, but should be removed in the postoperative period by day two [40].

7.4.5 How Do You Manage the Airway in these Patients and Discuss Their Pros and Cons?

Airway and isolation of the lung can be managed in patients for esophagectomy with the use of the following devices:

Double lumen tube (DLT): It is commonly used for lung isolation as alternating between one lung and two lungs ventilation is easier, suctioning is better, lung deflation is faster, and has lesser risk of malpositioning [84]. However, it is difficult to place in patients with difficult airways and may be traumatic. A recent advance in the design of DLT is VivaSight. It allows continuous monitoring of correct position with the help of the camera attached at the distal end of the DLT [85].

Bronchial blockers: Lung isolation in difficult airways, smaller bronchi, during awake intubation or unplanned OLV can be *accomplished using bronchial blockers.* The disadvantages of bronchial blockers are frequent malpositioning and the requirement of fiberoptic skills for placement [86]. Arndt wire-guided blocker [87], Cohen's tip deflecting blocker [88], Univent blocker [89], and Fogarty's catheter [90]*are the commonly available bronchial blockers.* EZ blocker is a Y-shaped blocker. It has two prongs each of which is placed in one main bronchus. Some advantages of this EZ blocker are easy to place, central lumen for both of the stems, separate inflation balloons making alternate lung isolation easier, radiopaque shaft, and feasibility of application of CPAP and suction [90, 91].

Single lumen tube (SLT): SLT is a good choice due to its easy placement, lesser chance of malposition, ease of suction, and no FOB skills required. However, the OLV may be difficult due to high airway pressure [92].

7.4.6 Discuss the Intraoperative Ventilatory Strategies in These Patients

During surgery the dissection of abdominal esophagus and anastomosis requires traditional two-lung ventilation (TLV) whereas the thoracotomy needs one-lung ventilation (OLV). There is no definitive evidence to support the use of pressure-controlled ventilation over volume-controlled ventilation [93, 94]. The lung-protective ventilation reduces local and systemic inflammation and reduces postoperative pulmonary complications [95]. Evidences are more robust for the beneficial effects of lung protective ventilation for TLV than OLV [96].

During TLV, using a low tidal volume during ventilation (6–8 mL/kg IBW) has been shown to improve pulmonary outcomes [40, 96]. A PEEP

>2 cm of H_2O and recruitment maneuvers can be used while monitoring for hypotension [40]. For OLV, a low tidal volume of 4–5 mL/kg IBW: and PEEP of 5 cm of H_2O in the ventilated lung improves oxygenation [40, 97]. A CPAP OF 5 cm of H_2O to the non-ventilated lung also improves the oxygenation but may interrupt the surgery. The lowest FiO_2 to maintain $SPO_2 > 92\%$ should be used to avoid hyperoxia [96] and allow mild hypercapnia ($PaCO_2 < 60$ mmHg) [97] [evidence: high, level of recommendation: moderate].

7.4.7 Outline the Management of Intraoperative Hypoxia During One-Lung Ventilation

Hypoxia during OLV is a common occurrence due to reduced oxygen reserve, ventilation -perfusion mismatch, and dissociation of oxygen from hemoglobin. If the desaturation occurs suddenly and rapidly immediately abandon OLV and resume TLV. If the desaturation occurs gradually a stepwise approach is needed to manage the hypoxia [98]:

- Increase the FiO_2 to 100%.
- Ensure the patency and correct positioning of DLT by performing a check bronchoscopy.
- Ensure euvolemia. Maintain volatile anesthetics concentration of <1MAC.
- A recruitment maneuver should be applied to the ventilated lung followed by the application of PEEP of 5 cm of H_2O.
- CPAP (1–2 cm of H_2O) should be applied to the lung which is not ventilated after a recruitment maneuver.
- Partial ventilation strategies can be used for the lung that is non-ventilating, e.g. intermittent partial pressure ventilation, fiberoptic lobar insufflation, etc.
- The pulmonary artery can be clamped to cause mechanical restriction of blood flow to the non-ventilated lung.
- ECMO.

7.4.8 Discuss the Intraoperative Fluid and Blood Products Management Strategies

Fluid therapy in esophageal surgery is a complex concept as it involves both abdominal and thoracic surgery. Fluid overload and pulmonary complications can occur, whereas restrictive fluid therapy can lead to AKI, which has a high incidence in esophagectomy surgeries (10–35.3%) [99–101]. Unreliability of dynamic markers of fluid responsiveness in open thorax [102, 103] and lung protective ventilation with low tidal volume [104] makes it more challenging to administer fluid precisely. An elderly patient with multiple comorbidities and preoperative chemoradiation are also major concerns which anesthesiologists need to take into concern.

Overall, one should not use more than 4 L fluid intraoperatively. ERAS guidelines recommend that there should not be a daily weight gain of more than 2 kg/day. Balanced salt solutions are the preferred type of fluid for intraoperative use. For low-risk patients, a "zero balance" fluid therapy [105] should be practiced with monitoring of urine output, intra-abdominal pressure, mixed venous oxygen saturation, and dynamic parameters such as stroke volume variation, and pulse pressure variation [106]. Fluid administration at a rate of 1–3 mL/kg/h usually achieves a "zero balance" at the end of surgery [106]. It is preferable to use goal-directed fluid (GDT) therapy in high-risk patients [107]. A GDT should aim for supranormal oxygen delivery to tissues ($DOI_2 > 600$ mL/min/m^2) [106]. Early use of vasopressors is encouraged in patients having hypotension associated with anesthetic drugs.

With the use of minimally invasive techniques of surgery, blood loss is often minimal in esophagectomy. Overzealous transfusion of PRBC in the perioperative period can increase pulmonary complications and mortality in postoperative patients [108, 109]. Thus, a lower threshold for blood transfusion (Hb <7 gm% with deranged oxygen perfusion to organs [110] or Hb < 9gm% in patients with cardiac diseases) is advocated in these surgeries.

7.4.9 What Will Be Your Extubation Strategy and Place for Postoperative Care?

The postoperative pulmonary complications may increase with delayed extubation [111, 112]. A safe and uneventful extubation at the end of esophagectomy is feasible in patients with stable hemodynamics, adequate reversal from muscle relaxants, and maintained oxygenation parameters. In patients requiring prolonged ventilation a DLT must be exchanged with a SLT.

The need for ICU care in the postoperative management of patients after esophagectomy should be individualized [113]. A low-risk patient (ASA 1 or 2) can be shifted to HDU postoperatively, whereas a high-risk patient (ASA 3 or ASA 4, cardiac conditions, surgical factors, hemodynamically unstable, requiring prolonged ventilation) needs to be shifted to ICU.

7.5 Postoperative Management

7.5.1 Describe the Pain Management in Esophagectomy Patients

Analgesia for esophagectomy is challenging as it involves two different body cavities: thorax and abdomen. The plan for analgesia depends on the surgical approach and site of incisions. A multimodal approach combining regional anesthesia with non-opioid analgesics helps to reduce perioperative opioid consumption [114]. Breakthrough pain can be managed using a rescue dose of opioids. Regional anesthesia is the backbone of this multimodal approach. Thoracic epidural has shown excellent analgesia in esophagectomy [115]. A continuous infusion of low concentration of local anesthetics with opioids as adjuvant is preferred as it causes minimal motor blockade and hypotension. Thoracic epidural infusion helps to reduce postoperative pulmonary complications [116]. The development of chronic post-thoracotomy pain may not be prevented by pre-emptive epidural infusion [117].

The paravertebral block with its lesser incidence of side effects like urinary retention and hypotension can be an effective alternative to thoracic epidural [118–120]. Ultrasound-guided ESP block at the level of T5 has also been found to have good efficacy for postoperative analgesia with opioid-sparing effect in open esophagectomy [121, 122]. USG-guided Serratus plane block (SAP) with continuous infusion may be useful for minimally invasive thoracoscopic esophagectomy] [123, 124]. A surgeon-guided SAP block seems to be also a feasible option for hybrid technique of esophagectomy (laparoscopy and thoracoscopy), especially where thoracic epidural fails or contraindicated [125].

Adjuvant analgesics are used in esophagectomy weighing their side effect profiles in individual patients. The most commonly used drug is acetaminophen, which has anti-inflammatory, antipyretic, and analgesic action. It is administered at 20 mg/kg sixth hourly via IV, oral, or rectal route. It is also effective for providing pre-emptive analgesia [126] and reducing perioperative opioid consumption. NSAIDS (e.g., Ketorolac, Parecoxib) should be used with an individualized approach based on the age, comorbidities, and complications of the surgery [40]. As esophagectomy increases the incidence of postoperative acute kidney injury (AKI), NSAIDS must be started after the surgery only after excluding the possibility of AKI. Gabapentine [127], Ketamine [128], magnesium sulfate [129], and lignocaine IV infusion [130] can also be used in esophagectomy patients but more studies are required to conclude about their efficacy and side effects. Opioids are used for rescue analgesics in breakthrough pain. Patient-controlled analgesia without a basal infusion of opioids can serve this purpose.

7.5.2 How Will You Manage the Drains, Tubes, Catheters, Feeding, and Thromboprophylaxis in the Postoperative Period?

Drains, Tubes, and Catheters: As per the ERAS recommendations [40], a minimal number of drains and tubes should be used for a minimum period to enhance early ambulation and better pain control. Insertion of only one chest drain instead of 2 drains is equally effective and causes less tissue damage and pain. The chest tube must be removed as early as possible whenever the drain is less than 200 mL/day without any chyle or air. Separate perianastomotic drainage should not be used for cervical anastomosis. Nasogastric tubes must be used before esophageal resection and be removed by postoperative day two. Foleys catheters also should be removed early by postoperative day two with a cautious assessment of the bladder in patients with in situ epidural catheters. If any patient requires bladder catheterization for more than 4 days, suprapubic catheterization should be considered.

Feeding: Esophagectomy patients are prone to malnutrition due to poor intake, exposure to chemoradiation, and advanced age. Thus, they need adequate nutritional support even up to many days after surgery. Enteral nutrition as early as postoperative day one [131] is recommended over parenteral nutrition, as it improves postoperative morbidities and hospital stay [40, 131]. Oral feeding though is the most preferred route for enteral feeding, risk of vomiting and aspiration may be increased. In case of inability to start oral feeds, NJ tube or feeding jejunostomy may be used.

Antithrombotic prophylaxis: Thromboprophylaxis is achieved with the use of both mechanical and pharmacological means [40]. Thromboprophylaxis with LMWH (80-100 IU/kg OD) has to be started 2–12 h before surgery and it should be continued in the postoperative period for 4 weeks post-surgery. The epidural catheter placement should be avoided for 12 h after a prophylactic dose of LMWH. LMWH is restarted 4 h after the removal of epidural catheter.

7.5.3 What Are the Postoperative Complications That You Can Expect in Esophagectomy Patients?

7.5.3.1 Early Complications

- *Anastomotic leakage: Anastomotic leakage is a common complication after esophagectomy (3.3–71%)* [132] Major leakage usually occurs within the first 5 days, whereas minor leakages may occur after 7–8 days of surgery. Patients with multiple comorbidities, exposure to neoadjuvant therapies, severe malnutrition, prolonged surgery, vasopressor support, prolonged ventilation, intraoperative fluid overload, and hypoxia are prone to major leaks [132]. Epidural anesthesia by its vasodilatory effect improves the blood flow to the anastomotic site thereby reducing the risk of anastomotic leakages after esophagectomy [133]. Patients with major leaks present with deteriorating general condition, unexplained tachycardia, hypotension, arrhythmias, pleural effusion, or hydropneumothorax. These patients are managed with reexploration along with supportive measures. In case of necrosis of thoracic anastomosis, conduit should be taken down followed by cervical esophagostomy and gastrostomy. A staged surgery with colonic conduit reconstruction and anastomosis is performed later on those patients.
  Almost 50% of the leakages are minor leaks usually and can be managed with conservative approach only, e.g., keeping patient nil per oral, starting IV fluids and parenteral nutrition, nasogastric tube drainage, antibiotics, USG/CT guided aspiration of collection and chest physiotherapy [134]. Some minimally invasive techniques, e.g., drain placement, endoscopic stents for 2–4 weeks, transnasal double elementary diet tube, endoscopic suturing, EVAC, application of human dermal patch (AlloDerm patch) have also been described as a part of conservative managements of postoperative anastomotic leakages [135].
- *Pulmonary complications*: Postoperative pulmonary complications may occur in early postoperative period after esophagectomy, e.g., pleural effusion, hydropneumothorax, atelectasis, aspiration pneumonia, acute lung injury (ALI), bronchopleural fistula, etc. The incidence of postoperative pulmonary complications following esophagectomy varies from 10% to 30% with pneumonia being the most common complication [136–139]. A low FEV1 in PFT, advanced age, preoperative chemoradiation, proximal tumor, and pro-

longed duration of surgery are risk factors for developing postoperative pulmonary complications after esophagectomy [136, 137, 140].

Postoperative oxygen therapy may be administered via high-flow nasal cannula (HFNC) or CPAP. It maintains better oxygenation, causes increased clearance of sputum, and decreases the risk of anastomotic leakages, as compared to traditional facemasks [141]. Non-invasive ventilation (NIV) may be a feasible method of oxygenation after esophagectomy, though the risk of aspiration and anastomotic dehiscence associated with NIV must be considered [145, 146].

- *Cardiovascular complications*: Esophagectomy involves right thoracotomy and is associated with various arrhythmias, e.g., atrial fibrillation, atrial flutter, and paroxysmal supraventricular tachycardia. Advanced age, cardiac comorbidities, preoperative chemoradiation, patients with COPD, perioperative use of theophylline, hemodynamic instability, prolonged surgery, prolonged OLV, and intraoperative hypoxia increase the risk of developing these arrhythmias [147]. Atrial fibrillation must be identified and managed promptly as it increases the rate of pulmonary complications, anastomotic leakage, and sepsis [142, 148]. In most cases, atrial fibrillation develops within the first 48–72 h after surgery [143]. Prophylactic amiodarone may reduce postoperative arrhythmias but it does not influence the length of hospital stay and postoperative mortalities [151]. Successful management of these arrhythmias includes correction of the underlying cause if any and a patient-specific systemic approach.

  Acute myocardial infarction is also common after esophagectomy (1–2%). Esophagectomies are considered an intermediate risk (1–5%) of surgeries [144, 145]. Acute postoperative MI should be evaluated and managed as per ACC AHA guidelines [146].
- *Renal complications*: Esophagectomies have a high incidence of postoperative AKI (10–35.3%) [155–157]. Advanced age, male sex, intraoperative hypotension, and use of vasopressors are prone to development of postoperative AKI.
- *Neurological complications*: Many elderly patients can develop postoperative cognitive dysfunction.
- *Iatrogenic complications*: Chylothorax, recurrent laryngeal nerve injury.

7.5.3.2 Late Complications

- Wound infection.
- Anastomotic strictures: This is the most common complications occurring in the late postoperative period. The incidence can vary from 0% to 63% [147–149]. It is more common with gastric pull-up conduit. A careful surgical technique, adequate place for anastomosis, and use of large diameter staple can avoid conduit ischemia and stricture formation [150]. Though dilation is feasible but may need multiple sessions.
- Chronic post-thoracotomy pain: Chronic post-thoracotomy pain has an incidence of 57% after 3 months and 47% after 6 months of surgery [151]. Central and peripheral hypersensitization in the perioperative period leads to chronic post-thoracotomy pain [152]. A posterolateral thoracotomy incision, muscle cutting approach, female sex, preoperative anxiety, and history of chemoradiation increase the risk of chronic postsurgical pain [153]. A combined method with pharmacological methods (gabapentin, amitriptyline, ketamine, and opioids), peripheral nerve blocks (erector spinae block, serratus anterior plane block, intercostal radiofrequency ablation) and non-pharmacological methods (cryo-analgesia, TENS and spinal cord stimulation) are beneficial in post-thoracotomy pain.

7.5.4 How Do You Manage Postoperative Atrial Fibrillation Following Esophagectomy

Atrial fibrillation in the postoperative period can occur quite commonly (12–37%) [154]. Pathophysiology of developing new atrial fibrillation may be multifactorial e.g. advanced age, preexisting cardiac diseases, preoperative chemoradiation, direct manipulation of pericardial surface, hypothermia, electrolyte imbalance, hypoxia, and postoperative sepsis [155]. The management of atrial fibrillation includes prevention and treatment of the arrhythmia.

7.5.4.1 Prevention of Arrhythmia

- Identify the patients at risk.
- Manage hemodynamic instability.
- Correct hypoxia.
- Identify sepsis and manage it at earliest.
- Correct electrolyte imbalances.
- Patients on preoperative beta blockers must continue to receive it in the post-operative period. New administration of beta blockers in preoperative period is not recommended for non-cardiac surgeries due to an increase in the risk of low blood pressure, stroke, and morbidity. It should be only initiated in patients with coronary artery disease for are considered as high risk at least 1 week before surgery [40, 156].
- Starting an infusion of amiodarone at the rate of 43.75 mg/h for 96 h in the preoperative period has been shown to reduce the risk of developing atrial fibrillation, but can lead to bradycardia, QT prolongation, and hypotension [151]. The duration of hospital stay, overall mortalities, and morbidities are not affected by the amiodarone infusion.

7.5.4.2 Treatment of Arrhythmia

- Asymptomatic and hemodynamically stable patients should receive rate control therapy [157]. Rate control therapy should target a heart rate below 110 beats per minute [158, 159]. For rate control in patients with preserved ejection fraction, digoxin, beta blocker, or calcium channel blockers; whereas in the setting of reduced ejection fraction, calcium channel blockers should be avoided [157]. As an antiarrhythmic agent, amiodarone should be added for maintenance of rhythm and rate [157].
- If the patient is symptomatic and hemodynamically unstable, the first step is electric cardioversion. Systemic anticoagulation should be considered for the prevention of stroke, especially if atrial fibrillation is there for more than 48 h [157]. Once the rhythm is converted to sinus one, it should be maintained with rate control drugs and antiarrhythmic as described before.

  Dosages of common drugs used for the treatment of atrial fibrillation:

(a) Rate control drugs:
  - Beta-blockers:
    - Esmolol: 500 microgram/kg over 1 min(loading dose) followed by 50 microgram/kg/min every 5–15 min.
    - Metoprolol: Intravenous bolus of 2.5 mg–5 mg over 2 min, to a maximum of 3 doses.
    - Propranolol: 0.15 mg/kg IV.
  - Calcium channel blockers:
    - Diltiazem: It is administered at a dose of 0.25 mg/kg over 2 min.
    - Verapamil: It is administered as 0.075–0.15 mg/kg IV over 2 min.
  - Digoxin: It is administered in a dose of 0.25 mg every second hour, to a maximum dose of 1.5 mg.

(b) Antiarrhythmic drug:

Amiodarone: It is administered as 150 mg IV over the first 10 min, followed by an infusion of 1 mg/min infusion for the next 6 h and an infusion of 0.5 mg/min infusion over the next 18 h.

7.5.5 Enumerate the Principles of ERAS in Esophagectomy

The ERAS Society published a set of recommendations in the year of 2018 for perioperative care for esophagectomy surgery [40]. These are multidisciplinary protocols that enable the maintenance of homeostasis by reducing the stress response during surgery and post-operative organ dysfunction and enhancing recovery. The major recommendations are summarized below:

Recommendations
Preoperative:
(a) *Procedure-specific recommendations*
• A multidisciplinary team should evaluate the patients to improve the treatment outcomes.
• Asses risk of nutritional risk in all patients and optimize accordingly. Enteral nutritional support needs to be provided along with the use of feeding tubes as needed.
• Immunonutrition should not be routinely used.
• Patients should undergo multimodal prehabilitation program which may improve the outcome after esophagectomy.
(b) *Non-procedure-specific recommendations*
• All patients and their caregivers must be counseled preoperatively with detailed information about perioperative care protocols and their targets.
• Smoking cessation and abstinence from alcohol for a minimum period of 4 weeks before surgery.
• CPET should be used for preoperative risk stratification for perioperative cardiopulmonary complications.
• Routine mechanical bowel preparations should be avoided specially for gastric conduit reconstructions.
• Prolonged fasting should be avoided.
• A carbohydrate-rich drink should be allowed 2 h before surgery (with caution in patients with dysphagia or obstruction).
• Short-acting anxiolytics may be used instead of long-acting anxiolytics.
• A multimodal therapy for PONV should be used in high-risk cases.
• A thromboprophylaxis with both pharmacological and mechanical therapy must be used in all patients. An extended duration of thromboprophylaxis for 4 weeks should be continued after surgery.
• Beta blockers must be continued until surgery. High-risk patients with CAD who require beta blockers must be started the drugs at least 7 days before surgery.
• Prophylactic amiodarone decreases the atrial fibrillation in the perioperative period, but has no effect on the duration of stay in the hospital and overall mortalities.
Intraoperative
(a) *Surgery-related*
• A recovery time of 3–6 weeks following the last session of chemotherapy and 6–10 weeks from the last radiotherapy must be allowed prior to surgery.
• A minimally invasive approach should be used over invasive approach whenever possible.
• Gastric conduits are preferred over jejunum or colonic conduits due to rich vascularity.
• The role of pyloroplasty is not certain.
• The role of pyloroplasty is yet not certain.
• In patients with loco regional disease of middle and lower esophagus, a two-field lymphadenectomy should be used sparing recurrent laryngeal nodes. A three-field lymphadenectomy should be reserved only for upper esophageal tumor or for a patient with early-stage tumor and a good performance status.
• No need of perianastomotic drain for cervical anastomosis.
• A single mid position chest tube is as effective as two tubes.
• A nasogastric tube must be placed before esophageal resection and should be removed by day two in the postoperative period.
(b) *Anesthesia-related*
• Volatile and intravenous anesthesia are equally effective for maintenance of anesthesia.
• Intermediate-acting muscle relaxants should be used along with BIS monitoring for depth of anesthesia.
• Lung protective ventilation should be used for two lung ventilation. The optimal settings for two lung ventilation are as follows.
– Tidal volume: 6–8 mL/kg IBW.
– High PEEP (>2cmH_2O) and recruitment maneuver not fully defined yet.
• Evidence for lung protective ventilation during OLV is not conclusive yet. The optimal settings for one-lung ventilation are as follows:
– Low VT (4–5 mL/kg IBW).
– PEEP (5 cm H2O) ventilated lung.
– CPAP (5 cm H2O) non-ventilated lung.
– Avoid hyperoxia; allow mild hypercapnia.
• Intraoperative hypothermia must be prevented with a target temperature of >36 °C.
• Blood sugar should be checked regularly in the perioperative period. A blood sugar >180 mg/dL must be treated.
• Optimal fluid therapy avoiding fluid overload is warranted. A weight gain of more than 2 kg/day is to be avoided.
• Goal-directed fluid therapy should be reserved only for high-risk patients.
• Balanced salt solutions are the fluid of choice for perioperative use.

Recommendations
Postoperative • Place for postoperative care should be individualized in esophagectomy patients. HDU care should be used for low-risk patients. • Thoracic epidural analgesia is the first line of therapy for postoperative pain management. Paravertebral block is considered as effective as thoracic epidural. • Acetaminophen should be used routinely, whereas use of NSAIDs should be individualized. • Gabapentinoids, ketamine, magnesium sulfate and IV lignocaine infusion may be applicable, but require more robust evidences. • Early oral nutrition is beneficial for the patients. • Early ambulation is advised. • NG tube should be removed by second postoperative day. • Foley catheter should be removed as early as possible, preferably within 48 h after surgery. Careful bladder monitoring is mandatory for patients with epidural infusion of local anesthetics. • Patients who require bladder catheterization more than 4 days should undergo suprapubic catheterization. • A multidisciplinary standardized protocol at every institute should be formed. • A regular audit improves compliance to the protocol. • The role of pyloroplasty is not yet certain. • Patients with loco-regional disease of middle and lower esophagus should undergo two-field lymphadenectomy sparing the recurrent laryngeal nodes. A three-field lymphadenectomy should be reserved only for upper esophageal tumors or for a patient with an early disease or a good performance status. • Perianastamotic drain is not required for cervical anastomosis. • A single mid-position chest tube is as effective as two tubes. • A nasogastric tube must be placed before esophageal resection and removed by POD 2.
Anesthesia-related • The maintenance of anesthesia can be done by either TIVA or volatile agents both of which are equally effective. • Muscle relaxants with an intermediate duration of action are to be used along with BIS for depth of anesthesia monitoring. • During two lung ventilation, protective lung strategies should be used. This includes a tidal volume of 6-8 mL/kg IBW, high PEEP(>2 cm H_2O), and recruitment maneuvers (not yet defined fully). • The evidence for lung protective ventilation during OLV is not conclusive yet. The optimal settings for OLV are as follows: A low tidal volume of 4-5 mL/kg, application of PEEP of 5 cm H_2O in the ventilated lung and CPAP of 5 cm H_2O in the non-ventilated lung, avoiding hyperoxia while mild hypercapnia is permissible. • Inraoperative hypothermia must be prevented with a target temperature > 36 C. • Regular monitoring of blood glucose should be done and blood sugar>180 mg/dl must be treated. • Optimal fluid therapy while avoiding fluid overload is warranted. In high-risk patients, goal-directed fluid therapy should be used. • Balanced salt solutions are preferred in the perioperative period.
Postoperative • Postoperative care plan should be individualized. HDU care should be used in low-risk patients. • Thoracic epidural analgesia is the first line of analgesia in postoperative pain management. Paravertebral blocks are as effective as thoracic epidurals. • Acetaminophen should be used as a part of multi-modal analgesia. Use of NSAIDS should be individualized. • Gabapentin, ketamine, lidocaine, magnesium sulphate may be used but lack robust evidence. • Early start of enteral feeding should be encouraged. • Early ambulation is beneficial. • NG tube should be removed by POD2. • Removal of Foley's catheter preferably within 48 h of surgery is recommended. • Patients requiring bladder catheterization>4 days should undergo suprapubic catheterization. • A multidisciplinary standardized protocol should be developed at each institute. • Regular audits should be conducted.

References

1. Hermanek P. Pathologic classification of the esophageal carcinoma. In: Surgery of the Esophagus. Steinkopff; 2009. https://doi.org/10.1007/978-3-7985-1743-1_9.
2. Sarpel U. Esophagectomy. In: Surgery. Cham: Springer; 2021. https://doi.org/10.1007/978-3-030-65074-2_5.
3. Abbas G, Krasna M. Overview of esophageal cancer. Ann Cardiothorac Surg. 2017;6(2):131–6. https://doi.org/10.21037/acs.2017.03.03.
4. Survival rates for esophageal cancer https://www.cancer.org/cancer/esophagus-cancer/detection-diagnosis-staging/survival-rates.html. Accessed 15 Jun 2022.
5. Rice TW, Patil DT, Blackstone EH. 8th edition AJCC/UICC staging of cancers of the esophagus and esophagogastric junction: application to clinical practice. Ann Cardiothorac Surg. 2017;6(2):119–30. https://doi.org/10.21037/acs.2017.03.14.
6. Berry MF. Esophageal cancer: staging system and guidelines for staging and treatment. J Thorac Dis. 2014;6 Suppl 3(Suppl 3):S289–97. https://doi.org/10.3978/j.issn.2072-1439.2014.03.11.
7. van Vliet EP, Heijenbrok-Kal MH, Hunink MG, Kuipers EJ, Siersema PD. Staging investigations for oesophageal cancer: a meta-analysis. Br J Cancer. 2008;98(3):547–57. https://doi.org/10.1038/sj.bjc.6604200.
8. Lordick F, Mariette C, Haustermans K, Obermannová R, Arnold D, Guidelines ESMO, Committee. Oesophageal cancer: ESMO clinical practice Guidelines for diagnosis, treatment and follow-up. Ann Oncol. 2016;27(suppl 5):v50–7. https://doi.org/10.1093/annonc/mdw329.
9. Shapiro J, van Lanschot JJB, Hulshof MCCM, et al. Neoadjuvant chemoradiotherapy plus surgery versus surgery alone for oesophageal or junctional cancer (CROSS): long-term results of a randomised controlled trial. Lancet Oncol. 2015;16(9):1090–8. https://doi.org/10.1016/S1470-2045(15)00040-6.
10. Pultrum BB, Bosch DJ, Nijsten MW, et al. Extended esophagectomy in elderly patients with esophageal cancer: minor effect of age alone in determining the postoperative course and survival. Ann Surg Oncol. 2010;17(6):1572–80. https://doi.org/10.1245/s10434-010-0966-7.
11. Ilson DH. Esophageal cancer chemotherapy: recent advances. Gastrointest Cancer Res. 2008;2(2):85–92.
12. Callejo A, Sedó-Cabezón L, Juan ID, Llorens J. Cisplatin-Induced Ototoxicity: Effects, Mechanisms and Protection Strategies. Toxics. 2015;3(3):268–93. https://doi.org/10.3390/toxics3030268.
13. Gregg RW, Molepo JM, Monpetit VJA, et al. Cisplatin neurotoxicity: the relationship between dosage, time, and platinum concentration in neurologic tissues, and morphologic evidence of toxicity. J Clin Oncol. 1992;10(5):795–803.
14. Ozols RF, Young RC. High-dose cisplatin therapy in ovarian cancer. Semin Oncol. 1985;12(4):21–30.
15. van der Hoop RG, van der Burg MEL, ten Bokkel Huinink WW, van Houwelingen JC, Neijt JP. Incidence of neuropathy in 395 patients with ovarian cancer treated with or without cisplatin. Cancer. 1990;66(8):1697–702.
16. von Schlippe M, Fowler CJ, Harland SJ. Cisplatin neurotoxicity in the treatment of metastatic germ cell tumour: time course and prognosis. Br J Cancer. 2001;85(6):823–6.
17. Finley RS, Fortner CL, Grove WR. Cisplatin nephrotoxicity: a summary of preventative interventions. Drug Intell Clin Pharm. 1985;19(5):362–7. https://doi.org/10.1177/106002808501900505.
18. Hayati F, Hossainzadeh M, Shayanpour S, Abedi-Gheshlaghi Z, Beladi Mousavi SS. Prevention of cisplatin nephrotoxicity. J Nephropharmacol. 2015;5(1):57–60.
19. Farrar MC, Jacobs TF. Paclitaxel. In: StatPearls. Treasure Island (FL): StatPearls Publishing; 2022. https://www.ncbi.nlm.nih.gov/books/NBK536917/.
20. Alter P, Herzum M, Soufi M, Schaefer JR, Maisch B. Cardiotoxicity of 5-fluorouracil. Cardiovasc Hematol Agents Med Chem. 2006;4(1):1–5. https://doi.org/10.2174/187152506775268785.
21. Kishi P, Price CJ. Life-threatening reaction with topical 5-Fluorouracil. Drug Saf Case Rep. 2018;5(1):4. https://doi.org/10.1007/s40800-017-0068-6.
22. Saif MW, Katirtzoglou NA, Syrigos KN. Capecitabine: an overview of the side effects and their management. Anti-Cancer Drugs. 2008;19(5):447–64. https://doi.org/10.1097/CAD.0b013e3282f945aa.
23. Walko CM, Lindley C. Capecitabine: a review. Clin Ther. 2005;27(1):23–44. https://doi.org/10.1016/j.clinthera.2005.01.005.
24. Bradley J, Movsas B. Radiation pneumonitis and esophagitis in thoracic irradiation. Cancer Treat Res. 2006;128:43–64. https://doi.org/10.1007/0-387-25354-8_4.
25. Hanania AN, Mainwaring W, Ghebre YT, Hanania NA, Ludwig M. Radiation-induced lung injury: assessment and management. Chest. 2019;156(1):150–62. https://doi.org/10.1016/j.chest.2019.03.033.
26. Ozturk B, Egehan I, Atavci S, Kitapci M. Pentoxifylline in prevention of radiation-induced lung toxicity in patients with breast and lung cancer: a double-blind randomized trial. Int J Radiat Oncol Biol Phys. 2004;58:213–9. https://doi.org/10.1016/S0360-3016(03)01444-5.
27. Robbins ME, Diz DI. Pathogenic role of the renin-angiotensin system in modulating radiation-induced late effects. Int J Radiat Oncol Biol Phys. 2006;64:6–12. https://doi.org/10.1016/j.ijrobp.2005.08.033.
28. Medhora M, Gao F, Jacobs ER, Moulder JE. Radiation damage to the lung: mitigation by angiotensin-converting enzyme (ACE) inhibi-

tors. Respirology. 2012;17:66–71. https://doi.org/10.1111/j.1440-1843.2011.02092.x.
29. Muraoka T, Bandoh S, Fujita J, Horiike A, Ishii T, Tojo Y, et al. Corticosteroid refractory radiation pneumonitis that remarkably responded to cyclosporin a. Intern Med. 2002;41:730–3. https://doi.org/10.2169/internalmedicine.41.730.
30. Frandsen J, Boothe D, Gaffney DK, Wilson BD, Lloyd S. Increased risk of death due to heart disease after radiotherapy for esophageal cancer. J Gastrointest Oncol. 2015;6:516–23.
31. Gharzai L, Verma V, Denniston KA, Bhirud AR, Bennion NR, Lin C. Radiation therapy and cardiac death in long-term survivors of esophageal cancer: an analysis of the surveillance, epidemiology, and end result database. PLoS One. 2016;11:e0158916.
32. Vošmik M, Hodek M, Buka D, et al. Cardiotoxicity of radiation therapy in esophageal cancer. Rep Pract Oncol Radiother. 2020;25(3):318–22. https://doi.org/10.1016/j.rpor.2020.02.005.
33. Beukema JC, van Luijk P, Widder J, Langendijk JA, Muijs CT. Is cardiac toxicity a relevant issue in the radiation treatment of esophageal cancer. Radiother Oncol. 2015;114:85–90.
34. Gayed IW, Liu HH, Yusuf SW, et al. The prevalence of myocardial ischemia after concurrent chemoradiation therapy as detected by gated myocardial perfusion imaging in patients with esophageal cancer. J Nucl Med. 2006;47(11):1756–62.
35. Brosius FC, Waller BF, Roberts WC. Radiation heart disease. Analysis of 16 young (aged 15 to 33 years) necropsy patients who received over 3,500 rads to the heart. Am J Med. 1981;70(3):519–30.
36. Nakao T, Kanaya H, Namura M, et al. Complete atrioventricular block following radiation therapy for malignant thymoma. Jpn J Med. 1990;29(1):104–10.
37. Eisbruch A, Lyden T, Bradford CR, et al. Objective assessment of swallowing dysfunction and aspiration after radiation concurrent with chemotherapy for head-and-neck cancer. International journal of radiation oncology* biology*. Physics. 2002;53(1):23–8.
38. Tolentino Ede S, Centurion BS, LHC F, de Souza AP, Damante JH, IRF R-B. Oral adverse effects of head and neck radiotherapy: literature review and suggestion of a clinical oral care guideline for irradiated patients. J Appl Oral Sci. 2011;19(5):448–54.
39. Balakrishnan M, Kuriakose R, Koshy RC. Radiation induced changes in the airway—anaesthetic implications. South Afr J Anaesth Analg. 2004;10(2):19–21.
40. Pisarska M, Małczak P, Major P, Wysocki M, Budzyński A, Pędziwiatr M. Enhanced recovery after surgery protocol in oesophageal cancer surgery: systematic review and meta-analysis. PLoS One. 2017;12(3):e0174382. Published 2017 Mar 28. https://doi.org/10.1371/journal.pone.0174382.
41. Nagatsuka Y, Sugimura K, Miyata H, et al. Predictive value of preoperative echocardiographic assessment for postoperative atrial fibrillation after esophagectomy for esophageal cancer. Esophagus. 2021;18:496–503. https://doi.org/10.1007/s10388-020-00804-y.
42. Lund M, Tsai JA, Nilsson M, et al. Effects of neoadjuvant chemo or chemoradiotherapy for oesophageal cancer on perioperative haemodynamics: a prospective cohort study within a randomised clinical trial. Eur J Anaesthesiol. 2016;33:653–61. https://doi.org/10.1097/EJA.0000000000000480.
43. Levett DZH, Jack S, Swart M, et al. Perioperative cardiopulmonary exercise testing (CPET): consensus clinical guidelines on indications, organization, conduct, and physiological interpretation. Br J Anaesth. 2018;120:484–500. https://doi.org/10.1016/j.bja.2017.10.020.
44. Reeh M, Metze J, Uzunoglu FG, et al. The PER (preoperative Esophagectomy risk) score: a simple risk score to predict short-term and Long-term outcome in patients with surgically treated esophageal cancer. Medicine (Baltimore). 2016;95(7):e2724. https://doi.org/10.1097/MD.0000000000002724.
45. Forshaw MJ, Strauss DC, Davies AR, et al. Is cardiopulmonary exercise testing a useful test before esophagectomy? Ann Thorac Surg. 2008;85(1):294–9. https://doi.org/10.1016/j.athoracsur.2007.05.062.
46. Patel N, Powell AG, Wheat JR, et al. Cardiopulmonary fitness predicts postoperative major morbidity after esophagectomy for patients with cancer. Physiol Rep. 2019;7(14):e14174. https://doi.org/10.14814/phy2.14174.
47. Chmelo J, Khaw RA, Sinclair RCF, Navidi M, Phillips AW. Does cardiopulmonary testing help predict Long-term survival after Esophagectomy? Ann Surg Oncol. 2021;28(12):7291–7. https://doi.org/10.1245/s10434-021-10136-5.
48. Arends J, Bachmann P, Baracos V, et al. ESPEN guidelines on nutrition in cancer patients. Clin Nutr. 2017;36(1):11–48. https://doi.org/10.1016/j.clnu.2016.07.015.
49. Wynter-Blyth V, Moorthy K. Prehabilitation: preparing patients for surgery. BMJ. 2017;358:j3702. https://doi.org/10.1136/bmj.j3702.
50. Tew GA, Ayyash R, Durrand J, Danjoux GR. Clinical guideline and recommendations on pre-operative exercise training in patients awaiting major noncardiac surgery. Anaesthesia. 2018;73(6):750–68. https://doi.org/10.1111/anae.14177.
51. Moran J, Guinan E, McCormick P, et al. The ability of prehabilitation to influence postoperative outcome after intra-abdominal operation: a systematic review and meta-analysis. Surgery. 2016;160:1189–201. https://doi.org/10.1016/j.surg.2016.05.014.
52. Michael CM, Lehrer EJ, Schmitz KH, Zaorsky NG. Prehabilitation exercise therapy for cancer: a systematic review and meta-analysis. Cancer Med. 2021;10(13):4195–205. https://doi.org/10.1002/cam4.4021.
53. Levett DZ, Grocott MP. Cardiopulmonary exercise testing, prehabilitation, and enhanced recovery after surgery (ERAS). Can J Anaesth. 2015;62(2):131–42. https://doi.org/10.1007/s12630-014-0307-6.

54. Dettling DS, van der Schaaf M, Blom RL, et al. Feasibility and effectiveness of pre-operative inspiratory muscle training in patients undergoing oesophagectomy: a pilot study. Physiother Res Int. 2013;18:16–26. https://doi.org/10.1002/pri.1524.
55. Ferreira V, Agnihotram RV, Bergdahl A, et al. Maximizing patient adherence to prehabilitation: what do the patients say? Support Care Cancer. 2018;26:2717–23. https://doi.org/10.1007/s00520-018-4109-1.
56. Chen K, Yao F, Chen X, Lin Y, Kang M. Effectiveness of telerehabilitation on short-term quality of life of patients after esophageal cancer surgery during COVID-19: a single-center, randomized, controlled study. J Gastrointest Oncol. 2021;12(4):1255–64. https://doi.org/10.21037/jgo-21-385.
57. Piraux E, Caty G, Reychler G, et al. Feasibility and preliminary effectiveness of a tele-Prehabilitation program in Esophagogastric cancer patients. J Clin Med. 2020;9:2176. https://doi.org/10.3390/jcm9072176.
58. Svanfeldt M, Thorell A, Hausel J, Soop M, Nygren J, Ljungqvist O. Effect of "preoperative" oral carbohydrate treatment on insulin action--a randomised cross-over unblinded study in healthy subjects. Clin Nutr. 2005;24:815–21.
59. Marik PE, Lemson J. Fluid responsiveness: an evolution of our understanding. Br J Anaesth. 2014;112:617–20. https://doi.org/10.1093/bja/aet590.
60. Sekandarzad MW, van Zundert AAJ, Lirk PB, Doornebal CW, Hollmann MW. Perioperative anesthesia care and tumor progression. Anesth Analg. 2017;124:1697–708.
61. Yang W, Cai J, Zabkiewicz C, Zhang H, Ruge F, Jiang WG. The effects of anesthetics on recurrence and metastasis of cancer, and clinical implications. World J Oncol. 2017;8:63–70.
62. Stollings LM, Jia LJ, Tang P, et al. Immune modulation by volatile anesthetics. Anesthesiology. 2016;125:399–411. https://doi.org/10.1097/ALN.0000000000001195.
63. Egeblad M, Werb Z. New functions for the matrix metalloproteinases in cancer progression. Nat Rev Cancer. 2002;2:161–74.
64. Jun IJ, Jo JY, Kim JI, et al. Impact of anesthetic agents on overall and recurrence-free survival in patients undergoing esophageal cancer surgery: a retrospective observational study. Sci Rep. 2017;7:14020. https://doi.org/10.1038/s41598-017-14147-9.
65. de la Gala F, Piñeiro P, Reyes A, et al. Postoperative pulmonary complications, pulmonary and systemic inflammatory responses after lung resection surgery with prolonged one-lung ventilation. Randomized controlled trial comparing intravenous and inhalational anaesthesia. Br J Anaesth. 2017;119(4):655–63. https://doi.org/10.1093/bja/aex230.
66. Lee S, Cho JS, Kim E, Kim Y, Lee J. Effects of inhalation versus Total intravenous anesthesia on postoperative pulmonary complications after anatomic pulmonary resection. J Chest Surg. 2022;55(1):30–6. https://doi.org/10.5090/jcs.21.119.
67. Parab S, Gaikwad S, Majeti S. Inhalational versus intravenous anesthetics during one lung ventilation in elective thoracic surgeries: a narrative review. Saudi J Anaesth. 2021;15(3):312–23. https://doi.org/10.4103/sja.sja_1106_20.
68. Liu S, Carpenter RL, Neal JM. Epidural anesthesia and analgesia: their role in postoperative outcome. Anesthesiology. 1995;82:1474–506.
69. Ahlers O, Nachtigall I, Lenze J, et al. Intraoperative thoracic epidural anaesthesia attenuates stress-induced immunosuppression in patients undergoing major abdominal surgery. Br J Anaesth. 2008;101:781–7.
70. Lucchinetti E, Awad AE, Rahman M, et al. Antiproliferative effects of local anesthetics on mesenchymal stem cells: potential implications for tumor spreading and wound healing. Anesthesiology. 2012;116:841–56.
71. Wang J, Yin Y, Zhu Y, et al. Thoracic epidural anaesthesia and analgesia ameliorates surgery-induced stress response and postoperative pain in patients undergoing radical oesophagectomy. J Int Med Res. 2019;47(12):6160–70. https://doi.org/10.1177/0300060519866943.
72. Li XQ, Tan WF, Wang J, Fang B, Ma H. The effects of thoracic epidural analgesia on oxygenation and pulmonary shunt fraction during one-lung ventilation: an meta-analysis. BMC Anesthesiol. 2015;15:166. Published 2015 Nov 19. https://doi.org/10.1186/s12871-015-0142-5.
73. Jung SM, Cho CK, Kim YJ, et al. The effect of thoracic epidural anesthesia on pulmonary shunt fraction and arterial oxygenation during one-lung ventilation. J Cardiothorac Vasc Anesth. 2010;24(3):456–62. https://doi.org/10.1053/j.jvca.2009.09.011.
74. Xu Y, Tan Z, Wang S, Shao H, Zhu X. Effect of thoracic epidural anesthesia with different concentrations of ropivacaine on arterial oxygenation during one-lung ventilation. Anesthesiology. 2010;112(5):1146–54. https://doi.org/10.1097/ALN.0b013e3181d40347.
75. Kakegawa T, Fujita H. A history of esophageal surgery in the twentieth century. Gen Thorac Cardiovasc Surg. 2009;57:55–63. https://doi.org/10.1007/s11748-008-0381-1.
76. The Association of Upper Gastrointestinal Surgeons (AUGIS). A consensus view and recommendations on the development and practise of minimally invasive oesophagectomy. The Association of Upper Gastrointestinal Surgeons (AUGIS); 2009. www.augis.org/news/documents/MIO_Consensus.pdf.
77. McKeown KC. Total three-stage oesophagectomy for cancer of the oesophagus. Br J Surg. 1976;63:259–62. https://doi.org/10.1002/bjs.1800630403.
78. Papenfuss WA, Kukar M, Attwood K, et al. Transhiatal versus transthoracic esophagectomy

for esophageal cancer: a 2005-2011 NSQIP comparison of modern multicenter results. J Surg Oncol. 2014;110:298–301. https://doi.org/10.1002/jso.23637.
79. Straatman J, van der Wielen N, Cuesta MA, et al. Minimally invasive versus open esophageal resection: three-year follow-up of the previously reported randomized controlled trial: the TIME trial. Ann Surg. 2017;266:232–6. https://doi.org/10.1097/SLA.0000000000002171.
80. Rucklidge M, Sanders D, Martin A. Anaesthesia for minimally invasive oesophagectomy. Continuing Educ Anaesth Crit Care Pain. 2010;10(2):43–7.
81. Tsunoda S, Obama K, Hisamori S, et al. Lower incidence of postoperative pulmonary complications following robot-assisted minimally invasive Esophagectomy for esophageal cancer: propensity score-matched comparison to conventional minimally invasive Esophagectomy. Ann Surg Oncol. 2021;28:639–47. https://doi.org/10.1245/s10434-020-09081-6.
82. Campos J, Ueda K. Update on anesthetic complications of robotic thoracic surgery. Minerva Anestesiol. 2014;80(1):83–8.
83. Langiano N, Fiorelli S, Deana C, et al. Airway management in anesthesia for thoracic surgery: a "real life" observational study. J Thorac Dis. 2019;11:3257–69. https://doi.org/10.21037/jtd.2019.08.57.
84. Larsen S, Holm JH, Sauer TN, et al. A cost-effectiveness analysis comparing the VivaSight double-lumen tube and a conventional double-lumen tube in adult patients undergoing thoracic surgery involving one-lung ventilation. Pharmacoecon Open. 2020;4:159–69. https://doi.org/10.1007/s41669-019-0163-y.
85. Merli G, Guarino A, Della Rocca G, et al. Recommendations for airway control and difficult airway management in thoracic anesthesia and lung separation procedures. Minerva Anestesiol. 2009;75(59–78):79–96.
86. Arndt GA, Buchika S, Kranner PW, DeLessio ST. Wire-guided endobronchial blockade in a patient with a limited mouth opening. Can J Anaesth. 1999;46:87–9.
87. Cohen E. The Cohen flexitip endobronchial blocker: an alternative to a double lumen tube. Anesth Analg. 2005;101:1877–9.
88. Inoue H, Shohtsu A, Ogawa J, Koide S, Kawada S. Endotracheal tube with movable blocker to prevent aspiration of intratracheal bleeding. Ann Thorac Surg. 1984;37:497–9.
89. Purohit A, Bhargava S, Mangal V, Parashar VK. Lung isolation, one-lung ventilation and hypoxaemia during lung isolation. Indian J Anaesth. 2015;59(9):606–17. https://doi.org/10.4103/0019-5049.165855.
90. Moritz A, Irouschek A, Birkholz T, Prottengeier J, Sirbu H, Schmidt J. The EZ-blocker for one-lung ventilation in patients undergoing thoracic surgery: clinical applications and experience in 100 cases in a routine clinical setting. J Cardiothorac Surg. 2018;13(1):77. https://doi.org/10.1186/s13019-018-0767-9.
91. Ashok V, Francis J. A practical approach to adult one-lung ventilation. BJA Educ. 2018;18(3):69–74. https://doi.org/10.1016/j.bjae.2017.11.007.
92. Young CC, Harris EM, Vacchiano C, et al. Lung-protective ventilation for the surgical patient: international expert panel-based consensus recommendations. Br J Anaesth. 2019;123:898–913. https://doi.org/10.1016/j.bja.2019.08.017.
93. Choi YS, Shim JK, Na S, et al. Pressure-controlled versus volume-controlled ventilation during one-lung ventilation in the prone position for robot-assisted esophagectomy. Surg Endosc. 2009;23:2286–91. https://doi.org/10.1007/s00464-008-0310-5.
94. Güldner A, Kiss T, Serpa Neto A, et al. Intraoperative protective mechanical ventilation for prevention of postoperative pulmonary complications: a comprehensive review of the role of tidal volume, positive end-expiratory pressure, and lung recruitment maneuver. Anesthesiology. 2015;123:692–713. https://doi.org/10.1097/ALN.0000000000000754.
95. Şentürk M, Slinger P, Cohen E. Intraoperative mechanical ventilation strategies for one-lung ventilation. Best Pract Res Clin Anaesthesiol. 2015;29:357–69. https://doi.org/10.1016/j.bpa.2015.08.001.
96. Forkin KT, Nemergut EC. Miller's Anesthesia. Anesthesiology. 2016;124:977–8. https://doi.org/10.1097/ALN.0000000000001020.
97. Corsini EM, Zhou N, Antonoff MB, et al. Postoperative bleeding and acute kidney injury in esophageal cancer patients receiving ketorolac. Ann Thorac Surg. 2021;111(4):1111–7. https://doi.org/10.1016/j.athoracsur.2020.07.028.
98. Konda P, Ai D, Guerra CE, et al. Identification of risk factors associated with postoperative acute kidney injury after Esophagectomy for esophageal cancer. J Cardiothorac Vasc Anesth. 2017;31(2):474–81. https://doi.org/10.1053/j.jvca.2016.07.030.
99. Lee EH, Kim HR, Baek SH, et al. Risk factors of postoperative acute kidney injury in patients undergoing esophageal cancer surgery. J Cardiothorac Vasc Anesth. 2014;28(4):936–42. https://doi.org/10.1053/j.jvca.2013.12.006.
100. Wyffels PA, Sergeant P, Wouters PF. The value of pulse pressure and stroke volume variation as predictors of fluid responsiveness during open chest surgery. Anaesthesia. 2010;65(7):704–9. https://doi.org/10.1111/j.1365-2044.2010.06371.x.
101. Perez Nieto OR, Wong A, Lopez Fermin J, et al. Aiming for zero fluid accumulation: first, do no harm. Anaesthesiol Intensive Ther. 2021;53:162–78. https://doi.org/10.5114/ait.2021.105252.
102. Deana C, Vetrugno L, Bignami E, Bassi F. Perioperative approach to esophagectomy: a narrative review from the anesthesiological standpoint.

J Thorac Dis. 2021;13(10):6037–51. https://doi.org/10.21037/jtd-21-940.
103. Klevebro F, Boshier PR, Low DE. Application of standardized hemodynamic protocols within enhanced recovery after surgery programs to improve outcomes associated with anastomotic leak and conduit necrosis in patients undergoing esophagectomy. J Thorac Dis. 2019;11:S692–701. https://doi.org/10.21037/jtd.2018.11.141.
104. Lee J, Chin JH, Kim JI, et al. Association between red blood cell transfusion and long-term mortality in patients with cancer of the esophagus after esophagectomy. Dis Esophagus. 2018;31(2):dox123. https://doi.org/10.1093/dote/dox123.
105. Kaufmann KB, Baar W, Glatz T, et al. Epidural analgesia and avoidance of blood transfusion are associated with reduced mortality in patients with postoperative pulmonary complications following thoracotomic esophagectomy: a retrospective cohort study of 335 patients. BMC Anesthesiol. 2019;19:162. https://doi.org/10.1186/s12871-019-0832-5.
106. Spahn DR, Spahn GH, Stein P. Evidence base for restrictive transfusion triggers in high-risk patients. Transfus Med Hemother. 2015;42(2):110–4. https://doi.org/10.1159/000381509.
107. Whooley BP, Law S, Murthy SC, Alexandrou A, Wong J. Analysis of reduced death and complication rates after esophageal resection. Ann Surg. 2001;233:338–44.
108. Lanuti M, de Delva PE, Maher A, Wright CD, Gaissert HA, Wain JC, Donahue DM, Mathisen DJ. Feasibility and outcomes of an early extubation policy after esophagectomy. Ann Thorac Surg. 2006;82:2037–41.
109. O'Grady M, Firth R, Roberts R. Intensive care unit utilisation post-oesophagectomy. N Z Med J. 2020;133:56–61.
110. Thota RS, Ramkiran S, Garg R, Goswami J, Baxi V, Thomas M. Opioid free onco-anesthesia: is it time to convict opioids? A systematic review of literature. J Anaesthesiol Clin Pharmacol. 2019;35(4):441–52. https://doi.org/10.4103/joacp.JOACP_128_19.
111. Flisberg P, Törnebrandt K, Walther B, Lundberg J. Pain relief after esophagectomy: thoracic epidural analgesia is better than parenteral opioids. J Cardiothorac Vasc Anesth. 2001;15(3):282–7. https://doi.org/10.1053/jcan.2001.23270.
112. Sentürk M, Ozcan PE, Talu GK, et al. The effects of three different analgesia techniques on long-term postthoracotomy pain. Anesth Analg. 2002;94(1):11. https://doi.org/10.1213/00000539-200201000-00003.
113. Bong CL, Samuel M, Ng JM, Ip-Yam C. Effects of preemptive epidural analgesia on post-thoracotomy pain. J Cardiothorac Vasc Anesth. 2005;19(6):786–93.
114. Michelet P, D'Journo XB, Roch A, et al. Perioperative risk factors for anastomotic leakage after esophagectomy: influence of thoracic epidural analgesia. Chest. 2005;128(5):3461–6.
115. Davies RG, Myles PS, Graham JM. A comparison of the analgesic efficacy and side-effects of paravertebral vs epidural blockade for thoracotomy—a systematic review and meta-analysis of randomized trials [published correction appears in Br J Anaesth. 2007 Nov;99(5):768]. Br J Anaesth. 2006;96(4):418–26. https://doi.org/10.1093/bja/ael020.
116. Ding X, Jin S, Niu X, Ren H, Fu S, Li Q. A comparison of the analgesia efficacy and side effects of paravertebral compared with epidural blockade for thoracotomy: an updated meta-analysis. PLoS One. 2014;9(5):e96233. https://doi.org/10.1371/journal.pone.0096233.
117. Baidya DK, Khanna P, Maitra S. Analgesic efficacy and safety of thoracic paravertebral and epidural analgesia for thoracic surgery: a systematic review and meta-analysis. Interact Cardiovasc Thorac Surg. 2014;18(5):626–35. https://doi.org/10.1093/icvts/ivt551.
118. Zengin M, Baldemir R, Ulger G, Sazak H, Alagoz A. Postoperative analgesic efficacy of thoracic paravertebral block and erector Spinae plane block combination in video-assisted thoracic surgery. Cureus. 2021;13(6):e15614. Published 2021 Jun 12. https://doi.org/10.7759/cureus.15614.
119. Chen G, Li Y, Zhang Y, Fang X. Effects of serratus anterior plane block for postoperativeanalgesia after thoracoscopic surgery compared with local anesthetic infiltration: a randomized clinical trial. J Pain Res. 2019;12:2411–7. https://doi.org/10.2147/JPR.S207116.
120. Wang L, Wang Y, Zhang X, Zhu X, Wang G. Serratus anterior plane block or thoracic paravertebral block for postoperative pain treatment after uniportal video-assisted thoracoscopic surgery: a retrospective propensity-matched study. J Pain Res. 2019;12:2231–8. https://doi.org/10.2147/JPR.S209012.
121. Barbera C, Milito P, Punturieri M, Asti E, Bonavina L. Serratus anterior plane block for hybrid transthoracic esophagectomy: a pilot study. J Pain Res. 2017;10:73–7. https://doi.org/10.2147/JPR.S121441.
122. Xuan C, Yan W, Wang D, Mueller A, Ma H, Wang J. Effect of preemptive acetaminophen on opioid consumption: a meta-analysis. Pain Physician. 2021;24(2):E153–60.
123. Schmidt PC, Ruchelli G, Mackey SC, Carroll IR. Perioperative gabapentinoids: choice of agent, dose, timing, and effects on chronic postsurgical pain. Anesthesiology. 2013;119(5):1215–21. https://doi.org/10.1097/ALN.0b013e3182a9a896.
124. Laskowski K, Stirling A, McKay WP, Lim HJ. A systematic review of intravenous ketamine for postoperative analgesia. Can J Anaesth. 2011;58(10):911–23. https://doi.org/10.1007/s12630-011-9560-0.
125. De Oliveira GS Jr, Castro-Alves LJ, Khan JH, McCarthy RJ. Perioperative systemic magnesium

to minimize postoperative pain: a meta-analysis of randomized controlled trials. Anesthesiology. 2013;119(1):178–90. https://doi.org/10.1097/ALN.0b013e318297630d.
126. Masic D, Liang E, Long C, Sterk EJ, Barbas B, Rech MA. Intravenous lidocaine for acute pain: a systematic review. Pharmacotherapy. 2018;38(12):1250–9. https://doi.org/10.1002/phar.2189.
127. Xiao-Bo Y, Qiang L, Xiong Q, et al. Efficacy of early postoperative enteral nutrition in supporting patients after esophagectomy. Minerva Chir. 2014;69(1):37–46.
128. Martin LW, Hofstetter W, Swisher SG, Roth JA. Management of intrathoracic leaks following esophagectomy. Adv Surg. 2006;40:173–90.
129. Manghelli JL, Ceppa DP, Greenberg JW, et al. Management of anastomotic leaks following esophagectomy: when to intervene? J Thorac Dis. 2019;11(1):131–7. https://doi.org/10.21037/jtd.2018.12.13.
130. Famiglietti A, Lazar JF, Henderson H, et al. Management of anastomotic leaks after esophagectomy and gastric pull-up. J Thorac Dis. 2020;12(3):1022–30. https://doi.org/10.21037/jtd.2020.01.15.
131. Law S, Wong KH, Kwok KF, Chu KM, Wong J. Predictive factors for postoperative pulmonary complications and mortality after esophagectomy for cancer. Ann Surg. 2004;240(5):791–800.
132. Ferguson MK, Durkin AE. Preoperative prediction of the risk of pulmonary complications after esophagectomy for cancer. J Thorac Cardiovasc Surg. 2002;123(4):661–9.
133. Bailey SH, Bull DA, Harpole DH, et al. Outcomes after esophagectomy: a ten-year prospective cohort. Ann Thorac Surg. 2003;75(1):217–22. discussion 222.
134. Muller JM, Erasmi H, Stelzner M, Zieren U, Pichlmaier H. Surgical therapy of oesophageal carcinoma. Br J Surg. 1990;77(8):845–57.
135. Avendano CE, Flume PA, Silvestri GA, King LB, Reed CE. Pulmonary complications after esophagectomy. Ann Thorac Surg. 2002;73(3):922–6. https://doi.org/10.1016/s0003-4975(01)03584-6.
136. Xia M, Li W, Yao J, et al. A postoperative comparison of high-flow nasal cannula therapy and conventional oxygen therapy for esophageal cancer patients. Ann. Palliat Med. 2021;10:2530–9. https://doi.org/10.21037/apm-20-1539.
137. Yu KY, Zhao L, Chen Z, et al. Noninvasive positive pressure ventilation for the treatment of acute respiratory distress syndrome following esophagectomy for esophageal cancer: a clinical comparative study. J Thorac Dis. 2013;5:777–82.
138. Michelet P, Blayac D, Jaber S. Case scenario: management of postesophagectomy respiratory failure with noninvasive ventilation. Anesthesiology. 2010;113:454–61. https://doi.org/10.1097/ALN.0b013e3181e7fa81.
139. Ma JY, Wang Y, Zhao YF, et al. Atrial fibrillation after surgery for esophageal carcinoma: clinical and prognostic significance. World J Gastroenterol. 2006;12(3):449–52.
140. Murthy SC, Law S, Whooley BP, Alexandrou A, Chu KM, Wong J. Atrial fibrillation after esophagectomy is a marker for postoperative morbidity and mortality. J Thorac Cardiovasc Surg. 2003;126(4):1162–7.
141. Amar D, Burt ME, Bains MS, Leung DH. Symptomatic tachydysrhythmias after esophagectomy: incidence and outcome measures. Ann Thorac Surg. 1996;61(5):1506–9.
142. Stawicki SP, Prosciak MP, Gerlach AT, et al. Atrial fibrillation after esophagectomy: an indicator of postoperative morbidity. Gen Thorac Cardiovasc Surg. 2011;59(6):399–405. https://doi.org/10.1007/s11748-010-0713-9.
143. Tisdale JE, Jaynes HA, Watson MR, Corya AL, Shen C, Kesler KA. Amiodarone for prevention of atrial fibrillation following esophagectomy. J Thorac Cardiovasc Surg. 2019;158(1):301–310.e1. https://doi.org/10.1016/j.jtcvs.2019.01.095.
144. Low DE, Kuppusamy MK, Alderson D, et al. Benchmarking complications associated with Esophagectomy. Ann Surg. 2019;269:291–8. https://doi.org/10.1097/SLA.0000000000002611.
145. Kristensen SD, Knuuti J, Saraste A, et al. 2014 ESC/ESA Guidelines on non-cardiac surgery: cardiovascular assessment and management: the joint task force on non-cardiac surgery: cardiovascular assessment and management of the European Society of Cardiology (ESC) and the European Society of Anaesthesiology (ESA). Eur Heart J. 2014;35:2383–431. https://doi.org/10.1093/eurheartj/ehu282.
146. Fleisher LA, Fleischmann KE, Auerbach AD, et al. 2014 ACC/AHA guideline on perioperative cardiovascular evaluation and management of patients undergoing noncardiac surgery: executive summary: a report of the American College of Cardiology/American Heart Association task force on practice Guidelines. Circulation. 2014;130(24):2215–45. https://doi.org/10.1161/CIR.0000000000000105.
147. De Giacomo T, Francioni F, Venuta F, et al. Complete mechanical cervical anastomosis using a narrow gastric tube after esophagectomy for cancer. Eur J Cardiothorac Surg. 2004;26:881–4.
148. Okushiba S, Kawarada Y, Shichinohe T, et al. Esophageal delta-shaped anastomosis: a new method of stapled anastomosis for the cervical esophagus and digestive tract. Surg Today. 2005;35:341–4.
149. Petrin G, Ruol A, Battaglia G, et al. Anastomotic stenoses occurring after circular stapling in esophageal cancer surgery. Surg Endosc. 2000;14:670–4.
150. Rice TW. Anastomotic stricture complicating esophagectomy. Thorac Surg Clin. 2006;16(1):63–73. https://doi.org/10.1016/j.thorsurg.2006.02.002.
151. Bayman EO, Brennan TJ. Incidence and severity of chronic pain at 3 and 6 months after thoracotomy: meta-analysis. J Pain. 2014;15(9):887–97. https://doi.org/10.1016/j.jpain.2014.06.005.
152. Ji RR, Nackley A, Huh Y, Terrando N, Maixner W. Neuroinflammation and central sensitization

in chronic and widespread pain. Anesthesiology. 2018;129(2):343–66. https://doi.org/10.1097/ALN.0000000000002130.
153. Mesbah A, Yeung J, Gao F. Pain after thoracotomy. BJA Education. 2016;16:1–7. https://doi.org/10.1093/bjaceaccp/mkv005.
154. Seesing MFJ, Borggreve AS, Ruurda JP, van Hillegersberg R. New-onset atrial fibrillation after esophagectomy for cancer. J Thorac Dis. 2019;11(Suppl 5):S831–4. https://doi.org/10.21037/jtd.2019.02.03.
155. Vaporciyan AA, Correa AM, Rice DC, et al. Risk factors associated with atrial fibrillation after noncardiac thoracic surgery: analysis of 2588 patients. J Thorac Cardiovasc Surg. 2004;127:779–86. https://doi.org/10.1016/j.jtcvs.2003.07.011.
156. POISE Study Group, Devereaux PJ, Yang H, Yusuf S, Guyatt G, Leslie K, Villar JC, Xavier D, Chrolavicius S, Greenspan L, Pogue J, Pais P, Liu L, Xu S, Málaga G, Avezum A, Chan M, Montori VM, Jacka M, Choi P. Effects of extended-release metoprolol succinate in patients undergoing non-cardiac surgery (POISE trial): a randomised controlled trial. Lancet. 2008;371:1839–47. https://doi.org/10.1016/S0140-6736(08)60601-7.
157. McCallum CJ, Raja DC, Pathak RK. Atrial fibrillation: an update on management. Aust Prescr. 2019;42(6):186–91. https://doi.org/10.18773/austprescr.2019.067.
158. Van Gelder IC, Groenveld HF, Crijns HJ, Tuininga YS, Tijssen JG, Alings AM, et al. RACE II investigators lenient versus strict rate control in patients with atrial fibrillation. N Engl J Med. 2010;362:1363–73. https://doi.org/10.1056/NEJMoa1001337.
159. Omae T, Kanmura Y. Management of postoperative atrial fibrillation. J Anesth. 2012;26(3):429–37. https://doi.org/10.1007/s00540-012-1330-9.

Chondrosarcoma Pelvis for Internal Hemipelvectomy

8

Rajiv Chawla and Shagun Bhatia Shah

8.1 Case Scenario

A 49-year-old male patient presented with a painful swelling over his left gluteal region which was expanding for the past 8 months. On physical examination, a lobular, firm, painful mass of dimensions 12 × 10cm^2 fixed to the underlying ilium was palpated. The neurovascular bundle in the left hip was preserved, with a good functional range of motion. A plain X-ray of the pelvis showed popcorn-shaped calcifications on the background of lysis over the left iliac bone, indicative of chondrosarcoma (Fig. 8.1) [1]. Routine blood investigations were done. MRI revealed an exophytic tumor with heterogeneous intensity arising from the gluteal surface of the left iliac bone, suggesting chondrosarcoma. Sacroiliac joint and neurovascular structures remain uninvolved. Wide-bore needle biopsy yielded a histopathology report confirming the diagnosis of chondrosarcoma of intermediate grade. Metastatic assessment did not reveal distant metastasis. The patient was scheduled for internal hemipelvectomy.

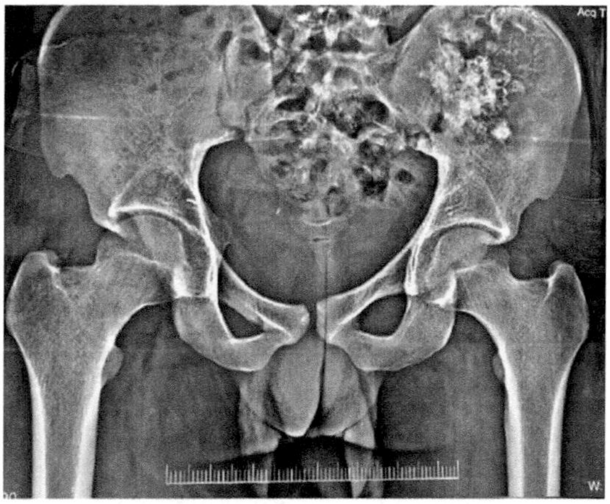

Fig. 8.1 Preoperative radiograph showing popcorn calcifications on the background of lysis over the left ilium. (Adapted from Kar B K, Kumar Yadav S, Venishetty N, et al. (July 10, 2021) Internal Hemipelvectomy and Pelvic Reconstruction With Non-Vascularized Fibular Graft for Chondrosarcoma Ilium. Cureus 13(7): e16292. DOI 10.7759/cureus.16292)

Q1

What is a chondrosarcoma? What are the common sites of occurrence?

Chondrosarcoma is one of the commonest solid bone malignancies [2]. It is frequently seen in the fifth to seventh decades [3, 4]. The commonest primary sites comprise the proximal humerus, proximal femur, and pelvis. Long-standing swelling and/or pain are the common presentations. Mostly chondrosarcomas (90%) are low/intermediate grade, but the 10% of high-grade tumors have a much higher metastatic potential [3].

R. Chawla · S. B. Shah (✉)
Department of Anesthesiology, Rajiv Gandhi Cancer Hospital, New Delhi, India

N. Gupta et al. (eds.), *Problem Based Learning Discussions in Onco-Anesthesia and Onco-Critical Care*, https://doi.org/10.1007/978-981-99-6339-3_8

Q2

What are the treatment options available for chondrosarcoma?

For over five decades surgical resection is considered the cornerstone of treatment [2]. The surgical options comprise internal and external hemipelvectomy. Internal hemipelvectomy constitutes a limb-sparing procedure entailing resection of the innominate bone with preservation of the ipsilateral limb. External hemipelvectomy comprises resection of the innominate bone accompanied by amputation of the ipsilateral limb.

Chondrosarcomas are not sensitive to the chemotherapy administered for dedifferentiated, mesenchymal, and metastatic forms. Radiotherapy comprises a substitute therapy to incomplete surgery.

Q3

What are the radiological imaging findings of chondrosarcoma?

Radiological imaging frequently displays a typical "ring-and-arc" mineralization of the chondroid matrix (denoting enchondral calcification). Deep endosteal scalloping and soft-tissue extension denote an aggressive nature which is mostly assessed with CT scan or MRI just like lesion staging [5, 6]. Subtle matrix mineralization and lesions situated in anatomically complex areas are optimally detected by CT. Both of these imaging (CT and MRI) reveal high water content of these lesions as low attenuation and very high signal intensity with T2-weighting, respectively.

Q4

What are the important anesthetic concerns for hemipelvectomy?

Surgery for hemipelvectomy is often complex and difficult. Generally, pelvic tumors are massive, distort the normal anatomy, and lie juxtaposed to major neurovascular bundles and pelvic viscera. An understanding of the type, location, and size of tumor helps the anesthesiologist assess the possible extent of surgery required [7].

The surgeon–anesthesiologist discussion prior to surgery allows the anesthesiologist to appreciate the details of proposed procedure and permits appropriate planning for monitoring and access [4].

The procedure often requires major neurovascular dissection, significant bone and muscle resection, replacement of large segments of bone and adjacent joints, significant bone-cement boluses for fixation, and rotational/free flaps. A thorough understanding of the surgical procedure allows for proper patient positioning, airway management, intraoperative monitoring, and postoperative arrangements. Detailed pre-anesthetic check and preparedness is essential for a favorable outcome.

Q5

How would you perform the pre-anesthetic evaluation of this patient?

Pre-anesthetic assessment starts 2–3 weeks before the scheduled surgery. Preoperative assessment includes determination of functional status of various organ systems prior to surgery. Additionally, of particular importance is knowledge of site and pathology and type and impact of preoperative adjuvant therapy. In patients who have received chemotherapy or radiotherapy, it is important to assess status of bone marrow functions (significant anemia and thrombocytopenia) [7]. Erythropoietin administration, packed red blood cell (PRBC), and platelet transfusions in preoperative period have proven beneficial [4].

In patients with co-morbidities like hypertension, coronary artery disease, or diabetes mellitus, a prehabilitation program is adopted to optimize the patient's condition in the preoperative period.

Q6

Which anesthetic technique would you prefer in this patient?

In view of prolonged duration and extensive surgery, combined general anesthesia with neuraxial block (epidural or combined spinal-epidural) after preoperative optimization is the preferred technique. The basic premise is that hemipelvectomy is a complex surgery with severe postoperative pain and high complication rate.

Q7

What is the role of prehabilitation and ERAS protocol in hemipelvectomy?

Prehabilitation plays a key role in optimization and improves outcome.

The operational, critical control, and interventional phases for an elective orthopedic surgery [8] are given by the blue, grey, and red boxes respectively, in Fig. 8.2.

Enhanced recovery after surgery (ERAS) refers to the rapid recovery of patient. It involves optimizing the key treatment elements in the preoperative, intraoperative, and postoperative periods as with multidisciplinary coordination. It intends to provide preoperative education, reduce the stress response (mental and physical), reduce the complications, reduce the length of hospital stay, reduce the risk of readmission, decrease costs, reduce morbidity, and mortality.

Malnutrition is a preoperative risk. It includes poor protein intake, iron deficiency anemia, hypovitaminosis D, and recent weight loss resulting in higher complications. Sarcopenia is another risk with manifestations like decreased muscle mass, diminished gait speed, and poor handgrip strength culminating in a delayed recovery.

In the absence of specific guidelines for hemipelvectomy, the current ERAS Society guidelines for total hip and knee replacement [9] may be extrapolated to hemipelvectomy patients. Table 8.1 depicts the ERAS template for hemipelvectomy.

The role of preoperative physiotherapy as an essential intervention is equivocal [10]. Similarly, gabapentinoids as an adjunct in a multimodal analgesia regime are not currently recommended although further studies are indicated [9, 11].

No conclusive evidence exists indicating that choice of surgical approach accelerates the achievement of discharge criteria. Usage of objective discharge criteria (ability to dress independently, move in and out of bed, sit and rise

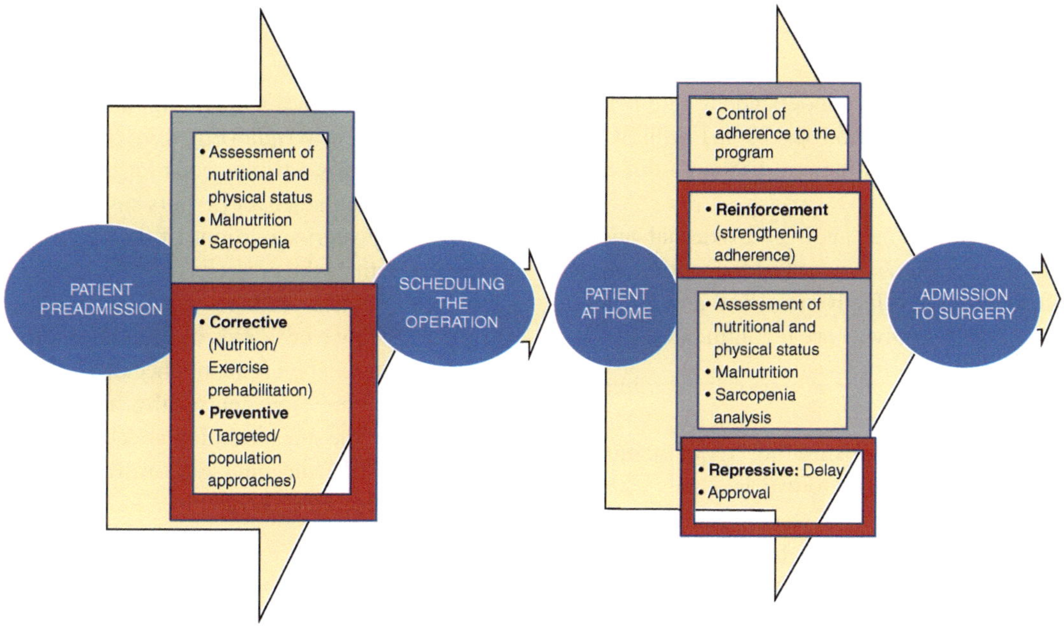

Fig. 8.2 Prehabilitation in a hemipelvectomy patient

Table 8.1 The ERAS template for hemipelvectomy

ERAS protocol template for hemipelvectomy
• Preoperative patient information, education, and counseling is recommended
• Four weeks or more smoking cessation is recommended before planned surgery
• Alcohol cessation programs are recommended before surgery
• Preoperative anemia should be identified, investigated, and corrected prior to surgery. Interventions such as preoperative iron or erythropoietin therapy
• Intake of clear fluids until 2 h before the induction of anesthesia, and a 6-h fast for solid food is recommended
• Carbohydrate loading may improve patient Well-being and metabolism, but it has not been shown to accelerate the achievement of discharge criteria or reduce complications, and so it is not currently recommended as an essential routine intervention
• The routine administration of sedatives to reduce anxiety preoperatively is not recommended
• General anesthesia and neuraxial techniques in combination are used as part of multimodal anesthetic regimes
• Epidural analgesia through indwelling epidural catheter is recommended for intraoperative and postoperative pain relief. Regional analgesia could be epidural or combined spinal epidural anesthesia technique
• Evidence supports the use of screening for and multimodal PONV prophylaxis and treatment for patients undergoing hip replacement
• Tranexamic acid is recommended to reduce perioperative blood loss and the requirement for postoperative allogenic blood transfusion
• The routine use of paracetamol is recommended
• The routine use of NSAIDS is recommended for patients without contraindications
• ERAS programs seek to minimize the use of opioids. However, opioids such as oxycodone may be used when required as part of a multimodal approach
• Normal body temperature should be maintained peri- and postoperatively through pre-warming and the active warming of patients intraoperatively. Measures include pre-warming and humidification of anesthetic gases, warming IV and irrigation fluids and forced air warming blankets and devices. In addition, the ambient temperature should be at least 21 °C while the patient is exposed prior to active warming starting
• Patients should receive systemic antimicrobial prophylaxis in accordance with local policy and availability. Antibiotic-loaded bone cement may reduce infection rates after joint replacement
• Patients should be mobilized as soon as possible post-surgery and receive antithrombotic prophylaxis treatment
• It is recommended that intravenous fluids should be used judiciously and postoperative intravenous fluids discouraged in favor of early oral intake
• An early return to normal diet is recommended and should be promoted
• Patients should be mobilized as early as they are able to in order to facilitate early achievement of discharge criteria

from a chair/toilet, be independent with personal care, and mobilization (> 70 m) with walker/crutches) facilitates patient discharge directly to their home.

Regular internal audit and external audit of process measures, patient satisfaction, clinical outcomes, cost-effectiveness, and any alterations to the ERAS pathway are recommended.

Q8

What are the positioning requirements for internal hemipelvectomy?

The patient's position for surgery is a loose lateral position, assisted by OT table side supports placed widely apart [7]. This allows the patient's body to move through an arc of 90° (−45° to 45°), when the operating table is rolled laterally from left to right (Fig. 8.3).

This position is advantageous for the surgeon since the rolling maneuver permits easy access to anterior and posterior portions of the pelvis. The patients benefit as the pressure points of potential nerve compression change with every rolling movement. However, a risk of breathing circuit disconnection exists. Frequent checking of areas at risk of compression neuropathy needs to be performed by the anesthesiologist each time the patient is rolled from one side to the other and appropriate precautions taken [4].

Q9

What monitoring techniques should be adopted?

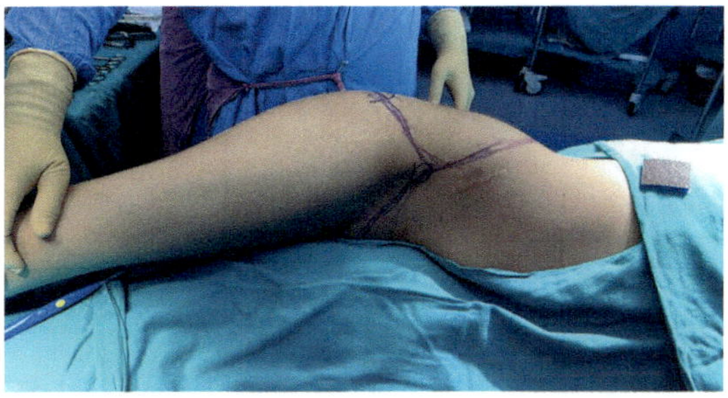

Fig. 8.3 Lateral positioning for hemipelvectomy

Standard monitoring: Pulse oximetery, capnography, electrocardiography, and blood pressure (BP).

Hemodynamic monitoring: Since the procedure requires extensive dissection, there is likelihood of severe blood loss. Invasive arterial BP monitoring and central venous monitoring are therefore essential. Urine output may be used as an indicator of perfusion. Serial arterial blood gas (ABG) analysis (including serum lactate levels) informs about the metabolic status. Advanced hemodynamic monitoring based on plethysmographic stroke volume variation (Vigileo; EV 1000; Capstesia; MostCareUP, etc.) is required for patients with low ejection fraction post-chemotherapy or with vascular tumors and anticipated massive blood loss.

Temperature: Every patient receiving anesthesia must have temperature monitoring when clinically significant changes in body temperature are intended, anticipated, or suspected. Hypothermia is conducive to arrhythmias, impairs clotting mechanisms, and increases blood loss. Hemipelvectomy patients often require massive blood transfusion which can cause hypothermia. All blood transfusions should employ an active warming device to minimize hypothermia. In accordance with the Outcomes Research Consortium guidelines, core temperature monitoring at 15 min intervals is required to maintain intraoperative core temperatures >36 °C.

Blood loss: Since less than half of the blood is collected in the surgical sucker container or contained within the surgical packs, monitoring intraoperative blood loss is difficult. The remainder of the blood is spilt onto the drapes and floor which is concealed by application of fresh drapes over the blood-soaked ones by the surgeon. Serial hematocrit assessment might be useful. The ABG reports inform hemoglobin which can be a good indicator of blood lost.

Coagulopathy: Massive blood transfusion-induced coagulopathy occurs frequently. Blood sampling for prothrombin time, activated partial thromboplastin time, platelets, and serum fibrinogen level each hour is, therefore, recommended. Point-of-care intraoperative viscoelastic hemostatic assays are useful in patients with major blood loss, commonest being thromboelastography (TEG) and rotational thromboelastometry (ROTEM). These assays have quick processing time, and evaluate all stages of clot formation as well as clot lysis. Coagulopathy is treated with platelet and fresh frozen plasma transfusion.

ABG analysis: Baseline ABG analysis is often done at the start of surgery once arterial cannula is placed in situ for IABP monitoring. It provides important information on ventilation, hemoglobin, and serum lactate which serves as a guide for further blood infusion, fluid therapy, and electrolyte correction.

Q10

What are the modalities to control pain?

Hemipelvectomy requires extensive tissue dissection and mobilization. Therefore, patients experience severe pain both in the intraoperative period and postoperative period. A multidisciplinary team approach is adopted. A team, comprising an anesthesiologist, surgeon, pain specialist, and physiotherapist, should develop a strategy to minimize the hemipelvectomy patient's postoperative discomfort.

8.2 Pain Relief: Intraoperative

The use of neuraxial anesthesia for intraoperative and postoperative analgesia may be considered for patients with pelvic tumor. [12–14] Administration of preservative-free morphine by epidural route is highly efficacious for postoperative pain relief [4]. Intraoperative single dose of dexamethasone provides excellent pain relief and reduces postoperative nausea and vomiting [15].

Conforming to the ERAS protocol, an opioid-sparing, multimodal analgesia (MMA) approach is becoming the benchmark standard for perioperative pain management. This includes a variety of systemic pharmacological agents as well as targeted analgesia techniques [12, 13]. Although opioids continue to be effective analgesics, they are accompanied with side effects like respiratory depression, pruritis, sedation, nausea, vomiting, constipation, ileus, and abuse potential.

Non-opioid medications for controlling postoperative pain include intravenous (IV) acetaminophen, non-steroidal anti-inflammatory drugs (NSAIDs), magnesium, ketamine, and dexmedetomidine. Liposomal bupivacaine, and newer neuraxial and peripheral regional techniques are also used for patient-controlled analgesia. Although gabapentinoids have gained popularity, recent meta-analyses have cast a shadow on their routine perioperative use. IV oxycodone, sublingual sufentanil, and iontophoretic transdermal fentanyl patches are some newer modalities. Acupuncture and transcutaneous electrical nerve stimulation (TENS) are other adjuncts in MMA bundles [14, 15]. IV patient-controlled analgesia is also an option when epidural analgesia is contra-indicated.

Q11

How would you manage massive intraoperative blood loss?

Unanticipated massive blood loss is a major concern in hemipelvectomy. Sites of intraoperative bleeding include the oozing from minor blood vessels, bone margins, besides major arteries and veins of the pelvis. In the postoperative period further bleeding often occurs. It may need transfusion which can be about a third of that given intraoperatively [7].

A targeted approach to transfusion is followed. It requires multidisciplinary approach requiring collaboration between laboratories and clinical departments enabling a timely component therapy. Specific major hemorrhage protocols can be adopted [16].

8.3 Component Therapy

8.3.1 Red Blood Cells

While RBC transfusion is potentially lifesaving, there are associated risks. One must, therefore, be cautious and avoid unwarranted excessive RBC transfusion.

RBC transfusion is indicated whenever 30–40% of blood volume is lost (1500 mL in 70 kg male). Blood loss greater than 40% volume (1500–2000 mL) is considered life threatening, and requires prompt blood transfusion. The rate of blood loss and the degree of hemodynamic compromise guide the rates of RBC/plasma transfusion. One aims at maintaining critical perfusion and tissue oxygenation. RBC transfusion serves to maintain hemoglobin at a level high enough to support tissue oxygen delivery (target range 60–100 g/L). When major bleeding is encountered, infusion devices designed for the purpose of rapid infusion over 5–10 min may be used [15].

8.3.2 Fresh Frozen Plasma (FFP)

Plasma not only serves as a reliable source of clotting factors, but also helps in volume expansion. The blood component of choice to manage the coagulopathy of bleeding has universally been FFP, although it does not constitute optimal therapy for hypofibrinogenemia correction. In the absence of any coagulation tests, low ratios of empirical RBC to FFP (>2:1), with a marked excess of RBC units, should be avoided in major bleeding. Ideally, transfusion should be guided by serial coagulation/point-of-care tests.

The hospital blood bank should be notified about anticipated major blood loss during surgery. An order for 40 units of packed RBCs, 20 units of FFP, and 20 units of platelets may be made.

8.4 Techniques to Reduce Blood Loss

Since major hemorrhage is anticipated, it is prudent to adopt various blood loss reduction strategies. Organizational (preoperative history, risk stratification, management of antiplatelet and anticoagulant therapies), surgical (using antifibrinolytics, cell salvage system, diathermy, topical agents), anesthetic (permissive hypotension, neuraxial anesthesia, patient positioning, normothermia, adequate ventilation), and hemostatic (desmopressin, procoagulant factors viscoelastic hemostatic assays) measures go a long way in reducing blood loss [15].

8.4.1 Anesthetic Strategies to Reduce Blood Loss

8.4.1.1 Permissive Hypotension Central Neuraxial Block

Central neuraxial techniques are safe. Subarachnoid/epidural anesthesia or combined spinal-epidural blocks that cause preganglionic sympathetic nerve fibers blockade result in arterial hypotension and reduced peripheral venous pressures ensuing less blood loss and fewer transfusions. [16]

8.4.1.2 Patient Positioning

Proper positioning of patient is a valuable intervention to decrease intraoperative blood loss. The surgical site should not be a dependent site.

8.4.1.3 Avoidance of Hypothermia

Intraoperative hypothermia (core body temperature < 36 °C) has multifactorial etiology. Low operating theatre temperature, evaporation from body cavities, cold intravenous fluids and anesthetic gases, reduced metabolic activity, and anesthesia-induced impairment of thermoregulation (such as shivering) are common factors causing hypothermia.

Temperature-dependent enzymatic reactions are reversibly hampered by hypothermia, adversely affecting the thrombocyte function and the coagulation cascade. In a study, 16% increase in blood loss and 22% increase in relative risk of red blood cell transfusion have been reported even after mild hypothermia [15].

8.4.1.4 Ventilation Strategies

Intermittent positive pressure ventilation using the least amount of positive end-expiratory pressure (PEEP) required, keeping tidal volumes low enhances venous return and serves to minimize blood loss.

8.4.2 Other Strategies to Reduce Blood Loss

8.4.2.1 Role of Antifibrinolytics

Antifibrinolytics like tranexamic acid and synthetic lysine analogs inhibit plasminogen activation and provide clot stabilization. Tranexamic acid has been shown to reduce the rate of allogeneic blood transfusion by up to 69% after hip and knee surgery, with no increase in risk of complications, including thromboembolic events. The same benefit has been observed by the authors in hemipelvectomy.

Tranexamic acid by intravenous, intra-articular, oral, or in combination can be administered. Weight-adjusted doses of 10–20 mg/kg, with top up during the intraoperative and postoperative phase may be required.

Topical delivery of tranexamic acid is seen to overcome its contraindications like renal disease owing to lower plasma levels. Repeat doses to maintain therapeutic levels may play a greater role in prolonged surgery or massive blood loss [15].

Preoperative tumor embolization is beneficial in highly vascular tumor where major blood loss is expected [3, 17].

Intra-aortic balloon occlusion: During resections of huge pelvic and sacral tumors, this technique is effective to control bleeding [18].

Autologous transfusion and normovolemic hemodilution may be useful [3].

8.4.2.2 Diathermy

Radiofrequency electrosurgery (both monopolar and bipolar) are key tools for achieving intraoperative hemostasis. Various new devices are available (bipolar sealing systems), suggesting to result in less damage to adjacent healthy tissue. There is limited evidence that they reduce blood loss and factors such as surgical technique are likely to be more important.

8.4.2.3 Topical Agents

Topical agents like fibrin sealants (fibrinogen and thrombin), gelatine–thrombin matrices, and oxidized cellulose are applied to bleeding areas to reduce bleeding. These agents are expensive and their role in reduction of blood loss is equivocal.

Q12

What is cell salvage technique? Can it be used in the present case?

Cell salvage is a technique in which blood is recovered from the surgical field during the intraoperative or immediate postoperative phase and then reinfused after anticoagulation and filtration. Blood collected intraoperatively (via a suction system) is normally washed followed by resuspension in normal saline and reinfusion. Blood collected postoperatively via surgical drains is typically unwashed. There is mounting evidence to support cell salvage use in infection and malignancy which was traditionally contraindicated. The use of a leucocyte depletion filter (40 μm) causes a 99% reduction in bacterial contamination in blood following resuspension in normal saline. The potentially augmented risks of bacterial contamination during cell salvage must be weighed against the raised risk of infection posed by allogeneic blood transfusion and secondary immunomodulation. Studies have not confirmed any association between the use of cell salvage and increased risk of cancer metastasis following surgery. The reinfused tumor cells do not have metastatic potential [19].

Q13

Describe the fluid management in this patient

Goal-directed fluid therapy keeping CVP > 10 cmH_2O or stroke volume variation (SVV) <10 or pleth variability index (PVI) <10 as a goal using crystalloids as a baseline infusion supplemented with colloid in aliquots of 100 mL whenever SVV/PVI exceeded 10 constitutes ideal fluid therapy in this patient. The type and amount of fluid administered can have a significant effect on outcomes. Couto et al. [20] studied 35 hemipelvectomy patients. Intraoperative requirement of colloids was 0.5 L in 12 patients, 1 L in 7 patients, and 1.5 L in 3 patients. Average intraoperative crystalloid requirement was 3500 mL (1000–8500 mL). Six patients received intraoperative albumin infusion. More than half of the patients required an intraoperative blood transfusion averaging 2 units and ranging from 1 to 6 units of packed red cells. Three patients received fresh frozen plasma and one received cryoprecipitate. In another study on 49 consecutive hemipelvectomy patients, the median crystalloid requirement was 8500 mL (range 1000–42,000 mL) and a median of 7 units of packed red blood cells were transfused (range 0–44 units) [7].

Owing to a much larger molecular size than that of crystalloids, colloids remain in the vasculature, producing more effective expansion of the circulatory volume. Peripheral and pulmonary edema, cardiac failure, and renal damage are reported following excessive use of colloids. Crystalloids produce more nausea and vomiting, but score higher on cost-effectiveness [21].

Q14

What VTE prophylaxis measures would you employ in this patient?

ASCO clinical practice guidelines are followed for venous thromboembolism prophylaxis and treatment in patients with cancer [22]. The salient features are

- All cancer patients undergoing major surgical intervention should be offered pharmacologic thromboprophylaxis with either unfractionated heparin (UFH) or LMWH unless contraindicated.

- Prophylaxis should be commenced preoperatively.
- Mechanical thromboprophylaxis may be added to pharmacothromboprophylaxis but not used as monotherapy for VTE prevention unless pharmacologic methods are contraindicated (active bleeding/high bleeding risk).
- A combination regimen of pharmacologic and mechanical prophylaxis may improve efficacy.
- Pharmacologic thromboprophylaxis should be continued for at least 7–10 days. Extended prophylaxis with LMWH for up to 4 weeks postoperatively is recommended for patients undergoing major pelvis surgery.
- Initial anticoagulation may involve LMWH, UFH, fondaparinux, or rivaroxaban. For patients initiating treatment with parenteral anticoagulation, LMWH is preferred over UFH for the initial 5–10 days of anticoagulation for the patient with cancer with newly diagnosed VTE who does not have severe renal impairment (creatinine clearance <30 mL/min).
- For long-term anticoagulation, LMWH, edoxaban, or rivaroxaban for at least 6 months are preferred because of improved efficacy over vitamin-K antagonists.
- The insertion of a venacaval filter may be offered as an adjunct to anticoagulation in patients with progression of thrombosis (recurrent VTE or extension of existing thrombus) despite optimal anticoagulant therapy.

Q15

Are there any contraindications for pharmacological DVT prophylaxis?

Patients with active bleeding, high risk for bleeding, or recent bleeding.

Thrombocytopenia (less than 50,000).

Patients with altered coagulation profile (INR > 1.5).

Bleeding disorders.

Q16

How would you manage postoperative nausea and vomiting?

Postoperative nausea and vomiting (PONV) is multifactorial in etiology. The type of surgery, duration of exposure to inhalational anesthetics, use of nitrous oxide, opioids, and specific patient factors may affect the incidence of PONV. Preoperatively, cancer patients frequently become opioid-dependent/tolerant. Escalated intraoperative opioid doses for adequate analgesia or the presence of pain could lead to PONV.

Large variety of medications have been used for PONV, the most commonly used being serotonin (5HT3) inhibitors (ondansetron, granisetron, dolasetron, palonosetron). Dopamine-antagonists like metoclopramide, droperidol, promethazine, and prochlorperazine are effective adjuvants and antiemetics. Dexamethasone which acts by decreasing prostaglandin synthesis is also effective for PONV prophylaxis.

Q17

What is bone cement implantation syndrome? How will you manage it?

Bone cement is polymethyl methacrylate (90%) and minute quantities of radio-opaque crystals (Barium sulfate/Zirconia), initiator (Benzoyl peroxide), and accelerator (N, N-Dimethyl para-toluidine). Various antibiotic-loaded bone cements (containing Gentamycin, Tobramycin, Erythromycin, Cefuroxime, Vancomycin, or Colistin) when combined with systemic antibiotics provide good prophylaxis against postoperative infection.

The exothermic free-radical polymerization process heats up the cement reaching temperatures of up to 86 °C. The cause of the low polymerization temperature in the body is the relatively thin cement coating (≤5 mm), and the temperature dissipation via the large prosthesis surface and the flow of blood.

Clinical features of bone implantation syndrome include hypoxia, hypotension, cardiac arrhythmias, and cardiac arrest. These cardiopulmonary effects can be reduced by the recognition of high-risk patients and modifications of surgical technique. Management is mainly focused toward treating pulmonary arterial hypertension and right ventricular failure [23].

Q18

What are the expected postoperative complications after hemipelvectomy?

While there is a considerable decrease in the mortality rate (currently 0–10%), the complications remain very high (30–80%). Postoperative blood transfusion, acute postoperative pain (VAS > 7), acute renal failure, neurological disorders, arrhythmias, chronic pain 3 months after surgery, and surgical wound complications (infection, flap necrosis, urethrocutaneous fistula) are the reported post-operative complications. Aseptic loosening, fractures, and pseudarthrosis often cause reconstruction failures. Nerve lesions, thrombosis, visceral injuries, and functional disability have also been frequently reported [24, 25]. The leading causes of death are blood loss, infections, and multiple organ failure.

References

1. Kar BK, Yadav SK, Venishetty N, Kowshik S. Internal Hemipelvectomy and pelvic reconstruction with non-vascularized fibular graft for chondrosarcoma ilium. Cureus. 2021;13(7):e16292.
2. Sinardja CD, Senapathi TG, Suarjaya IP, Suranadi IW, Kusuma OI, Asterina DH. Anaesthesia management of patient at 16 weeks pregnancy with primary malignant bone tumour underwent hemipelvectomy surgery. Bali J Anesthesiol. 2018;2:41.
3. Doroshow JH. Malignant tumors of bone, sarcomas, and other soft tissue neoplasms. In: Goldman-Cecil medicine. 25th ed. Philadelphia, PA: Elsevier; 2016. p. 1370–3.
4. Anderson MR, Jeng CL, Wittig JC, Rosenblatt MA. Anesthesia for patients undergoing orthopedic oncologic surgeries. J Clin Anesth. 2010;22:565–72.
5. Murphey MD, Walker EA, Wilson AJ, Kransdorf MJ, Temple HT, Gannon FH. From the archives of the AFIP: imaging of primary chondrosarcoma: radiologic-pathologic correlation. Radiographics. 2003;23:1245–78.
6. Ollivier L, Vanel D, Leclère J. Imaging of chondrosarcomas. Cancer Imag. 2003;4:36–8.
7. Molnar R, Emery G, Choong PF. Anaesthesia for hemipelvectomy—a series of 49 cases. Anaesth Intensive Care. 2007;35:536–43.
8. Briguglio M, Wainwright TW. Nutritional and physical Prehabilitation in elective orthopedic surgery: rationale and proposal for implementation. Ther Clin Risk Manag. 2022;18:21–30.
9. Wainwright TW, Gill M, McDonald DA, Middleton RG, Reed M, Sahota O, et al. Consensus statement for perioperative care in total hip replacement and total knee replacement surgery: enhanced recovery after surgery (ERAS®) society recommendations. Acta Orthop. 2020;91:3–19.
10. Ghimire N, Yan ZK, Fang Y, Chirume WM, Yang Y. Management of traumatic hemipelvectomy through ERAS pathway: a case report. Medicine. 2018;97:1–5.
11. Mao Y, Wu L, Ding W. The efficacy of preoperative administration of gabapentin/pregabalin in improving pain after total hip arthroplasty: a meta-analysis. BMC Musculoskelet Disord. 2016;17:1–11.
12. Chen Q, Chen E, Qian X. A narrative review on perioperative pain management strategies in enhanced recovery pathways—the past, present and future. J Clin Med. 2021;10:2568.
13. Wick EC, Grant MC, Wu CL. Postoperative multimodal analgesia pain management with nonopioid analgesics and techniques: a review. JAMA Surg. 2017;152:691–7.
14. Mitra S, Carlyle D, Kodumudi G, Kodumudi V, Vadivelu N. New advances in acute postoperative pain management. Cur Pain Headache Rep. 2018;22:1–11.
15. Joshi GP, Kehlet H. Postoperative pain management in the era of ERAS: an overview. Best Pract Res Clin Anaesthesiol. 2019;33:259–67.
16. Shah A, Palmer AJR, Klein AA. Strategies to minimize intraoperative blood loss during major surgery. Br J Surg. 2020;107:26–38.
17. Jha R, Sharma R, Rastogi S, Khan SA, Jayaswal A, Gamanagatti S. Preoperative embolization of primary bone tumors: a case control study. World J Radiol. 2016;8:378–89.
18. Ratto N, Boffano M, Pellegrino P, Conti A, Rossi L, Verna V. The intraoperative use of aortic balloon occlusion technique for sacral and pelvic tumor resections: a case-control study. Surg Oncol. 2020;32:69–74.
19. Rajasekaran RB, Palmer AJ, Whitwell D, Cosker TD, Pigott D, Zsolt O. The role of intraoperative cell salvage for musculoskeletal sarcoma surgery. J Bone Oncol. 2021;30:100390.
20. Couto AG, Araújo B, Torres de Vasconcelos RA, Renni MJ, Da Fonseca CO, Cavalcanti IL. Survival rate and perioperative data of patients who have undergone hemipelvectomy: a retrospective case series. World J Surg Oncol. 2016;14:1–7.
21. Key NS, Khorana AA, Kuderer NM, Bohlke K, Lee AY, Arcelus JI. Venous thromboembolism prophylaxis and treatment in patients with cancer: ASCO clinical practice guideline update. J Clin Oncol. 2020;38:496–520.
22. National Guideline Centre (UK). Evidence review for intravenous fluid management strategy: perioperative care in adults: evidence review I. London: National Institute for Health and Care Excellence (NICE);

2020. (NICE Guideline, No. 180). https://www.ncbi.nlm.nih.gov/books/NBK561981/.
23. Vaishya R, Chauhan M, Vaish A. Bone cement. J Clin Orthop. Trauma. 2013;4:157–63.
24. Umer M, Ali M, Rashid RH, Mohib Y, Rashid HU. Outcomes of internal hemipelvectomy for pelvic tumors: a developing country's prospective. Int J Surg Oncol. 2017;2:1–5.
25. Benatto MT, Hussein AM, Gava NF, Maranho DA, Engel EE. Complications and cost analysis of hemipelvectomy for the treatment of pelvic tumors. Acta Ortop Bras. 2019;27:104–7.

Periampullary Carcinoma for Whipple's Procedure

9

Tanveer Singh

9.1 Case

A 70-year-old male chronic alcoholic and smoker presents with gradual onset, painless jaundice. On investigations, his bilirubin is 8.2 mg% with direct bilirubin of 7.8 mg%. Contrast-enhanced CT scan of abdomen reveals growth in the periampullary area.

Q1

What is the most likely diagnosis and what is the best treatment modality for these patients?

Ans: The most likely diagnosis in this case would be periampullary carcinoma. Periampullary area has a complex anatomy with various important structures in close vicinity (Fig. 9.1). Either the pancreas, duodenum, distal common bile duct (CBD) or the structures of the ampullary complex may be afflicted by the neoplastic growth. These tumours are quite aggressive and carry a dismal prognosis; hence radical surgical excision via pancreaticoduodenectomy (Whipple's procedure) is preferred when feasible. In this procedure, resection of the proximal pancreas, the distal stomach, duodenum, distal bile duct and gall bladder is performed and this is followed by multiple anastomoses to maintain intestinal continuity.

T. Singh (✉)
DMC Ludhiana, Ludhiana, Punjab, India

Q2

Describe the functional anatomy of pancreas in brief.

Pancreas is a solid organ serving both endocrine as well as exocrine functions. Anatomically, it has been divided into four parts: head, neck, body and tail. 99% of the pancreas is an exocrine gland having secretory functions and 1% is endocrine. The pancreatic parenchyma is made up of Acinar cells secreting digestive proteolytic enzymes (exocrine product) which aid in digestion of proteins, carbohydrates and lipids. The pancreatic duct carries the exocrine secretions. It runs through the body of pancreas and is joined by the CBD and both open together into duodenum forming 'Ampulla of Water'. The endocrine cells form the Islets of Langerhans, in which beta cells secrete insulin while the Alpha cells secrete glucagon. It is important to note that the beta cells are located throughout the islet of Langerhans while the alpha cells are around the periphery of the islet. The primary function of the pancreas is to aid in digestion of food and control of blood glucose.

Both the coeliac artery and superior mesenteric artery supply blood to the pancreas through their branches. The head of pancreas receives its blood supply from superior and inferior pancreaticoduodenal arteries which run along the anterior and posterior surfaces of the head of the pancreas. The pancreatic branches of splenic

N. Gupta et al. (eds.), *Problem Based Learning Discussions in Onco-Anesthesia and Onco-Critical Care*, https://doi.org/10.1007/978-981-99-6339-3_9

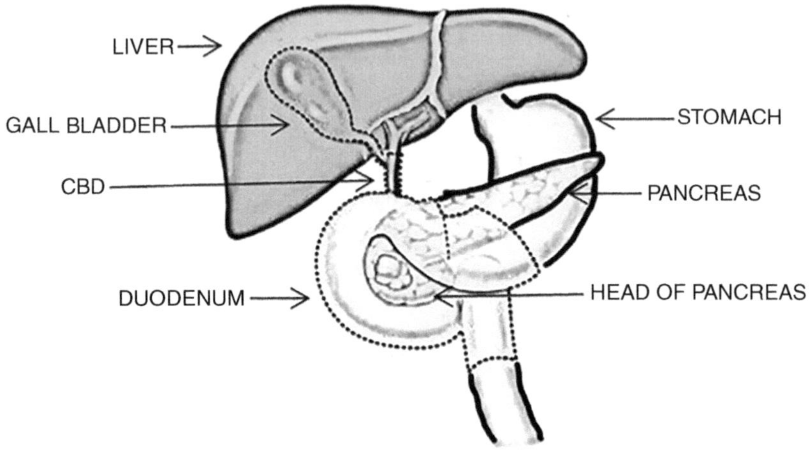

Fig. 9.1 The area marked as dotted line is resected during Whipple's procedure

artery supply the left part of the body and the tail of the pancreas. The head of pancreas drains into the superior mesenteric and portal veins, via the pancreaticoduodenal veins while splenic vein drains body and neck of the pancreas [1].

Q3

What is the likely prognosis for such patients?

Pancreatic malignancies have a relatively poor prognosis with survival rate lowest among all the solid cancers. In fact, it is the fourth leading cause of deaths due to cancer in the USA and the sixth in Europe despite being the 11th most common cancer overall. The poor prognosis is due to the fact that these tumours are often detected late and have often spread by the time symptomatology appears. In less than 15% of the patients are the tumours potentially resectable. The only potentially curative treatment for pancreatic cancer is surgical resection, but the postoperative 5-year survival is also only 15-25%. It is often difficult to distinguish between primary ampullary carcinoma and other periampullary tumours preoperatively. The prognosis of true ampullary malignancy, however, is better than periampullary cancers of pancreatic or bile duct origin. In patients with limited lymph node involvement, resectability rates are higher and 5-year survival rates are approximately 30-50%. Therefore, in such patients, an aggressive approach involving early diagnosis and optimal management is the key to ensure a favourable prognosis [2, 3].

Q4

What are the presenting symptoms?

Initially, the tumours grow without causing any symptoms. Later on, patients may report non-specific abdominal pain and jaundice or both. Jaundice occurs due to obstruction of outflow of bile by the cancer. Palpable gallbladder in the presence of painless jaundice (Courvoisier sign) is seen in less than 25% of patients. Other less common symptoms include unexplained weight loss, steatorrhea, pancreatitis, diabetes or recurrent venous thrombosis. The tumour may compress upon the duodenum or stomach resulting in symptoms of gastric outlet obstruction such as nausea, vomiting and early satiety [4].

Q5

What are the pathophysiological changes due to jaundice on various body systems?

Increased bilirubin in obstructive jaundice affects almost all body systems. There are pathophysiological changes in cardiovascular system, gastrointestinal system, renal system, changes in blood biochemistry and coagulation, predisposition to infection, and immunosuppression.

9.2 Pathophysiological Changes in the Gastrointestinal Tract

1. Malnutrition: Malnutrition occurs as obstructive jaundice leads to malabsorption of proteins and fats. Steatorrhea leads to deficiency of fat-soluble vitamins, i.e. Vit A, D, E and K. Vit K deficiency often results in prolonged prothrombin time.
2. Stress ulcer: Hyperbilirubinemia led decrease in appetite and poor intestinal absorption due to bile salt deficiency causes an increase in incidence of peptic ulcer in obstructive jaundice.
3. Intestinal barrier dysfunction leading to bacterial translocation: The normal intestinal mucosal barrier is damaged in obstructive jaundice, which enables bacterial translocation. In addition, there is inhibition of cell-mediated immunity. Both these factors predispose patients to bacterial endotoxemia and bacterial sepsis [5, 6].

9.3 Renal System

Obstructive jaundice may result in renal dysfunction without any pathological disease of the kidney itself. The incidence and severity of acute renal failure in such cases seems to be directly related to the severity of jaundice. Though the exact aetiology is poorly understood but gram-negative sepsis, decreased extracellular fluid volume, hypotension, myocardial dysfunction, hypoproteinaemia and dyselectrolytaemia (hyponatremia and hypokalaemia) are some of the contributing factors towards the development of renal failure in these patients [7].

9.4 Hepatic System

Obstructive jaundice may lead to hepatic injury which is seen microscopically as hepatocellular necrosis, apoptosis and liver fibrosis. Though the exact pathogenesis of obstructive jaundice-related hepatic injury is unknown but endotoxemia, microvascular perfusion failure, Toll-like receptor (TLR) activation and inflammatory factors, such as tumour necrosis factor-α, interleukin-1β and interleukin-6, are believed to be causative factors [8].

9.5 Cardiovascular Effects

1. Cardiac depression (jaundiced heart).

   Jaundice often leads to suppression of cardiac function, a condition described as 'jaundiced heart'. Bile acids have direct inhibitory effect on myocytes inhibiting both myocardial conduction as well as contraction. At cellular level, negative inotropic and chronotropic effect is caused by the alteration of membrane currents, down-regulation of cardiac β- adrenoceptor affinity and density, vagal stimulation and membrane fluidity.
2. Vascular hypo-reactivity.

   Impaired responsiveness of blood vessels to vasoactive substances is seen in obstructive jaundice. Bile salts, endotoxin release, endogenous opioid peptides and prostaglandin all contribute to reduced vascular reactivity. These result in increased synthesis of nitric oxide contributing to peripheral vasodilation. In addition, accumulation of bradykinin, substance P, vasoactive intestinal peptide (VIP), glucagon and prostacyclin cause vasodilatation predisposing to hypotension.
3. Volume depletion.

   Obstructive jaundice is associated with decreased extracellular fluid volume (ECF). This ECF depletion may be related to the following factors:
   (a) Increased atrial natriuretic peptide (ANP) and brain natriuretic peptide (BNP).
   (b) The diuretic and natriuretic effects of bile salts [9–11].

Q6

How will you evaluate this patient in the pre-anaesthetic clinic?

Preoperative evaluation includes detailed history, thorough clinical examination and laboratory investigations. Usual investigations include complete blood count, serum electrolytes, blood urea, serum creatinine, coagulation profile, liver function test and electrocardiogram. The etiological factors of pancreatic cancers and lung cancer are common so it is essential to get a chest X-ray and evaluate these patients for pulmonary functions. In addition, a detailed cardiovascular evaluation is also warranted especially in elderly patients.

Q7

Discuss preoperative preparation and optimization before surgery.

This surgery for obstructive jaundiced patient is an urgent one so usually there is paucity of time for a thorough optimization. Nevertheless, optimization should be attempted in whatever time is available before taking up these patients for surgery. Preoperative optimization even for few days prior to surgery has been shown to favourably affect the postoperative outcome. Smokers should quit smoking and alcohol consumption should be stopped. For best results, the abstinence should be exercised for 4-6 weeks.

9.6 Optimization of Pulmonary Function

In patients with reversible airflow obstruction, antibiotic and bronchodilator therapy should be instituted. Patients should be educated regarding deep breathing exercises and lung-expansion manoeuvres like incentive spirometry. All these measures have been found to be helpful in preventing pulmonary complications in postoperative period.

9.7 Correction of Dehydration and Malnutrition

Jaundiced patients are often dehydrated so adequate hydration should be ensured, often necessitating use of IV fluids. Another important problem that needs to be addressed in these patients is malnutrition. These patients often suffer from protein and fat malabsorption due to the obstruction of CBD. Therefore, preoperative supplementation with diet rich in proteins and carbohydrates but low in fats should be started through the enteral route to improve the poor nutritional status of patients. If feeding via enteral route is not possible due to gastric dilatation, one can consider nasojejunal tube feeding. Parenteral nutrition should be started only if enteral is not possible and only in patients with severe malnutrition. The malnutrition universal screening tool (MUST) can be used to identify patients at high risk for major complications due to malnutrition. Serum total protein ≥60 g/L, and albumin ≥30 g/L is desirable prior to surgery. Low albumin level is an independent risk factor for perioperative morbidity and mortality. More recently, enteral formulas supplemented with arginine and glutamine, nucleotides or omega-3 fatty acids are being used to modulate the immune system. The benefits of this concept of immunonutrition are, however, debatable [12–13].

9.8 Correcting Coagulation Profile

Deranged coagulation can be treated with intramuscular vitamin K (started 3 days before surgery) or fresh frozen plasma.

9.9 Anti-Thrombotic Prophylaxis

The risk of venous thromboembolism (VTE) is increased due to malignancy and nature of surgery. So use of low molecular weight heparin (LMWH) 12 hr. prior to surgery till the patient becomes mobile after surgery is recommended for prevention of VTE. In addition to pharmacological measures, use of mechanical prophylaxis using compression stockings and intermittent pneumatic leg compression reduces the risk of VTE [14].

Q8

Is there a role of preoperative biliary drainage in the preoperative preparation of patients?

Preoperative biliary drainage (PBD) was introduced to improve the postoperative outcomes by alleviating the negative effects of jaundice. However, several studies concluded that PBD had no beneficial effect on the outcome after surgery rather it being an invasive procedure carries a risk of procedure-related complications. PBD was associated with increased incidence of drainage-induced complications, surgical site infections and delayed gastric emptying thus worsening postoperative outcomes. Recent studies have suggested that PBD should not be a routine prior to surgery and should be limited to cases with profound jaundice, pruritus, cholangitis or delayed surgery due to neoadjuvant treatment or rarely while awaiting surgery at a busy tertiary care hospital [15, 16].

Q9

How will you plan anaesthesia for this patient?

General anaesthesia with endotracheal intubation is the technique of choice. Regional analgesic technique like epidural analgesia can be planned for intraoperative analgesia supplementation and postoperative pain relief. However, regional anaesthesia as a sole anaesthetic technique is not advisable due to long duration of surgery, high level of sensory blockade required and the massive fluid shifts associated with this major surgery. At least two units of typed and cross-matched blood should be kept preoperatively.

Antibiotic prophylaxis should be given within 30-60 min of incision. Intraoperative repeat dose is recommended when surgery is prolonged more than the half-life of the antibiotic used or in case of major blood loss. Attempt should be made to maintain normothermia as these patients are prone to hypothermia due to long duration of surgery and exposure of peritoneal cavity. This can be accomplished by pre-warming, use of forced hot air devices, warm IV fluids and warm irrigation fluids.

Inside the operating room, standard monitoring in the form of pulse oximetry, electrocardiogram, non-invasive blood pressure, temperature, urine output monitoring and capnography should be followed. Additionally, invasive arterial pressure monitoring is helpful in these patients who might present with wide fluctuations in the pressures and also require repeated ABG analysis for acid-base balance. Also, central venous pressure monitoring, trans-oesophageal echocardiography and neuromuscular blockade monitoring can be used when deemed necessary. At least two large-bore peripheral intravenous lines are required for resuscitation in case of sudden massive blood loss which can occur in these cases. Though central line is not indicated routinely, but can be inserted in case of complicated resections.

One has to be extremely careful about the choice of anaesthetic agents in these patients because the pharmacological effects of many drugs which are dependent on hepatic metabolism may get prolonged. In general, phase I drug reactions like oxidation, reduction, and hydrolysis are less affected as compared to phase II reactions like conjugation. Keeping this in view, the drugs which are eliminated by redistribution or undergo renal clearance (e.g. propofol, etomidate, fentanyl) are preferred over those undergoing hepatic metabolism (e.g. thiopental, alfentanil).

9.10 Premedication

Benzodiazepines like midazolam and diazepam are metabolized in liver so in patients with hepatic compromise, duration of action is increased which leads to delayed recovery. But drugs like oxazepam and temazepam which undergo conjugation without hepatic metabolism may be considered [17].

9.11 Induction Agents/ Intravenous Anaesthetics

Thiopental is metabolized in liver via cytochrome P450 to active metabolite pentobarbital which has longer half-life. Therefore, it is not a preferred agent in these patients. The clearance of a single dose of propofol is not affected by moderate degree of liver dysfunction; therefore, it can be used as an induction agent. However, one must be cautious because there are increased chances of hypotension in these patients with the use of propofol. Therefore, small aliquots of propofol, titrated to effect may be used for induction. Etomidate can also be chosen as an alternative induction agent with the advantage of having stable cardiovascular profile [13, 18].

9.12 Inhalation Anaesthetics

Halothane use is associated with production of hepatotoxic metabolite trifluoroacetic acid, so should be avoided in obstructive jaundice. Enflurane does not have any significant adverse effect on liver function and can be used. Volatile anaesthetic agents such as isoflurane or desflurane which are poorly metabolized can be safely used for maintenance of anaesthesia. MACawake of desflurane is reduced in patients with obstructive jaundice and is probably due to hyperbilirubinemia. Use of isoflurane might improve hepatic blood flow and hepatic oxygen supply. However, it has been observed that sensitivity to isoflurane is increased in jaundiced patients making them susceptible to hypotension and bradycardia. There is prolongation of recovery time with sevoflurane in patients with obstructive jaundice. Therefore, the dosage of inhalation anaesthetics needs to be reduced with careful titration in these patients and vigilant intraoperative monitoring is required. Some studies have suggested beneficial effect of volatile agents over intravenous anaesthetic agents in terms of postoperative inflammatory response and hepatocellular injury but it remains debatable [19, 20].

9.13 Neuromuscular Blocking Drugs

The neuromuscular blocking agents which undergo hepatic metabolism or are excreted via the biliary tract or can decrease the heart rate should be avoided in jaundiced patients. Succinylcholine can cause bradycardia or ventricular arrhythmia by exciting the vagus nerve. Atracurium and cisatracurium which undergo Hoffman elimination (non-hepatic metabolism) are muscle relaxants of choice for jaundiced patients. They are preferred over vecuronium and rocuronium which are dependent on liver and kidney for their elimination. Atracurium or cisatracurium does not accumulate in the body even when administered by continuous infusion. Prolonged duration of neuromuscular blockade is seen with the use of rocuronium in patients with obstructive jaundice. The use of neuromuscular monitoring is desirable as it helps in reducing postoperative residual neuromuscular blockade and consequent complications. Neostigmine being a cholinergic drug may cause serious arrhythmia or even cardiac arrest and hence should be used cautiously [21, 22].

9.14 Analgesics

The requirements of analgesics are reduced in patients with obstructive jaundice, probably due to cholestasis-induced increased release of endogenous encephalin. Studies have also found that the pain threshold is increased in jaundiced patients as compared with normal patients.

9.14.1 Opioids

Morphine is metabolized to active metabolite morphine-6-glucuronide and inactive metabolite morphine-3-glucuronide in the liver. Therefore, it will have prolonged duration of action and thus should be avoided. Shorter acting opioids are preferred over morphine for this reason. Fentanyl, alfentanil and sufentanil are primarily metabolized in the liver and clearance of all these drugs is decreased in presence of hepatic dysfunction. This reduced elimination prolongs the effect of the drug after administration of either a single or repeated dose. Thus, the initial dose of all these opioids needs to be decreased and the dosing interval increased in patients with liver dysfunction. Remifentanil is a synthetic μ opioid agonist which undergoes extrahepatic metabolism by the blood and tissue-nonspecific esterases to inactive metabolites which are excreted via kidneys. Metabolism or excretion of remifentanil is not affected in patients with hepatic disease of any severity. No dose modification of remifentanil is required in these patients as it does not accumulate even when administered by continuous infusion. All opioid analgesics can cause spasm of Oddi's sphincter and an increase in bile duct pressure; however, studies have shown that it is of not much clinical significance [18, 23, 24].

In liver dysfunction, metabolism of hydromorphone is decreased which prolongs its duration of action. Therefore, in patients with moderate to severe liver dysfunction, the initial dose of hydromorphone should be reduced by 25–50%. Meperidine undergoes metabolism in the liver to normeperidine which is further hydrolysed to meperidinic acid. Normeperidine is neurotoxic and it can lead to neuromuscular irritability and seizures when accumulated. So, dose needs to be reduced and dosing intervals increased while using meperidine in patients with liver disease [25].

9.14.2 Acetaminophen

N-acetyl-p-benzoquinone imine (NAPQI) is a hepatotoxic metabolite of acetaminophen and conjugation with glutathione makes it non-hepatotoxic. But in patients with liver disease, levels of glutathione are decreased which leads to increased levels of NAPQI in these patients. Literature about the perioperative use of acetaminophen in patients with liver disease is conflicting. Short-term use seems to be safe, however dose reduction as per severity of hepatic impairment is advised [24].

9.14.3 Nonsteroidal Anti-Inflammatory Drugs (NSAIDs)

In patients with mild to moderate liver dysfunction, NSAIDs like ibuprofen, etodolac and diclofenac can be administered in the usual doses as their pharmacokinetics is not altered. However, others like naproxen, sulindac and celecoxib need to be prescribed in reduced doses. In patients with severe liver dysfunction use of NSAIDS can have serious adverse effects and should be avoided [24, 25].

9.15 Intraoperative Fluid Management

Optimal fluid management is very important because both inadequate and over-zealous fluid administration can lead to complications. The problem of excessive fluid administration is that it can predispose to tissue oedema and anastomotic breakdown while excessive fluid restriction can lead to renal hypoperfusion. Goal-directed fluid management ensures appropriate use of fluids, better tissue oxygen tension and perfusion and hence, improved outcomes. Stroke volume variation or pulse pressure variation are the two dynamic parameters which provide good prediction of fluid responsiveness and are recommended for fluid management in the perioperative period [7, 26–28].

Q10

How will you plan for management of post-operative pain of these patients?

Ans: Postoperative pain management in these patients is challenging due to a large abdominal incision and altered metabolism of analgesic agents due to derangements of hepatic function.

On the other hand, untreated pain can interfere with respiratory function predisposing to basal atelectasis and pulmonary complications. Therefore, a multimodal approach is often adopted as this technique provides analgesia while minimizing adverse effects that may result due to excess dose of any single agent.

Continuous thoracic epidural analgesia with local anaesthetics provides good analgesia with an opioid-sparing effect and aids in early mobilisation, reducing postoperative ileus and pulmonary complications. Addition of small dose of an opioid in the epidural infusion has a synergistic analgesic effect, thereby reducing the dose of both the agents. In case of breakthrough pain, NSAIDS and a bolus of epidural are helpful.

Other alternatives include abdominal wound catheters, patient-controlled analgesia with intravenous opioids and fascial plane blocks. In cases of coagulation abnormality, both wound catheters and fascial plane blocks are much safer than epidural [29, 30].

Q11

What are the complications that one can anticipate in these patients?

Ans: The patients are exposed to a variety of postoperative complications which lead to increased morbidity, mortality, duration of hospital stay and hospital costs. Leakage from pancreatic anastomosis can lead to life-threatening sepsis. Delayed gastric emptying is commonly seen to cause discomfort in the postoperative period and prolong duration of hospital stay. Post pancreatic resection there may occur insufficiency of exocrine function leading to fat malabsorption. Other complications like bleeding, pulmonary complications, wound infection and thromboembolic events are also seen like in any other abdominal surgery [31, 32].

References

1. Moore KL, Dalley AF, Agur AMR. Clinically oriented anatomy. 7th ed. Philadelphia, PA: Lippincott Williams & Wilkins; 2014.
2. Michaud DS. Epidemiology of pancreatic cancer. Minerva Chir. 2004;59:99–111.
3. Kedra B, Popiela T, Sierzega M, Precht A. Prognostic factors of long-term survival after resective procedures for pancreatic cancer. Hepato-Gastroenterology. 2001;48:1762–6.
4. Bond-Smith G, Banga N, Hammond TM, Imber CJ. Pancreatic adenocarcinoma. BMJ. 2012;344:e2476.
5. Abbas Z, Khan AH, Jafri SM, Hamid SS, Shah SH, Abid S, et al. Duodenal erosions and ulcers in patients with pancreatobiliary obstruction. J Gastroenterol Hepatol. 1997;12(11):70.
6. Assimakopoulos SF, Scopa CD, Vagianos CE. Pathophysiology of increased intestinal permeability in obstructive jaundice. World J Gastroenterol. 2007;13(48):6458–64.
7. Sitges-Serra A, Carulla X, Piera C, Martinez-Rodenas F, Franch G, Pereira J, et al. Body water compartments in patients with obstructive jaundice. Br J Surg. 1992;79(6):553–6.
8. Gujral JS, Farhood A, Bajt ML, Jaeschke H. Neutrophils aggravate acute liver injury during obstructive cholestasis in bile duct-ligated mice. Hepatology. 2003;38(2):355–63.
9. Ma Z, Miyamoto A, Lee SS. Role of altered betaadrenoceptor signal transduction in the pathogenesis of cirrhotic cardiomyopathy in rats. Gastroenterology. 1996;110(4):1191–8.
10. Finberg JP, Syrop HA, Better OS. Blunted pressor response to angiotensin and sympathomimetic amines in bile-duct ligated dogs. Clin Sci (Lond). 1981;61(5):535–9.
11. Song JG, Cao YF, Sun YM, Ge YH, Xu XW, Yang LQ, et al. Baroreflex sensitivity is impaired in patients with obstructive jaundice. Anesthesiology. 2009;111(3):561–5.
12. White JV, Guenter P, Jensen G, Malone A, Schofield M. Consensus statement: academy of nutrition and dietetics and American Society for Parenteral and Enteral Nutrition: characteristics recommended for the identification and documentation of adult malnutrition (undernutrition). J Parenter Enter Nutr. 2012;36:275–83.
13. Long Y, Mi W, Weifeng Y. Anesthesia for patients with obstructive jaundice. J Anesth Perioper Med. 2018;5:149–60.
14. Bozzato S, Galli L, Ageno W. Thromboprophylaxis in surgical and medical patients. Semin Respir Crit Care Med. 2012;33:163–75.
15. Lassen K, Coolsen MM, Slim K, Carli F, de Aguilar-Nascimento JE, Schäfer M, et al. Guidelines for perioperative care for pancreaticoduodenectomy: enhanced recovery after surgery (ERAS®) society recommendations. Clin Nutr. 2012;31(6):817–30.
16. Blacker S, Lahiri RP, Phillips M, Pinn G, Pencavel TD, Kumar R, et al. Which patients benefit from preoperative biliary drainage in resectable pancreatic cancer? Expert Rev Gastroenterol Hepatol. 2021;15(8):855–63.

17. Hanje AJ, Patel T. Preoperative evaluation of patients with liver disease. Nat Clin Pract Gastroenterol Hepatol. 2007;4(5):266–76.
18. Marandola M, Albante A. Anaesthesia and pancreatic surgery: techniques, clinical practice and pain management. World J Anesthesiol. 2014;3(1):1–11.
19. Song JG, Cao YF, Yang LQ, Yu WF, Li Q, Song JC, et al. Awakening concentration of desflurane is decreased in patients with obstructive jaundice. Anesthesiology. 2005;102:562e5.
20. Yang LQ, Song JC, Irwin MG, Song JG, Sun YM, Yu WF. A clinical prospective comparison of anesthetics sensitivity and hemodynamic effect among patients with or without obstructive jaundice. Acta Anaesthesiol Scand. 2010;54:871e7.
21. Wang ZM, Zhang P, Lin MJ, Tan B, Qiu HB, Yu WF. Influence of obstructive jaundice on pharmacodynamics of rocuronium. PLoS One. 2013;8(10):e78052.
22. Chiu JW, White PF. The pharmacoeconomics of neuromuscular blocking drugs. Anesth Analg. 2000;90:S19–23.
23. Dershwitz M, Hoke JF, Rosow CE, Michałowski P, Connors PM, Muir KT, Dienstag JL. Pharmacokinetics and pharmacodynamics of remifentanil in volunteer subjects with severe liver disease. Anesthesiology. 1996;84:812–20.
24. Bosilkovska M, Walder B, Besson M, Daali Y, Desmeules J. Analgesics in patients with hepatic impairment: pharmacology and clinical implications. Drugs. 2012;72(12):1645–69.
25. Marinella MA. Meperidine-induced generalized seizures with normal renal function. South Med J. 1997 May;90(5):556–8.
26. Lobo DN, Bostock KA, Neal KR, Perkins AC, Rowlands BJ, Allison SP. Effect of salt and water balance on recovery of gastrointestinal function after elective colonic resection: a randomised controlled trial. Lancet. 2002;359:1812–8.
27. Gurgel ST, do Nascimento P. Maintaining tissue perfusion in high-risk surgical patients: a systematic review of randomized clinical trials. Anesth Analg. 2011;112:1384–91.
28. Jacob M, Chappell D, Rehm M. Clinical update: perioperative fluid management. Lancet. 2007;369:1984–6.
29. Aloia TA, Kim BJ, Segraves-Chun YS, Cata JP, Truty MJ, Shi Q, et al. A randomized controlled trial of postoperative thoracic epidural analgesia versus intravenous patient-controlled analgesia after major hepatopancreatobiliary surgery. Ann Surg. 2017;266(3):545–54.
30. Soliz JM, Lipski I, Hancher-Hodges S, Speer BB, Popat K. Subcostal transverse abdominis plane block for acute pain management: a review. Anesth Pain Med. 2017;7(5):e12923.
31. Pietri LD, Montali R, Begliomini B. Anaesthetic perioperative management of patients with pancreatic cancer. World J Gastroenterol. 2014;20:2304–20.
32. Karim SAM, Abdulla KS, Abdulkarim QH, Rahim FH. The outcomes and complications of pancreaticoduodenectomy (Whipple procedure): cross sectional study. Int J Surg. 2018;52:383–7.

10 Anaesthetic Considerations in Patients with Carcinoma Prostate for Robot-Assisted Laparoscopic Radical Prostatectomy

Balbir Kumar and Rohini Dattatri

10.1 Case Vignette

A 68-year-old male presented to the outpatient department with a history of difficulty in micturition, and poor urinary stream for the past 2 months. He also complained of low back pain for the past 1 month. Digital rectal examination revealed nodularity. On further evaluation patient was diagnosed with carcinoma (Ca) prostate. He has been posted for robot-assisted laparoscopic radical prostatectomy.

10.2 What Are the Risk Factors and Clinical Features of Ca Prostate?

Prostate cancer is the second most common cancer in men worldwide. Most of the cases occur in men over 65 years of age [1]. Various risk factors attributed include advancing age (more than 70% in men older than 65 years) ethnicity, genetic mutations, history of malignancy in the family, and insulin-like growth factors [2]. Diet, obesity, sedentary lifestyle, cigarette smoking, alcohol consumption, ionizing radiation, and occupational exposure to certain chemicals have also been associated with an increased risk of Prostate cancer.

> Ca prostate can be asymptomatic in the initial stages. However, later stages can present with symptoms like difficulty in micturition, poor urinary stream, haematuria. Metastatic carcinoma can present with low back pain, anemia and weight loss. Stages can present with symptoms like difficulty in urination, increased frequency, poor urinary stream, and haematuria.

10.3 Briefly Describe the Da Vinci System

The *da Vinci Surgical System* consists of three components, namely a surgical cart, an optical 3D-vision tower, and a console [3]. The four arms of the surgical cart can be manipulated by the surgeon in a console in real time through the computer. The instruments are held by the first two arms which represent the right and left arm of the surgeon while the endoscope is positioned by the third arm. The fourth arm is optional and is used to hold instrument or provide counter-traction eliminating the need of a surgeon the patent side. The bulky and heavier surgical cart is in proximity to the cart and hence, inadvertent contact with the patient due to the movement of robotic arms should be avoided.

Instruments in the surgical cart can have 7° of freedom which is far more than the ability of a

B. Kumar (✉) · R. Dattatri
Department of Onco-anaesthesia and Palliative Medicine, NCI AIIMS, New Delhi, India

Department of Anaesthesiology and Critical care, AIIMS Bibinagar, Bibinagar, India

N. Gupta et al. (eds.), *Problem Based Learning Discussions in Onco-Anesthesia and Onco-Critical Care*, https://doi.org/10.1007/978-981-99-6339-3_10

surgeon's hand. It also helps to filter >6 Hz tremors. Two surgeons are present in most of the cases. One surgeon at the console where he sits to view the operating field and manipulated the robotic arms. The assistant helps to place the trocar and connects the arms of the robot to the trocars. As the surgeon uses the manipulator, it translates the hand movement into the movement of the instruments. Foot pedals are used to disengage the motion of the robot, adjust the camera, alternate between the arms as well as control the electric cautery. The stereoscopic vision is provided by integrating the right and the left optical channels optical by using computer in the optical tower. The software required to control the movement of robotic arms is present in optical tower.

The major advantages of use of robots in surgery include provision of 3D stereoscopic view along with ability to adjust magnification. The camera platform is stable and can be controlled directly. Tremor filtering, motion scaling, and extra degrees of motion are additional benefits [4]. Smaller incision, lesser postoperative pain, reduced blood loss, lesser incidence of urinary incontinence, and positive margins preservation of neurovascular bundle and decreased length of hospital stay are a few benefits of RALRP [5].

The robotic systems also have limitations such as prohibitive costs, long operating time, limited access to the patient, precarious positioning, absence of tactile feedback, and high maintenance costs. It requires specialized training and skills and larger operating room to accommodate bulky equipment.

10.4 What Are the Goals in Robotic Surgeries? What Are the Measures to Reduce the Complications?

- Ensuring the patient safety by minimizing robotic arms collision, maximizing the exposure of operative field and improving the efficiency of surgical team.
- A thorough understanding of the docking, the console and the safety measures to be followed by all the team members. Training should be imparted by using simulation, assisting the procedures and visiting the high-volume centres so as to improve the confidence.
- It has been proposed that the operating room should be square shaped with at least an area of 60 m^2 with a central operating table which can be rotated [6]. The console should be preferably placed at the less frequented corners of the OR. The cables used for connection should be detangled and placed at places that is ergonomically correct.
- Positioning of the patient requires diligent planning to prevent neurological and physical injuries.
- Closed loop communication is essential so as to prevent any untoward incidents as the operating room would be dark.

10.5 What Is Docking of the Robot?

In robotic surgeries, once the patient is positioned and ports are inserted, the patient cart instrument arms is attached to the patient. This is termed as docking.

- Once the robot is docked, it is extremely difficult to adjust the patient or operating table.
- Placement of vascular access or performing any anaesthetic manoeuvre is onerous. It is the collective responsibility of the team to ensure accurate positioning of the patient.
- The anaesthesia monitors should be clearly visible along with ensuring access to the anaesthesia equipment.
- The decision for temporary or permanent interruption of the robotic approach in an emergency scenario should be taken after an effective communication among the team members.
- An institutional protocol for emergency undocking should be developed, and all the team members should undergo training in a simulated environment.

10.6 Describe the Preoperative Assessment Patients Posted for Robotic Prostatectomy

The preoperative preparation of the patient includes preoperative assessment and preparation of ergonomics.

10.6.1 Preoperative Assessment

- Routine preoperative assessment should be done with a focus on identifying high-risk patients (severe ischemic or valvular heart disease, significant respiratory disease, morbid obesity, or patient with raised ICP and IOP). Patients with significant cardiac disease should be further evaluated by cardiologist. Surgery is contra-indicated in patients with a recent history of myocardial infarction, severe valvular heart disease, decompensated heart failure, congenital heart disease, and significant arrhythmias will not tolerate pneumoperitoneum [7].
- Patients with severe COPD develop high peak airway pressures during mechanical ventilation due to steep trendelenberg position (30^0 to 40^0 head down position) and pneumoperitoneum [8]. Hypoxaemia can occur due to V/Q mismatch. RALRP is a relative contraindication in patients with lung bullae as it can rupture leading to complications.
- Higher incidence of ischemic heart disease, obstructive sleep apnoea, diabetes, and difficult airway is seen in obese patients with BMI > 30 kg/m^2.Ventilation difficulties can occur in these patients. Careful positioning must be done to prevent neurological injury.
- The anaesthesiologist should be aware of the adverse impact on the physiology due to extreme position required during the surgery. Most of the patients undergoing prostatectomy are elderly. Hence, physiological changes associated with ageing can make the perioperative period more challenging.
- These patients could be on antiplatelets and anticoagulants which needs to be discontinued prior to the surgery.
- Patients with compromised renal function should be carefully managed due to further reduction of renal perfusion during intraoperative period.
- Enhanced recovery after surgery protocols should be followed to improve the outcomes and reduced morbidity [9].
- Preoperative counselling and education help to improve the patient compliance and reduce the anxiety.
- Prehabilitation in the form of medical optimisation, nutritional support, physical exercise, and psychological support fastens the postoperative recovery.

10.6.2 Ergonomics

- Limited access to the patient due to bulky equipment [10] Hence, two-wide bore intravenous access should be obtained and secured. Airway should be carefully secured. Institutional protocol should be in place to manage emergency.
- Intraoperative removal of robot in the event of any emergency is a multi-step process and is time-consuming. This is of importance during cardiopulmonary resuscitation. Adequate training should be provided by simulation for rapid removal of robot. It has been noted that with practice of emergency drill, it is possible to remove the robot within 30 s. In case of need, DC shock can be delivered with the robot docked in position [11].
- Absolute immobility is required in the intraoperative period to prevent any catastrophic events resulting in vascular or visceral injuries.
- The table position should be changed only after surgical equipment has been disengaged.

10.7 Describe the Intraoperative Management of a Patient Posted for Robotic Prostatectomy

10.7.1 Intraoperative Management

The intraoperative challenges faced in RALRP and troubleshooting have been summarized in Table 10.1.

- General anaesthesia with standard induction and airway control with a tracheal tube is preferred in RALRP.
- Preferably two-wide bore cannulae should be secured prior to tucking the arms and docking the robot. Arterial line should be secured in indicated cases [12].
- Short acting anaesthetic agents should be used. Volatile agent with a favourable recovery profile should be used.

Table 10.1 Challenges in the perioperative period and troubleshooting in patients undergoing RALRP

Systems	Challenges	Trouble shooting
Positioning	Access to airway and extremities limited Risk of nerve injuries and compartment syndrome Postoperative corneal abrasion and vision loss Reflux of stomach acid High venous pressure over ear lobe causing erroneous reading	Secure iv and intraarterial access before positioning Padding the pressure points Use antiskid bedding and cross-torso straps to decrease the skidding risk Minimize the duration and degree of Trendelenburg position Proper protection of the eyes Placement of nasogastric tube Pulse oximeter to be placed over finger instead of ear lobe
Heavy and bulky robot	Not positioned properly can contact the head of the patient	Ensure face is visible
Robot is over chest and abdomen of the patient	Delay in case of cardiovascular or airway issues	Close communication between team members Simulation training
Airway	Airway edema, cerebral edema Subcutaneous emphysema Displacement of the ETT → mainstem intubation	Reduce the amount of CO_2 insufflation Carefully secure ET tube recheck the endotracheal tube after positioning Prior to extubation cuff leak test may be performed Meticulous attention to fluid administration
Cardiovascular	Decreased venous output, cardiac output Increased mean arterial pressure, systemic vascular resisnce	Recognize high-risk cases and obtain cardiologist opinion CO_2 insufflation should be slow Maintain optimal volume status Early use of pressors Adequate DVT prophylaxis
Respiratory	Hypercapnia Hypoxemia	Use lowest peritoneal insufflation pressure Use lung protective ventilation strategy-pressure-controlled ventilation, optimize PEEP
Nervous system	Increased ICP Raised IOP	Ensure that there is no external pressure on eyes, head/neck due to equipment Ensure adequate MAP for cerebral and ocular perfusion Neurologist consultation if at risk of raised ICP OR IOP
Others	Hypothermia Subcutaneous emphysema Pneumothorax, pneumomediastinum, pneumopericardium	Use forced air warmer Be vigilant

- Ensure complete immobility of the patient by continuous infusion of non-depolarising neuromuscular agent. Neuromuscular monitor can be used.
- Pulse oximeter should be placed on the finger as high venous pressure in ear lobe due to Trendelenburg position can result in erroneous readings.

10.7.2 Airway Management

Endotracheal tube position should be checked prior to and after pneumoperitoneum and after placing the patient is Trendelenburg position due to high chance of endobronchial intubation.

10.7.3 Patient Positioning

- Care should be taken to ensure proper positioning to prevent neuropathies in view of long surgical duration.
- Diabetes, thin body habitus, improper placement, or inadequate padding of the robot's immobile arms on the patient's lower extremities [13].
- Commonly injured nerves are common peroneal nervefemoral nerve and brachial plexus.
- Proper padding of pressure points specially elbow, back, shoulders, and axilla should be done. Upper limbs should be placed in neutral position.
- Prolonged lithotomy position can lead to decrease in pao2 and increase in paCO2 and shunt fraction [14, 15]. It can also increase the risk of compartment syndrome, rhabdomyolysis, and renal failure. Prolonged hypotension should be avoided as it can exacerbate pressure sores and neurological injuries [16]. Care should be taken to prevent corneal abrasions.
- Physiological changes associated with pneumoperitoneum are shown in Table 10.2. Injury to the hollow structures and blood vessels can occur during insertion of Veress needle. Slow

Table 10.2 Physiological effects of pneumoperitoneum

System	Increase↑	Decrease ↓
Respiratory system	Peak airway pressure Hypercarbia and acidosis Ventilation perfusion mismatch Surgical emphysema Pulmonary congestion and edema	Vital capacity Functional residual capacity Compliance Pao2
Airway	Tracheal tube displacement Facial/airway edema	
Cardiovascular	Systemic vascular resistance Venous air embolism Mean arterial pressure Oxygen consumption	Venous return Cardiac output
Neurological	Intraocular pressure Cerebral blood volume Intracranial pressure Peripheral nerve injury	
Endocrine	Activation of renin–angiotensin–aldosterone system Catecholamine release	
Renal		Renal and splanchnic blood flow Glomerular filtration rate Urine output
Gastro-intestinal	Regurgitation	
Others	Hypothermia Occult blood loss Postoperative corneal abrasion and vision loss Periorbital edema Venous air embolism	

insufflation and use of lower pressures are advocated. Careful patient selection is important. Considerable amount of CO_2 is stored in the extracellular compartment which is slowly redistributed, metabolized, and exhaled resulting in elevated levels of CO_2 despite release of pneumoperitoneum. End tidal carbon dioxide should be maintained at normal level to prevent increase in ICP leading to cerebral edema.

- Venous air embolism, subcutaneous emphysema, pneumothorax, pneumopericardium, and pneumomediastinum are rare complications resulting in haemodynamic collapse [17, 18].
- The steep Trendelenburg position results in a decrease in functional residual capacity and compliance. It also affects arterial oxygen tension. An increase in central venous pressure, pulmonary artery pressure, and pulmonary capillary wedge pressure occurs.
- Adjuncts used such as shoulder braces, leg suspension, and iliac support are not recommended due to risk of neuropathic injuries [19].

Use of antiskid material (egg-crate pink foam) prevents the shift of the patient without resulting in skin or neurologic injuries [20].

10.7.4 Pulmonary Considerations

Trendelenburg position and pneumoperitoneum can lead to hypercarbia and the need for higher airway pressures which can lead to barotrauma exacerbating the lung injury [21]. Pressure controlled ventilation and optimization of PEEP are preferable to improve the lung mechanics and arterial oxygenation [22]. A PEEP of 7 cm H_2O was found to increase the arterial oxygenation without increase in peak airway pressure [23]. Use of recruitment manoeuvre and prolonging the inspiratory phase to 2:1 and 1:1 could also provide better oxygenation and help in CO_2 elimination [24, 25].

10.7.5 Haemodynamic Considerations

- Intraoperative haemodynamics is affected by steep Trendelenburg position, lithotomy position, and pneumoperitoneum. In addition, blood loss during surgery also affects the haemodynamic parameters. It results in decrease in venous return and cardiac output, increase in systemic vascular resistance, and mean arterial pressure. .
- Urine output may not be a suitable marker for adequacy of perfusion as bladder will be opened during the surgery and hence drains into the surgical field. It can result in overestimation of blood loss due to mixing of blood and urine. .
- A carefully designed fluid strategy balancing haemodynamic goals individual to the patient and minimizing facial and airway edema is important. Excess fluid administration can affect the surgical field by excessive urine production.
- Vasopressors should be used early in case of hypotension to avoid fluid overload.

10.7.6 Monitoring

Intraoperative monitoring should include all ASA standard monitors such as electrocardiogram, non-invasive blood pressure, pulse oximetry, capnography, and temperature. In addition, monitoring of urine output, depth of anaesthesia (BIS), respiratory gas monitoring, and neuromuscular monitoring should also be done. Invasive blood pressure, cardiac output, and central venous monitoring should be done on case-to-case basis.

10.7.7 Intraoperative Fluid Therapy

An individualized fluid therapy balancing the haemodynamic goals is to be followed. Care should be taken to minimize facial and airway edema. Goal-directed fluid therapy (GDFT) aims to optimize the cardiac preload and the tissue oxygen therapy by using specific haemodynamic parameters, thereby minimizing both hypovolemia and fluid excess [26]. Transesophageal echocardiography, arterial waveform analysis-based techniques, and transesophageal Doppler are the commonly used techniques to measure key parameters including cardiac index, stroke volume variation (SVV), mixed venous oxygen saturation (SvO2), and systemic vascular resistance.

10.8 What Are the Postoperative Issues and How Will You Manage Them?

Postoperative concerns include airways management, postoperative pain management, and prevention of deep vein thrombosis.

10.8.1 Airway Management

Neuromuscular blockade is reversed once the robotic arms have been removed from the patient. Patients should be assessed for the presence of airway edema prior to extubation. Airway edema can occur due to venous congestion that can develop in steep trendelenburg position maintained for a prolonged duration. Cuff leak test can be done prior to extubation to detect ant airway edema. Delayed emergence can occur due to cerebral edema following prolonged Trendelenburg position.

10.8.2 Pain Management

The main benefit of RALRP is the reduced incidence of postoperative pain as compared to open radical prostatectomy. However, pain can still occur due to multiple factors such as pneumoperitoneum leading to peritoneal irritation, diaphragmatic stretching causing referred pain, visceral pain, trocar incisional pain, or pain at the site of extraction on the abdominal wall extraction site. Inadequate pain relief can result in an increase in cardiopulmonary complications, autonomic dysfunction, deep vein thrombosis, increased duration of paralytic ileus, and longer length of hospital stay. There is paucity of data suggesting the most suitable analgesic technique as this is a relatively newer procedure.

Treatment options vary depending on the origin and mechanism of the pain. Shoulder tip pain due to residual CO_2 from pneumoperitoneum can be reduced by lowering the pneumoperitoneum pressures [27]. Yet another way to minimize shoulder pain is to place the patient in a 30° Trendelenburg position at the end of surgery and manually inflating the lungs 5 times by means of recruitment manoeuvre [28].It has been noted that the size of CO2 bubble has a linear correlation with the severity of shoulder pain.

Multimodal modal analgesia using non-opiate systemic analgesics plus regional techniques is beneficial by providing superior pain relief and reducing opioid related side effects. The regional techniques that are found to be beneficial in robotic urological surgeries are neuraxial analgesia, transversus abdominal plane block, rectus sheath block (RSB), paravertebral block, quadratus lumborum(QL), and intercostals block [29]. Each technique has its own advantages and disadvantages as described in Table 10.3. Talwar et al. presented a tailor made pain management program for patients undergoing robotic urologic surgeries at American Society of Surgical Oncology [30]. In this program, patients were administered only non-opioids initially which was supplemented with opioids in those with inadequate pain relief. Gabapentin and acetaminophen in the preoperative period followed by eighth hourly administration of the same drugs along with intravenous ketorolac in the postoperative period. Tramadol 50 mg or 100 mg sixth hourly was added in severe pain which was escalated to oxycodone if required. Amongst 170 patients in the program, 115 (68%) were managed without opioids, 41 (24%) patients required tramadol while only 14 (8%) were administered oxycodone. No significant difference in pain scores was noted in the three groups.

Table 10.3 Different regional techniques used in robotic urological surgeries

Technique	Analgesia covered	Advantage	Disadvantage
Neuraxial block	Below umbilicus	Rapid onset of blockade—motor, sensory, and autonomic (sympathetic) blockade	Hypotension, urinary retention, PDPH
Intercostal block	Intercostal nerves on the same side are blocked	Easy technique	Only somatic pain relief; risk of pneumothorax
TAP block	Nerves supplying anterior abdominal wall (T6—L4)	Simple technique	Does not provide visceral analgesia
QL block	Abdominal wall (T12—L1)	Provides both somatic and visceral analgesia	Technical difficulty

Various adjuvant mediations used include acetaminophen, dexamethasone, NSAIDS,COX-2 inhibitors, intravenous lidocaine, and magnesium [31–34].

10.8.3 Deep Venous Thrombosis(DVT) Prophylaxis

Venous thromboembolism (VTE) can be categorized into low risk, medium risk, and high risk based on patient risk factors. Some of the risk factors for VTE include immobility, duration of surgery, malignancy, use of oral contraception, spinal cord injury, and inheritable blood disorders such as antiphospholipid antibody syndromes, factor V Leiden, antithrombin, and protein C or S deficiencies. Low risk for VTE patients are those with no risk factors. Medium risk is when any of the following is present: age 75 years or more; BMI $\geq$ 35 or VTE in first degree relative (parent, full sibling, or child) [35]. High risk is when two or more risk factors are present or a prior history of VTE is positive. Guidelines recommend against the use of mechanical and pharmacological thromboprophylaxis in low-risk patients undergoing robotic radical prostatectomy without PLND, mechanical thromboprophylaxis until ambulation is recommended in medium- and high-risk patients. Patients undergoing robotic radical prostatectomy with standard PLN, pharmacological prophylaxis should be administered to high-risk patients only while mechanical thromboprophylaxis is given to all the patients. In medium- and high-risk patients undergoing extended pelvic lymph node dissection, pharmacological prophylaxis should be given and mechanical thromboprophylaxis should be used until ambulation irrespective of the VTE risk [35].

The most common complication seen in the postoperative period is paralytic ileus which occurs secondary to pelvic haematoma and anastomotic leakage. The risk of intraoperative blood loss requiring blood transfusion is low. Blood transfusion is not normally required as intraoperative blood loss is very low, but patient should be carefully monitored for the occurrence of significant haemorrhage which may be insidious. Compartment syndrome may occur after prolonged lithotomy position and careful attention should be paid for the presence of calf tightness and tenderness.

10.9 Describe the Enhanced Recovery After Surgery ERAS Protocols for Robotic Radical Prostatectomy

ERAS pathways are multimodal multidisciplinary care pathways addressing the entire patient journey from the referral to the discharge. This standardized perioperative care helps to achieve early recovery by maintaining homeossis and reducing the surgical stress response [36]. The main components of ERAS are summarized in table. At present, radical cystectomy is the only urological procedure having official ERAS guidelines. However, recent evidence suggests that adoption of ERAS protocol can decrease the duration of hospital stay as well as also shown to

Table 10.4 Components of ERAS [39]

Preoperative	Intraoperative	Postoperative
Preoperative counselling and education Prehabilitation No mechanical bowel preparation Pharmacological thromboprophylaxis 12 h prior to surgery Clear liquids until 2 h and solids until 6 h prior to surgery Carbohydrate loading 2 h prior to surgery Use short acting anxiolytics if required Antimicrobial prophylaxis atleast 60 min prior to surgery	Skin preparation using chlorhexidine Use of mechanical thromboprophylaxis Epidural anaesthesia to be avoided Rectus sheath catheters to be inserted and (0.125% bupivacaine) administered for 48 h Optimal perioperative fluid management-goal directed fluid therapy Nasogastric intubation should be avoided Preventing intraoperative hypothermia Minimally invasive approach to be used Resection site drainage Urinary drainage Wound closure using 2/0 polydioxanone suture to rectus sheath 3/0 subcuticular Monocryl suture to skin	Postoperative diet Early oral diet Prevention of postoperative ileus (use of peripheral μ receptor antagonist Alvimopan to accelerate GI recovery) Prevention of PONV Postoperative analgesia that Includes rectus sheath catheters (0.125% bupivacaine) Early mobilization Audit

shorten hospital stay and improve abdominal symptoms in patients who received robot-assisted radical prostatectomy (RARP) [37]. A retrospective analysis of 70 patients who underwent laparoscopic transperitoneal radical prostatectomy with ERAS and conventional approach showed that adoption of ERAS decreased the duration of hospital stay, start of enteral feeds and antibiotics use. The rate of paralytic ileus and time to first defecation was not statistically significant between two groups [38] (Table 10.4).

10.10 Summary

- RALRP is challenging due to the difficulties with patient positioning, reduced access to the patient, possibility of airway oedema, prolonged duration of surgery, physiological effects of pneumoperitoneum and steep trendelenburg, elderly patients.
- Careful preoperative assessment to identify high-risk patients helps to reduce complications in the perioperative period. A meticulous attention should be paid to positioning in the intraoperative period. Pressure points should be padded. Judicious administration of fluids should be followed.
- Adoption of ERAS protocol reduces the surgical stress response and hastens the recovery.
- Close communication between the team members is essential to reduce the complication rate.
- Emergency drill must be conducted to train the theatre staff for urgent removal of robots if the situation demands.

References

1. Global Burden, of Disease Cancer Collaboration, Fitzmaurice C, Allen C, et al. Global, Regional, and National Cancer Incidence, Morality, Years of Life Lost, Years Lived With Disability, and Disability-Adjusted Life-years for 32 Cancer Groups, 1990 to 2015: A Systematic Analysis for the Global Burden of Disease Study. JAMA. Oncologia. 2017;3:524.
2. https://seer.cancer.gov/statfacts/html/prost.html . Accessed 12 Jun 2018.
3. Tameze Y, Low YH. Outpatient robotic surgery: considerations for the anesthesiologist. Adv Anesth. 2022;40(1):15–32. https://doi.org/10.1016/j.aan.2022.06.001.

4. Du Y, Long Q, Guan B, Mu L, Tian J, Jiang Y, Bai X, Wu D. Robot-assisted radical prostatectomy is more beneficial for prostate cancer patients: a system review and me-analysis. Med Sci Monit. 2018;24:272–87. https://doi.org/10.12659/msm.907092.
5. Papachristos A, Basto M, Te Marvelde L, Moon D. Laparoscopic versus robotic-assisted radical prostatectomy: an Australian single-surgeon series. ANZ J Surg. 2015;85:154–8.
6. Bačak Kocman I, Mihaljević S, Goluža E, Peršin Beraković A, Margaretić Piljek N, Kuliš T, Hudolin T, Knežević N, Kaštelan Ž. Anesthesia for robot-assisted radical prostatectomy—a challenge for anaesthesiologist. Acta Clin Croa. 2022;61(suppl 3):76–80. https://doi.org/10.20471/acc.2022.61.s3.11.
7. Aceto P, Beretta L, Cariello C, et al. Joint consensus on anesthesia in urologic and gynecologic robotic surgery: specific issues in management from a task force of the SIAARTI, SIGO, and SIU. Minerva Anestesiol. 2019;85(8):871–85.
8. Phong SV, Koh LK. Anaesthesia for robotic-assisted radical prostatectomy: considerations for laparoscopy in the Trendelenburg position. Anaesth Intensive Care. 2007;35(2):281–5.
9. Ploussard G, Almeras C, Beauval JB, Gautier JR, Garnault V, Frémont N, Dallemagne S, Loison G, Salin A, Tollon C. A combination of enhanced recovery after surgery and prehabilitation pathways improves perioperative outcomes and costs for robotic radical prostatectomy. Cancer. 2020;126(18):4148–55. https://doi.org/10.1002/cncr.33061.
10. Mills JT, Burris MB, Warburton DJ, Conaway MR, Schenkman NS, Krupski TL. Positioning injuries associated with robotic assisted urological surgery. J Urol. 2013;190:580–4.
11. Irvine M, Patil V. Anaesthesia for robot-assisted laparoscopic surgery, continuing education. Anaesth Crit Care Pain. 2009;9(4):125–9. https://doi.org/10.1093/bjaceaccp/mkp020.
12. Lee JR. Anesthetic considerations for robotic surgery. Korean J Anesthesiol. 2014;66(1):3–11.
13. Warner MA, Martin JT, Schroeder DR, Offord KP, Chute CG. Lower- extremity motor neuropathy associated with surgery performed on patients in a lithotomy position. Anesthesiology. 1994;81:6–12.
14. Berryhill R Jr, Jhaveri J, Yadav R, et al. Robotic prostatectomy: a review of outcomes compared with laparoscopic and open approaches. Urology. 2008;72:15–23.
15. Ryniak S, Brännstedt S, Blomqvist H. Effects of exaggerated lithotomy position on ventilation and hemodynamics during radical perineal prostatectomy. Scand J Urol Nephrol. 1998;32:200–3.
16. Biswas S, Gnanasekaran I, Ivatury RR, Simon R, Patel AN. Exaggerated lithotomy position-related rhabdomyolysis. Am Surg. 1997;63:361–4.
17. Hong JY, Kim JY, Choi YD, et al. Incidence of venous gas embolism during robotic-assisted laparoscopic radical prostatectomy is lower than that during radical retropubic prostatectomy. Br J Anaesth. 2010;105(6):777–81.
18. Miller RD, Eriksson LI, Fleisher LA, et al. Vol. 1647. Elsevier Churchill Livingstone; Philadelphia: 2005. (Miller's anesthesia). Pneumothorax after laparoscopic robotic-assisted supracervical hysterectomy and sacrocolpopexy. Female Pelvic Med Reconstr Surg. 2017;23(3):e22–4.
19. Irwin W, Anderson W, Rice L. Minimizing the risk of injury in gynaecologic surgery. Obstet Gynaecol. 2004;103(2):374–82.
20. Klauschie J, Wechter ME, Jacob K, et al. Use of anti-skid material and patient-positioning to prevent patient shifting during robotic-assisted gynecologic procedures. J Minim Invasive Gynecol. 2010;17(4):504–7.
21. Carry PY, Gallet D, François Y, et al. Respiratory mechanics during laparoscopic cholecystectomy: the effects of the abdominal wall lift. Anesth Analg. 1998;87(6):1393–7.
22. Lee HJ, Kim KS, Jeong JS, Shim JC, Cho ES. Optimal positive end-expiratory pressure during robot-assisted laparoscopic radical prostatectomy. Korean J Anesthesiol. 2013;65:244–50.
23. Kwak HJ. What is the proper ventilation strategy during laparoscopic surgery? Korean J Anesthesiol. 2017;70:596–600.
24. Ahn S, Byun SH, Chang H, Koo YB, Kim JC. Effect of recruitment maneuver on arterial oxygenation in patients undergoing robot-assisted laparoscopic prostatectomy with intraoperative 15 cmH2O positive end expiratory pressure. Korean J Anesthesiol. 2016;69:592–8.
25. Kim WH, Hahm TS, Kim JA, Sim WS, Choi DH, Lee EK, et al. Prolonged inspiratory time produces better gas exchange in patients undergoing laparoscopic surgery: a randomised trial. Acta Anaesthesiol Scand. 2013;57:613–22.
26. Danic MJ, Chow M, Alexander G, et al. Anesthesia considerations for robotic-assisted laparoscopic prostatectomy: a review of 1,500 cases. J Robot Surg. 2007;1(2):119–23.
27. Phelps P, Cakmakkaya OS, Apfel CC, Radke OC. A simple clinical manuever to reduce laparoscopy-induced shoulder pain: a randomized controlled trial. Obstet Gynecol. 2008;111:1155–60.
28. Esmat ME, Elsebae MM, Nasr MM, Elsebaie SB. Combined low pressure pneumoperitoneum and intraperitoneal infusion of normal saline for reducing shoulder tip pain following laparoscopic chole- cystectomy. World J Surg. 2006;30:1.
29. Khater N, Comardelle NJ, Domingue NM, Borroto WJ, Cornett EM, Imani F, Rajabi M, Kaye AD. Current strategies in pain regimens for robotic urologic surgery: a comprehensive review.

Anesth Pain Med. 2022;12(3):e127911. https://doi.org/10.5812/aapm-127911.
30. The ASCO Post. 2019 ASCO: pain management program for patients undergoing robotic urologic surgery. New York, USA: The ASCO Post; 2019. https://ascopost.com/News/60118.
31. Imani F, Varrassi G. Ketamine as adjuvant for acute pain management. Anesth Pain Med. 2019;9(6):e100178. https://doi.org/10.5812/aapm.100178.
32. Urits I, Jung JW, Amgalan A, Fortier L, Anya A, Wesp B, et al. Utilization of magnesium for the treatment of chronic pain. Anesth Pain Med. 2021;11(1):e112348. https://doi.org/10.5812/aapm.112348.
33. Soleimanpour H, Imani F, Dolati S, Soleimanpour M, Shahsavarinia K. Management of pain using magnesium sulphate: a narrative review. Postgrad Med. 2022;134(3):260–6. https://doi.org/10.1080/00325481.2022.2035092.
34. Tully J, Jung JW, Patel A, Tukan A, Kandula S, Doan A, et al. Utilization of intravenous lidocaine infusion for the treatment of refractory chronic pain. Anesth Pain Med. 2020;10(6):e112290. https://doi.org/10.5812/aapm.112290.
35. Violette PD, Cartwright R, Briel M, Tikkinen KA, Guyatt GH. Guideline of guidelines: thromboprophylaxis for urological surgery. BJU Int. 2016;118(3):351–8. https://doi.org/10.1111/bju.13496.
36. Fearon KC, Ljungqvist O, Von Meyenfeldt M, Revhaug A, Dejong CH, Lassen K, Nygren J, Hausel J, Soop M, Andersen J, Kehlet H. Enhanced recovery after surgery: a consensus review of clinical care for patients undergoing colonic resection. Clin Nutr. 2005;24(3):466–77. https://doi.org/10.1016/j.clnu.2005.02.002.
37. Lv Z, Cai Y, Jiang H, Yang C, Tang C, Xu H, Li Z, Fan B, Li Y. Impact of enhanced recovery after surgery or fast track surgery pathways in minimally invasive radical prostatectomy: a systematic review and meta-analysis. Transl Androl Urol. 2020;9(3):1037–52. https://doi.org/10.21037/tau-19-884.
38. Guleser AS, Basaga Y, Karadag MA. Comparison of enhanceds recovery after surgery protocol and conventional approach after laparoscopic transperitoneal radical prostatectomy: a retrospective analysis. Afr J Urol. 2021;27:129. https://doi.org/10.1186/s12301-021-00233-y.
39. Lee G, Patel HV, Srivastava A, Ghodoussipour S. Updates on enhanced recovery after surgery for radical cystectomy. Ther Adv Urol. 2022;14:17562872221109022. https://doi.org/10.1177/17562872221109022.

Carcinoma Urinary Bladder for Cystectomy and Ileal Conduit

11

Manpreet Kaur, Nisha Jain, and Prabhjot Singh

11.1 What Are Different Available Treatment Options for Carcinoma Urinary Bladder?

Noninvasive bladder cancer is treated with complete transurethral resection of visible bladder tumor (TURBT). Patient with intermediate or high-risk non-muscle invasive disease intravesical therapy such as chemotherapy or BCG may be indicated. For locally advanced bladder cancer chemoradiation with cystectomy is the option.

11.2 What Is Neoadjuvant Chemotherapy? What Are the Side Effects of Cisplatin?

Neoadjuvant chemotherapy for bladder carcinoma patients is methotrexate, vinblastine, doxorubicin, and cisplatin. Cisplatin is associated with nephrotoxicity and neurotoxicities including peripheral neuropathy, ototoxicity, vestibulopathy, and encephalopathy. Eligibility criteria for cisplatin-based chemotherapy are as follows:

1. Creatinine clearance (crcl) $\geq$ 60.
2. Eastern Cooperative Oncology Group (ECOG) performance status <2.
3. Grade < 2 neuropathy.
4. No significant hearing loss.
5. No clinical evidence of congestive heart failure.

11.3 Describe Radical Cystectomy. How Do You Define Ileal Conduit? What Are Alternative Diversion Procedures Available?

Radical cystectomy involves removal of entire urinary bladder, lower ureters, and regional lymph nodes for invasive bladder tumors (Fig. 11.1a). In RC, bilateral pelvic lymphadenectomy includes removal of external and internal iliac and obturator nodes. In men, it includes removal of prostate, seminal vesicle also. In women, standard approach involves removal of entire urethra, adjacent vagina, and uterus. Pelvic organ-preserving techniques are used to preserve neurovascular bundle, vagina, uterus, and ovaries. RC is always obliged to a companion surgery that allows future urine collection. This involves redirecting ureters to a bowel segment,

M. Kaur (✉)
Department of Anesthesiology and Perioperative Medicine, Penn State Milton S Hershey Med Center, Hershey, PA, USA

N. Jain
Department of Anaesthesiology, Pain Medicine and Critical Care, New Delhi, India

P. Singh
Department of Urology, Penn State Milton S Hershey Med Center, Hershey, PA, USA

N. Gupta et al. (eds.), *Problem Based Learning Discussions in Onco-Anesthesia and Onco-Critical Care*, https://doi.org/10.1007/978-981-99-6339-3_11

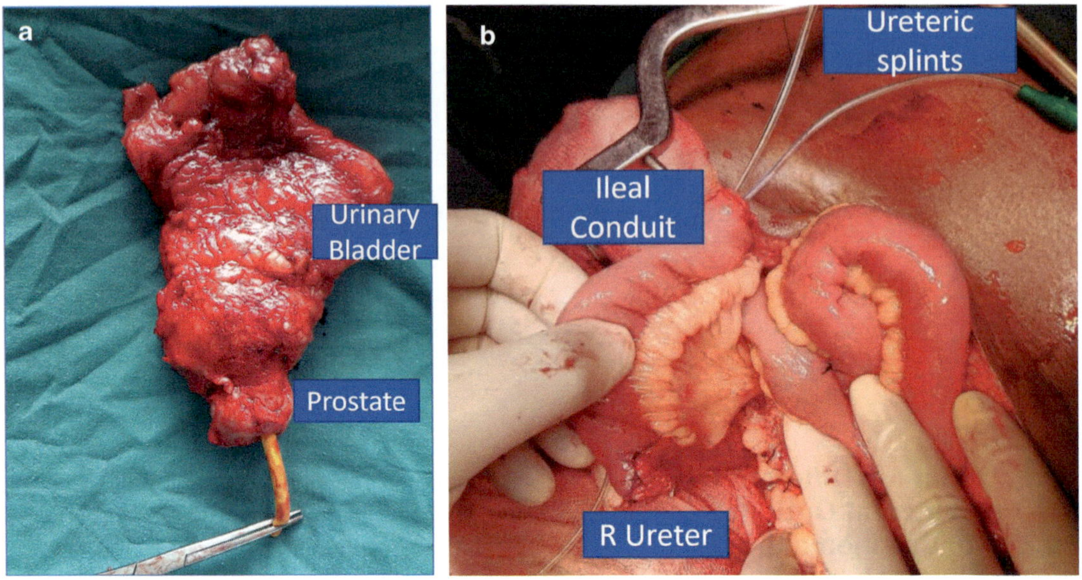

Fig. 11.1 (**a**) Cystectomy specimen (**b**) Ileal conduit

most commonly to ileum pouch (ileal conduit) (Fig. 11.1b), that passively drain urine to a bag through a stoma on patient's abdominal wall. Alternative options are continent diversion reconstructive procedures categorized as ureterosigmoidostomy, continent cutaneous diversions, and neobladder diversions.

11.4 Preoperative Evaluation and Optimization

11.4.1 How Would You Evaluate the Patient Preoperatively? What Preoperative Work-Up Is Required?

It involves assessment, optimization of medical conditions, and reduction of risk factors that affect perioperative homeostasis. Bladder tumors are generally diagnosed by hematuria (microscopic or macroscopic) with or without voiding symptoms such as urgency, frequency, and dysuria. Occasionally these patients present with urinary retention. Radical cystectomy (RC) and urinary diversion is a major resection surgery with increased risk of bleeding, perioperative transfusion, and high frequency of postoperative complications. Prior to cystectomy patients have usually undergone several cystoscopies for biopsy or resection and many have received radiotherapy or chemotherapy.

These patients are usually elderly with cardiovascular and other comorbidities, anemia, possible infection, and malnutrition. Comprehensive geriatric assessment (CGA) is required for older patients if surgery is being considered. The key domains of CGA include functional status, comorbidity, cognition, nutrition, psychological state, social support, and medication review.

Physiological changes in elderly and their anesthetic implications are tabulated in Table 11.1.

Perioperative concerns for radical cystectomy have been summarized in Table 11.2.

Table 11.1 Perioperative concerns in radical cystectomy with ileal conduit

Preoperative	Intraoperative	Postoperative
Elderly	Positioning	Pain
Co-morbidities & its optimization	Blood loss	Thermoregulation
Specific history related to risk factors and their effects on body	Thermoregulation	Bacteremia
Presenting signs and symptoms	Major fluid shifts	Post-op ileus
Paraneoplastic syndrome	Analgesia	Electrolyte imbalance (hyperchloremic metabolic acidosis)
	Duration of surgery	
	Inability to measure urine output	

Table 11.2 Physiological changes in elderly and its anesthetic implications

	Physiological changes	Anaesthetic implications
Nervous system	Decreased cerebral blood flow and conduction velocity	– Increased cephalad spread of local anesthetics – less requirement of anesthetics
CV system	– Increased myocardial and vascular stiffness leading to increased BP – Decreased beta receptor responsiveness	– Hypotension on induction – Increased sensitivity to hypovolemia
Respiratory system	– decreased elasticity and compliance – poor gas exchange	Increased chances of post-op respiratory failure
Renal function	Decreased GFR, renal mass, concentrating and diluting ability	Accumulation of renal clearance-dependent drugs
GI & endocrine system	Decreased gastric emptying and insulin secretion	Increased risk of aspiration and DM
Musculoskeletal system	Arthritis, osteoporosis	– Airway difficulty – Difficult positioning

11.4.2 What Are the Common Types of Bladder Cancer? Describe the Risk Factors Associated with Bladder Cancer?

Urothelial carcinoma/transitional cell carcinoma, squamous cell carcinoma, and adenocarcinoma are three main types of bladder cancer. Among them urothelial carcinoma is the most common type.

Risk factors for bladder cancer and atherosclerosis are overlapping. History of smoking causing hyperactive airway, occupational exposures to dye, leather, rubber industry, and drinking water with high arsenic levels are common contributing factors.

Paraneoplastic syndromes such as tumor lysis syndrome, Cushing syndrome, etc. associated with bladder cancer are rare but have been reported.

Eighty percent of radical cystectomy cases are current or former smokers. Preoperative smoking cessation for more than 48 h might reduce the risk of pneumonia and mechanical ventilation. According to a study by Turan et al. [1] active smokers have higher rates of myocardial infarction, postoperative cardiac arrest, stroke, deep vein thrombosis, and sepsis. Systemic review [2] which included urological and genitourinary patients revealed that intensive smoking cessation, 4–8 weeks before surgery with individual counseling and pharmacotherapy, reduced the risk of postoperative complications.

Daily more than two to three drinks intake decreases the immune response, prolongs the bleeding time, and increases endocrine stress response to surgery [3]. Preoperative 4 weeks long abstinence from alcohol reduces exaggerated surgical stress response in alcohol abusers [4].

Routine blood investigations include Hb, complete blood count (CBC), renal function test (RFT), liver function test (LFT), serum electrolytes, and coagulation profile which can be deranged in chronic smokers. Other additional investigations include pulmonary function test (PFT), electrocardiogram (ECG), chest X-ray, and assessment of effort tolerance.

11.4.2.1 Thromboprophylaxis

Patients undergoing RC are considered to be at high risk of venous thromboembolism (VTE) because of cancer disease and surgical procedure lasting for more than 120 min [5]. European guidelines on perioperative VTE prophylaxis recommend the first dose of LMWH 12 H before procedure or 6–8 hrs after the procedure. According to a study done by Sachdeva et al., graduated compression stockings or compressive stockings enables effective thromboprophylaxis [6].

11.4.2.2 Preoperative Fasting

The European Society of Anaesthesiology fasting guidelines encourage to drink clear liquids (tea, coffee without milk, and water) up to 2 hr. before the elective surgery. With the highest level of evidence, recommendation is prohibition of solid food 6 hr. before the elective operation. Preoperative carbohydrate loading 2 hr before surgery reduce patient anxiety, improve hydration, reduce insulin resistance, inflammatory response, and improve outcome from surgery [7].

11.4.2.3 Antimicrobial Prophylaxis

In RC patients, prophylaxis for both aerobic and anaerobic pathogens is recommended. Combination of cefuroxime and aminopenicillin/beta-lactamase inhibitors together with metronidazole is recommended. In case of prolonged operation or important morbidity factors, antimicrobial prophylaxis might be prolonged to <72 h.

11.4.2.4 Prevention of PONV

PONV may intensify postoperative pain, wound dehiscence, hematoma and hence increase patient distress. For preoperative and postoperative phases, rescue antiemetics are advised. Histamine antagonists (Tab ranitidine 150 mg before shifting to OT), ondansetron and dexamethasone, during intraoperative period are used as rescue antiemetics.

11.5 Intraoperative Period

11.5.1 Discuss Monitoring and Anesthesia Plan for these Patients. What Are Intraoperative Considerations?

After completion of preanesthetic checklist and obtaining informed written consent, ASA standard monitors (E.C.G, NIBP, Pulse-oximeter) are attached to the patient and baseline readings are noted. Two wide-bore venous cannula are required because of the possibility of excessive blood loss. After induction and intubation arterial cannula is placed for invasive blood pressure monitoring and repeated blood gas assessment with serum lactate levels for adequacy of end organ perfusion. Central venous catheter should be used for inotropes and transfusion purpose. Temperature monitoring and capnometry are also part of the standard care. At least one intraoperative blood glucose should be documented. Maintain it <180 mg/dL.

Supine or modified lithotomy position is common in RC and ileal conduit surgeries. Improper positioning can result in local structures injury such as obturator nerve injury leading to adductor palsy, gait disturbances, and impaired lymph drainage (lymphocele, leg edema). Proper patient positioning with pressure point padding is essential to prevent these injuries.

11.5.2 How to Prevent Intraoperative Hypothermia in These Extensive Surgeries?

Maintenance of normothermia during surgery reduces oxygen consumption, risks of wound infection, bleeding, and pain. Intraoperative hypothermia under general anesthesia results in delayed recovery, increased ICU admission, and prolonged hospital stay [8]. The active warming strategies, such as use of warm fluids using hot-lines and forced air warming, are more effective than passive warming in maintaining stable intraoperative hemodynamics and core temperature [9].

11.5.3 How to Monitor Urine Output in Genitourological Surgeries?

In most of the major surgeries, urine output is used to measure the fluid status, which is however not possible in radical cystectomy surgery. Though adequacy of urine output is difficult to access but inquiry from the surgeon to determine whether urine is flowing from cut ends of ureters can aid in determining that patient does not have anuria.

11.5.4 Enumerate the Different Anesthetic Plans Available and Discuss Their Pros and Cons

Anesthesia techniques for radical cystectomy can be either general anesthesia with endotracheal intubation alone or combined with epidural neuraxial technique. General anesthesia can be with total intravenous anesthesia (TIVA) or inhalational agents.

Combined general anesthesia with endotracheal intubation and neuraxial technique is the preferred choice. Level of insertion of epidural catheter in radical cystectomy cases is generally around thoracic Th 9–11 targeting sensory block around Th6. Epidural has various positive effects on the general perioperative status of patients (Table 11.3). Several studies have revealed decrease in mortality [10, 11] as well as decrease in the risk of cardiovascular and respiratory [12] events in abdominal surgery due to epidural effects. It is also associated with reduced intraoperative blood loss [12], earlier recovery of gastrointestinal peristalsis [13], and postoperative pain control [12]. Some studies suggest TIVA is beneficial in oncological surgeries due to its antimetastatic effect [14].

Table 11.3 Advantages of epidural anesthesia

• Decrease in mortality
• Decrease in the risk of cardiovascular and respiratory events
• Reduced intraoperative blood loss
• Earlier recovery of gastrointestinal peristalsis
• Postoperative pain control

11.5.5 Discuss the Fluid Management in these Patients

Optimization of fluid therapy aims at "zero balance," maintaining preoperative fluid composition and weight. Isotonic fluid is recommended in urological surgeries. Estimated blood loss in RC is 560–3000 mL which makes the need for transfusion common [15]. Intraoperative cell salvage (IOCS) blood management strategy is safe in various urologic malignancies without risk of tumor spread. It sustains intraoperative patient blood volume and minimizes allogenic blood transfusion [16]. Target hemoglobin should be >8 g/dL for all patients.

Dynamic variables guided "Goal-directed" fluid therapy is safe and helps in early recovery as it results in less estimated blood loss and less intraoperative blood transfusion [17]. Several newer automated devices (FloTrac, LiDCO) allow measurement of continuous cardiac output and stroke volume variation. Existing arterial line helps in measurement of pulse pressure variation and respiratory variation of systolic pressure. According to Gupta and Gan [18], maintenance fluid therapy in adult patients during major abdominal surgery should be accomplished with 1–3 mL/kg/h.

11.5.6 Discuss all Available Options for Perioperative Analgesia

Epidural neuraxial anesthesia provides excellent intraoperative and postoperative analgesia which helps in early recovery of the patient and reduces morbidity. Epidurally local anesthetic agents with or without opioids (PCEA) can be used for analgesic purpose.

Intravenous patient-controlled analgesia (IV PCA) using hydromorphone or morphine or fentanyl is also an available tool for perioperative analgesia but on lower rank than PCEA in terms of early recovery.

Intrathecal opioids provide excellent analgesia in laparoscopic or robotic RC.

IV paracetamol every sixth hourly is part of multimodal analgesia. IV ketorolac 0.5 mg/kg at conclusion of case (GFR > 35) can be given after discussing with surgeons.

Alternatively, rectus sheath block can also be used for perioperative analgesia which offers the advantages of patient safety and feasibility in patients on antiplatelet medications.

11.6 Postoperative Period

11.6.1 Enumerate the Postoperative Complications that May Arise in Immediate Postoperative Period in these Patients. Discuss the Principles of Enhanced Recovery after Genitourinary Surgery

Extensive surgery with longer duration can result in many postoperative complications such as pain, bacteremia, metabolic disturbances, and postoperative ileus. Various metabolic complications may arise following urinary diversion [19]:

- Altered bowel function.
- Malabsorption.
- Acid-base imbalance.
- Electrolyte abnormality.
- Bone demineralization.
- Calculi formation.
- Renal and hepatic malfunction.
- Impaired drug metabolism.

Hyperchloremic metabolic acidosis is a consequence of intestinal fluid and electrolyte exchange between intestinal mucosa and urine (absorption of ammonium and chloride from urine). Long-term chronic metabolic acidosis may lead to impaired bone metabolism and osteomalacia. Regular monitoring of PH, chlorine, bicarbonate, and calcium-phosphorus metabolism is essential for early diagnosis and treatment.

Enhanced recovery after surgery (ERAS) protocols define multimodal approach to surgical patients which aims at improvement of patient preoperative status and the perioperative maintenance of homeostasis, by minimizing stress response and inflammation [8].

Components of ERAS:

- Early nasogastric tube (NGT) removal and allow oral clear liquids on second post-op day.
- Post-op analgesia—epidural analgesia is given for 2–3 days post-op with local anesthetic agent bupivacaine/ropivacaine 0.2% or epidural opioids. Alternatively, TAP block/ rectus sheath block can also be given. Intravenous paracetamol Q.I.D can be used as a part of multimodal analgesia.
- Prevention of post-op ileus (POI). It is defined as inability to tolerate solid food by post-op day five, need to place NGT or need to stop oral intake due to abdominal distension, nausea, or emesis. Proposed mechanisms include components of ERAS including fluid overload, electrolyte imbalance, bowel manipulation, and opioid use. Prevention of POI can be achieved by perioperative epidural analgesia, optimized intraoperative fluid therapy, minimal invasive approach of surgery, early NGT removal with early oral intake, and early mobilization.
- Early oral intake and nutrition. ERAS guidelines suggest for normal diet establishment as soon as possible in RC cases. Clear fluids should be initiated within hours after surgery.

- Early mobilization. This helps in reducing hospital stay and reduces associated complications of prolonged bed rest like respiratory, musculoskeletal changes.
- Surgery type. Compared with open surgery, minimal invasive robotic RC enhances patient recovery. It has reduced blood loss and transfusion rate, inpatient narcotic requirement, time to regular diet, and length of hospital stay.

11.6.2 Components of ERAS Protocol in Radical Cystectomy

Preoperative phase
• Education and counseling • Medical optimization • Preoperative fasting and carbohydrate loading • No mechanical bowel preparation • Pain management (epidural/TAP/rectus sheath block) • Antimicrobial prophylaxis • Venous thromboembolism prophylaxis
Intraoperative phase
• Goal-directed fluid therapy • Hypothermia prevention • Analgesic protocol
Postoperative phase
• Early removal of nasogastric tube • Prevention of nausea, vomiting • Prevention of postoperative ileus • Early feeding • Pain management • Early mobilization

11.6.3 Describe the Risk Factors Associated with Morbidity and Mortality Following Radical Cystectomy

1. Elderly.
2. Comorbidities—hypertension, diabetes, coronary artery disease, etc.
3. High American Society of Anaesthesiology grade.
4. Addiction chronic smokers, alcoholic.
5. Preoperative nutrition, thrombotic status.
6. Intraoperative blood loss and rate of transfusion.
7. Postoperative complications like gastrointestinal, infection, wound-related complications.

References

1. Turan A, Mascha EJ, Roberman D, Turner PL, You J, Kurz A, et al. Smoking and perioperative outcomes. Anesthesiology. 2011;114:837–46.
2. Thomsen T, Tonnesen H, Moller AM. Effect of preoperative smoking cessation interventions on postoperative complications and smoking cessation. Br J Surg. 2009;96:451–61.
3. Tonnesen H, Nielsen PR, Lauritzen JB, Moller AM. Smoking and alcohol intervention before surgery: evidence for best practice. Br J Anaesth. 2009;102:297–306.
4. Tonnesen H, Rosenberg J, Nielsen HJ, Rasmussen V, Hauge C, Pedersen IK, et al. Outcome in alcohol misusers: randomized controlled trial. BMJ. 1999;318:1311–6.
5. Venclauskas L, Llau JV, Jenny JY, Kjaersgaard-Andersen P. European guidelines on perioperative venous thromboembolism prophylaxis: day surgery and fast-track surgery. Eur J Anaesthesiol. 2017;34(1–5):10.
6. Sachdeva A, Dalton M, Amaragiri SV, Lees T. Elastic compression stockings for prevention of deep vein thrombosis. Cochrane Database Syst Rev. 2010;7:CD001484.
7. Noblett SE, Watson DS, Huong H, Davison B, Hainsworth PJ, Horgan AF. Pre-operative oral carbohydrate loading in colorectal surgery: a randomized controlled trial. Color Dis. 2006;8(7):563–9.
8. Vukovic N, Dinic L. Enhanced recovery after surgery protocols in major urologic surgery. FrontMed. 2018;5:93.
9. Moola S, Lockwood C. Effectiveness of strategies for the management and/or prevention of hypothermia within the adult perioperative environment. Int J Evid Based Healthcare. 2011;9:337–45.
10. Chou R, Gordon DB, de Leon-Casasola OA, Rosenberg JM, Bickler S, Brennan T, et al. Management of postoperative pain: a clinical practice guideline from the American pain society, the American Society of Regional Anesthesia and Pain Medicine, and the American Society of Anesthesiologists' committee on regional anesthesia, executive committee, and administrative council. J Pain. 2016;17:131–57.
11. Popping DM, Elia N, Marret E, Remy C, Tramer MR. Protective effects of epidural analgesia on pulmonary complications after abdominal and thoracic surgery: a meta-analysis. Arch Surg. 2008;143:990–9.
12. Shir Y, Raja SN, Frank SM, Brendler CB. Intraoperative blood loss during radical retropubic prostatectomy: epidural versus general anesthesia. Urology. 1995;45:993–9.
13. Mazul-Sunko B, Gilja I, Jelisavac M, Kozul I, Troha D, Osmancevic N, et al. Thoracic epidural analgesia for radical cystectomy improves bowel function even in traditional perioperative care: a retrospective study in eighty-five patients. Acta Clin Croat. 2014;53:319–25.

14. Edward ZE, Kelliher LJS. Propofol-TIVA versus inhalational anaesthesia for cancer surgery. Dig Med Res. 2020;3:15.
15. Barash PG. Clinical anaesthesia. 7th ed. Library of congress publication; 2012. p. 1423.
16. Ferroni MC, Correa AF, Lyon TD, Davies BJ, Ost MC. The use of intraoperative cell salvage in urologic oncology. Rev Urol. 2017;19:89–96.
17. Ghoreifi A, Basin M, Ghodoussipour S, Bazargani S, Erfan A, Aslzare M, Cai J.etal. Perioperative outcomes of goal-directed versus conventional fluid therapy in radical cystectomy with enhanced recovery protocol. Int Urol Nephrol. 2021;53:1827–33.
18. Gupta R, Gan TJ. Peri-operative fluid management to enhance recovery. Anaesthesia. 2016;71:40–5.
19. Vasdev N, Moon A, Thorpe AC. Metabolic complications of urinary intestinal diversion. Indian J Urol. 2013;29:310–5.

12 Renal Cell Carcinoma for Laparoscopic Nephrectomy

Brajesh Kumar Ratre

12.1 Case

A 55-year-old male patient presented with complaints of right-side abdominal pain and fullness in the right-side loin region for the last 2 months, pain was gradually increasing and associated with weight loss and decreased appetite. On examination tenderness was there in right lumber region. CECT chest, abdomen, and pelvis show right renal mass of size 6.5 cm. Biopsy confirmed the diagnosis of renal cell carcinoma.

Question 1

What are the risk factors and presentation of renal cell carcinoma?

The most common form of urogenital malignancy is renal cell carcinoma which accounts for more than 90% of urogenital malignancies [1]. The established risk factors for renal cell carcinoma include cigarette smoking, hypertension, obesity, and acquired cystic kidney disease [2]. Hereditary renal cell carcinoma develops early in life and is usually bilateral or multiple.

Around 50% of renal cell carcinoma is detected incidentally in abdominal scan. Most common presentation is hematuria, fullness in frank, and frank pain [3]. The non-specific symptoms are weight loss, fever, anorexia, malaise, hematuria, hypertension, etc. Patients with venous tumor thrombus may present with ascites, lower limb edema, deep vein thrombosis, and feature of pulmonary embolism [3].

Question 2

Describe TMN staging of renal cell carcinoma and concern in relation to stage?

The TNM staging of renal cell carcinoma is given in Table 12.1 [4].

Stage group:

- Stage I: T1 N0M0
- Stage II: T2 N0M0
- Stage III: T3 or N1 with M0
- Stage IV: T4 or M1

Patients with T1 and T2 stage require radical nephrectomy but patients with T3 or T4 disease require a multidisciplinary team approach. Renal cell carcinoma has a tendency of venous extension and approximately 5–10% of patients have renal vein involvement or extension to IVC at the time of presentation [5, 6].

B. K. Ratre (✉)
Department of Onco-Anesthesiology and Palliative Medicine, Dr. BRAIRCH, AIIMS, New Delhi, India

N. Gupta et al. (eds.), *Problem Based Learning Discussions in Onco-Anesthesia and Onco-Critical Care*, https://doi.org/10.1007/978-981-99-6339-3_12

Table 12.1 TNM staging of renal cell carcinoma

T		Description
T1	T1a	Tumor confined to kidney, <4 cm
	T1b	Tumor confined to kidney, >4 cm but <7 cm
T2	T2a	Tumor confined to kidney, >7 cm but not >10 cm
	T2b	Tumor confined to kidney, >10 cm
T3	T3a	Tumor grossly extends into the renal vein or its segmental (muscle-containing) branches, or tumor invades perirenal and/or renal sinus fat but not beyond Gerota's fascia
	T3b	Spread to infra-diaphragmatic IVC
	T3c	Spread to supra-diaphragmatic IVC or invades the wall of the IVC
T4		Involves ipsilateral adrenal gland or invades beyond Gerota's fascia
N	N0	No nodal involvement
	N1	Metastatic involvement of regional lymph node(s)
M	M0	No distant metastases
	M1	Distant metastases

Question 3

What are the treatment modalities for renal cell carcinoma?

Surgical resection is the treatment of choice for renal cell carcinoma. Even patient with venous extension and distance metastasis surgical resection improves the prognosis and quality of life [7]. Tumor confined to kidney require radical nephrectomy and laparoscopic nephrectomy is standard surgical modality.

For stage III and IV disease the level of surgical dissection depends upon tumor extension. Tumor extended to inferior vena cava may require liver mobilization or resection of liver or reconstruction of inferior vena cava. So, a multidisciplinary team approach with gastrointestinal and vascular surgeon may give a better outcome in extended venous tumor thrombus renal cell carcinoma [8].

Question 4

What preoperative evaluation are required for this patient?

A thorough history will be taken for the assessment of co-morbid condition, routine ASA recommended preoperative investigation should include complete blood count with renal and liver function test, coagulation status, chest X-ray, and ECG. Blood grouping and cross-match should be done in all patients because there may be possibility of intraoperative blood loss [9].

Transthoracic echocardiography (TTE) can be helpful in providing cardiac and volume tolerance status in patients with cardiac co-morbidity or with poor performance status, TTE will also provide information regarding tumor thrombus and thrombus emboli. If patients have poor exercise tolerance and have risk factor for ischemic heart disease standard AHA/ACC guideline should be followed [10]. Lower extremity Doppler study is indicated in patient with lower limb swelling and pain. Patients who are on anticoagulant therapy for deep vein thrombosis should discontinue it according to peri-operative anticoagulant guidelines and restart as soon as possible after surgery. Low molecular weight heparin (LMWH) is preferred over warfarin because HMWH is associated with increased survival and decreased incidence of thromboembolism. Bridging should be done if the patient is on warfarin [11].

Question 5

What special consideration to be taken preoperatively?

Renal cell carcinoma has tendency to extend through venous invasion so a thorough preoperative imaging study is required for adequate planning of surgical steps and the imaging should be performed within 30 days of surgery [12].

Magnetic resonance imaging is the modality of choice but multi-detector CT imaging is equally accurate in diagnosing extend of disease, venous invasion, and collaterals around tumor mass. A discussion with radiologist should also be done prior to planning to rule out any possibility of vascular invasion by tumor. Renal Doppler is helpful to find attachment of tumor to renal vein and inferior vena cava. Few imaging finding may suggest vascular invasion by tumor, i.e., contrast filling defect due to presence of tumor thrombus, inferior vena cava diameter more than 40 mm, renal vein diameter more than 18 mm, tumor signal both inside and outside of vessels in MRI [8].

Question 6

Discuss the different surgical approach and positioning for laparoscopic nephrectomy?

There are different techniques for laparoscopic nephrectomy and patient position depends upon the surgeon's approach. In trans-peritoneal approach patient is placed in lateral position and at the edge of the table so the abdomen is hanging down and back is supported by bolsters. This approach gives a good working space specially with large size kidney [13, 14].

Retroperitoneal approach provides direct access to renal hilum and avoids transabdominal fats, but this approach will not provide a good space for dissection. For this approach the patient is placed in modified flank position in which the patient is placed in lateral decubitus position with lower leg flexed upper leg extended and arm abducted to 90° [14]. One must take care to provide optimal patient position and avoid nerve or organ injury.

Question 7

Describe the physiological effect due to pneumoperitoneum and positioning?

Standard position for laparoscopic radical nephrectomy is lateral decubitus position with flank break in table. This position causes the following changes:

Cardiovascular changes: As compared to lateral decubitus position kidney bridge position has a significant change in the hemodynamics of the patient. There is venous pooling because the level of lower limb is significantly below the heart which causes decrease in mean arterial pressure, right atrial pressure, pulmonary artery mean pressure, pulmonary capillary wedge pressure, cardiac output, stroke volume index, and cardiac index [15].

The physiological changes in different organ system due to pneumoperitoneum are given in below flow diagram [16] (Fig. 12.1).

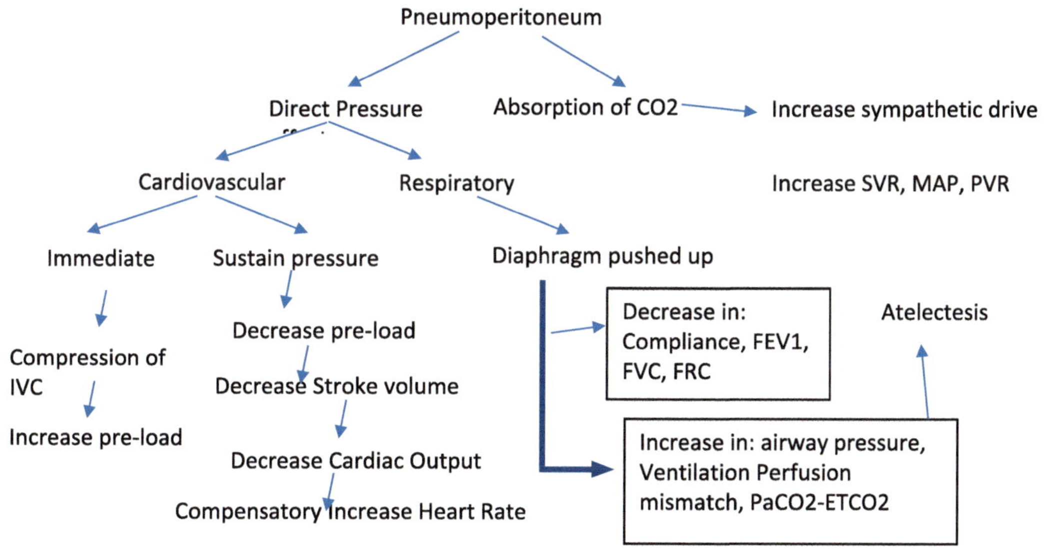

Fig. 12.1 Physiological changes in pneumoperitoneum

CO_2 gas insufflation should be done slowly as bradycardia may occur just after gas insufflation, if still there is sympathetic response then deepening the plain of anaesthesia, extra dose opioids may be helpful. In case of severe bradycardia gas insufflation should be stopped for few minutes [17]. Mild hypercarbia is acceptable in laparoscopic surgery as it causes vasodilatation and rightward shift of oxygen dissociation curve and improves the tissue oxygenation [16].

Question 8

Discuss the intraoperative consideration for this surgery.

Advancement in surgical technique will make them less invasive, laparoscopic nephrectomy is the standard operative procedure for early stage of renal cell carcinoma. General anesthesia with short-acting drugs for early recovery, prevention of postoperative nausea vomiting, use of multimodal analgesia and preservation of renal function is the goal of anesthesia for laparoscopic nephrectomy. General anesthesia provides better control on ventilation and anesthesiologist can adjust the ventilator settings according to patient position and end-tidal CO_2 Level [18]. Endo-tracheal intubation should be preferred over supra-glottic airway devices because there may be possibility of aspiration with high abdominal pressure. In few studies second-generation supra-glottic airway devices (LMA-Proseal) are found to be an effective alternative to endotracheal intubation in laparoscopic gynecological and cholecystectomy [19–21]. However, in laparoscopic nephrectomy patient position is lateral decubitus and there is increased intra-abdominal pressure due to pneumoperitoneum, so the use of supra-glottic airway devices is still debatable.

Standard ASA-recommended monitoring should be used. Pulse oximetry probe should be place in dependent arm, it will help in early detection of any mismatch in peripheral perfusion [18]. Invasive hemodynamic monitoring is recommended only in high-risk patients with cardiac co-morbidity [22]. The risk of bleeding is less during laparoscopic surgery, two large bore intravenous cannulas are sufficient for fluid resuscitation. Ideally peripheral intravenous access will be taken in non-dependent side (side of operation). Active warming should be initiated early to prevent hypothermia. In low-risk patients for venous thromboembolism intermittent pneumatic compression prophylaxis should be used, for moderate to high-risk patients venous thromboembolism prophylaxis guideline should be followed and low molecular weight heparin or unfractionated heparin should be initiated preoperatively [23].

The blood loss during surgery is dependent upon the skill of surgeon and the approach which is used for surgery. In retroperitoneal approach the expected blood loss is 600 mL and 800 mL for transperitoneal approach. However, the surgery is around the vicinity of major vessels so anesthesiologist should be ready for any mishaps [18].

Question 9

What will be your intraoperative fluid management plan?

In laparoscopic surgery, two things that may affect the perioperative outcome. One is the preoperative hypovolemic status and the second is pneumoperitoneum which causes pressure-induced mechanical compression of renal vasculature [16]. Renal vasculature compression is more in patient with hypovolemic state. Both these factors decrease the renal blood flow and oxygen delivery which may further cause ischemic renal injury. Hemodynamic stability is important to maintain renal perfusion. Hydration after gas insufflation is less effective to counteract the hemodynamic instability. Preoperatively intravascular volume status should be assessed and if required preoperatively fluid bolus given to maintain adequate renal perfusion. Intraoperatively the target urine output should be kept above 1 mL/kg/h. Sudden hemodynamic instability should be avoided and ephedrine should be preferred over phenylephrine as later causes more constriction of renal vasculature. Intraoperative crystalloid/5% albumin/colloid is considered to maintain intravascular volume. After hemostasis major blood loss should be replaced with red blood cells [22].

Question 10

What are the complications that you may encounter after laparoscopic radical nephrectomy?

Apart from surgery-related complication there are two other factors that may cause complication: one is the positioning related and second due to pneumoperitoneum. Surgical procedure-related complication includes bleeding, injury to organs or major vessels, pneumothorax, pneumomediastinum, and subcutaneous emphysema.

Position-related complication includes nerve damage, injury to dependent eye and pressure sores. Lateral decubitus position with flank bridge or flexed flank position may cause venous stasis. This position creates pressure on gravity-dependent body parts and compromises the circulation of that part. Prolonged surgery in Flank position is associated with rhabdomyolysis [24, 25]. Other risk factor for rhabdomyolysis includes hypovolemia, and obesity [24]. To avoid such complication rotated supine position or little flexed position can be considered. Elevated level of creatinine kinase and presence of myoglobin in serum indicate rhabdomyolysis, treatment is to maintain high urine output, mannitol to promote diuresis, and avoid cast formation in renal tubules [26].

Prolonged pneumoperitoneum may cause hemodynamic instability in high-risk patient like those with hypovolemic state. In case of severe hemodynamic instability it is advisable to rule out any vascular injury and intraabdominal pressure should be less than 15 mm of Hg. Carbon dioxide embolism is a fatal complication that may cause cardiovascular collapse. Measures to protect against complication due to pneumoperitoneum include short surgical time, low flow rate of carbon dioxide, intraabdominal pressure less than 15 mm of Hg, and continuous monitoring of end-tidal CO_2 [16, 17].

Question 11

Discuss the etiopathogenesis of postoperative pain in this patient.

Patient who underwent laparoscopic nephrectomy experiences less pain as compared to open nephrectomy. There are two major factors for postoperative pain in laparoscopic nephrectomy. One is due to surgery related, i.e., port site, organ irritation, retrieval incision size, site, and presence of drain.

Second cause is due to pneumoperitoneum which further depends upon type, temperature of gas used, duration of surgery, and residual gas volume. Pneumoperitoneum leads to neuroprexia of phrenic nerve, irritation of diaphragm, and causes postoperative shoulder and upper abdominal pain [27]. The duration of surgery is also important as carbon dioxide used for creating pneumoperitoneum forms acidic medium (carbonic acid) in peritoneum which decrease the pH of peritoneum and irritates the peritoneum, diaphragmatic nerves and causes pain [27, 28].

The negative pressure of peritoneum is lost due to presence of remaining carbon dioxide after the laparoscopic surgery and presence of carbon dioxide pocket between liver and diaphragm provides traction to ligaments of liver with produces sub-diaphragmatic pain [29, 30].

Question 12

Discuss the postoperative pain management plan other than regional analgesia techniques

As discussed in the previous question patient experiences both nociceptive and neuropathic pain. Tissue trauma and irritation of peritoneum also causes inflammatory pain [31]. Multimodal analgesia practice will give good pain relief because of multifactorial mechanism of pain origin in laparoscopic nephrectomy [32].

For immediate postoperative period, intravenous opioids are standard of care either bolus or through patient controlled analgesia system (PCA pump) [33]. The use of multimodal analgesia technique will reduce the requirement of opioids and its undesirable side effects, i.e., sedation, ileus, and respiratory depression. Along with opioids, paracetamol in a dose of 1 g intravenous provides good pain relief in immediate postoperative period and this should be continued in subsequent postoperative days [34]. Use of non-steroidal anti-inflammatory drugs (NSAIDs) or cyclooxygenase 2 (COX 2) inhibitors can relieve inflammatory pain due to tissue injury and local site inflammatory response [35]. NSAIDs further decrease the requirement of opioids. However, nephrotoxicity is well well-known complication of NSAIDs so one should be very cautious before using NSAIDs in nephrectomy patients.

Preemptive analgesia can be given in the form of preoperative oral gabapentin. Oral gabapentin in dose 600 mg preoperative reduces the postoperative pain, nausea, vomiting and also decreases the requirement of opioids in laparoscopic ovarian cystectomy [36]. Intravenous ketamine prior to incision can decrease postoperative pain and opioids requirement. Postoperative infusion of ketamine can also decrease the postoperative pain, nausea vomiting, and opioid requirement [37]. Port site subfascial infiltration with long-acting local anesthetic reduces postoperative pain.

Other techniques that give good postoperative pain relief are intravenous lignocaine infusion in postoperative period [38]. Co-analgesics, i.e., parenteral magnesium, Alpha-2 agonist (clonidine, dexmedetomidine) infusion and parenteral glucocorticoids can also provide postoperative pain relief and reduce the need of opioids [39].

Question 13

Describe the regional analgesia and peripheral nerve blocks for perioperative pain management in this patient.

A regional analgesia (RA) technique provides better pain relief in perioperative period. In laparoscopic nephrectomy, apart from port site incision the other incision is 4–5 cm for the extraction of resected kidney and specimen. Polish society of anesthesiology and intensive care recommend the use of RA technique with multimodal pain management approach for nephrectomy surgeries [40]. Pre-emptive RA with local anesthetic covering T6–T12 dermatomal levels prevents the nociceptive response and central sensitization. This provides good analgesia in perioperative period [41]. Sole spinal anesthesia and epidural anesthesia are not recommended for laparoscopic nephrectomy due to lateral decubitus position, increased risk of cardiovascular instability and poor control over ventilation. Addition of RA technique with general anesthesia reduces the requirement of opioids in perioperative period and associated side effect, i.e., PONV, respiratory depression, sedation, etc. [42].

Different regional analgesia technique with their effective dermatomal level are given in Table 12.2.

Table 12.2 RA techniques for effective analgesia in nephrectomy patients

S. no.	Technique	Dermatomes/action
1.	Spinal opioids (morphine)	Spinal or epidural opioids act on spinal opioids receptor and provide good analgesia. Analgesic effect lasts up to 24 h
2.	Thoracic epidural	T4–T12, long-acting local anesthetic (bupivacaine, ropivacaine) provides 6–8 h of good pain relief
3.	Paravertebral block	Covers both somatic and visceral pain
4.	Erector spinae plane block	Covers both somatic and visceral pain
5.	Transverse abdominis plane block	Somatic pain only
6.	Rectus sheath block	Somatic pain only
7.	Quadratus lumborum block	T7–T12, L1; Covers both somatic and visceral pain

References

1. Gupta K, Miller JD, Li JZ, Russell MW, Charbonneau C. Epidemiologic and socioeconomic burden of metastatic renal cell carcinoma (mRCC): a literature review. Cancer Treat Rev. 2008;34:193–205.
2. Chow WH, Dong LM, Devesa SS. Epidemiology and risk factors for kidney cancer. Nat Rev Urol. 2010;7(5):245–57.
3. Lee CT, Katz J, Fearn PA, Russo P. Mode of presentation of renal cell carcinoma provides prognostic information. Urol Oncol. 2002;7(4):135–40.
4. Swami U, Nussenzveig RH, Haaland B, Agarwal N. Revisiting AJCC TNM staging for renal cell carcinoma: quest for improvement. Ann Transl Med. 2019;7(Suppl 1):S18.
5. Lardas M, Stewart F, Scrimgeour D, Hofmann F, Marconi L, Dabestani S, et al. Systematic review of surgical management of nonmetastatic renal cell carcinoma with vena caval thrombus. Eur Urol. 2016;70:265–80.
6. Blute ML, Leibovich BC, Lohse CM, Cheville JC, Zincke H. The Mayo Clinic experience with surgical management, complications and outcome for patients with renal cell carcinoma and venous tumour thrombus. BJU Int. 2004;94:33–41.
7. Kirkali Z, Van Poppel H. A critical analysis of surgery for kidney cancer with vena cava invasion. Eur Urol. 2007;52(3):658–62.
8. Evans MA, Wolf FA. Anesthesia for nephrectomy with vena cava thrombectomy. In: Anesthesiology: a practical approach. Springer International Publishing; 2018. p. 635–644.
9. Henny CP, Hofland J. Laparoscopic surgery: pitfalls due to anesthesia, positioning, and pneumoperitoneum. Surg Endosc. 2005;19(9):1163–71.
10. Fleisher LA, Fleischmann KE, Auerbach AD, Barnason SA, Beckman JA, Bozkurt B, Davila-Roman VG, Gerhard-Herman MD, Holly TA, Kane GC, Marine JE, Nelson MT, Spencer CC, Thompson A, Ting HH, Uretsky BF, Wijeysundera DN. 2014 ACC/AHA guideline on perioperative cardiovascular evaluation and management of patients undergoing noncardiac surgery: a report of the American College of Cardiology/American Heart Association task force on practice guidelines. Circulation. 2014;130:e278–333.
11. Matar CF, Kahale LA, Hakoum MB, Tsolakian IG, Etxeandia-Ikobaltzeta I, Yosuico VE, Terrenato I, Sperati F, Barba M, Schünemann H, Akl EA. Anticoagulation for perioperative thromboprophylaxis in people with cancer. Cochrane Database Syst Rev. 2018;7(7):CD009447.
12. Dominik J, Moravek P, Zacek P, Vojacek J, Brtko M, Podhola M, et al. Long-term survival after radical surgery for renal cell carcinoma with tumour thrombus extension into the right atrium. BJU Int. 2013;111:E59–64.
13. Mikhail D, Tabibzadeh A, Rai A, Richstone L. Laparoscopic radical nephrectomy. J Endourol. 2021;35(S2):S83–92.
14. Matin SF, Gill IS. Laparoscopic radical nephrectomy: retroperitoneal versus transperitoneal approach. Curr Urol Rep. 2002;3(2):164–71.
15. Yokoyama M, Ueda W, Hirakawa M. Haemodynamic effects of the lateral decubitus position and the kidney rest lateral decubitus position during anaesthesia. Br J Anaesth. 2000;84(6):753–7.
16. Atkinson TM, Giraud GD, Togioka BM, Jones DB, Cigarroa JE. Cardiovascular and ventilatory consequences of laparoscopic surgery. Circulation. 2017;135(7):700–10.
17. Jung KT, Kim SH, Kim JW, So KY. Bradycardia during laparoscopic surgery due to high flow rate of CO2 insufflation. Korean J Anesthesiol. 2013;65(3):276–7.
18. Nasrallah G, Souki FG. Perianesthetic management of laparoscopic kidney surgery. Curr Urol Rep. 2018;19(1):1.
19. Park SK, Ko G, Choi GJ, Ahn EJ, Kang H. Comparison between supraglottic airway devices and endotracheal tubes in patients undergoing laparoscopic surgery: a systematic review and meta-analysis. Medicine (Baltimore). 2016;95(33):e4598.
20. Beleña JM, Ochoa EJ, Núñez M, Gilsanz C, Vidal A. Role of laryngeal mask airway in laparoscopic cholecystectomy. World J Gastrointest Surg. 2015;7(11):319–25.
21. Ahn H, Min SK, Park JY, Seo WS, Kim JY. Safety and efficacy of the Baska mask versus endotracheal intubation in 64 women undergoing elective laparoscopic gynecological surgery under general anesthesia: a prospective single-center study. Med Sci Monit. 2022;28:e937630.
22. Evans MA, Wolf FA. Anesthesia for nephrectomy with vena cava thrombectomy. 2018.
23. Anderson DR, Morgano GP, Bennett C, Dentali F, Francis CW, Garcia DA, Kahn SR, Rahman M, Rajasekhar A, Rogers FB, Smythe MA, Tikkinen KAO, Yates AJ, Baldeh T, Balduzzi S, Brożek JL, Ikobaltzeta IE, Johal H, Neumann I, Wiercioch W, Yepes-Nuñez JJ, Schünemann HJ, Dahm P. American Society of Hematology 2019 guidelines for management of venous thromboembolism: prevention of venous thromboembolism in surgical hospitalized patients. Blood Adv. 2019;3(23):3898–944.
24. Reisiger KE, Landman J, Kibel A, Clayman RV. Laparoscopic renal surgery and the risk of rhabdomyolysis: diagnosis and treatment. Urology. 2005;66(5 Suppl):29–35.
25. Halvachizadeh S, Jensen KO, Pape HC. Chapter 12. Compartment syndrome due to patient positioning. In: Mauffrey C, Hak DJ, Martin III MP, editors. Compartment syndrome: a guide to diagnosis and management [Internet]. Cham: Springer; 2019.
26. Fabuel Deltoro M, Ramos de Campos M, Juan Escudero J, de la Cruz Torrijos FS, Montoliu García A, Marqués Vida E, Navalón VP. Rabdomiolisis tras nefrectomía laparoscópica; a propósito de un caso [Rhabdomyolysis after laparoscopic nephrectomy: case report]. Arch Esp Urol. 2008;61(7):823–825.
27. Chih-Hsuan S, Chan-Tiopianco M, Chung K-C, Chen Y-J, Huann-Cheng H, Lee W-L, Wang P-H. Pain after

laparoscopic surgery: focus on shoulder-tip pain after gynecological laparoscopic surgery. Crit Care Med. 2019;82(11):819–26.
28. Riedel HH, Semm K. [The post-laparoscopic pain syndrome (author's syndrome)]. Geburtshilfe Frauenheilkd. 1980;40:635–643.
29. Donatsky AM, Bjerrum F, Gögenur I. Intraperitoneal instillation of saline and local anesthesia for prevention of shoulder pain after laparoscopic cholecystectomy: a systematic review. Surg Endosc. 2013;27:2283–92.
30. Kaloo P, Armstrong S, Kaloo C, Jordan V. Interventions to reduce shoulder pain following gynaecological laparoscopic procedures. Cochrane Database Syst Rev. 2019;1:CD011101.
31. Talbot K, Madden VJ, Jones SL, Moseley GL. The sensory and affective components of pain: are they differentially modifiable dimensions or inseparable aspects of a unitary experience? A systematic review. Br J Anaesth. 2019;123:e263–72.
32. Golzari SEJ, Nader ND, Mahmoodpoor A. Underlying mechanisms of postoperative pain after laparoscopic surgery. JAMA Surg. 2016;151(3):295–6.
33. Hager B, Herzog SA, Hager B, Sandner-Kiesling A, Zigeuner R, Pummer K. Comparison of early postoperative pain after partial tumour nephrectomy by flank, transabdominal or laparoscopic access. Br J Pain. 2019;13(3):177–84.
34. Gousheh SM, Nesioonpour S, Foroosh FJ, Akhondzadeh R, Sahafi SA, Alizadeh Z. Intravenous paracetamol for postoperative analgesia in laparoscopic cholecystectomy. Anesth Pain Med. 2013;3:214–8.
35. Smith HS. Perioperative intravenous acetaminophen and NSAIDs. Pain Med. 2011;12(6):961–81.
36. Valadan M, Banifatemi S, Yousefshahi F. Preoperative gabapentin to prevent postoperative shoulder pain after laparoscopic ovarian cystectomy: a randomized clinical trial. Anesth Pain Med. 2015;5:e31524.
37. Radvansky BM, Shah K, Parikh A, Sifonios AN, Le V, Eloy JD. Role of ketamine in acute postoperative pain management: a narrative review. Biomed Res Int. 2015;2015:749837.
38. Tauzin-Fin P, Bernard O, Sesay M, Biais M, Richebe P, Quinart A, Revel P, Sztark F. Benefits of intravenous lidocaine on post-operative pain and acute rehabilitation after laparoscopic nephrectomy. J Anaesthesiol Clin Pharmacol. 2014;30(3):366–72.
39. Raeder J, Dahl V. Clinical application of glucocorticoids, antineuropathics, and other analgesic adjuvants for acute pain management. In: McQuay H, Sinatra R, De Leon-Cassasola O, Viscusi E, Ginsberg B, editors. Acute pain management. Cambridge: Cambridge University Press; 2009. p. 377–90.
40. Wordliczek J, Zajączkowska R, Dziki A, et al. Postoperative pain relief in general surgery—recommendations of the Association of Polish Surgeons, Polish Society of Anaesthesiology and Intensive Therapy, Polish Association for the Study of Pain and Polish Association of Regional Anaesthesia and Pain Treatment. Pol Przegl Chir. 2019;91(1):47–68.
41. Macías AA, Finneran JJ. Regional anesthesia techniques for pain management for laparoscopic surgery: a review of the current literature. Curr Pain Headache Rep. 2022;26(1):33–42.
42. Róziewska A, Klukowski M, Jureczko L. New techniques of regional anaesthesia for renal laparoscopic surgeries. Urologia. 2022;89(4):610–5.

Carcinoma Cervix for Pelvic Exenteration

13

Prashant Sirohiya

13.1 Case

A 55-year-old woman has recurrent carcinoma of the cervix. She had received chemoradiation 2 years ago. She has been posted for pelvic exenteration surgery. How will you manage this case perioperatively? What are the anaesthetic considerations?

13.2 What Is Pelvic Exenteration?

Pelvic exenteration (PE), a highly radical surgical procedure, was pioneered at Ellis Fischel Cancer Centre in the 1940s. Brunschwig further detailed this approach in 1948, specifically for patients facing advanced pelvic malignancies. It is crucial to acknowledge that this procedure poses a substantial risk of both morbidity and mortality. It is typically considered as a viable course of action only when there are no remaining curative alternatives for addressing advanced localized pelvic malignancy [1, 2]. The types of PE are mentioned in Table 13.1.

Table 13.1 Types of pelvic exenteration

Total exenteration	Anterior exenteration	Posterior exenteration
Resection of • Fallopian tubes • Ovaries • Uterus • Parametrium • Urinary bladder • Urethra • Vagina • Rectum/rectal segment • Portion of the levator muscles	• Resection of all structures mentioned in total exenteration with preservation of the rectum	• Resection of all structures mentioned in total exenteration with preservation of the urinary bladder and urethra

P. Sirohiya (✉)
Department of Onco-Anaesthesia and Palliative Medicine, NCI, AIIMS, New Delhi, India
e-mail: prashantsirohiya@aiims.edu

N. Gupta et al. (eds.), *Problem Based Learning Discussions in Onco-Anesthesia and Onco-Critical Care*, https://doi.org/10.1007/978-981-99-6339-3_13

Table 13.2 Indications and contraindications for pelvic exenteration

Indications	Contraindications
Classical indication – Centrally recurrent cervical cancer after primary radiation therapy (RT) or after surgery followed by RT **Newer indications** – In selected cases, pelvic exenteration may be considered for locally advanced primary or recurrent carcinomas of the endometrium, vagina, vulva, and ovaries **Occasionally** – As a palliative procedure to control localized disease-causing severe fistulas or other intolerable symptoms	**Absolute** – Peritoneal metastasis – Skip metastasis to bowel – Distant metastases (extra-pelvic) such as lung metastases **Relative** – Retroperitoneal lymph node metastasis – Tumour invaded directly to adherent bowel loops – Obstructive uropathy (hydroureter or hydronephrosis) *NOTE: Involvement of the sidewall on examination is not a contraindication*

13.3 What Are the Indications and Contraindications for PE?

The indications and contraindications for PE are mentioned in Table 13.2 [3].

13.4 How Will you Evaluate and Prepare for this Patient Prior to Surgery?

The anaesthesiologist involved during the case should pre-evaluate the patient and assess the risk involved and prepare a perioperative management plan to

- Determine the level of surgical fitness because PE is a prolonged duration surgery with extensive fluid shifts that may require vasopressors, inotropes and blood product transfusion.
- Know the cardiopulmonary reserve if the patient can withstand periods of significant stress of surgery.
- Identify, evaluate and manage medical comorbidities such as heart disease, lung disease, diabetes mellitus, etc. that may affect overall patient outcomes.
- Anticipate possible difficulties that may occur in the perioperative course.

If available, the patient's functional capacity can be assessed preoperatively using a cardiopulmonary exercise testing (CPET). Patients with maximum oxygen consumption (VO_2max) of more than 20 mL/kg/min and metabolic equivalents (METs) greater than 4 have a low risk of major perioperative morbidity. The Revised Cardiac Risk Index (RCRI) can be used to assess perioperative cardiac risk. This includes 6 independent predictors of major cardiovascular complications (1 procedural and 5 clinical). In an otherwise fit patient, routine evaluation by a cardiologist is usually not required. If a patient presents with two clinical cardiac risk factors and limited functional capacity (equal to or less than 4 METs), it is recommended that they undergo image stress-testing and myocardial perfusion imaging before proceeding with surgery [4].

The implementation of prehabilitation, involving preoperative physical exercise, nutritional management, psychological intervention, and lifestyle modifications (e.g., smoking cessation), has been shown to significantly enhance functional capacity, mitigate postoperative complications, and contribute to an improved quality of life for individuals undergoing colorectal cancer surgery. This holistic approach aims to optimize overall health and well-being, fostering better surgical outcomes and recovery [5, 6].

Patients presenting for PE may have anaemia which constitutes a risk for adverse events and increased mortality during the perioperative period. Correction of anaemia by iron replacement, if necessary, including parenteral iron therapy, may reduce the risk of allogeneic blood transfusion [4].

Informed consent for surgery should be taken. Comprehensive preoperative counselling of the patient and family should be done to reduce the anxiety and depression associated with surgery. Patient's medical condition should be optimized. Patients are instructed to remain well hydrated during mechanical and antibiotic bowel preparation. Consumption of clear fluids and carbohydrate-containing beverages 2 h before surgery has been shown to prevent surgery-induced immunodepression, reduce preoperative hunger and thirst, and reduce insulin resistance postoperatively [7].

13.5 What Are the Anaesthetic Considerations for PE?

PE can be done through

- Open abdominal approach—typically performed
- Laparoscopic and robotic techniques—for minimally invasive PE (performed less frequently) [8]

Anaesthesia technique—Since this is a radical and complicated surgery, general anaesthesia is mandatory. Regional anaesthesia techniques may be considered for postoperative analgesia [4, 8]. Eliciting a sympathetic blockade, epidural, or spinal anaesthesia plays a crucial role in alleviating the stress response commonly associated with surgery. Additional advantages include a decreased occurrence of cardiopulmonary and thromboembolic complications [9].

Avoid using pre-medication with midazolam to reduce the risk of postoperative sedation and respiratory depression [10]. Avoid the use of long-acting opioids and reduce the total intravenous opioid dose [7]. Concerning the maintenance of anaesthesia, emerging evidence suggests that volatile anaesthetics exhibit proinflammatory properties, potentially influencing the immune response to surgery. This effect may increase the risk of postoperative cancer recurrence and have adverse effects on overall survival [11, 12]. Total intravenous anaesthesia (TIVA) offers notable benefits, such as a decreased risk of postoperative nausea and vomiting, along with a prompt recovery of consciousness after anaesthesia [13]. Some studies claim that the TIVA group had better oncological outcomes than the volatile anaesthetic group [14, 15]. Similarly, some studies have also shown the TIVA group to have similar oncological outcomes as the volatile anaesthetic group [16, 17]. The disadvantages of TIVA are machine errors, underdosing, and overdosing and the use of TIVA requires more skill and training [18]. Therefore, there is no consensus on the appropriateness of TIVA in PE. Utilizing Bispectral Index (BIS) or entropy monitoring can serve as a preventive measure against both awareness and excessive administration of anaesthetic drugs [18].

To prevent profound muscle paralysis, it is recommended to avoid the use of long-acting neuromuscular blocking agents and instead employ peripheral nerve stimulator-guided dosing for neuromuscular blocking agents [19].

Urine output measurement is not meaningful, especially in patients undergoing resection of the bladder and/or ureters, as it may not accurately reflect renal function in such cases. Placement of an arterial line is recommended for continuous invasive blood pressure monitoring, conducting arterial blood gas analysis, and periodically checking haemoglobin levels. Target for maintaining plasma lactate levels is below 1 mmol/L, or as low as possible. In cases where resuscitation with significant volumes of fluid and blood products is necessary, and for the administration of vasopressors and inotropes, it is advisable to secure a central venous line and a large-bore venous catheter [20].

Further assistance from another anaesthesia consultant should be considered, particularly in long-duration surgery (>12–18 h) or high-risk surgery [4].

13.6 How Will you Ensure Smooth Coordination of Care?

Advocating for standardized protocols and heightened patient safety, the imperative is to universally implement the World Health Organization's surgical checklist across healthcare settings worldwide. Elevating patient outcomes requires the establishment of effective, multidisciplinary collaboration and seamless inter-professional coordination in the delivery of healthcare services. Implementing regular, combined and structured preoperative team briefings has proven effective in significantly reducing disruptions to the workflow during surgery. Encouraging open communication and the exchange of critical surgical, anaesthetic, nursing, and logistical concerns is vital for comprehensive and effective patient care [21, 22].

13.7 What Is the Role of Mechanical and Pharmacological Thromboprophylaxis?

Given the heightened risk of postoperative venous thromboembolic (VTE) complications in individuals undergoing extensive abdominal and pelvic procedures, the appropriateness of using pharmacological methods for preventing thromboembolism during the perioperative period is a subject of ongoing debate. This discussion is particularly pertinent in the case of Asian surgical patients, who, notably, exhibit a substantially lower risk of developing VTE complications compared to other populations [4, 23]. Routine mechanical thromboprophylaxis, employing appropriately sized compression stockings and/or intermittent pneumatic compression devices, should be consistently administered until the patient is discharged from the medical care facility [24]. There is a lack of widespread agreement on the routine administration of LMWH within the first 24 h of the perioperative period [4]. Administering routine antibiotic prophylaxis within 60 min before the incision is recommended, ensuring broad coverage for both aerobic and anaerobic microorganisms. This approach should be guided by the patient's allergic status [25].

13.8 What Is the Correct Positioning of the Patient During PE?

The surgical table should possess complete manoeuvrability and adaptability while ensuring optimal stability. Place the patient in a low dorsal lithotomy position. Support the hips, knees and thighs using the stirrups. Operating table mattresses can be paired with non-slip warming gel pads to ensure increased stability and offer protection against hypothermia. Prudent utilization of protective padding, particularly in the sacral region, is essential to prevent the occurrence of pressure ulcers. Careful positioning also helps in the prevention of peripheral nerve injuries that can be caused by stretching, compression, ischemia, or trauma [4, 8].

13.9 What Are Your Strategies for Intraoperative Fluid Management?

Intraoperative fluid management aims to restore and maintain euvolemia. The strategies commonly involved are:

- Restrictive fluid therapy: This approach, characterized by maintaining a zero-fluid balance, aims to prevent fluid overload by replenishing only the amount lost during surgery. In a multicentre randomized controlled trial (RCT) involving patients undergoing elective colorectal surgery, comparable postoperative outcomes were observed between restrictive fluid therapy and goal-directed fluid therapy (GDFT) [26].
- In a meta-analysis involving patients undergoing elective major abdominal surgery, the authors found no benefit of GDFT compared to a fixed-volume regimen in the setting of the ERAS protocol. GDFT is recommended primarily for high-risk patients and in surgeries where substantial intravascular fluid loss is anticipated [7, 27]. As pelvic exenteration is a high-risk surgery with large fluid shifts anticipated and patients often have significant comorbidities, GDFT should be considered. GDFT allows for the dynamic adjustment of fluid administration based on real-time hemodynamic monitoring, optimizing patient outcomes by maintaining euvolemia and ensuring adequate tissue perfusion during this complex procedure [4].
- GDFT aims to optimize hemodynamic status by ensuring effective oxygen supply to tissues through prudent fluid administration and inotropic support. This optimization is guided by monitoring variables such as cardiac output, stroke

volume variation, and cardiac index. Inotropes should be used when there is low cardiac contractility (cardiac index <2.5 L/min/m^2) [26].
- Fixed-volume approach: This represents a conventional approach wherein fluid administration relies on predefined formulas (e.g., the 4-2-1 rule). Such practices may result in volume overload and have adverse effects on patient outcomes [28].

13.10 How Will you Prevent Intraoperative Hypothermia?

To maintain normothermia, accurate measurement of temperature is required. Various sites are used to measure core temperature, such as the nasopharynx (with probe inserted 10–20 cm into the nares), distal oesophagus, etc. Intraoperative hypothermia may lead to coagulopathy, suppression of immune function, cardiovascular challenges, and an augmented vulnerability to infectious complications. Hypothermia is more prone to occur during extended surgical procedures, in individuals with low body fat, and in patients with concurrent medical conditions, especially in the elderly [29].

The methods described to prevent intraoperative hypothermia are:

- Prewarming before induction of anaesthesia to ameliorate redistribution hypothermia
- Anaesthetic gas humidification
- Warming intravenous and irrigation fluids
- Implementing forced-air warming blankets and devices for enhanced thermal control [30]

13.11 How Do you Anticipate Possible Massive Haemorrhage?

In PE, avoiding haemodynamic instability due to massive haemorrhage is a major challenge for the anaesthetist. The extent of blood loss is contingent upon the tumour's location and its association with surrounding structures or fibrosis.

Sudden and substantial haemorrhage from the iliac vasculature and the sacral venous plexus may occur. Swift and vigorous resuscitation with intravenous fluids and blood products is imperative to avert complications. Preoperative haemoglobin optimization is crucial, though there is a lack of consensus regarding the cut-off haemoglobin level. Intravenous iron infusion to replenish iron stores may decrease the likelihood of requiring allogeneic blood transfusions and reduce the potential for perioperative morbidity. The utilization of antifibrinolytic agents, such as tranexamic acid, during surgery can diminish the probability and magnitude of bleeding throughout the procedure. It is recommended to have multiple (at least two) units of blood cross-matched for each patient. Each institution should establish a robust massive transfusion protocol, routinely audited to ensure logistical readiness when necessary [4, 31].

In situations of active massive haemorrhage, it is advisable to tailor blood transfusion strategies dynamically based on evolving circumstances and point-of-care testing of blood, such as thromboelastography.

This facilitates precise blood component therapy and enhances the efficient utilization of components [32]. Implementing bundled intervention has been tried to optimize blood transfusion practices [33]. This comprehensive bundle comprised the standardization of blood transfusion practices in accordance with validated institutional guidelines, incorporating recommendations from reputable organizations such as the American Association of Blood Banks and the American Society of Anesthesiologists. Additionally, it included the systematic use of an intraoperative haemostasis checklist before closure, uniform communication of intraoperative fluid status for every 500 mL of fluid in the suction canister, and evidence-based administration of tranexamic acid (15 mg/kg) within 30 min of incision to optimize surgical outcomes.

13.12 What Are your Strategies for Pain Management?

There should be a multi-modal pain management plan. There is increasing evidence about opioid-sparing approaches that result in

- Quicker restoration of gastrointestinal function.
- Shortened hospitalization duration, contributing to a more efficient recovery process.
- Decreased occurrence of postoperative complications [34].

Various opioid-sparing modalities may be used such as

- Epidural analgesia
  - Attenuate the autonomic response through neuraxial blockade. A decrease in postoperative morbidity and mortality is linked to a lowered incidence of complications in the cardiopulmonary and gastrointestinal systems, contributing to improved overall patient outcomes. Tunnelling the epidural catheter is advisable to potentially extend its duration. Potential adverse effects may include hypotension, itching, inadequate block, and, in rare instances, serious neurological complications.
- Spinal analgesia
- Intravenous lignocaine infusion
- Intravenous ketamine infusion
- Gabapentanoids
- Transverse abdominis plane block
- Continuous infusion of local anaesthetics into the wound through a catheter [4, 35]

13.13 How Would you Manage Stress Responses and What Are Your Strategies for Postoperative Care?

A significant systemic inflammatory response (SIR) may ensue, resulting in hemodynamic instability necessitating the use of vasopressors and inotropes. The first drug recommended is noradrenaline. Patients who develop major SIR and are on vasopressors and inotropes should be shifted to the critical care unit prior to extubation. Postoperatively, admission to a critical care unit is typically necessary for invasive monitoring and/or measurement of organ support. Although preoperative assessment is very important, the SIR encountered cannot be predicted from it. The stress response related to surgery can be reduced through:

- Neuraxial blockade
- Early identification and timely recognition of systemic inflammatory response syndrome (SIRS)
- Judicious fluid administration. GDFT in high-risk cases to optimize hemodynamic status [4].

To maintain a stable postoperative course, the following strategies should be followed:

- Maintain a stable haematocrit level
- Maintain normal prothrombin and partial thromboplastin levels
- Measure serum protein levels
- Frequent blood count and electrolyte measurements
- Adequate pain control
- Ambulation or at least out of bed within 48 h

With regard to postoperative nutrition, if bowel integrity is confirmed, early oral feeding can be started in stable, alert patients. Chronic malnourished patients may be started on total parenteral nutrition after surgery and continued until bowel integrity is confirmed and oral intake is adequate [4, 5, 8].

13.14 What Are the Postoperative Complications?

The postoperative complications are mentioned in Table 13.3 [3, 36].

Table 13.3 Postoperative complications of pelvic exenteration

Early complications	Late complications	Other complications
– Haemorrhage – Sepsis – Wound dehiscence – Anastomotic breakdown	– Gastrointestinal fistula – Genitourinary fistula – Ileus/bowel obstruction – Strictures – Kidney failure – Pyelonephritis – Stomal stenosis	– Deep venous thrombosis – Pulmonary embolism – Flap and stomal necrosis

References

1. Brunschwig A. Complete excision of pelvic viscera for advanced carcinoma; a one-stage abdominoperineal operation with end colostomy and bilateral ureteral implantation into the colon above the colostomy. Cancer. 1948;1:177–83.
2. Kim J. Pelvic exenteration: surgical approaches. J Korean Soc Coloproctol. 2012;28:286–93.
3. Grimes WR, Stratton M. Pelvic exenteration. StatPearls; 2022.
4. Perioperative management and anaesthetic considerations in pelvic exenterations using Delphi methodology: results from the PelvEx Collaborative. BJS Open. 2021;5:zraa055.
5. Ng K-S, Lee PJM. Pelvic exenteration: pre-, intra-, and post-operative considerations. Surg Oncol. 2021;37:101546.
6. Molenaar CJ, van Rooijen SJ, Fokkenrood HJ, Roumen RM, Janssen L, Slooter GD. Prehabilitation versus no prehabilitation to improve functional capacity, reduce postoperative complications and improve quality of life in colorectal cancer surgery. Cochrane Database Syst Rev. 2022;5:CD013259.
7. Gustafsson UO, Scott MJ, Hubner M, et al. Guidelines for perioperative care in elective colorectal surgery: enhanced recovery after surgery (ERAS®) society recommendations: 2018. World J Surg. 2019;43:659–95.
8. Diver EJ, Rauh-Hain JA, Del Carmen MG. Total pelvic exenteration for gynecologic malignancies. Int J Surg Oncol. 2012;2012:693535.
9. Salicath JH, Yeoh EC, Bennett MH. Epidural analgesia versus patient-controlled intravenous analgesia for pain following intra-abdominal surgery in adults. Cochrane Database Syst Rev. 2018;8:CD010434.
10. Garcia A, Clark EA, Rana S, Preciado D, Jeha GM, Viswanath O, Urits I, Kaye AD, Abdallah C. Effects of premedication with midazolam on recovery and discharge times after tonsillectomy and adenoidectomy. Cureus. 13:e13101.
11. Lee JH, Kang SH, Kim Y, Kim HA, Kim BS. Effects of propofol-based total intravenous anesthesia on recurrence and overall survival in patients after modified radical mastectomy: a retrospective study. Korean J Anesthesiol. 2016;69:126–32.
12. Lai H-C, Lee M-S, Lin C, Lin K-T, Huang Y-H, Wong C-S, Chan S-M, Wu Z-F. Propofol-based total intravenous anaesthesia is associated with better survival than desflurane anaesthesia in hepatectomy for hepatocellular carcinoma: a retrospective cohort study. Br J Anaesth. 2019;123:151–60.
13. Yoo Y-C, Bai S-J, Lee K-Y, Shin S, Choi EK, Lee JW. Total intravenous anesthesia with Propofol reduces postoperative nausea and vomiting in patients undergoing robot-assisted laparoscopic radical prostatectomy: a prospective randomized trial. Yonsei Med J. 2012;53:1197–202.
14. Enlund M, Berglund A, Ahlstrand R, Walldén J, Lundberg J, Wärnberg F, Ekman A, Sjöblom Widfeldt N, Enlund A, Bergkvist L. Survival after primary breast cancer surgery following propofol or sevoflurane general anesthesia—A retrospective, multicenter, database analysis of 6305 Swedish patients. Acta Anaesthesiol Scand. 2020;64:1048–54.
15. Wigmore TJ, Mohammed K, Jhanji S. Long-term survival for patients undergoing volatile versus IV anesthesia for cancer surgery: a retrospective analysis. Anesthesiology. 2016;124:69–79.
16. Makito K, Matsui H, Fushimi K, Yasunaga H. Volatile versus total intravenous anesthesia for cancer prognosis in patients having digestive cancer surgery. Anesthesiology. 2020;133:764–73.
17. Yoo S, Lee H-B, Han W, Noh D-Y, Park S-K, Kim WH, Kim J-T. Total intravenous anesthesia versus inhalation anesthesia for breast cancer surgery: a retrospective cohort study. Anesthesiology. 2019;130:31–40.
18. Nimmo AF, Absalom AR, Bagshaw O, et al. Guidelines for the safe practice of total intravenous anaesthesia (TIVA): joint guidelines from the Association of Anaesthetists and the Society for Intravenous Anaesthesia. Anaesthesia. 2019;74:211–24.
19. Adeyinka A, Layer DA. Neuromuscular blocking agents. StatPearls; 2022.
20. Brienza N, Biancofiore G, Cavaliere F, et al. Clinical guidelines for perioperative hemodynamic management of non cardiac surgical adult patients. Minerva Anestesiol. 2019;85:1315–33.
21. Russ S, Rout S, Sevdalis N, Moorthy K, Darzi A, Vincent C. Do safety checklists improve teamwork and communication in the operating room? A systematic review. Ann Surg. 2013;258:856–71.

22. Henrickson SE, Wadhera RK, Elbardissi AW, Wiegmann DA, Sundt TM. Development and pilot evaluation of a preoperative briefing protocol for cardiovascular surgery. J Am Coll Surg. 2009;208:1115–23.
23. Ngarmukos S, Kim K-I, Wongsak S, Chotanaphuti T, Inaba Y, Chen C-F, Liu D. Asia-Pacific venous thromboembolism consensus in knee and hip arthroplasty and hip fracture surgery: part 1. Diagnosis and risk factors. Knee Surg Relat Res. 2021;33:18.
24. Sachdeva A, Dalton M, Lees T. Graduated compression stockings for prevention of deep vein thrombosis. Cochrane Database Syst Rev. 2018;2018:CD001484.
25. Perioperative antibiotics. J Orthop Res. 2014;32:S31–S59.
26. Brandstrup B, Svendsen PE, Rasmussen M, et al. Which goal for fluid therapy during colorectal surgery is followed by the best outcome: near-maximal stroke volume or zero fluid balance? Br J Anaesth. 2012;109:191–9.
27. Rollins KE, Lobo DN. Intraoperative goal-directed fluid therapy in elective major abdominal surgery: a meta-analysis of randomized controlled trials. Ann Surg. 2016;263:465–76.
28. Malbrain MLNG, Langer T, Annane D, et al. Intravenous fluid therapy in the perioperative and critical care setting: executive summary of the international fluid academy (IFA). Ann Intensive Care. 2020;10:64.
29. Sessler DI. Temperature monitoring and perioperative thermoregulation. Anesthesiology. 2008;109:318–38.
30. Simegn GD, Bayable SD, Fetene MB. Prevention and management of perioperative hypothermia in adult elective surgical patients: a systematic review. Ann Med Surg (Lond). 2021;72:103059.
31. Thomas D, Wee M, Clyburn P, Walker I, Brohi K, Collins P, Doughty H, Isaac J, Mahoney P, Shewry L. Blood transfusion and the anaesthetist: management of massive haemorrhage. Anaesthesia. 2010;65:1153–61.
32. Sirohiya P, Kumar V. Transfusion therapy: when to give it and how to minimize it. 2022. pp. 195–204.
33. Wallace SK, Halverson JW, Jankowski CJ, DeJong SR, Weaver AL, Weinhold MR, Borah BJ, Moriarty JP, Cliby WA, Kor DJ, Higgins AA, Otto HA, Dowdy SC, Bakkum-Gamez JN. Optimizing blood transfusion practices through bundled intervention implementation in patients with gynecologic cancer undergoing laparotomy. Obstet Gynecol. 2018;131(5):891–8. https://doi.org/10.1097/AOG.0000000000002463.
34. Kaye AD, Urman RD, Rappaport Y, Siddaiah H, Cornett EM, Belani K, Salinas OJ, Fox CJ. Multimodal analgesia as an essential part of enhanced recovery protocols in the ambulatory settings. J Anaesthesiol Clin Pharmacol. 2019;35:S40–5.
35. Bauer M, George JE, Seif J, Farag E. Recent advances in epidural analgesia. Anesthesiol Res Pract. 2012;2012:309219.
36. Exenteration for gynecologic cancer—UpToDate. https://www.uptodate.com/contents/exenteration-for-gynecologic-cancer?search=anesthesia%20for%20pelvic%20exenteration&source=search_result&selectedTitle=2~150&usage_type=default&display_rank=2#H23. Accessed 21 Aug 2022.

14 Anaesthetic Management of Cytoreductive Surgery and Hyperthermic Intraperitoneal Chemotherapy

Anuja Pandit

14.1 Case

A 53-year-old male k/c/o of ca colon post NACT is posted for CRS + HIPEC surgery. He is a known diabetic for 2 years. At presentation he has a history of abdominal pain and distension—3 months, loss of weight 15 kg in 3 months and altered bowel habits. How do we proceed?

14.2 HIPEC

Cytoreductive surgery (CRS) entails removing the macroscopic disease whereas HIPEC is the instillation of chemotherapy at high temperature inside the peritoneal cavity to eliminate microscopic disease, after CRS [1].

14.2.1 What Are the Indications/Contraindications for HIPEC?

The indications and contraindications for HIPEC are mentioned in Table 14.1.

A. Pandit (✉)
Department of Oncoanaesthesia and Palliative Medicine, National Cancer Institute, AIIMS, New Delhi, India

14.2.2 What Are the Criteria for Patient Selection for These Procedures

Factors taken into consideration for appropriately selecting patients for this procedure are mentioned in Table 14.2 [2].

14.2.3 What Are the Disease Scoring Systems Used for Patient Selection/Prognostication in HIPEC?

The scoring systems PCI and CC [3] are used as intraoperative prognostic indicators in peritoneal surface malignancy by quantifying the amount of disease in the peritoneum at the beginning of the surgery and the macroscopic residual disease after cytoreduction.

PCI: Peritoneal Cancer Index [3]

- It illustrates the extent of disease burden.
- For each lesion, a score is given based on its size.
- Abdomen and pelvis are assigned 9 regions and intestines are allotted 4 regions.
- PCI score is estimated by totalling scores for each region to get score from 1 to 39
- If PCI > 20
- **5-year survival**: 50% for PCI < 10, 20% for 11–20 and 0% for PCI > 20.

N. Gupta et al. (eds.), *Problem Based Learning Discussions in Onco-Anesthesia and Onco-Critical Care*, https://doi.org/10.1007/978-981-99-6339-3_14

Table 14.1 Indications and contraindications for HIPEC

Indications	Contraindications
Classical indications • **Pseudomyxoma peritonei** • Peritoneal malignant mesothelioma • Peritoneal sarcomatosis • **Peritoneal carcinomatosis** of ovarian or colorectal origin • Appendicular tumours • Absence of extra abdominal metastasis • High probability of complete macroscopic surgical resection **Relative** • **Palliation** of malignant ascites • **Prophylactic procedure** in patients with high risk of acquiring peritoneal metastases • **Perforated gastrointestinal tumours** or invading adjacent organs • Gastric, hepatobiliary, and pancreatic tumours	**Absolute** • Extra abdominal metastasis • Substantial extraperitoneal spread, for example, more than three liver metastases • Sizeable retroperitoneal lymph nodes • Infiltrative tumour deposits at the root of mesentery and porta hepatis • Unknown primary tumour **Relative** • Age of patient >70 years • Multiple co-morbidities • Grade 3 adenocarcinoma • Synchronic peritoneal carcinomatosis following diagnosis of primary adenocarcinoma • Frozen pelvis owing to a rectal cancer recurrence • Pancreatic, biliary and hepatic origin • PCI > 20 • Clinical aggravation with systemic chemotherapy

Table 14.2 Factors for patient selection

Patient-related Factors	Disease-related factors
1. Performance status—ECOG **0/1** 2. Age: • **<70 years** • Patients >**65** years of age without comorbidities, with a low PCI and a low-grade malignancy • Age less than **65** years with medical comorbidities in control 3. BMI <**35** (Preferably) 4. Preoperative serum albumin level > **3 g/dL** 5. Prior systemic chemotherapy • Based on drug type and response to therapy • Platinum-based, needs dose modification • Stable disease • Early recurrence (<6 months) • Progressive disease is a poor predictor of CRS-HIPEC 6. Written/informed consent with an understanding of risk involved	1. Low PCI (Peritoneal Cancer Index) • Colorectal cancer: PCI < 15 • Gastric cancer PCI < 6 2. Predicted CC Score (Sugar baker's Completeness of Cytoreduction) –0/1 3. Less than three intraoperative anastomoses

- PCI >20, HIPEC should not be done. Palliation is the goal of treatment, relative contraindication for elective intervention for colon cancer.

CC: Sugarbaker's Completeness of Cytoreduction [3]

CCR 0	No residual peritoneal seeding following cytoreduction
CCR 1	<2.5 mm diameter of tumour nodules remaining after cytoreduction
CCR 2	>2.5 mm to <2.5 cm diameter of tumour nodules after cytoreduction
CCR 3	>2.5 cm diameter of tumour nodules after cytoreduction or a confluence of unresectable tumour nodules

14.2.4 What Is the Rationale Behind HIPEC?

1. ***The pharmacokinetic benefit of intraperitoneal chemotherapy administration***
   - Cytotoxic medicines can be delivered intraperitoneally to obtain high localized concentrations while maintaining low systemic level of drug. A 'Three Compartment Model' elucidates a pharmacokinetic advantage where the drug is absorbed by tissue penetration into the tumour-bearing peritoneum where a high concentration gradient of chemotherapeutic drug is

achieved. This 'peritoneal-plasma barrier' acts as a third compartment between the two compartments of peritoneal cavity and the plasma [4, 5]

- Additionally, the liver receives peritoneal surface drainage through the portal vein, which has a first-pass (detoxifying) effect and improves the exposure of possible hepatic micrometastases to cytotoxic medications [6]
- *Pharmacokinetic advantage of* HIPEC PLUS: Third compartment is also accessible via systemic drug administration through subperitoneal capillaries; which supports 'bidirectional" chemotherapy regimen.

2. ***Tissue penetration***

Drugs administered intraperitoneally have a maximum penetration depth of 3–5 mm [7, 8]. A satisfactory cytoreductive surgery should therefore be achieved before the intraperitoneal delivery of drugs.

3. ***Hyperthermia***

The rationale for the use of hyperthermia is summarized in Fig. 14.1.

Hyperthermia between 41 and 43 °C selectively kills malignant cells [9, 10]

- Hyperthermia reversibly and nonselectively inhibits synthesis of RNA and halts mitosis.
- Hyperthermia selectively increases the number of lysosomes and lysosomal enzyme activity in malignant cells, which thereby increases their destruction.
- Moreover, in response to heat, microcirculation of most malignant tumours shows a reduction in blood flow or vascular stasis (contrary to an increased flow in normal tissues) [11]. As a result, anaerobic glycolysis is unaffected and oxidative metabolism is inhibited, which lowers pH and affects buildup of lactic acid in the malignant cell's microenvironment. The intracellular acidosis augments the activity of the lysosomes, which triggers cell death of the more friable malignant cells exposed to hyperthermia in comparison to normal cells [10]
- ***Increased cytotoxicity due to heat:*** Heat and cytotoxic drugs work synergistically to improve membrane permeability and transport, which increases drug uptake in malignant cells. Greater tumour penetration—with heat 3–6 mm, without heat 1–3 mm.
- Heat alters drug pharmacokinetics and excretion as well as the cellular metabolism, thereby enhancing the cytotoxicity of some chemotherapeutic drugs [12]

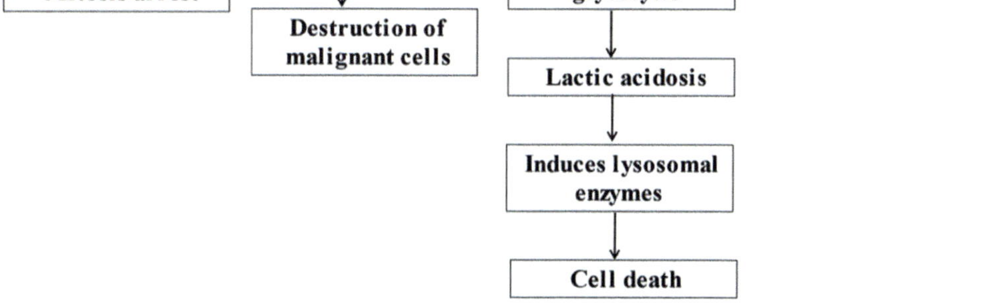

Fig. 14.1 Mechanism of hyperthermic destruction of malignant cells

- ***Other considerations*** consist of enhanced drug penetration in tissue, temperature-dependent rise in drug activity and inhibition of healing processes.
- Hyperthermia also reduced the cellular resistance to cisplatin.

14.2.5 What Are the Methods/Techniques for Intraperitoneal Administration of Hyperthermic Chemotherapy?

- Closed abdomen technique
- Open abdomen technique
- PCE—peritoneal cavity expander
- PIPAC

1. ***Open abdomen technique***
   - Sugarbaker's 'Coliseum method' is typically used to perform it. Through the Tenckhoff catheter, a roller pump drives chemotherapy perfusion into the abdomen at a flow rate of roughly 1 L/min, and draws it out through the drains.
   - Recirculating the medication and perfusate into and out of the peritoneal cavity requires maintaining an intraperitoneal temperature minimum of 41.5 °C. A heat exchanger maintains the temperature of infusate at 43–45 °C so that the intraperitoneal fluid is preserved at 41–43 °C.
2. **Closed abdomen technique**
   - Temperature probes and catheters are inserted and laparotomy skin edges are sutured firm and perfusion is carried out in a closed circuit. During the perfusion period, abdomen is physically agitated in an effort to enhance an even heat distribution.
   - The abdomen is reopened after perfusion, and the perfusate is removed.
3. **Peritoneal cavity expander**
   - PCE is a modification of the open abdomen technique. It is secured over the incision and consists of an acrylic cylinder with in- and out-flow catheters within. The small intestine can fit inside the PCE when it is filled with heated perfusate, permitting it to float easily and be handled in the perfusate.
   - Advantage—Compared to a closed approach, an advantage is a more even drug and heat distribution.
4. **Pressurized intraperitoneal aerosol chemotherapy**
   - A method of administering normothermic chemotherapy as an aerosol under pressure into the abdominal cavity, which has been shown to be helpful by compensating for the higher interstitial fluid pressure in the tumour [13–15] and improving drug penetration and distribution.

14.2.6 What Are the Advantages and Disadvantages of Open and Closed Technique?

The advantages and disadvantages of the two common techniques are discussed in Table 14.3.

14.2.7 What Is the Choice of Chemotherapeutic Drug and Drug Dosaging for HIPEC? What Are its Implications on Perioperative Period?

- Drug ought to *have a well-recognized action against the malignancy being treated.*
- Following intraperitoneal administration, *the drug should not cause severe direct local toxicity.*
- It is recommended to use standard doses of the medication based on body surface area as well as the volume of the carrier solution [12]
- TARGET—Maximize the implicated tissue's exposure to high chemotherapeutic drug concentrations (20–1000 times higher than plasma levels) and reducing the contact of healthy tissue.

Table 14.3 Advantages and disadvantages of open and closed abdomen techniques

Open abdomen technique	Closed abdomen technique
Advantages • There is no temperature or chemotherapy pooling and the heated drug is evenly disseminated across the abdominal cavity	***Advantages*** • Hyperthermia is rapidly achieved • Heat loss is minimal • Minimal chemotherapeutic aerosol exposure of the personnel present in operating room • When the abdomen is closed, intraabdominal pressure increases, facilitating the drug's deeper absorption • Minimal drug spillage
Disadvantages • Heat dissipation—more challenging to initially reach and retain hyperthermic state • Increased risk of chemotherapeutic aerosol exposure of the operating room crew • Potential for contact exposure • Risk of spillage of cytotoxic drugs	***Disadvantages*** • The chemotherapy may not be distributed evenly. Increased risk of intra-abdominal complications due to varied dissemination within the closed abdomen • Pooling of drug causes foci of hyperthermic injury in dependent parts of the abdominal cavity leading to bowel perforation or fistula, postoperative ileus • Increased risk of systemic absorption and toxicity

14.2.8 What Are Adverse Effects of Specific Chemotherapeutic Agents Used for HIPEC?

Adverse effects from intraperitoneal chemotherapeutic medicines might result from both the drug's and its carrier solution's absorption. These may include postoperative nausea, effects on wound healing, bone marrow suppression, and organ toxicity. The adverse effects of chemotherapy agents used for HIPEC are shown in Table 14.4.

14.2.9 What Different Evaluations/Preoperative Risk Assessment Are Required for This Patient Apart from Routine Assessment?

Besides routine operative risk assessment for a major surgery, preoperative management of CRS-HIPEC patients should be individualized depending on patient and disease-related factors [17]. Identifiable risk factors should be evaluated and addressed.

- **Patient-related factors**
  - Patients' age, Body mass index, the patient's height, weight, and body surface area should be recorded in order to determine the anaesthesia and chemotherapy dosages. Functional status, ASA classification, ECOG performance status
  - Comorbid diseases
- **Disease-related factors**
  - Disease burden
  - Nutritional status-BMI, Albumin, SGA
  - Presence or absence of hypoalbuminemia/malnutrition
  - Presence or absence of anaemia preoperatively
  - Previous chemotherapy received, their response and toxicity should be recorded
  - Altered renal, liver & cardiac function that may require dose adjustments
  - Organ-specific preoperative concerns are summarized in Table 14.5

Table 14.4 Chemotherapy agents commonly used for heated intraperitoneal chemotherapy [16]

Class	Chemotherapy		Carrier solution	Adverse effects
Platinum-based chemotherapy	Cisplatin	Ovary stomach mesothelioma	0.9% sodium chloride/ peritoneal dialysate solution	• Nephrotoxicity/AKI • Peripheral neuropathy • Myelotoxicity • Prolonged QT, pulseless VT, hyponatremia
	Oxaliplatin	Colon, appendix, rectum	5% dextrose	• Thrombocytopenia • Gastrointestinal haemorrhage • Electrolyte disturbances (hyponatremia, hyperglycaemia) • Neurotoxicity (laryngeal/ pharyngeal dysesthesias)
	Carboplatin		0.9% sodium chloride	• Postoperative nausea • Thrombocytopenia
Non-platinum-based chemotherapy	Mitomycin (alkylating tumour antibiotic)	Colorectal cancer Pseudomyxoma peritonei	1.5% dextrose dialysis solution	• Neutropenia • Nephrotoxicity • Pulmotoxicity interstitial lung disease (dose-dependent) • Myelosuppression • Neurotoxicity
	Doxorubicin (anthracycline antibiotic)	Ovary stomach mesothelioma	1.5% dextrose dialysis solution	• Cardiotoxicity (arrhythmias, cardiomyopathy) • Myelotoxicity • Neurotoxicity

Table 14.5 Systemic alterations and preoperative concerns

Expected alterations	Concerns—preoperative
Respiratory function	
• Ascites • Pleural effusion • Basal atelectasis • Diaphragmatic splinting • Decreased FRC	• Patients at risk of hypoxia • Inv-Chest X-ray, ABG, PFT, CPET • Optimization and incentive spirometry • Prehabilitation • Preoxygenation at induction of anaesthesia • Abstinence from smoking and alcohol
CVS	
• Comorbidities	• ECHO indicated in h/o heart failure and chemotherapy-induced cardiotoxicity • CPET
Coagulation homeostasis	
• Decreased platelet count due to preoperative chemotherapy • Deranged INR due to preoperative nutritional deficiencies	• PT, INR and aPTT testing preoperatively [18] Epidural to be placed only if INR and platelet counts are WNL
Renal function and electrolyte balance	
Risk of AKI due to major fluid loss and chemotherapy-induced nephrotoxicity	• Baseline KFT and electrolytes to be done • In gross ascites and raised IAP, ureteric stenting to be done prophylactically preoperatively
Abdomen	
• Increased abdominal girth • Increased IAP due to ascites • Decreased FRC	• Risk of regurgitation and aspiration at induction of anaesthesia, RSI • Premedication with H2 blocker and prokinetic

Table 14.5 (continued)

Expected alterations	Concerns—preoperative
QoL perspective	
	• Preoperative counselling • Pros and cons of the procedure • Need of systemic chemotherapy • Marking and counselling for stoma
Multisystem involvement	
	• High risk explained and postoperative mechanical ventilation consent to be taken, arranging ICU bed
DVT prophylaxis	
• Patients at increased risk of VTE	• LMWH or mechanical pneumatic compression stockings can be started preoperative as per institution protocol
Pain management	
• Large incision • Lots of tissue manipulation and dissection • h/o pain medication	• Thoracic epidural/PCA/PCEA to be explained • IVPCA to be explained if epidural is contraindicated • Timing of regional/epidural placement may have to be timed according to anticoagulant regimen

14.2.10 What Is the Role of Prehabilitation in This Patient?

Prior to surgery, prehabilitation aims to improve the patient's functional ability so that he or she would be better able better withstand a stressful event.

The components of prehabilitation include

1. **Medical optimization**
   - Preoperative diagnosis and correction of anaemia is indicated. Patients should undergo an anaemia screening at least 30 days before surgery in order to allow time for treatment.
   - For iron deficiency anaemia, oral or intravenous iron supplementation can be taken into consideration; to improve haemoglobin by 0.5–1 g/dL per week.
   - Treatment with folate/vitamin B12 replacement or erythropoietin where indicated.
   - Preoperative blood transfusions for difficult refractory anaemia.
   - It is recommended to stop smoking and alcohol consumption (alcohol abusers) 4 weeks prior to surgery.
     - Alcohol—Moderate to excessive alcohol intake impairs recovery, weakens the immune system, increases the risk of bleeding complications, infections, cardiovascular events, and causes alcohol withdrawal symptoms postoperatively.
     - Weekly counselling and nicotine substitution or abstinence are beneficial for postoperative recovery.
2. **Physical exercise/prehabilitation**
   - Prehabilitation with a physical exercise program ought to be recommended.
   - Respiratory exercise training, aerobic and resistance training should be included.
3. **Nutritional support**
   - Preoperative nutritional assessment utilizing a validated tool, and serum albumin measurement should be done.
   - Nutritional correction and protein supplements are indicated in situations of malnutrition.
   - Correction: minimal treatment of 7–14 days.
   - Patients with inadequate oral intake or with severe malnutrition, should receive parenteral nourishment.
4. **Psychological support**
   - Preoperative education, information, and counselling are indicated to alleviate anxiety, better pain control and improve patient satisfaction.
   - Prior to surgery, patient-reported outcome indicators, such as quality of life, physical

symptoms, and psychological outcomes, may improve with psychological pre-habilitation.
- Plan for pain management should be discussed preoperatively with the patient.
- Stoma counselling & marking should be done in upright position

14.2.11 What Are the Anaesthetic Considerations for CRS + HIPEC?

The goals of intraoperative management specific to CRS with HIPEC are to minimize complications from chemotherapy agents and to maintain end-organ perfusion in the face of major fluid and hemodynamic shifts. To achieve these goals, anaesthesiologists must anticipate and manage the hemodynamic changes throughout HIPEC. We divide the anaesthetic management into three major phases: pre-HIPEC, HIPEC, and post-HIPEC phases

14.2.12 Enumerate the Physiological Alterations That May Occur During HIPEC, and Its Anaesthetic Implications

The anticipated physiological alterations that may occur during HIPEC, and its anaesthetic implications are enumerated in Table 14.6.

Table 14.6 Physiological alterations during HIPEC and their anaesthetic implications

Physiological alteration	Anaesthetic implication
Cardiac	
• Hyperdynamic state in HIPEC phase • Increased heart rate and central venous pressure, wedge pressure, pulmonary artery pressure, and cardiac index [19] • Systemic vascular resistance and Mean arterial pressure are reduced during HIPEC phase [19] • A decrease in the abdominal blood volume and a rise in splanchnic vascular resistance leads to reduction in the venous return	• Goal-directed fluid therapy • Vasopressor and inotropes guided by physiologic parameters
Respiratory	
• Increased end-tidal CO_2 levels • Decreased PaO_2/FiO_2 ratio • Increased peak airway pressures • Filling the abdomen with a perfusate-drug solution causes the diaphragm to shift cranially, which lowers functional residual capacity and raises airway pressure • On ABG, increased $PaCO_2$ and a simultaneous decrease in A-a gradient and arterial pH indicate deterioration in gas exchanges • Hypermetabolic state due to hyperthermia leading to increase in oxygen extraction and consumption and increased end-tidal CO_2	• Low FRC, lower apnoea time • Minute ventilation should be increased during the HIPEC phase to normalize $EtCO_2$ • Serial ABGs during HIPEC phase to assess adequacy of ventilation and oxygenation
Renal	
• Reduced renal perfusion • Metabolic acidosis and raised lactate levels • Nephrotoxicity due to platinum-based compounds • Systemic hypoperfusion due to inadequate fluid resuscitation may lead to acute renal failure leading to lactic acidosis • Chemotherapeutic agents like mitomycin-c and cisplatin aggravate nephrotoxicity	• Urinary output of at least 0.5 (CRS phase), 2–4 (HIPEC phase), and 1–2 (reconstruction phase) mL/kg/h • Preoperative KFT should be done • Maintenance of adequate intravascular volume before the beginning of the HIPEC phase

Table 14.6 (continued)

Physiological alteration	Anaesthetic implication
Coagulation	

• Hyperthermia-associated coagulopathy
  • Decreased platelet count
  • Increased prothrombin time (PT) and international normalized ratio (INR)
• Aetiology
  • Massive fluid shift and bleeding
  • Massive ascites-protein loss
  • Hyperthermia
  • Chemotherapeutic toxicity
  • Nutritional deficiency
• Coagulopathy peaks within 24–48 h after surgery, and coagulation profile returns to normal within 72 h
• Various studies have reported the prolongation of prothrombin time (PT), activated partial thromboplastin time (PTT), and/or pathological reduction of platelets count over the baseline
	• Preoperative coagulation tests to be done
	• Point of care coagulation function testing—TEG, thrombocyte function analyser, ROTEM (rotational thromboelastometry) may be used if available
	• If blood loss exceeds 50% of the total volume of blood, PT, aPTT, and INR tests should be done during the intraoperative phase and following the HIPEC phase [18]

Hyperthermia	
• Peripheral vasodilatation • Increased metabolic rate • Increased O_2 demand • Increased HR • Increased $ETCO_2$ • Metabolic acidosis • Increased lactate, dyselectrolytemia	• Core temperature monitoring (oesophageal) • Switch off forced air warmers • Cooled infusions • Increase minute ventilation, lactic acid and electrolyte measurement—serial ABGs

14.2.13 What Risks Are Present During Induction of This Patient? How Are They Planned for?

- The ascites-related abdominal distension that these patients typically experience reduces their functional residual capacity.
- The patient is at risk for increased aspiration and desaturation.
- During induction of anaesthesia, rapid sequence induction may be used.
- The above-mentioned case is a diabetic and may present with difficult airway.

14.2.14 What Precautions/Premedications Would You Take Before Incision?

- PONV prophylaxis: Use of at least 2 anti-emetic drugs (ondansetron, dexamethasone, droperidol)
- Antimicrobial prophylaxis: Prophylactic antibiotics to be administered within 1 h before incision (preferred cephalosporins)
- Chlorhexidine-alcohol as skin disinfectant is preferred over povidone-iodine
- Shaving, antiseptic shower, and adhesive drapes are some other preventive measures

14.2.15 Discuss the Various Intraoperative Monitoring Options

- Standardized monitoring tools (electrocardiogram, pulse oximetry, noninvasive blood pressure, core-body temperature, end-tidal CO_2 monitoring and, BIS monitor)
- Additional hemodynamic monitoring:
  – An arterial catheter should be placed for continuous monitoring of blood pressure, dynamic fluid responsiveness, and frequent blood sampling to evaluate gas exchange,

  - electrolyte and lactate levels, and 1–2 hourly blood glucose levels [20]
  - The anaesthesiology team must closely monitor dynamic fluid responsiveness and cardiac preload indicators including CO, SVV, and SVR to preserve normovolemia and avoid acute renal failure [21]
  - Cardiac output monitoring: During the HIPEC procedure, the FloTrac/Vigileo system offers a simple-to-use, dependable and noninvasive instrument for monitoring hemodynamic changes.
  - Central venous catheters: can be used for administering vasopressors/inotropes.
  - Placement of central venous lines/PA catheters is not required routinely. Central venous pressure is a static parameter. Moreover, due to the raised intraabdominal pressure and alterations in the inclination of the operating table during HIPEC, central venous pressure is an unreliable indicator of cardiac preload.
  - Routine application of advanced invasive hemodynamic monitoring, such as Swan-Ganz catheters or transoesophageal echocardiography, is not recommended.
- Point-of-care coagulation monitoring-TEG.
- Nasopharyngeal/oesophageal temperature probe for core temperature monitoring.
- Urine output monitoring.

14.2.16 Describe the Anaesthetic Drugs of Choice for This Procedure

- Choice of drugs depends upon the patient's comorbidities.
- TIVA is preferred due to its antiemetic effect as these patients are at high risk of PONV. Also, TIVA has been found to cause less inflammation compared to volatile anaesthetics in cancer surgeries and HIPEC.
- Nephrotoxic drugs and analgesics should be avoided.

14.2.17 Discuss the Essential Principles for Fluid Management and Blood Product Transfusion in These Patients

- Fluid management is aimed to achieve normovolemia. Targets may vary during the distinct phases of CRS, HIPEC and post-HIPEC phase (Fig. 14.2).
- During CRS phase—intraoperative 8–12 mL/kg blood loss related to major debulking surgery as well as the evaporative fluid losses related to the open abdomen.
- Significant fluid shifts are caused by a capillary leak that causes large fluid, blood, and protein losses during CRS + HIPEC.
- During surgery, patients may exhibit hyperdynamic circulatory states and vasodilation due to the release of elevated inflammatory mediators [19]
- Monitoring of fluid status is a major part of the anaesthetic plan for preservation of acceptable systemic as well as regional perfusion. The goal is to safeguard end-organ perfusion and preserve hemodynamic targets without producing volume overload.
- In addition to invasive blood pressure monitoring, noninvasive cardiac output monitoring options include arterial-pressure-based cardiac output monitoring [18]
- Use of goal-directed fluid therapy and catecholamine infusions should be guided by advanced/invasive monitoring [22]
- Replacement of losses (fluids and protein) by use of crystalloids may be indicated. 9–12 mL/kg/h fluids have been advocated, in particular if platinum derivatives are used to safeguard a reasonable urinary output (at least 1 mL/kg/h) [22]
- Balanced salt solutions like Ringer's lactate and acetate-based solution are preferred [18]. Albumin must be used as the colloid of choice [18]. Patients with low serum protein levels may benefit from albumin, which has been

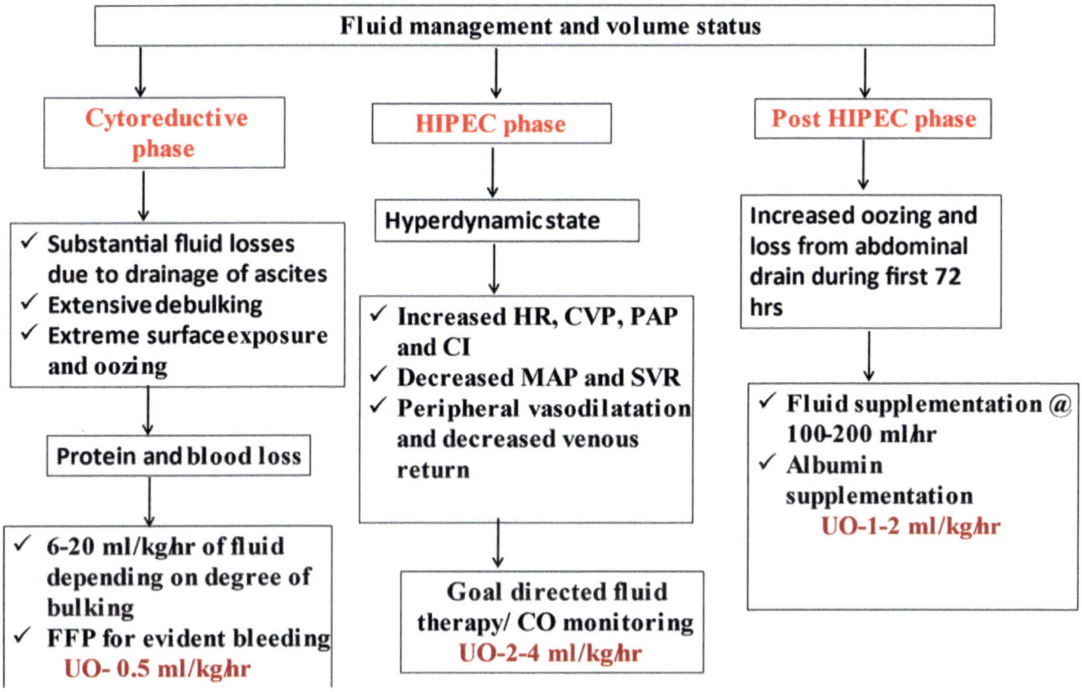

Fig. 14.2 Fluid management during CRS, HIPEC and post-HIPEC phase

demonstrated to be helpful in cases requiring large-volume ascites drainage and substantial surgical debulking.

- Postoperative fluid-related weight gain should be monitored [23]. It should be limited (target: <3.5 kg on postoperative day 3) to lower morbidity, hospital and ICU length of stay and time to recovery of bowel function.
- In certain situations when urine output is inadequate despite sufficient intravascular fluid therapy, diuretics may be necessary [18]
- Sodium thiosulphate has been used to prevent cisplatin-induced nephrotoxicity (under investigation) [24]

14.2.18 What Will Be Your Approach Towards Transfusion of Blood Products During This Surgery?

- Restrictive transfusion practices should be adopted [22] (with a transfusion Hb threshold level of 8 g/dL).
- Tranexemic acid alone or with cryoprecipitate may be administered if indicated [22] to lower the risk of bleeding during CRS ± HIPEC.
- Prothrombin complex concentrate may be administered [22] to reverse the anticoagulant effects of vitamin K antagonists.
- Survival benefits were imparted by a high FFP:RBC ratio, with a ratio of 1:1.5 being the highest survival benefit [25]

14.2.19 Why Is It Important to Monitor Coagulation Status of These Patients in the Perioperative Period?

- CAUSE of coagulopathy: preoperative nutritional deficiencies, hypoalbuminemia or prior chemotherapy.
- Depends on the duration of surgery, blood loss and degree of haemodilution, and extent of resection (PCI).
- Peaks around 24 h and may persist up to 72 h postoperatively period [19]

- If blood loss exceeds 50% of the total volume of blood, PT, aPTT, and INR tests should be done during the intraoperative phase and following the HIPEC phase [18]
- Preemptive/prophylactic treatment of coagulopathy with fresh frozen plasma is not indicated.
- PT, aPTT, and INR testing should be done in the postoperative period.
- Placement and removal of neuraxial catheter should be done keeping the coagulation status in mind.

14.2.20 What Is the Role of Monitoring Urine Output During This Surgery?

- As several chemotherapy drugs are nephrotoxic, measuring urine output is a crucial monitoring parameter. Euvolemia should be ensured.
- Setting a urine output goal of 1 mL/kg/h during CRS and reconstructive phases and 2 mL/kg/h during HIPEC phase [18]
- Urine output goal should be accomplished by use of intravenous fluids and if required diuretics based on clinical scenario [18]. After achieving euvolemia and adequate renal perfusion, a diuretic challenge may be attempted [26]. Furosemide should be administered only when urine output is inadequate despite confirmation of adequate intravascular volume and renal perfusion [27]

14.2.21 Why Do We Need to Cautiously Monitor for Electrolyte Imbalance?

- Dyselectrolytemia tend to differ depending on the agent used for chemotherapy [28, 29] ABGs, biochemistry and haemoglobin should be done 15 min prior to surgery and before the start of heated chemotherapeutic infusion. Rechecking electrolytes after the chemotherapy phase of the procedure is critical.
- When a perfusate of 5% dextrose is used as a carrier for oxaliplatin, hyperglycaemia may lead to intravascular fluid shift and dilutional hyponatremia.
- Cisplatin causes hypomagnesaemia which may lead to cardiac arrhythmias [30]
- Electrolyte disturbances like magnesium, calcium, potassium should be corrected [20]

14.2.22 Why Is Glycaemic Control Difficult in These Patients?

- Barrier to adequate glycaemic control
- Surgery itself (surgical stress causes insulin resistance, fasting induces a catabolic response, fluid administration).
- HIPEC (hyperthermia can lead to high lactate levels leading to acidosis, chemotherapy diluted in dextrose 5% solution, intraperitoneal carrier used).
- Glycaemic changes are very rapid and short lived thereby making glycaemic control more challenging. Thus, it is common practice to periodically monitor electrolytes and blood glucose during and up to 2 h after the treatment phase.

14.2.23 Enumerate the Various Options for Intraoperative and Postoperative Analgesia

- Regular use of epidural analgesia (T5–T11, low doses of local anaesthetic and opioids) for 72 h following CRS/HIPEC is recommended in order to relieve pain, spare opioids, and accelerate the restoration of bowel function [23]. The recommended daily check of coagulation tests is advised until the fourth postoperative day or upon clinical request, with a median length of epidural use of 5 days. It may be necessary to use one or more drugs (dexmedetomidine, magnesium sulphate, lidocaine, and ketamine) in multimodal analgesia [23]

- If it is not contraindicated, a lower thoracic epidural catheter should be inserted prior to surgery [18]
- Intraoperative use of epidural analgesia is recommended [18]
- For the first 4–5 days following surgery, intravenous paracetamol should be given in conjunction with local anaesthetic and opioid-based epidural analgesia [18]
- If TEA does not provide adequate pain relief or if all dermatomes are not covered, IVPCA should be given for a longer period of time [18]
- IVPCA should be used in patients with contraindications for placement of an epidural catheter, or discontinued epidural catheter [18]

14.2.24 Describe the Implications in Intraoperative Temperature Control

- Monitor core body temperature. Temperature management is different during the different phases (Fig. 14.3).

CRS

- Risk of hypothermia as a result of extensive surgical resection and exposure, significant fluid loss and long duration of surgery. It can lead to coagulation and metabolic derangements
- Aim to maintain normothermia during the CRS phase.
- Intraoperative hypothermia should be prevented by use of active warming measures [22]
  - Convective warming equipment like forced-air warming blankets (Bair Hugger)
  - Raised ambient operating room temperature
  - Warm intravenous fluids

HIPEC

- Risk of hyperthermia of up to 40.5 °C due to the hyperthermic perfusion.
- Hypermetabolic phase and hyperdynamic circulation and peripheral vasodilatation occur during systemic hyperthermia.
- Active interventions for preventing intraoperative hyperthermia could be taken [22]
- Passive cooling methods (switching-off warming equipments) before starting HIPEC (35–36 °C).

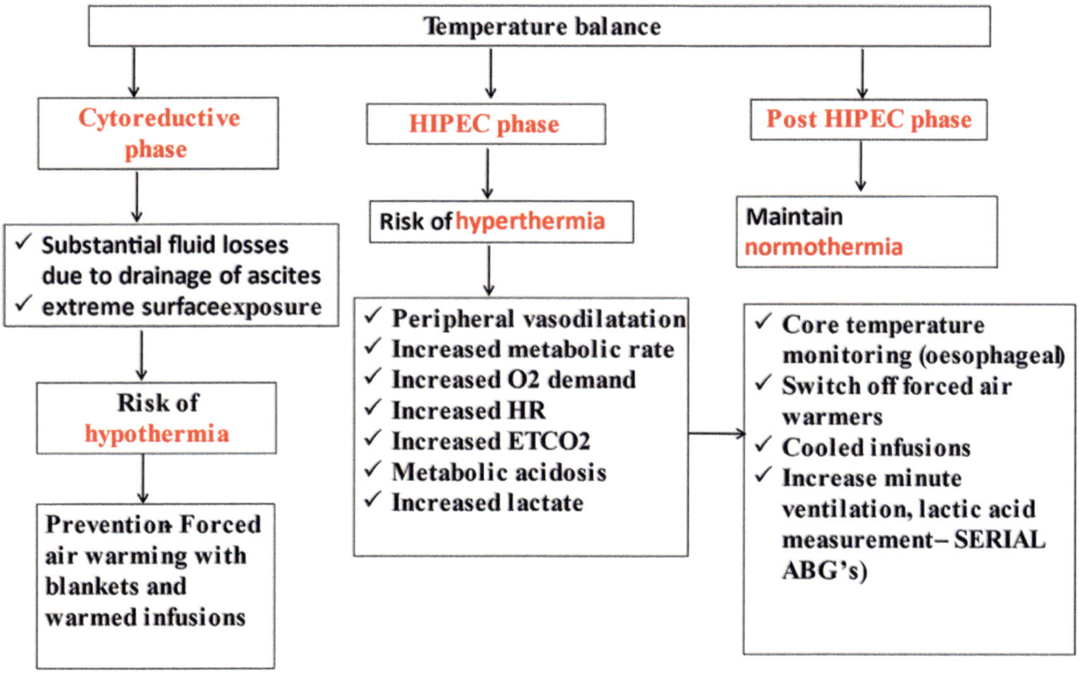

Fig. 14.3 Temperature changes and management during CRS, HIPEC and post-HIPEC phase

- Core body temperature should be kept below 39 °C [18]
- Temperature control during HIPEC phase can be accomplished by [18]
  - Use of cold crystalloids at around 6 °C during HIPEC phase.
  - Use of cool air circulating blankets during HIPEC.
- The perfusionist should be advised to reduce the instillate temperature if despite all these measures, core body rises to ≥39 °C then.

14.2.25 Enumerate the Physiological Alterations and Its Implications in the Postoperative Period

The physiological alterations and their anaesthetic implications are mentioned in Table 14.7.

Table 14.7 Postoperative management

System involved	Pathophysiological alterations	Postoperative management
Fluid and haemodynamics	• Fluid loss of 4 L/day during initial 72 h due to oozing from raw surface area • Decrease in albumin levels	• Requirement of vasopressors • Transfusion of blood and blood products • Albumin supplementation if (<3 g/dL)
Coagulation [19]	• Thrombocytopenia due to cytotoxic drugs • Dilutional coagulopathy	• TEG to diagnose • Platelet and FFP transfusion
Electrolyte imbalance	Due to massive fluid shifts, metabolic derangement	Correction and supplementation
Analgesia	Increase pain due to extensive surgery	• Multimodal analgesia-Epidural, intrathecal, iv opioids, acetaminophen • Avoid NSAIDS • Coagulation profile should be normal before removal of epidural catheter
Stress ulcer prophylaxis	Risk of stress ulcer due to requirement of mechanical ventilation, vasopressors and coagulopathy	PPI/H2 receptor antagonists to all patients
Thromboprophylaxis	Increased risk of thrombosis due to malignancy, prolonged surgery and female gender	• Mechanical or pharmacological • Once coagulation profile is WNL and risk of bleeding is minimal
Feeding/Nutrition	Nutrition promotes wound healing and improves intestinal transit	• Orally allowed POD 2 • Enteral preferred over TPN • Parenteral nutrition in postoperative stress ulcer, ileus, or anastomotic leak
Respiratory support	• Requirement of postop ventilation due to hemodynamic instability • Basal lung collapse due to ascites or HIPEC procedure or prolonged mechanical ventilation	• Weaning trial and early extubation • Incentive spirometry, deep breathing exercises, physiotherapy, propped up position • Continuous positive pressure (CPAP) after extubation may be required
Infection control	Risk of infection due to leucopenia after chemotherapy	• Aseptic precaution • Low threshold to escalate higher antibiotics
Renal status	Risk of chemotherapy-induced nephrotoxicity	KFT and urine output monitoring
Glycaemic control	Risk of hyperglycaemia	Standard care, insulin if required
Ambulation	Risk of thrombosis, atelectasis, delirium	As early as possible
Stoma care		Education and care of stoma
Watch for complications	Anastomotic leaks, intestinal fistula, intra-abdominal sepsis, haematological Toxicity, pancreatitis and, renal failure	

14.2.26 What Are the Occupational Safety Concerns for Professionals Involved in the Perioperative Care of This Patient?

- The personnel doing HIPEC surgery have to be informed on the consequences of drug exposure and how to clean up leaks [31]. Aerosol and vapour inhalation as well as direct touch are frequent exposure routes. Hair loss, headache, acute irritation, hypersensitivity, increased fetal loss, congenital malformations, low birth weight, infertility and increased risk of leukaemia
- Cisplatin—anaphylactic reaction, irritates eye, skin and airway and toxic effect on kidney, bone marrow and inner ear
- Doxorubicin—mucosal inflammation, leucopenia and dilated CMP
- Carcinogenic to humans

The following subgroups should be excluded from a HIPEC team [20]

1. Individuals planning a pregnancy (men/women).
2. Pregnant/nursing women.
3. Prior chemotherapy/radiotherapy treatment.
4. History of abortions/congenital malformations.
5. Hematologic/teratogenic history.
6. History of allergic reactions to cytotoxic drugs/latex.
7. Radiographers/people working with radiotherapy.
8. Patients on immunosuppressive therapy.
9. Severe dermatologic disease.

Safety measures

- Nobody to remain in OR.
- Zero flow of CO_2—System airtight with no leak.
- Laminar airflow in OR.
- Chemotherapy aerosols to be exhausted into hospital air—waste system.
- Bodily fluids of patients are considered to be chemotherapy contaminated for 48 h.
- Cytotoxic precaution should be displayed on OT doors prior to the start of perfusion.
- Polyethylene-coated polypropylene disposable gowns, protective glasses, and double gloving.
- N 95 masks—block 95% of particles 0.3 μm and larger.
- Remote monitoring.
- HIPEC equipment tubing and chemotherapeutic medication containers need to be disposed of properly.

References

1. González-Moreno S. Peritoneal surface oncology: a progress report. Eur J Surg Oncol. 2006;32(6):593–6.
2. Elias D, Goéré D, Dumont F, Honoré C, Dartigues P, Stoclin A, et al. Role of hyperthermic intraoperative peritoneal chemotherapy in the management of peritoneal metastases. Eur J Cancer. 2014;50(2):332–40.
3. Jacquet P, Sugarbaker PH. Clinical research methodologies in diagnosis and staging of patients with peritoneal carcinomatosis. Cancer Treat Res. 1996;82:359–74.
4. Jacquet P, Sugarbaker PH. Peritoneal-plasma barrier. Cancer Treat Res. 1996;82:53–63.
5. Flessner MF. The transport barrier in intraperitoneal therapy. Am J Physiol Renal Physiol. 2005;288(3):F433–42.
6. Speyer JL, Sugarbaker PH, Collins JM, Dedrick RL, Klecker RW, Myers CE. Portal levels and hepatic clearance of 5-fluorouracil after intraperitoneal administration in humans. Cancer Res. 1981;41(5):1916–22.
7. El-Kareh AW, Secomb TW. A theoretical model for intraperitoneal delivery of cisplatin and the effect of hyperthermia on drug penetration distance. Neoplasia. 2004;6(2):117–27.
8. Fujimoto S, Takahashi M, Kobayashi K, Nagano K, Kure M, Mutoh T, et al. Cytohistologic assessment of antitumor effects of intraperitoneal hyperthermic perfusion with mitomycin C for patients with gastric cancer with peritoneal metastasis. Cancer. 1992;70(12):2754–60.
9. Sticca RP, Dach BW. Rationale for hyperthermia with intraoperative intraperitoneal chemotherapy agents. Surg Oncol Clin N Am. 2003;12(3):689–701.
10. Overgaard J. Effect of hyperthermia on malignant cells in vivo. A review and a hypothesis. Cancer. 1977;39(6):2637–46.
11. Dudar TE, Jain RK. Differential response of normal and tumor microcirculation to hyperthermia. Cancer Res. 1984;44(2):605–12.

12. de Bree E, Tsiftsis DD. Principles of perioperative intraperitoneal chemotherapy for peritoneal carcinomatosis. Recent Results Cancer Res. 2007;169:39–51.
13. Beckert S, Struller F, Grischke EM, Glatzle J, Zieker D, Königsrainer A, et al. [Surgical management of peritoneal surface malignancy with respect to tumour type, tumour stage and individual tumour biology]. Zentralbl Chir. 2016;141(4):415–420.
14. Minchinton AI, Tannock IF. Drug penetration in solid tumours. Nat Rev Cancer. 2006;6(8):583–92.
15. Jacquet P, Stuart OA, Chang D, Sugarbaker PH. Effects of intra-abdominal pressure on pharmacokinetics and tissue distribution of doxorubicin after intraperitoneal administration. Anticancer Drugs. 1996;7(5):596–603.
16. Raspé C, Flöther L, Schneider R, Bucher M, Piso P. Best practice for perioperative management of patients with cytoreductive surgery and HIPEC. Eur J Surg Oncol. 2017;43(6):1013–27.
17. Raspe C, Piso P, Wiesenack C, Bucher M. Anesthetic management in patients undergoing hyperthermic chemotherapy. Curr Opin Anaesthesiol. 2012;25(3):348–55.
18. Solanki SL, Mukherjee S, Agarwal V, Thota RS, Balakrishnan K, Shah SB, et al. Society of Onco-Anaesthesia and Perioperative Care consensus guidelines for perioperative management of patients for cytoreductive surgery and hyperthermic intraperitoneal chemotherapy (CRS-HIPEC). Indian J Anaesth. 2019;63(12):972–87. https://www.ncbi.nlm.nih.gov/pmc/articles/PMC6921319/.
19. Pandit A, Singh V, Bharati SJ, Mishra S, Deo SV, Bhatnagar S. A pilot randomised clinical trial comparing desflurane anaesthesia vs total intravenous anaesthesia, for changes in haemodynamic, inflammatory and coagulation parameters in patients undergoing hyperthermic intraperitoneal chemotherapy. Indian J Anaesth. 2020;64(8):688–95.
20. Ashvin R, Nikhilesh J. Preoperative preparation and patient selection for cytoreductive surgery and HIPEC. Indian J Surg Oncol. 2016;7(2):208–14.
21. Esquivel J, Sticca R, Sugarbaker P, Levine E, Yan TD, Alexander R, et al. Cytoreductive surgery and hyperthermic intraperitoneal chemotherapy in the management of peritoneal surface malignancies of colonic origin: a consensus statement. Society of Surgical Oncology. Ann Surg Oncol. 2007;14(1):128–33.
22. Hübner M, Kusamura S, Villeneuve L, Al-Niaimi A, Alyami M, Balonov K, et al. Guidelines for perioperative care in cytoreductive surgery (CRS) with or without hyperthermic intraperitoneal chemotherapy (HIPEC): enhanced recovery after surgery (ERAS®) society recommendations—Part I: preoperative and intraoperative management. Eur J Surg Oncol. 2020;46(12):2292–310.
23. Hübner M, Kusamura S, Villeneuve L, Al-Niaimi A, Alyami M, Balonov K, et al. Guidelines for perioperative care in cytoreductive surgery (CRS) with or without hyperthermic intraperitoneal chemotherapy (HIPEC): enhanced recovery after surgery (ERAS®) society recommendations—Part II: postoperative management and special considerations. Eur J Surg Oncol. 2020;46(12):2311–23.
24. Kurreck A, Gronau F, Alberto Vilchez ME, Abels W, Enghard P, Brandl A, et al. Sodium thiosulfate reduces acute kidney injury in patients undergoing cytoreductive surgery plus hyperthermic intraperitoneal chemotherapy with cisplatin: a single-center observational study. Ann Surg Oncol. 2022;29(1):152–62.
25. Rahouma M, Kamel M, Jodeh D, Kelley T, Ohmes LB, de Biasi AR, et al. Does a balanced transfusion ratio of plasma to packed red blood cells improve outcomes in both trauma and surgical patients? A meta-analysis of randomized controlled trials and observational studies. Am J Surg. 2018;216(2):342–50.
26. Owusu-Agyemang P, Arunkumar R, Green H, Hurst D, Landoski K, Hayes-Jordan A. Anesthetic management and renal function in pediatric patients undergoing cytoreductive surgery with continuous hyperthermic intraperitoneal chemotherapy (HIPEC) with cisplatin. Ann Surg Oncol. 2012;19(8):2652–6.
27. Rothfield KP, Crowley K. Anesthesia considerations during cytoreductive surgery and hyperthermic intraperitoneal chemotherapy. Surg Oncol Clin N Am. 2012;21(4):533–41.
28. Raft J, Parisot M, Marchal F, Tala S, Desandes E, Lalot JM, et al. [Impact of the hyperthermic intraperitoneal chemotherapy on the fluid-electrolytes changes and on the acid-base balance]. Ann Fr Anesth Reanim. 2010;29(10):676–681.
29. De Somer F, Ceelen W, Delanghe J, De Smet D, Vanackere M, Pattyn P, et al. Severe hyponatremia, hyperglycemia, and hyperlactatemia are associated with intraoperative hyperthermic intraperitoneal chemoperfusion with oxaliplatin. Perit Dial Int. 2008;28(1):61–6.
30. Thix CA, Königsrainer I, Kind R, Wied P, Schroeder TH. Ventricular tachycardia during hyperthermic intraperitoneal chemotherapy. Anaesthesia. 2009;64(10):1134–6.
31. Kyriazanos I, Kalles V, Stefanopoulos A, Spiliotis J, Mohamed F. Operating personnel safety during the administration of hyperthermic intraperitoneal chemotherapy (HIPEC). Surg Oncol. 2016;25(3):308–14.

Hepatic Metastases for Right Hepatectomy

15

Sana Y. Hussain, Rashmi Ramachandran, and Vimi Rewari

15.1 General Considerations

Q1.1

What are the indications of hepatic resection? What are contraindications to hepatic resection surgery in secondary liver metastasis?

Indications for hepatic resection are [1, 2]

1. Secondary liver metastases
2. Primary hepatic malignancy (hepatocellular carcinoma)
3. Primary biliary malignancy (cholangiocarcinoma)
4. Benign hepatic tumour
5. Trauma

Of these, liver metastasis is the most common indication with more than 50% of resections attributed to it.

The contraindications to hepatic resection surgery in secondary liver metastases are [2]

1. Not able to achieve complete resection of tumour
2. Future liver remnant after surgery is <30% and <40% (cirrhosis)
3. Unresectable primary tumour
4. Concomitant unresectable extrahepatic disease

Q1.2

What are the most common sites of primary tumour with liver metastasis?

Liver is a very common site for metastasis and various types of tumours are responsible for it. Colorectal adenocarcinomas are the most common cause of liver metastasis and 20–25% of all colorectal malignancies present with liver metastasis. Other primary malignancies with hepatic metastases are those of adrenal gland, skin, breast, neuroendocrine tumours, stomach and pancreas [3].

Q1.3

Which lobe of liver is more common for metastasis and why?

The right side is more commonly involved in secondary metastasis. There is no established reason for this and various theories have been postulated. The right lobe of liver has more weight and volume than left lobe, thus a greater chance of metastasis. Also, the right side receives larger portion of the portal blood flow, while hepatic arterial flow is less. This could lead to seeding of metastatic lesions from the gastrointestinal carcinomas [4].

S. Y. Hussain · R. Ramachandran · V. Rewari (✉)
Deaprtment of Anaesthesiology, Pain medicine and Critical care, All India Institute of Medical Sciences, New Delhi, India

N. Gupta et al. (eds.), *Problem Based Learning Discussions in Onco-Anesthesia and Onco-Critical Care*, https://doi.org/10.1007/978-981-99-6339-3_15

Q1.4

Describe in brief the segments and blood supply of liver? Outline the various types of hepatic resection?

The liver is divided into the right and left lobes by a line that extends from the inferior vena cava to the gall bladder bed. This is known as the Cantlie's line and it lies along the division of the portal vein. These are further divided into segments known as Couinad segments, depending on the vascular supply and biliary drainage.

The division of liver into four sectors is by the three hepatic veins into right anterior and posterior and left lateral and medial sectors. These are divided horizontally by branches of portal vein forming eight segments which are numbered clockwise. Left side of the liver is formed by segments II, III, IV (IVa, IVb); while the right side is formed by segments V, VI, VII, VIII. Caudate lobe forms segment I [5].

Liver resections are done along these segments as they have independent blood supply and biliary drainage.

Right hepatectomy is resection of segments V–VIII. Extended right hepatectomy, also known as right trisegmentectomy, is resection of segments IV to VIII. Resection of segments II, III and IV comprises left hepatectomy. Extended left hepatectomy or left trisegmentectomy includes resection of segment V and VIII as well [6].

Liver receives approximately one-fourth of the cardiac output. It has blood supply from both hepatic artery and the portal vein. Around 70% of the supply comes from the portal vein whereas 30% blood supply is from the hepatic artery. Venous outflow is via the three hepatic veins which separately drain the right and left side of the liver. They further drain into the inferior vena cava.

Flow of blood to the liver is determined by resistance of the hepatic artery, portal vein and flow in the splanchnic vessels. Decreased flow in the portal veins leads to an increase in hepatic artery flow which is also called as hepatic arterial buffer response [7].

15.2 Preoperative Management of Liver Resection

Q2.1

What are the various treatment modalities for metastatic hepatic tumours? Discuss about neoadjuvant chemotherapy?

Management of liver metastasis consists of

1. Surgery
2. Chemotherapy
3. Radioablative techniques

Hepatic resection is the best available treatment option for selected patients and can be performed laparoscopically or open resection.

Neoadjuvant chemotherapy is used to decrease tumour size and make it resectable before performing hepatectomy. The most common agents used are 5-flurouracil (5 FU), oxaliplatin, irinotecan, capecitabine and bevacuzimab. Systemic side effects include leucopenia, diarrhoea and hypertension. Other problems encountered with chemotherapy are steatosis, steatohepatitis and sinusoidal obstruction. This can compromise the liver function preoperatively leading to adverse postoperative outcomes [8].

Ablative therapies, like radiofrequency ablation, can be used for smaller lesions (<5 cm). It can be done intraoperatively or via percutaneous approach. It decreases the overall morbidity and mortality as compared to open resection of tumour [9].

Q2.2

What are the preoperative concerns and assessment in patients undergoing right hepatectomy?

Preoperative assessment for liver resection surgeries should focus on general comorbidities of patient and liver function. A standard hemogram, renal, liver function tests and coagulation profile should be obtained. Other preoperative investigations like pulmonary function test and echocardiography should be obtained depending upon the functional status and the comorbidities of the patient. Neoadjuvant chemotherapy may have adverse effects on organ systems which requires evaluation.

Liver imaging is an important part of preoperative management and includes magnetic resonance imaging (MRI) and computed tomography (CT) to evaluate liver metastasis, monitor response to neoadjuvant chemotherapy and help in surgical decision-making. Liver function assessment should be performed as these patients may have primary liver pathology or tumour infiltration and future liver remnant (FLR) needs to be calculated. Patients with low FLR and cirrhosis are at risk of developing post-hepatectomy liver failure. CT and MRI volumetry may be done to assess liver and tumour volume. Functional assessment of liver can also be performed by specialized tests like indocyanine green retention test which measures liver perfusion and biliary excretion. Patients with low FLR can be planned for staged hepatectomy, preoperative portal vein embolization (PVE) and portal vein ligation [10].

Q2.3

What is the role of preoperative portal vein embolization?

It is the elective obliteration of portal vein to a select part of the liver 4–6 weeks before liver resection surgeries. As a result the non-embolized portion of the liver hypertrophies. This results in an increase in the function and volume of future remnant liver (FLR). This will increase the functional capacity of the liver to a safe threshold and allow for liver resection surgeries in candidates who had marginal FLR volumes. It is indicated where FLR <20% (normal liver), <30% (cholestasis, hepatitis) and <40% (cirrhosis). PVE has shown to result in minimal postoperative liver dysfunction and increase the rate of curative liver resections [11]. Complications of this procedure include portal vein thrombosis, portal hypertension, necrosis and may result in accelerated tumour growth. It is commonly done via percutaneous approach and requires sedation during the procedure.

15.3 Intraoperative Management of Liver Resection

Q3.1

Outline the general principles of anaesthesia for liver resection

Anaesthesia management depends upon the comorbidities, pre-existing liver dysfunction, surgical technique (open vs laparoscopic), planned resection and anticipated blood loss.

General anaesthesia with endotracheal intubation is the standard technique. Use of regional or epidural anaesthesia is also common.

Standard monitoring including electrocardiogram, pulse oximetry, capnography, temperature, and blood pressure measurement are used.

Invasive arterial BP and central venous pressure (CVP) monitoring is usually done.

Maintenance of anaesthesia can be done by inhalational or intravenous agents. However, dose should be titrated taking into account the pharmacodynamics and pharmacokinetics of drugs during liver resection. Neuromuscular blocking drugs should be titrated using a neuromuscular monitor. Management of hemodynamic changes during vascular occlusion, transfusing blood products during blood loss, intravenous fluids, acid-base balance and maintaining normothermia is important.

Q3.2

What is the effect of anaesthesia on liver blood flow?

Hepatic arterial buffer response (HABR) is attenuated by volatile anaesthetics, thereby compromising the liver blood flow. Halothane has the maximum effect and sevoflurane has the least effect [12]. Intravenous agents like propofol exhibit minimal effect on HABR.

All anaesthetic agents can decrease the hepatic blood flow due to decrease in blood pressure and cardiac output. Epidural anaesthetics can also reduce the hepatic and splanchnic blood flow as a result of decrease in mean arterial pressure.

Q3.3

Describe the role of invasive monitoring during hepatectomy? What is the role of CVP?

Invasive arterial monitoring by cannulating the radial artery is common. It helps in close monitoring during massive blood loss or hemodynamic changes associated with vascular occlusion. It also helps in sampling blood for measurement of arterial blood gases.

Advanced hemodynamic monitoring like cardiac output, cardiac index, and stroke volume variation helps in guiding the fluid and vasopressor therapy.

Internal jugular vein is cannulated for giving vasopressors as well as measuring CVP. One of the key strategies to minimize blood loss is to maintain a low CVP (≤5 mmHg). Retrograde flow from the hepatic veins can cause increased bleeding during resection. Pressure in the hepatic veins is related to pressure in the inferior vena cava [13].

Methods to keep a low CVP include restricted fluid therapy. 1–2 mL/kg/h of intravenous balanced salt solutions can be used till resection is completed. Other methods include reverse Trendelenburg position, employing a ventilation strategy of low positive end-expiratory pressure (less than or equal to 5) and tidal volume of 4–6 mL per kg to avoid excessive increase in intrathoracic pressure. Pharmacological methods include furosemide boluses or intravenous nitroglycerin infusion.

However, a mean arterial pressure of more than or equal to 65 mmHg and a urine output more than 25 mL/h should be targeted to ensure adequate organ perfusion.

The problems of maintaining a low CVP include risk of organ hypoperfusion, air embolism and decreased reserve in the event of massive blood loss.

Q3.4

What are the blood loss-limiting surgical techniques?

Blood loss during hepatic resection can be reduced by a variety of techniques. Commonly performed techniques include

1. Performing surgery with low CVP (<5 mmHg)
2. Use of tranexamic acid [14]
3. Use of newer techniques such as heat coagulation, ultrasonic dissection, LigaSure Vessel Sealing System and ultrasonic coagulation devices
4. Hepatic vascular exclusion. These can be divided into occlusion of hepatic inflow or occlusion of both inflow and outflow vessels [15]

Inflow vascular occlusion	Inflow and outflow vascular occlusion
1. Occlusion of hepatic pedicle • Intermittent or continuous Pringle pringle manoeuvre	Total hepatic vascular exclusion (THVE)
1. Selective inflow occlusion • Segmental vascular clamping • Semihepatic vascular clamping	Occluding inflow by extraparenchymal control of hepatic veins

Pringle manoeuvre consists of placing vascular clamp or tourniquet in the porta hepatis with the aim of occluding the inflow of portal venous and hepatic arterial vessels. This results in cardiovascular changes in the form of decreased venous return, cardiac index and increased systemic vascular resistance. It is generally well tolerated, but one should remain cautious of cardiac dysfunction and air embolism. This manoeuvre can be applied continuously or intermittently. Inhalational anaesthetics especially sevoflurane have been shown to cause ischaemic pre- and post-conditioning during Pringle manoeuvre.

Total hepatic vascular exclusion (THVE) is performed by Pringle manoeuvre followed by clamps to infrahepatic (above renal veins) and suprahepatic inferior vena cava. This results in significant decrease in venous return and increase in systemic vascular resistance causing hemodynamic instability. In contrast, extraparenchymal control of hepatic veins does not affect the caval flow. Hence, hemodynamic changes are less drastic as compared to THVE.

Q3.5

What is acute normovolemic hemodilution?

Acute normovolemic hemodilution (ANH) is one of the techniques used for conserving blood and decreasing the need for allogenic blood transfusion. It is done by withdrawing blood before the start of surgery. A maximum of 3 L of blood is withdrawn or a haemoglobin of 8 g/dL is targeted. This is then replaced by isotonic crystalloids to maintain euvolemia. Since the diluted blood has lower haematocrit, lesser red blood cells are lost during hepatic resection. The collected blood is later transfused [16].

Q3.6

What are common acid-base abnormalities seen during hepatic resection?

Liver is an important organ for detoxifying metabolites and maintaining homeostasis of biochemical substances. This can be disturbed in patients undergoing liver resections due to pre-existing liver dysfunction, intraoperative vascular clamping and decreased liver volume after resection. Commonest derangement is metabolic acidosis. Accumulation of lactic acid leads to anion gap acidosis.

As liver is the major organ for metabolizing lactates, liver dysfunction and resection hampers it. Also, during vascular occlusion there is decreased lactate clearance along with increased production due to anaerobic metabolism. Hyperlactemia can also be due to significant blood loss, hypovolemia, use of vasopressors and blood transfusion. It may lead to reduction in cardiac contractility and risk of arrhythmia.

Increased serum lactate level is an independent marker of postoperative complications.

Adequate organ perfusion by maintaining mean arterial pressures should be targeted. Serum lactate levels usually tend to decline after the third postoperative hour. Sodium bicarbonate may not be useful to correct acidosis solely due to lactic acid accumulation. Tromethamine (THAM) may be used as it buffers protons. [THAM 0.3 M(mL) = body weight (kg) × base deficit×1.1] [17].

Adjustments in tidal volume or increase in respiratory rate can decrease the PCO_2.

15.4 Postoperative Management

Q4.1

What are the principles of post-operative management after liver resection surgery?

Most patients are extubated postoperatively, but need intensive monitoring and should be admitted in the intensive care unit. Postoperative management mainly focuses on the following parameters [17]:

1. Fluid management—Due to massive fluid shifts, blood loss and reduced oncotic pressure, patients are at risk of hypovolemia and extravascular fluid accumulation in lung. Fluid assessment should be done regularly and 20% albumin may be used for intravascular fluid expansion.
2. Thromboembolism prophylaxis using compression stockings or low molecular weight heparin (LMWH)—Cautious use with concomitant coagulopathy.
3. Early administration of enteral nutrition.
4. Hyperglycaemia is common after surgery due to insulin resistance.
5. Monitoring liver function—Due to substantial regenerative capacity of liver, there is hypertrophy of residual liver along with increased hepatic and splanchnic blood flow. However, functional and synthetic activity of liver may take time and is evident by improvement in laboratory parameters.

6. Postoperative analgesia and early ambulation.
7. Coagulopathy—may occur due to massive blood loss, pre-existing liver dysfunction, postoperative liver injury and hypothermia.
8. Electrolyte abnormalities—Hypophosphatemia is commonly seen post liver resection. Hypophosphatemia may be due to uptake by regenerating liver cells and urinary losses. Correction is done with oral or intravenous phosphate.

Q4.2

How will you manage postoperative pain in these patients?

Hepatic resection involves large upper abdominal incision and entails significant postoperative pain. Control of postoperative pain is a key principal of postoperative management to prevent further complications. Thoracic epidural analgesia (TEA) is commonly used for postoperative analgesia and results in decreased respiratory complications, efficient pain control and faster ambulation. However, the use of TEA is controversial in hepatic resection surgeries due to the following reasons:

1. Postoperative coagulopathy which can make catheter removal unsafe.
2. TEA may result in increased fluid requirement and hypotension due to sympathetic blockade. This may lead to an increased risk of acute injury to kidneys and other organs.

Other modalities for pain control like intravenous patient controlled analgesia (PCA) with opioids may be used [18]. It does not provide superior analgesia compared to TEA, but does not lead to increased hospital stay or complications. Recently, continuous wound infiltration (CWI) with a catheter in situ has become popular for providing postoperative analgesia. It has been compared to TEA and has shown to provide equivalent analgesia with faster recovery time. Also, it does not carry the risk of neuraxial hematoma seen with TEA [19]. For these reasons, enhanced recovery after surgery (ERAS) protocol too recommends CWI instead of TEA. Other regional analgesia techniques like transverse abdominis plane block, quadratus lumborum block, erector spinae plane block and intrathecal morphine have also been used. NSAIDS and paracetamol have also been utilized for effective pain control. However, dose should be titrated according to liver and renal function tests. Pain management following hepatectomies should involve multimodal analgesia techniques consisting of intravenous medications and regional analgesia [20].

Q4.3

What are the common postoperative complications in such patients?

Incidence of complications after hepatic resection surgeries ranges from 20 to 50%. Few common complications include post-resection liver failure, haemorrhage and development of biliary fistula [17].

Post- hepatectomy biliary fistula (PHBF) is a common complication increasing the morbidity in the postoperative period. It results in increased length of hospital stay and in severe cases may result in sepsis, liver failure and death. Biliary disease, preoperative chemotherapy and extensive hepatic resection are some of the predictive factors for developing PHBF.

Post hepatectomy liver failure (PHLF) is a critical complication with worsening of liver functions and inability of the liver to maintain its synthetic, detoxifying and excretory function. It is characterized by coagulopathy and hyperbilirubinemia on or after fifth postoperative day. The incidence can reach up to 5% after metastatic hepatectomy and mortality can reach >50% in severe cases [21]. The risk factors for developing PHLF are preoperative cirrhosis, hepatic steatosis and neoadjuvant chemotherapy. Extensive hepatic resections, excess blood loss and FLR < 20% also predict the development of PHLF.

The incidence of post-hepatectomy haemorrhage (PHH) ranges from 4 to 10%. The sources of PHH include bleeding from the surface of residual liver, incomplete haemostasis and loosening of vascular sutures. Coagulopathy due to massive blood loss, transfusion, sepsis and PHLF can result in increased bleeding. Viscoelastic tests can aid in the diagnosis and goal-directed management in post-operative bleeding.

Post-operative pulmonary complications can also result in significant morbidity and comprise of pleural effusion, pneumonia, atelectasis and pulmonary embolism. Other complications include incisional and intrabdominal infection, urinary tract infections and electrolyte abnormalities [22].

Q4.4

Discuss in brief the ERAS guidelines for hepatic resection?

The ERAS Society recommends various strategies for expedited recovery after liver surgery. These include the following [23]:

1. Preoperative counselling.
2. Perioperative nutrition—Oral nutrition supplements should be given for 7 days before surgery in high-risk patients (weight loss of more than 10–15% in 6 months, albumin less than 30 g/L and Body Mass Index less than 18.5 kg/m^2)
3. Avoid long-acting anxiolytic drugs
4. Anti-thrombotic prophylaxis—unfractionated heparin or LMWH can be started 2–12 h before surgery
5. In normal liver parenchyma, steroids can be used
6. Antimicrobial prophylaxis—intravenous antibiotic should be administered before skin incision as well as one hour before hepatectomy. Skin sterilization to be done with 2% chlorhexidine
7. Avoidance of Mercedes-type surgical skin incision
8. Minimally invasive approach like laparoscopy should be preferred
9. Avoid prophylactic nasogastric tube insertion
10. Maintain normothermia and normoglycemia
11. Use of omental flap to cover the cut surface of liver in left-sided hepatectomy may decrease the risk of delayed gastric emptying
12. Thoracic epidural analgesia is not recommended. This is due to concern of catheter removal in the presence of coagulopathy in the postoperative period. Instead, patients can be given intrathecal opioids or wound catheters for pain control
13. Low CVP (<5 mmHg) is preferred during hepatic resection
14. PONV prophylaxis should be given with 2 anti-emetic agents
15. Balanced crystalloid solution is preferred over normal saline (0.9% NS) or colloids due to risk of hyperchloremic acidosis or renal dysfunction

References

1. Dimick JB, Cowan JA, Knol JA, Upchurch GR. Hepatic resection in the United States: indications, outcomes, and hospital procedural volumes from a nationally representative database. Arch Surg. 2003;138(2):185–91.
2. Van Cutsem E, Cervantes A, Adam R, et al. ESMO consensus guidelines for the management of patients with metastatic colorectal cancer. Ann Oncol. 2016;27(8):1386–422.
3. Manfredi S, Lepage C, Hatem C, Coatmeur O, Faivre J, Bouvier AM. Epidemiology and management of liver metastases from colorectal cancer. Ann Surg. 2006;244(2):254–9.
4. Kadiyoran C, Cizmecioglu HA, Cure E, Yildirim MA, Yilmaz PD. Liver metastasis in colorectal cancer: evaluation of segmental distribution. Prz Gastroenterol. 2019;14(3):188–92.
5. Juza RM, Pauli EM. Clinical and surgical anatomy of the liver: a review for clinicians. Clin Anat. 2014;27(5):764–9.
6. Bismuth H. Revisiting liver anatomy and terminology of hepatectomies. Ann Surg. 2013;257(3):383–38.
7. Gülberg V, Haag K, Rössle M, Gerbes AL. Hepatic arterial buffer response in patients with advanced cirrhosis. Hepatology. 2002;35(3):630–4.
8. Guo M, Jin N, Pawlik T, Cloyd JM. Neoadjuvant chemotherapy for colorectal liver metastases: a contemporary review of the literature. World J Gastrointest Oncol. 2021;13(9):1043–61.
9. Gillams AR, Lees WR. Five year survival following radiofrequency ablation of small, solitary,

hepatic colorectal metastases. J Vasc Interv Radiol. 2008;19(5):712–7.
10. Mattar RE, Al-Alem F, Simoneau E, Hassanain M. Preoperative selection of patients with colorectal cancer liver metastasis for hepatic resection. World J Gastroenterol. 2016;22(2):567–81.
11. May BJ, Madoff DC. Portal vein embolization: rationale, technique, and current application. Semin Intervent Radiol. 2012;29(2):81–9.
12. Stümpfle R, Riga A, Deshpande R, Mudan SS, Baikady RR. Anaesthesia for metastatic liver resection surgery. Curr Anaesth Crit Care. 2009;20:3–7.
13. Melendez JA, Arslan V, Fischer ME, et al. Perioperative outcomes of major hepatic resections under low central venous pressure anesthesia: blood loss, blood transfusion, and the risk of postoperative renal dysfunction. J Am Coll Surg. 1998;187(6):620–5.
14. Wu CC, Ho WM, Cheng SB, Yeh DC, Wen MC, Liu TJ, P'eng FK. Perioperative parenteral tranexamic acid in liver tumor resection: a prospective randomized trial toward a "blood transfusion"-free hepatectomy. Ann Surg. 2006;243(2):173–80.
15. Smyrniotis V, Farantos C, Kostopanagiotou G, Arkadopoulos N. Vascular control during hepatectomy: review of methods and results. World J Surg. 2005;29(11):1384–96.
16. Jarnagin WR, Gonen M, Maithel SK, et al. A prospective randomized trial of acute normovolemic hemodilution compared to standard intraoperative management in patients undergoing major hepatic resection. Ann Surg. 2008;248(3):360–9.
17. Giustiniano E, Nisi F, Rocchi L, et al. Perioperative management of complex hepatectomy for colorectal liver metastases: the alliance between the surgeon and the anesthetist. Cancers (Basel). 2021;13(9):2203.
18. Aloia TA, Kim BJ, Segraves-Chun YS, et al. A randomized controlled trial of postoperative thoracic epidural analgesia versus intravenous patient-controlled analgesia after major hepatopancreatobiliary surgery. Ann Surg. 2017;266(3):545–54.
19. Hughes MJ, Harrison EM, Peel NJ, et al. Randomized clinical trial of perioperative nerve block and continuous local anaesthetic infiltration via wound catheter versus epidural analgesia in open liver resection (LIVER 2 trial). Br J Surg. 2015;102(13):1619–28.
20. Dudek P, Zawadka M, Andruszkiewicz P, Gelo R, Pugliese F, Bilotta F. Postoperative analgesia after open liver surgery: systematic review of clinical evidence. J Clin Med. 2021;10(16):3662.
21. Ray S, Mehta NN, Golhar A, Nundy S. Post hepatectomy liver failure—A comprehensive review of current concepts and controversies. Ann Med Surg (Lond). 2018;34:4–10.
22. Jin S, Fu Q, Wuyun G, Wuyun T. Management of post-hepatectomy complications. World J Gastroenterol. 2013;19(44):7983–91.
23. Melloul E, Hübner M, Scott M, et al. Guidelines for perioperative care for liver surgery: enhanced recovery after surgery (ERAS) society recommendations. World J Surg. 2016;40(10):2425–40.

16 Ca Rectum for Laparoscopic Abdomino-Perineal Resection

Sohan Lal Solanki and Debashree Pradipta Lahiri

16.1 Case Scenario

A 60-year-old male presented with complaints of altered bowel habits for 2 months, pain abdomen for 15 days and bleeding per rectum for 5 days. Colonoscopy and biopsy were done, and he was diagnosed to have adenocarcinoma of the rectum. He received a short-course radiotherapy followed by FOLFOX-based chemotherapy. He gives history of tingling and numbness in hands and legs following two cycles of chemotherapy and was treated with T. Pregabalin 75 mg twice daily. Now the symptoms have reduced. He was posted for laparoscopic APR.

Q1

What is the burden of colorectal cancers and the surgical treatment available?

The incidence and mortality of colorectal cancers (CRC) vary widely throughout the world. As per the WHO GLOBOCON database, CRC is the third most commonly detected cancers in males and second amongst females with the rates of incidence and mortality being substantially higher in males than females.

Despite of advances in sphincter-sparing procedures, abdominoperineal resection (APR) still remains an important tool in the treatment of rectal cancer. APR involves completely removing the distal colon, rectum and anal sphincter complex using both anterior abdominal and perineal incisions leading to a permanent colostomy. APR was first described by Miles in 1908 [1]. During these initial times, mortality was as high as 42%. Gabriel introduced the one-stage APR surgery, in which the abdominal part was done supine and the perineal part in left lateral position [2]. It was Lloyd–Davies who demonstrated the synchronous approach to both the abdomen and perineum with the patient in the lithotomy position [3]. Advances in operative techniques like total mesorectal excision, using minimally invasive techniques and improvements in perioperative care with implementation of ERAS, have drastically reduced the mortality rates associated with APR.

Laparoscopic APR provide the benefits of reduced postoperative pain, lesser opioid usage, smaller incisions, reduced stress related to surgery, decreased wound complications, faster recovery times, shorter hospital stays and overall reduction in healthcare costs. However, it brings along with it challenges associated with CO_2 insufflation and steep head low position like haemodynamic changes, reduced urine output and reduced lung function. Thus, proper patient selection, preoperative optimisation, intraoperative management and appropriate surgical

S. L. Solanki (✉) · D. P. Lahiri
Department of Anaesthesiology, Critical Care and Pain, Tata Memorial Hospital, Homi Bhabha National Institute, Mumbai, India

N. Gupta et al. (eds.), *Problem Based Learning Discussions in Onco-Anesthesia and Onco-Critical Care*, https://doi.org/10.1007/978-981-99-6339-3_16

technique along with good postoperative care are essential to improve the outcomes of the surgery.

Q2

What is AJCC TNM staging of colorectal cancer?

Stage	Tumour	Node	Metastases
Stage 0	TIS	N0	M0
Stage 1	T1 or T2	N0	M0
Stage 2A	T3	N0	M0
Stage 2B	T4a	N0	M0
Stage 2C	T4b	N0	M0

Q3

How will you evaluate and optimise a patient posted for laparoscopic APR?

A large number of patients who are planned for laparoscopic APR are elderly and have associated comorbidities which should be properly optimised before they get operated. Detailed history, thorough clinical examination and review of laboratory investigations are vital for proper optimisation of these patients. Almost one-third of these patients usually have significant cardiac and pulmonary problems [4]. Recently, cardiopulmonary exercise testing (CPET) has been widely performed for an objective assessment of patient's functional reserve. In high-risk patients, it has been found that CPET does have a high predictive value of cardiopulmonary complications in postoperative period [5]. Wilson et al. found that CPET is useful in predicting the risk of death in patients who did not have any history of ischaemic heart disease or any risk factors for it [6]. They concluded that ventilatory equivalent for carbon dioxide >34 and anaerobic threshold ≤10.9 mL/kg/min are significant predictors of 90 days as well as all-cause mortality [6]. Various risk indices based on history, physical examination, functional capacity and serum markers are used to predict the risk in patients undergoing gastrointestinal surgeries [7]. The Physiological and Operative Severity Score for the Enumeration of Mortality and Morbidity (POSSUM) is helpful in predicting complications and outcome. The CR-POSSUM specific to colorectal surgeries has been developed in 2004 and uses six physiological and four operative measures and is more accurate and easier to use [8]. An important reason of risk assessment is for proper patient selection. Due to the pressure of insufflation and steep Trendelenburg, laparoscopic surgery may be inappropriate in patients with raised intracranial or intraocular pressures. Though laparoscopy is considered safe in patients with renal dysfunction, it is advisable to keep the insufflation pressures lower than 15 mm of Hg in these patients. Also in obese patients, due to the insufflation pressures and the steep head low position, it may be difficult to generate adequate tidal volumes, thereby requiring adjustments of ventilator settings to minimise the peak airway pressures. The literature mentions various guidelines and algorithms for assessment, optimisation and reduction of perioperative risk related to diabetes [9], heart disease [10], anemia [11], lung complications [12], obesity [13] and obstructive sleep apnea [14]. In elderly patients, preoperative assessment should include evaluation of cognitive functions to evaluate the risk of postoperative delirium and postoperative falls and the patient's frailty [15].

A large number of patients diagnosed with rectal carcinoma are malnourished or undernourished due to reduced oral intake and weight loss. In cancer patients, the nutritional status is also being affected by neoadjuvant chemotherapy and cancer cachexia. It has been shown that poor nutritional status in preoperative period increases the morbidity after rectal surgeries [16]. Hypoalbuminemia has been associated with increased chances of postoperative infections [17], thereby increasing the length of hospital stay [18]. Patients experiencing 10–15% weight loss in 6 months or have a body mass index of <18.5 kg/m^2 and patients who have Subjective Global Assessment scoring of grade C or serum albumin 30 g/L without any underlying liver or kidney dysfunction have severe nutritional risk [19] and need nutritional optimisation before undergoing surgery. Patients in whom the nutritional risk is mild should be given nutritional supplements added to normal diet. In patients having moderate to severe nutritional risk, it is recommended to start enteral nutrition for 7–10 days, even if that needs surgery to be delayed [19]. Preoperative parenteral nutrition must be started in severely malnourished patients who cannot tolerate enteral feeding or if enteral feeding appears to be non-feasible [19]. For patients in whom >60% of caloric requirement is not be met by enteral feeding, combining parenteral nutrition along with enteral feeding can be beneficial. Role of immunonutrition in preoperative period is doubtful. Thus, it would be beneficial to involve the nutritionist in the preoperative period for optimisation of the patient's nutritional status.

Cessation of smoking in the preoperative period has shown to improve outcomes [17]; however, the optimum duration of preoperative abstinence is still not clear but some reports recommend cessation of smoking for 4–8 weeks as essential to reduce pulmonary and wound healing complications [17]. Cessation of alcohol consumption should also be stressed upon in the preoperative period.

Many patients scheduled for rectal surgeries have low haemoglobin levels due to multiple reasons including nutritional deficiencies, per rectal bleeding and cancer cachexia. Anaemia increases the need of blood transfusion, increases the risk of postoperative complications and mortality and thus may worsen long-term oncological outcomes [18–20]. Thus, it is essential to optimise their haemoglobin levels in the preoperative period. If not contraindicated, parental iron administration should be considered as early as during the first visit to the preanaesthesia checkup clinic. It is essential that every institute has its own perioperative blood management strategies depending on their requirements and available resources.

Neoadjuvant chemotherapy has several side effects and associated complications. These should be considered and treated in preoperative period to improve postoperative outcomes.

In recent times, prehabilitation in the preoperative period has gained attention and is considered safe [21]. Prehabilitation basically means implementing preoperative exercise along with nutritional supplementation to enable the body to cope with the surgical stress. Patients of rectal cancer have poor baseline functional capacity due to chemotherapy and cancer cachexia which increase the risk of perioperative complications and morbidity [22]. Thus, prehabilitation is important to improve the physical fitness before the surgery.

Preoperative evaluation and optimisation need time which may not be suitable in these patients due to the fear of cancer progression. However, more randomised trials assessing the effect of delaying surgery for proper optimisation on long-term outcomes of colorectal cancers are needed.

Q4

What are the familial cancer syndromes associated with colorectal malignancy?

Familial polyposis syndrome, Lynch syndrome, MUTYH-associated polyposis, juvenile polyposis syndrome, serrated polyposis syndrome and hereditary nonpolyposis colorectal cancer are few high-risk familial syndromes associated with colorectal malignancy.

Q5

What are the neo-adjuvant treatment options in patients with rectal malignancy?

Depending on the stage of the disease, patients receive either a short-course radiotherapy (RT) or a longer course of chemo-radiation to reduce the risk of local recurrence [NCCN guidelines version 6.2020]. The chemotherapeutic regimens used are the following:

1. FOLFOX (folinic acid, 5-FU, oxaliplatin)
2. CAPEOX (capecitabine, oxaliplatin)
3. FOLFOXIRI (folinic acid, 5-FU, oxaliplatin, irinotecan)
4. 5-Fluorouracil/leucovorin
5. Capecitabine +long-course RT

Chemotoxicities Associated with These Regimens

Chemotherapy agent	M	GI	C	CNS	PNS	R	E	H	D	HS	P
5-FU	+	+	++	+					+		
Oxaliplatin	++	+	–		+++ Common	++ Rare		++ Rare		++	++ Rare
Irinotecan	+	+++			+		+	+			+
Capecitabine	++	++	+		++			+			

M myelosuppression, *C* cardiotoxicity, *CNS* central nervous system, *R* renal toxicity, *E* electrolyte abnormalities, *H* hepatotoxicity, *D* dermatologic toxicity, *PN* peripheral nervous system, *GI* gastrointestinal, *HS* hypersensitivity reactions, *P* pulmonary toxicity

Toxicity	Manifestations
Myelosuppression	Neutropenia, thrombocytopenia and anaemia
GI	Diarrhoea, mucositis and vomiting
Cardiotoxicity	Dysrhythmias, angina, ischaemia/infarction, coronary vasospasm, cardiomyopathy, sudden death and ECG changes
Hepatotoxicity	Deranged LFT, steatosis, steatohepatitis, hepatic vascular damage (irinotecan), raised liver enzymes and hepatic sinusoidal injury (oxaliplatin)
CNS	Cerebellar dysfunction and multifocal leuco-encephalopathy
PNS	Paresthesias; dysesthesias of hands, feet and perioral region; unusual cold-induced pharyngolaryngeal dysesthesias; and muscle cramps and sensory, symmetric distal axonal neuropathy without motor involvement
Pulmonary	Pneumonitis, interstitial pneumonia, cryptogenic organising pneumonia, eosinophilic pneumonia and diffuse alveolar damage
Dermatotoxicity	Alopecia

Q6

What are the other chemotherapeutic agents that can be received by patients with advanced/metastatic colorectal cancer and can be posted for unrelated emergency surgery?

Metastatic colorectal cancer patients receive numerous agents as single agent or in combination with other targeted drug or chemotherapeutic agents like FOLFOX, FOLFIRI, capecitabine and others based on presence of RAS wild-type, BRAF mutant disease, mismatch repair/microsatellite instability high or high levels of tumour mutational burden, performance status, side of the tumour, HER2 overexpression and many other factors. These include bevacizumab, cetuximab, nivolumab, panitumumab, regorafenib, pembrolizumab, Ziv-aflibercept and ramucirumab [up to date].

(a) Bevacizumab
  - It is an angiogenesis inhibitor. It is a monoclonal antibody against vascular endothelial growth factor (VEGF) that inhibits the binding of normal VEGF ligand to its receptor.
  - Used for metastatic colorectal malignancy.
  - Adverse effects
    - Cardiotoxicity—hypertension, thromboembolism, left ventricular dysfunction and proteinuria
    - CNS toxicity (rare)—reversible posterior leukoencephalopathy
    - Bleeding, gastrointestinal perforation, delayed wound healing and fatigue
    - Rare—Osteonecrosis of the jaw, microangiopathic haemolytic anaemia and nasal septal perforation

(b) Cetuximab and Panitumumab
  - Mouse/human chimeric monoclonal antibody that targets the epidermal growth factor receptor (EGFR)—cetuximab
  - Human monoclonal antibody against EGFR—panitumumab

- It is used in metastatic colorectal cancer and is limited to patients in whom tumours do not have a mutation in one of the RAS or BRAF genes.
- Adverse effects
  - Hypomagnesemia due to renal magnesium wasting
  - Hypokalaemia
  - Hypophosphatemia and hyponatremia
  - Acute kidney injury
  - Weakness and malaise
  - Infusion reactions—less with panitumumab
  - Acneiform eruptions
  - Ocular toxicity—keratitis, conjunctivitis, corneal erosions, eyelash trichomegaly, blepharitis and eyelid dermatitis
  - Pruritus

(c) Regorafenib

Orally administered inhibitor of angiogenic (including VEGFR 1–3), stromal and oncogenic receptor tyrosine kinases

Adverse effects

- Hypertension
- Proteinuria
- Acute kidney injury
- hypophosphatemia, hypocalcaemia, hyponatremia and hypokalaemia

(d) Aflibercept

Aflibercept is a recombinant fusion protein made of the second immunoglobulin (Ig)-like domain of FLT1 (VEGFR 1) joined to the third Ig-like domain of KDR (VEGFR 2) fused to the Fc portion of human IgG1. It acts by inhibiting VEGF binding to all classes of VEGFR, including placenta growth factor (PlGF) binding to VEGFR1. This action of PIGF is proposed to be the advantage in using this drug in bevacizumab-resistant patients.

- It has been used in metastatic colorectal malignancy in combination with FOLFOX/FOLFIRI.
- Adverse effects
  - Neutropenia and leukopenia
  - Hypertension and proteinuria
  - Diarrhoea, stomatitis, fatigue, decreased weight, decreased appetite, abdominal pain, dysphonia, elevated liver enzymes and increased serum creatinine
  - Headache
  - Serious risk of bleeding
  - Gastrointestinal perforation and delayed wound healing

Q7

What is the role of preoperative patient education in a patient posted for laparoscopic APR?

The ERAS programme emphasises on patient education in the preoperative period. It has been shown that preoperative education not only reduces anxiety but it also reduces postoperative pain, nausea and vomiting and therefore increases overall patient satisfaction [23, 24]. The preoperative education is usually executed by ERAS nurse coordinator and should be started early in the preoperative period as soon as decision of the surgery is made. The preoperative education should provide a detailed outline about all aspects on preoperative and postoperative period to the patient as well as to the relative or caregiver in oral and written format. Another important aspect that needs to be discussed in the preoperative period is the presence of stoma after the surgery. The fear and psychological impact of stoma many a times far outweighs the fear of the disease and the pain of the surgery. These can be avoided by proper preoperative discussion and counselling of both the patient and the caregiver.

Q8

How will you prepare a patient posted for laparoscopic APR?

Latest evidence shows that overnight fasting is not beneficial and in fact can be harmful. The practice of overnight fasting increases insulin resistance [25], reduces glycogen reserves [26], causes increased patient discomfort [27] and depletes intravascular volume especially in patients receiving mechanical bowel preparation [28]. Thus, ERAS programme recommends that high concentration oral carbohydrate drinks containing up to 12.5% maltodextrin should be administered to the patient on the evening before the surgery. Also, clear fluid containing high concentration carbohydrate should be given 2 h before surgery.

For surgeries scheduled in the second half of the day, patients should be allowed to drink clear liquids up to 3 h prior to surgery, and they should be given clear, high concentration carbohydrate drink 2 h before induction of anaesthesia [29]. This practice reduces the catabolic stress response of surgery, reduces development of postoperative insulin resistance, reduces protein and improves muscle strength [30, 31]. Data from randomised control trial show that preoperative carbohydrate loading in patients undergoing colorectal surgery significantly reduces the postoperative hospital stay as compared to patients who follow routine preoperative fasting protocols [32]. However, in patients with intestinal obstruction or delayed gastric emptying, these recommendations should not be followed. In diabetics, these recommendations should be modified according to glycaemic control.

(a) *Mechanical bowel preparation:* For colonic surgeries, the currently available evidences do not back the routine use of mechanical bowel preparations, though there can be some benefits in low rectal surgery with colostomy [33]. The use of mechanical bowel preparation is in fact associated with preoperative dehydration, electrolyte abnormalities and increased patient anxiety [34]. Thus, care should be taken to maintain appropriate hydration with oral and intravenous fluids, and dyselectrolemia must be adequately corrected.
(b) *Venous thromboembolism (VTE) prophylaxis:* Current evidence recommends routine use of venous thromboembolism prophylaxis in all patients undergoing major surgeries. VTE prophylaxis is usually in the form of compression stocking and/or intermittent pneumatic compression, low molecular weight heparin or unfractionated heparin [35]. These should be continued throughout the hospital stay of the patient unless contraindicated.
(c) *Preoperative sedation:* Routine administration of anxiolytic medication is not recommended in the preoperative period. It is best to avoid using long-acting sedatives because they not only delay mobilisation and feeding in postoperative period but also increase the risk of delirium [36]. Some centres do administer pre-emptive analgesia to patients scheduled for laparoscopic APR on arrival to up to 2 h prior to the surgery. Patients usually receive acetaminophen and gabapentin orally with a sip of water. Their use and dose must be adjusted depending on patient's age, comorbidities and blood levels [29].

Q9

Discuss the intraoperative management of laparoscopic APR

(a) *Antibiotic prophylaxis:* Antibiotic prophylaxis in laparoscopic APR should cover both aerobic and anaerobic flora of bowel. Antibiotic must be administered 30–60 min before the beginning of surgery. The antibiotic should be repeated if the duration of surgery is more than two half-lives of the antibiotic and in major blood loss. The selection of antibiotic depends on the locally available microbiological data and institutional or national guidelines. For laparoscopic APR, cefazolin along with metronidazole, or a second-generation cephalosporin having aerobic as well as anaerobic activities, can be administered [37].
(b) *Anaesthetic management:* Some of the most important objectives of the ERAS programme in colorectal surgeries are to maintain adequate anaesthesia, preserve organ perfusion and expedite feeding and postoperative mobilisation. Thus, anaesthesia for laparoscopic APR is based on the "trimodal

approach" of attenuation of stress response due to surgery, proper fluid balance and analgesia [38].

Regional anaesthesia technique like combined spinal epidural or continuous spinal to achieve a block height of T6–T7 is possible for low anterior resections of the rectum [39]. However, in laparoscopic APR due to the need of prolonged steep Trendelenburg position, general anaesthesia is being preferred in majority of centres, and regional techniques are reserved for patients who are extremely high risk to receive general anaesthesia. Currently, there is no literature supporting the use of any specific anaesthetic or analgesic agent in colorectal surgeries. It would however be reasonable to use short-acting anaesthesia agents like propofol, cisatracurium, fentanyl or remifentanyl for induction of anaesthesia [29] and short-acting inhalation agents like desflurane or sevoflurane for anaesthesia maintenance in order to facilitate rapid emergence [37]. However, for patients at high risk of postoperative nausea and vomiting (PONV), it is advisable to use total intravenous anaesthesia [37]. Currently there is no recommendation on the advantage of using total intravenous anaesthesia over inhalational agent for laparoscopic colorectal surgeries. Recently, the concept of opioid sparing oncoanaesthesia has gained a lot of attention. Even though there is no concrete evidence available on opioid-induced immune-homeostasis disruption, this is a welcome shift. The concept of opioid sparing oncoanaesthesia emphasises on the use of regional techniques along with non-opioid multimodal pain management techniques.

Though the use of nitrous oxide has not been associated with recurrence of colorectal cancers [40], it is better to avoid it in laparoscopic AR because it can cause bowel distension, thereby affecting surgical handling and return of bowel functions [41], and N_2O also increases the risk of PONV.

Monitoring the depth of anaesthesia improves the post anaesthesia recovery and reduces the incidence of postoperative cognitive dysfunction and delirium in old patients [37].

It is recommended to use short-acting or intermediate-acting muscle relaxants. Neuromuscular junction function should be monitored using train-of-four, double-burst stimulation or tetanic stimulation to avoid residual paralysis and hypoxia at the time of extubation and hence reduce postoperative pulmonary complications.

(c) *Intraoperative ventilation:* In laparoscopic APR, pneumoperitoneum along with steep Trendelenburg position markedly increases the risk of basal lung atelectasis and ventilator-induced lung injury. Thus, using lung-protective ventilation strategy with low tidal volumes of 6–8 mL/kg and PEEP of 6–10 cm H_2O and using lung recruitment manoeuvres allowing permissible hypercapnia are recommended. A recent RCT has concluded that in high-risk patients undergoing laparoscopic colorectal cancer resection using low-tidal-volume ventilation, an open-lung strategy with a PEEP of 6–8 cm of H_2O and repeated lung recruitment manoeuvres reduces postoperative complications as compared to using zero PEEP without lung recruitment manoeuvres [42]. However, lung recruitment manoeuvres should be used cautiously in patients with haemodynamic instability.

(d) *Intraoperative temperature regulation:* In colorectal surgeries, hypothermia, that is, core body temperature less than 35 °C, is said to be associated with blood loss, increased incidence of myocardial ischaemia and cardiac arrhythmias and increased risk of surgical site infections and thus leads to prolonged PACU and hospital stay [43]. Also, prevention of hypothermia is necessary to reduce the surgical stress [43]. Intraoperative drop in temperature is mainly caused because of anaesthesia; thus laparoscopic surgeries do not prevent hypothermia [44]. It is recommended that during laparoscopic APR, the core body temperature should be monitored with nasopharyngeal or esophageal temperature probes. Various methods used to maintain core temperature of more than 36 °C are using forced air blankets and underbody warming mattresses, prewarming in preoperative patient holding area and using warm intravenous fluid and anaesthetic gases.

(e) *Intraoperative glycaemic control:* Perioperative raised blood sugar levels are associated with increased morbidity and mortality. Reducing surgical stress by decreasing the preoperative fasting period, preoperative carbohydrate loading and providing good analgesia facilitate glycaemic control by decreasing insulin resistance. It is recommended that intraoperatively blood sugar should be maintained lower than 10 mmol/L or less than 180 mg/dL.

(f) *Analgesia:* It is recommended to use short-acting opioids like fentanyl or remifentanyl for analgesia in the intraoperative period. Recent literature indicates that in laparoscopic colorectal surgeries, thoracic epidural analgesia (TEA) has no impact [45] and even delays hospital discharge [46, 47]. This could be because of higher incidence of hypotension, motor blockade and urinary retention with TEA [48]. However, there is some evidence to support the use of epidural analgesia in patients at high risk of postoperative pulmonary complications [49] and in patients who have a high probability of conversion to open surgery. The 2018 ERAS society guidelines for perioperative care in elective colorectal surgeries recommends that in patients undergoing laparoscopic surgery, TEA can be used, but it cannot be recommended over other alternative choices [50]. Other alternatives like intravenous lidocaine, ultrasound-guided truncal blocks, instillation of intraperitoneal local anaesthetic and direct laparoscopic vision TAP block have been successfully used [37]. Opioid-sparing multimodal analgesia regimens are recommended in the postoperative period. Nonsteroidal anti-inflammatory drugs (NSAIDs), including COX-2 inhibitors and acetaminophen, are the key components of the opioid-sparing regimen. With regard to the increase in incidence of anastomotic leakage with NSAIDs, current literature is inconclusive in order to avoid NSAIDs in colorectal surgeries other than the usual contraindications. The role of drugs like ketamine, dexmedetomidine, magnesium sulphate, gabapentinoids or high-dose steroids for pain relief in laparoscopic colorectal surgeries is still unclear [50].

(g) *Intravenous fluid management:* The primary objective of intravenous fluid therapy is to maintain fluid homeostasis by maintaining the intravascular volume, cardiac output and tissue perfusion without causing salt and water overload. The colonic blood flow has a very poor autoregulation and is mainly dependent on the mean arterial pressure. It is therefore very important to maintain optimal colonic perfusion to prevent bowel dysfunction and to protect the anastomosis [37]. It is very difficult to calculate the optimal fluid therapy because the range is very narrow, and both over- or under-hydrations are associated with complications. Previous studies on goal-directed fluid therapy (GDFT) have shown a statistically significant reduction in complications along with a significant reduction in duration of ileus and reduced total length of hospital stay. However, recent trials conducted with enhanced recovery programmes have shown no difference in outcome [51–53]. A recent meta-analysis has shown that GDFT is not much beneficial because low-risk patients treated in ERAS programme with a restrictive fluid regimen had morbidity and surgical recovery similar to those of patients treated with GDFT [54]. The 2018 ERAS society guidelines for perioperative care in elective colorectal surgeries strongly recommend that GDFT and advanced haemodynamic monitoring should be used in high-risk patients as well as in patients undergoing surgery with large intravascular fluid loss, that is, blood loss and fluid shift [50]. For laparoscopic APR, iso-oncotic crystalloids at the rate of 2 mL/kg/h are recommended [37]. 0.9% normal saline solutions should be avoided as its use is shown to be associated with kidney dysfunction, prolonged hospitalisation and also increased 30-day mortality [55–57]. The 2018 ERAS society guidelines recommend that in colorectal surgeries, perioperative weight gain of more than 2.5 kg due to fluids should be avoided, and a near-zero fluid balance approach is preferred. When intravenous fluid boluses do not improve the stroke volume significantly, hypotension should be treated with vasopressors [58, 59]. The 2018 ERAS society guidelines also recommend considering inotropes in patients with reduced contractility of the heart (cardiac index less than 2.5 L/min) for achieving adequate oxygen delivery [50].

Laparoscopic APR is associated with less blood loss, but if needed, the decision about blood transfusion should be individualised on the basis of clinical condition of the patient, co-existing morbidities, serum lactate levels and central venous oxygen saturation [37] if available.

(h) *Prevention of postoperative nausea and vomiting (PONV):* One of the essential components in ERAS pathway for colorectal surgeries is prevention of PONV. Severe PONV can lead to dehydration, delayed oral feeding and increase in intravenous fluid administration postoperatively, may need insertion of a nasogastric tube and thereby increase the length of hospital stay and overall healthcare costs. The 2018 ERAS society guidelines for perioperative care in elective colorectal surgeries strongly recommend multimodal approach for PONV prophylaxis [50]. Patients with one or two risk factors for PONV should receive a combination of two-drug comprising of first-line antiemetics like serotonin (5HT3) antagonists (e.g., ondansetron), dopamine (D2) antagonists (e.g., droperidol) and corticosteroids (e.g., dexamethasone). Patients undergoing laparoscopic APR and having more than two risk factors of PONV should be given 2–3 antiemetics. Despite giving prophylaxis, if patients have nausea and vomiting multimodal approach with various classes of drugs like antihistamines (e.g., promethazine), anticholinergics (e.g., scopolamine) and other D2 antagonists such as metoclopramide should be considered.

Q10

Give a detailed account of intraoperative complications of laparoscopic LAR

In laparoscopic APR, the use of pneumoperitoneum and extreme Trendelenburg position gives rise to some complications which should be immediately recognised and treated to avoid catastrophe.

(a) Endobronchial intubation due to cephalad shift of the carina caused by CO_2 insufflation and Trendelenburg positioning: this can lead to hypoxemia which can be prevented by prompt recognition and repositioning of the endotracheal tube.
(b) Cardiac dysrhythmias can occur due to a variety of reasons. Increased vagal tone due to peritoneal stretch at the time of insufflation can lead to bradycardia and arrest. Other reasons of cardiac dysrhythmias are CO_2 embolism, tension pneumothorax, respiratory acidosis and acute blood loss.
(c) Subcutaneous emphysema can occur due to the inadvertent extraperitoneal insufflation of CO_2 in subcutaneous, preperitoneal or retroperitoneal tissues. It is usually diagnosed by crepitus or a sudden increase in end tidal CO_2. Subcutaneous emphysema is usually self-limiting and resolves after the abdomen is deflated. However, sometimes CO_2 may track into the mediastinum, thorax or pericardium leading to tension capnothorax or cardiac tamponade which may lead to unexplained increased airway pressure, hypoxemia, hypercarbia and sudden cardiovascular collapse. Treatment includes immediate deflation of the abdomen and supportive care. Minimal capnothorax/cardiac tamponade can be treated conserva-

tively as CO_2 is rapidly absorbed. However, if haemodynamic instability occurs, placement of chest drain or cardiac pigtail may be necessary.

(d) CO_2 embolism during laparoscopic surgeries is quite common, but it usually does not cause significant cardiopulmonary compromise. Signs suggestive of CO_2 embolism are cardiac arrhythmia, hypoxemia, hypotension and a sudden decrease in $ETCO_2$. The presence of patent foramen ovale or atrial septal defect leads to paradoxical CO_2 embolism to the brain. If there is haemodynamic instability, immediate deflation of the abdomen, hyperventilation to promote rapid CO_2 washout and supportive care are necessary. Patient can be moved to the left lateral along with Trendelenburg position to prevent obstruction of pulmonary artery outflow.

(e) Upper airway oedema due to prolonged Trendelenburg position.

(f) The prolonged Trendelenburg position can lead to brachial plexus injury due to prolonged caudate displacement of the shoulders. This can be prevented by adequate padding of the shoulders. The lithotomy position needed in laparoscopic APR can lead to foot drop due to peroneal nerve injury. This can be prevented by proper padding of the bony prominences.

(g) Inadvertent injury to organ and vascular structures during trocar or the Veress needle placement can lead to intestinal or bladder perforation and acute blood loss, respectively. Any unexplained hypotension at the time of needle or trocar placement should immediately be communicated to the surgeon to rule out inadvertent vascular injury.

Q11

Describe the postoperative management of laparoscopic APR

The perioperative outcome of APR has improved over time due to implementation of evidence-based practices and enhanced recovery care principles to pre-, intra- and postoperative period to prevent as well as treat common and uncommon postoperative complications.

(a) *Nasogastric tube:* The 2018 ERAS society guidelines for perioperative care in elective colorectal surgeries do not recommend the routine use of nasogastric tubes in postoperative period. The guidelines strongly recommend removal of nasogastric tube if inserted during surgery before reversal of anaesthesia [50].

(b) *Postoperative analgesia:* Adequate and prompt treatment of postoperative pain attenuates the surgical stress and is a vital component of the ERAS pathway in colorectal surgeries. Opioid-sparing multimodal analgesia techniques are associated with early mobilisation, early return of bowel function, lesser number of complications and an overall reduction in length of hospital stay [50]. The multimodal analgesia strategy should ideally begin in the intraoperative period and later continued in the postoperative period. The various techniques of postoperative analgesia in laparoscopic APR have already being discussed earlier.

(c) *Thromboprophylaxis:* The 2018 ERAS society guidelines for perioperative care in elective colorectal surgeries recommends that patients who have undergone major colorectal surgery should have mechanical thromboprophylaxis in the form of well-fitting compression stockings and/or intermittent pneumatic compression until discharge [50]. Though the quality of evidence is low, the 2018 ERAS society guidelines recommend the use of pharmacological prophylaxis with LMWH once daily for 28 days after surgery [50].

(d) *Fluid and electrolyte therapy*: The 2018 ERAS society guidelines for perioperative care in elective colorectal surgeries recommend the following [50]:
- In the postoperative period, a net "near-zero" fluid and electrolyte balance to be maintained.
- For maintenance, hypotonic crystalloids should be used instead of isotonic crystalloids which contain high concentrations

of sodium and cations. Maintenance fluid are given at a rate of 25–30 mL per kg per day and should not contain more than 70–100 mmol sodium per day with potassium supplementation of up to1 mmol per kg per day.

- For replacement of losses like vomiting or high stoma output, balanced solutions are preferred. 0.9% saline and other saline-based solutions should be avoided.
- For patients on epidural analgesia, arterial hypotension should be treated with vasopressors after ensuring the patient is normovolemic.

(e) *Urinary drainage:* The 2018 ERAS society guidelines for perioperative care in elective colorectal surgeries recommend removal of urinary catheter on the first day after the surgery in patients who are at low risk of urinary retention. While in patients at high risk for retention like male gender, patients on epidural analgesia and in those who have undergone pelvic surgery, urinary catheter can be kept for up to 3 days.

(f) *Prevention of postoperative ileus:* Development of ileus in the postoperative period leads to patient discomfort and delays discharge thereby increasing hospital cost. Thus, the ERAS programme recognises prevention of postoperative ileus as a key component. Laparoscopic surgeries have lesser incidence postoperative ileus as compared to open surgery. The 2018 ERAS society guidelines for perioperative care in elective colorectal surgeries strongly recommend multimodal approach to minimise development of postoperative ileus [50]. This multimodal approach includes limiting the use of opioids in the intraoperative and postoperative period and when needed to use short-acting opioids reduces the practice of routine nasogastric tube placement. The evidence on use of peripherally acting μ opioid receptor antagonists like alvimopan for preventing postoperative ileus is moderate and may be used [50].

(g) *Postoperative nutritional care:* The 2018 ERAS society guidelines for perioperative care in elective colorectal surgeries strongly recommend early resumption of oral intake [50] as any postponement in the resumption of oral intake leads to increased rates of infectious complications and delayed recovery.

(h) *Early mobilisation:* Prolonged immobilisation after surgery leads to increased risk of pulmonary complications, thromboembolic complications, reduced muscle strength and insulin resistance. Early mobilisation after surgery is an essential step in enhanced recovery programme. The 2018 ERAS society guidelines for perioperative care in elective colorectal surgeries strongly recommend early mobilisation after colorectal surgeries [50]. Thus, any factor hindering early mobilisation like inadequate pain control, prolonged intravenous fluid and indwelling urinary catheter should be addressed to allow mobilisation.

References

1. Miles WE. A method of performing abdomino-perineal excision for carcinoma of the rectum and of the terminal portion of the pelvic colon. Lancet. 1908;2:1812–3.
2. Perry WB, Connaughton JC. Abdominoperineal resection: how is it done and what are the results? Clin Colon Rectal Surg. 2007;20(3):213–20.
3. Ruo L, Guillem JG. Major 20th-century advancements in the management of rectal cancer. Dis Colon Rectum. 1999;42(5):563–78.
4. Alves A, Panis Y, Mathieu P, Mantion G, Kwiatkowski F, Slim K, Association Française de Chirurgie. Postoperative mortality and morbidity in French patients undergoing colorectal surgery: results of a prospective multicenter study. Arch Surg. 2005;140:278–83.
5. Older P, Hall A, Hader R. Cardiopulmonary exercise testing as a in the elderly. Chest. 1999;116:355–62.
6. Wilson RJ, Davies S, Yates D, Redman J, Stone M. Impaired functional capacity is associated with all-cause mortality after major elective intra-abdominal surgery. Br J Anaesth. 2010;105:297–303.
7. Chandra A, Mangam S, Marzouk D. A review of risk scoring systems utilised in patients undergoing gastrointestinal surgery. J Gastrointest Surg. 2009;13:1529–38.
8. Ramkumar T, Ng V, Fowler L, Farouk R. A comparison of POSSUM, P-POSSUM and colorectal POSSUM for the prediction of postoperative mortality in patients undergoing colorectal resection. Dis Colon Rectum. 2006;49:330–5.

9. Moghissi ES, Korytkowski MT, DiNardo M, et al. American Association of Clinical Endocrinologists and American Diabetes Association consensus statement on inpatient glycemic control. Diabetes Care. 2009;32(6):1119–31.
10. Fleisher LA, Beckman JA, Brown KA, et al. 2014 ACC/AHA guideline on perioperative cardiovascular evaluation and management of patients undergoing noncardiac surgery. J Am Coll Cardiol. 2014;64(22):e77–e137.
11. Goodnough LT, Shander A. Patient blood management. Anesthesiology. 2012;116(6):1367–76.
12. Qaseem A, Snow V, Fitterman N, et al. Risk assessment for and strategies to reduce perioperative pulmonary complications for patients undergoing noncardiothoracic surgery: a guideline from the American College of Physicians. Ann Intern Med. 2006;144(8):575–80.
13. Ebert TJ, Shankar H, Haake RM. Perioperative considerations for patients with morbid obesity. Anesthesiol Clin. 2006;24(3):621–36.
14. American Society of Anesthesiologists Task Force on perioperative management of patients with obstructive sleep apnea. Practice guidelines for the perioperative management of patients with obstructive sleep apnea: an updated report by the American Society of Anesthesiologists Task Force on perioperative management of patients with obstructive sleep apnea. Anesthesiology. 2014;120(2):268–286.
15. Chow WB, Rosenthal RA, Merkow RP, et al. Optimal preoperative assessment of the geriatric surgical patient: a best practices guideline from the American College of Surgeons National Surgical Quality Improvement Program and the American Geriatrics Society. J Am Coll Surg. 2012;215(4):453–66.
16. Garth AK, Newsome CM, Simmance N, et al. Nutritional status, nutrition practices and postoperative complications in patients with gastrointestinal cancer. J Hum Nutr Diet. 2010;23(4):393–401.
17. Mills E, Eyawo O, Lockhart I, et al. Smoking cessation reduces postoperative complications: a systematic review and meta-analysis. Am J Med. 2011;124(2):144–54.
18. Baron D, Hochrieser H, Posch M, et al. Preoperative anaemia is associated with poor clinical outcome in non-cardiac surgery patients. Br J Anaesth. 2014;113(3):416–23.
19. Cata J. Perioperative anemia and blood transfusions in patients with cancer. Anesthesiology. 2015;122(1):3–4.
20. Muñoz M, Acheson A, Auerbach M, et al. International consensus statement on the peri-operative management of anaemia and iron deficiency. Anaesthesia. 2016;72(2):233–47.
21. O'Doherty AF, West M, Jack S, et al. Preoperative aerobic exercise training in elective intra-cavity surgery: a systematic review. Br J Anaesth. 2013;110(5):679–89.
22. Lee L, Schwartzman K, Carli F, et al. The association of the distance walked in 6 min with pre-operative peak oxygen consumption and complications 1 month after colorectal resection. Anaesthesia. 2013;68(8):811–6.
23. Chapman S, Helliwell J, Lonsdale M, et al. Patient education about recovery after colorectal surgery: systematic scoping review. Int J Color Dis. 2020;22(12):1842–9.
24. Wongkietkachorn A, Wongkietkachorn N, Rhunsiri P. Preoperative needs-based education to reduce anxiety, increase satisfaction, and decrease time spent in day surgery: a randomized controlled trial. World J Surg. 2017;42(3):666–74.
25. Ljungqvist O, Jonathan E. Rhoads lecture 2011: insulin resistance and enhanced recovery after surgery. JPEN. 2012;36(4):389–98.
26. Martindale RG, McClave SA, Taylor B, et al. Perioperative nutrition: what is the current landscape? JPEN. 2013;37(5 Suppl):5S–20S.
27. Hausel J, Nygren J, Lagerkranser M, et al. A carbohydrate-rich drink reduces preoperative discomfort in elective surgery patients. Anesth Analg. 2001;93(5):1344–50.
28. Holte K, Nielsen KG, Madsen JL, et al. Physiologic effects of bowel preparation. Dis Colon Rectum. 2004;47(8):1397–402.
29. Cavallaro P, Bordeianou L. Implementation of an ERAS pathway in colorectal surgery. Clin Colon Rectal Surg. 2019;32:102–8.
30. Ljungqvist O. Modulating postoperative insulin resistance by preoperative carbohydrate loading. Best Pract Res Clin Anaesthesiol. 2009;23:401–9.
31. Awad S, Varadhan KK, Ljungqvist O, et al. A meta-analysis of randomised controlled trials on preoperative oral carbohydrate treatment in elective surgery. Clin Nutr. 2013;32(1):34–44.
32. Noblett SE, Watson DS, Huong H, Davison B, Hainsworth PJ, Horgan AF. Pre-operative oral carbohydrate loading in colorectal surgery: a randomized controlled trial. Color Dis. 2006;8(7):563–9.
33. Abis G, Stockmann H, Bonjer H, et al. Randomized clinical trial of selective decontamination of the digestive tract in elective colorectal cancer surgery (SELECT trial). Br J Surg. 2019;106(4):355–63.
34. Rollins K, Javanmard-Emamghissi H, Lobo D. Impact of mechanical bowel preparation in elective colorectal surgery: a meta-analysis. World J Gastroenterol. 2018;24(4):519–36.
35. Gee E. The national VTE exemplar centres network response to implementation of updated NICE guidance: venous thromboembolism in over 16s: reducing the risk of hospital acquired deep vein thrombosis or pulmonary embolism (NG89). Br J Haematol. 2019;186(5):792–3.
36. Kassie G, Nguyen T, Kalisch E, et al. Preoperative medication use and postoperative delirium: a systematic review. BMC Geriatr. 2017;17(1):298.
37. Baldini G, Fawcett WJ. Anesthesia for colorectal surgery. Anesthesiol Clin. 2015;33:93–123.
38. Levy BF, Scott MJ, Fawcett WJ, Day A, Rockall TA. Optimizing patient outcomes in laparoscopic surgery. Color Dis. 2011;13(7):8–11.

39. Imbelloni LE, Fornasari M, Fialho JC. Combined spinal epidural anesthesia during colon surgery in a high-risk patient: case report. Rev Bras Anestesiol. 2009;59:741–5.
40. Fleischmann E, Marschalek C, Schlemitz K, Dalton JE, Gruenberger T, Herbst F, et al. Nitrous oxide may not increase the risk of cancer recurrence after colorectal surgery: a follow-up of a randomized controlled trial. BMC Anesthesiol. 2009;9:1.
41. Scheinin B, Lindgren L, Scheinin TM. Peroperative nitrous oxide delays bowel function after colonic surgery. Br J Anaesth. 1990;64(2):154–8.
42. LiM H, ZhengM Z-N, Zhang N-R, et al. Intra-operative open-lung ventilatory strategy reduces postoperative complications after laparoscopic colorectal cancer resection. Eur J Anaesthesiol. 2021;38:1042–51.
43. Billeter A, Hohmann S, Druen D, et al. Unintentional perioperative hypothermia is associated with severe complications and high mortality in elective operations. Surgery. 2014;156(5):1245–52.
44. Danelli G, Berti M, Perotti V, et al. Temperature control and recovery of bowel function after laparoscopic or laparotomic colorectal surgery in patients receiving combined epidural/general anesthesia and postoperative epidural analgesia. Anesth Analg. 2002;95(2):467–71.
45. Liu H, Hu X, Duan X, et al. Thoracic epidural analgesia (TEA) vs. patient controlled analgesia (PCA) in laparoscopic colectomy: a meta-analysis. Hepatogastroenterology. 2014;61:1213–9.
46. Borzellino G, Francis NK, Chapuis O, et al. Role of epidural analgesia within an ERAS program after laparoscopic colorectal surgery: a review and meta-analysis of randomised controlled studies. Surg Res Pract. 2016;2016:7543684.
47. Halabi WJ, Kang CY, Nguyen VQ, et al. Epidural analgesia in laparoscopic colorectal surgery: a nationwide analysis of use and outcomes. JAMA Surg. 2014;149:130–6.
48. Hanna MH, Jafari MD, Jafari F, et al. Randomized clinical trial of epidural compared with conventional analgesia after minimally invasive colorectal surgery. J Am Coll Surg. 2017;225:622–30.
49. Popping DM, Elia N, Marret E, et al. Protective effects of epidural analgesia on pulmonary complications after abdominal and thoracic surgery: a meta-analysis. Arch Surg. 2008;143(10):990–9. [discussion: 1000].
50. Gustafsson UO, Scott MJ, Hubner M, et al. Guidelines for perioperative care in elective colorectal surgery: enhanced recovery after surgery (ERAS) society recommendations: 2018. World J Surg. 2019;43:659–95.
51. Brandstrup B, Svendsen PE, Rasmussen M, et al. Which goal for fluid therapy during colorectal surgery is followed by the best outcome: near-maximal stroke volume or zero fluid balance? Br J Anaesth. 2012;109:191–9.
52. Gomez-Izquierdo JC, Trainito A, Mirzakandov D, et al. Goal-directed fluid therapy does not reduce primary postoperative ileus after elective laparoscopic colorectal surgery: a randomized controlled trial. Anesthesiology. 2017;127:36–49.
53. Srinivasa S, Taylor MH, Singh PP, et al. Randomized clinical trial of goal-directed fluid therapy within an enhanced recovery protocol for elective colectomy. Br J Surg. 2013;100:66–74.
54. Rollins KE, Lobo DN. Intraoperative goal-directed fluid therapy in elective major abdominal surgery: a meta-analysis of randomized controlled trials. Ann Surg. 2016;263:465–76.
55. McCluskey SA, Karkouti K, Wijeysundera D, et al. Hyperchloremia after noncardiac surgery is independently associated with increased morbidity and mortality: a propensity-matched cohort study. Anesth Analg. 2013;117(2):412–21.
56. Yunos NM, Bellomo R, Hegarty C, et al. Association between a chloride-liberal vs chloride-restrictive intravenous fluid administration strategy and kidney injury in critically ill adults. JAMA. 2012;308(15):1566–72.
57. Shaw AD, Bagshaw SM, Goldstein SL, et al. Major complications, mortality, and resource utilization after open abdominal surgery: 0.9% saline compared to plasma-lyte. Ann Surg. 2012;255(5):821–9.
58. Bijker JB, van Klei WA, Vergouwe Y, et al. Intraoperative hypotension and 1-year mortality after noncardiac surgery. Anesthesiology. 2009;111:1217–26.
59. Feldheiser A, Conroy P, Bonomo T, et al. Development and feasibility study of an algorithm for intraoperative goal directed haemodynamic management in noncardiac surgery. J Int Med Res. 2012;40:1227–41.

17 CA Osteosarcoma for Below-Knee Amputation

Shailendra Kumar and Amit Kumar

17.1 Introduction

Osteosarcoma or osteogenic sarcoma is a malignant neoplasm arising from primitive transformed cells of mesenchymal origin. This primary bone sarcoma has incidence of 4.6 per million people [1]. These cells have osteoblastic differentiation and produce malignant osteoid. It can be found in any age group but is prevalent in paediatric and adolescents. This tumour is more prevalent in fast-growing metaphyseal ends of long bones. This tumour frequently grows at proximal end of tibia, humerus or distal end of the femur. Osteosarcoma affects the knee in around 60% of cases whereas other areas are around the hip, shoulder and jaw with incidence of around 15%, 10% and 8%, respectively [2]. Osteosarcoma has male preponderance with male-to-female ratio of 2.3:1 [2]. The initial symptoms and signs may be night pain and tenderness around the knee, local mass, limited joint mobility and pathological fracture. X-ray imaging is an initial imaging of choice which shows sunburst appearance and Codman triangle while CT scan is useful to define anatomy and detect pathological fracture. Also, soft tissue and medullary cavity is better imaged with the help of MRI scan [3]. The tumour may metastasise to lungs and is seen as solitary or multiple nodular opacities on chest X-ray. The treatment of osteosarcoma is complete radical, en block surgical resection of tumour [4] and neoadjuvant or adjuvant chemotherapy. Surgery is usually done after neoadjuvant chemotherapy with an aim of limb salvage. Limb salvage surgery is possible in majority of patients [5] but may need amputation in case of complications, such as infection, non-union or loco-regional tumour recurrence. The patient present to the anaesthesiologists may present unique issues of post radiation and post chemotherapy status. The treatment requires close co-coordination between various specialists such as medical oncologists, orthopaedic surgeons, physical therapists, anaesthesiologists, critical care specialists and oncology nurses.

Q1

What are the various types of osteosarcomas?

Osteogenic sarcoma types
Low-grade central osteosarcoma
Conventional (high-grade) osteosarcoma (chondroblastic fibroblastic osteoblastic)
Telangiectatic osteosarcoma
Small cell osteosarcoma
Secondary osteosarcoma
Parosteal osteosarcoma
Periosteal osteosarcoma
High-grade surface osteosarcoma

S. Kumar (✉) · A. Kumar
Department of Anaesthesiology, Pain Medicine and Critical Care, AIIMS, Delhi, New Delhi, India

N. Gupta et al. (eds.), *Problem Based Learning Discussions in Onco-Anesthesia and Onco-Critical Care*, https://doi.org/10.1007/978-981-99-6339-3_17

Q2

Enumerate various modalities of treatment for osteosarcoma?

Osteosarcoma treatment modalities

Common surgeries	Common chemotherapy agents
Amputation, endoprosthetic replacement and metastasectomy	Methotrexate, cisplatin, doxorubicin, ifosfamide and etoposide

Q3

What are the common chemotherapeutic agents and their systemic toxicities?

Common chemotherapy drugs and their systemic toxicities in osteosarcoma

Drugs	Common systematic toxicities
Methotrexate	Pulmonary, renal, hepatic and CNS
Cisplatin	Renal, cardiac, CNS and hepatic
Doxorubicin	Cardiac and pulmonary
Ifosfamide	Acute tubular necrosis, renal failure, cerebellar dysfunction, hemiparesis, coma and extrapyramidal abnormalities
Etoposide	Hematologic and pulmonary

Q4

How will you evaluate, prepare and premedicate the patient for surgery?

The weight bearing on the affected limb is advised to be avoided as soon as diagnosis is made as it may lead to pathological fracture which is associated with adverse prognostication [6]. There is increased metastasis to lungs and bones in patients with pathological fracture as initial presentation [3]. Preoperatively patient may be trained in gait maintenance and walking assist devices by the physical therapist. Also, preoperative vascular embolisation may be considered in highly vascular tumour [7]. Previous oncological treatments may be responsible for difficult vascular access. Peroperative multidisciplinary planning and execution are important for better patient outcome. Preoperative optimisation also includes optimisation of risk factors such as alcohol consumption, smoking, nutritional status, anaemia, metabolic derangements and low physical activity. These factors might be responsible for complications and/or increased length of hospital stay [8].

Patients' well-being and metabolism may be improved with carbohydrate loading, but the early achievement of discharge criteria and reduced complications have not been shown in studies. So it is not routinely recommended [9].

17.2 Psychological Evaluation

Amputation can result in significant psychological burden on the patient especially in sole bread earner of their family. Depression can result from sudden disability following surgery, and so the patients should be counselled preoperatively keeping risk factors of major depression such as young age, pain, poor coping skills and neurotic personality in mind [9, 10].

17.3 Perioperative Antibiotics

All the patients undergoing below-knee amputation should be receiving antibiotic prophylaxis 1 h before surgery regardless of surgical wound classification [11, 12].

A systematic review on prophylactic antibiotic for infection prevention after major limb amputation identified four randomised control trials with heterogenous data agreed that prophylactic antibiotics are standard of care [13].

A recent randomised control trial showed surgical site infection (SSI) and impaired wound healing (IWH) were common in patients with lower limb amputation and have significant outcome impact. Also, compared to 24-h antibiotics, 5-day course of antibiotic prophylaxis showed to reduce SSI and IWH reducing further need of surgery [14].

17.4 Premedication

Preoperative anxiety may be associated with postoperative phantom limb pain (PLP) and residual limb pain (RLP) [15] which warrant anxiety control preoperatively with pharmacological and non-pharmacological interventions.

However, routine administration of sedatives to reduce anxiety preoperatively is not recommended [9].

Q5

What are the various intraoperative considerations for osteosarcoma patient posted for amputation?

The surgical treatment of osteosarcoma has wide variations and complexities. Amputations are usually avoided and limb-sparing surgeries are usually performed. These limb-sparing surgeries maintain functionality of the limb compared to amputations [16]. The anaesthetic management for these surgeries also has varied options such as regional techniques, general anaesthesia or combination of both. The peri-operative pain can also be managed with several options depending on patient's preference, medical conditions, contraindications, anaesthetic specialist proficiencies and judgements.

A systematic review by *Hanna von Plato* et al. [17] including 19 studies and 949 patients did not find concrete evidence for epidural analgesia or continuous perineural analgesia (CPI). Also, epidural was found to be having more adverse effects than CPI.

A randomised control trial by Weinbroum et al. [18] patient control epidural analgesia was more effective than intravenous morphine patient control analgesia after bone tumour resection done under combined epidural and general anaesthesia.

Overtime, the techniques for anaesthetic and analgesic management for amputation have evolved to decrease the complications and improve patient outcomes while taking care of patient satisfaction.

17.5 Positioning

Positioning for above-knee amputation is usually supine. To avoid brachial plexus (C8 and T1 nerve roots) injuries care must be taken to avoid hyper-abduction of upper limbs above 90°, keeping the hand pronated and keeping the head in neutral position. Also, the ulnar nerve is prone to injuries in the ulnar groove behind humeral medial epicondyle.

The supine position also leads to loss of lumbar lordosis which may result in postoperative low back pain in prolonged surgeries. Hence, a lumbar wedge or support may be placed during positioning. Adequate padding to the bony pressure points should be ensued.

Q6

Which anaesthetic plan to choose? general or neuraxial anaesthesia (NA)

In general, both general anaesthesia and regional anaesthesia have been given with or without peripheral regional techniques for below-knee amputation. Considering the surgical time for below-knee amputation, spinal anaesthesia is also a feasible option.

An enhanced recovery pathway for major limb amputation in vascular surgeries recommends goals of avoiding general anaesthesia, maintaining haemodynamic stability and avoiding postoperative delirium-causing medications [19]. This pathway emphasises the role of continuous peripheral nerve block (CPNB) with sedation (propofol or dexmedetomidine).

A systematic review and meta-analysis by Bosanquet et al. [20] show that there is evidence for peripheral nerve catheter to reduce opioid consumption following lower limb amputation without other outcome changes while grade of evidence is low.

General anaesthesia has been known to be associated with higher associations with postoperative nausea, vomiting and delirium. Also, adverse effects of polypharmacy have been well known, whereas regional anaesthesia can be associated with complications of block failure, high spinal, epidural hematoma, epidural abscess and nerve injuries [21].

Currently, no single mode of anaesthesia is evident to be superior to other for below-knee amputation in terms of cardiovascular and pulmonary morbidities and mortality. Literature has previously demonstrated various advantages of regional anaesthesia such as lesser pulmonary complications, reduced arterial and venous thrombosis, reduced post procedure mechanical ventilation needs and reduced requirement for blood transfusions [22–24]. However, these findings are largely found in patients undergoing orthopaedic, urologic, vascular and general surgery procedures [14, 25, 26].

Also, the surgical literature shows that outcomes in lower extremity amputations are improved with local anaesthesia and regional anaesthesia. The incidence of early amputation failure has been shown to be associated with the use of general anaesthesia [25], whereas the incidences of surgical site infection, acute kidney injury, major adverse cardiac events and hospital length of stay do not seem to be affected by the choice of anaesthesia.

There are multiple theoretical advantages of regional anaesthesia (neuraxial and peripheral nerve blockade) over general anaesthesia such as decreased neuro-endocrine stress response and reduced blood catecholamine and cortisol levels. The stress on the heart is also reduced due to the decrease in preload and afterload especially beneficial in patients with decreased cardiac function [27]. Patients at risk of postoperative pulmonary dysfunction after general anaesthesia also benefit with regional anaesthesia as it avoids the risks of endotracheal intubations and mechanical ventilation [10].

A large systemic review by Rodgers et al. including 141 trials with 9559 patients showed that neuraxial blockade decreases the mortality and occurrence of serious complications though further research was suggested to determine if these effects were solely due to neuraxial anaesthesia or because of avoiding general anaesthesia [28]. This review showed reduction of overall mortality by one-third in neuraxial anaesthesia compared to general anaesthesia (odds ratio—0.70).

There is scarcity of literature to compare neuraxial and general anaesthesia in osteosarcoma for below-knee amputation. A retrospective study in functionally impaired patients with age ≥75 years based on the American College of Surgeons National Surgical Quality Improvement Program (ACS-NSQIP) data set concluded that the type of anaesthesia did not have any significant effect on the peri-operative outcomes in lower extremity amputations.

Although the benefits of regional anaesthesia are evident, the argument in support of general anaesthesia is to avoid challenges of haemodynamic fluctuations in case of large blood loss together with sympathectomy with neuraxial anaesthesia. Many anaesthesia physicians prefer to place an epidural catheter for postoperative use followed by anaesthesia induction of anaesthesia for surgery. In cases of contraindications for neuraxial blockade and in high-risk patients, peripheral nerve blocks can be given such as combination of femoral and popliteal-sciatic nerve block with or without catheter for below-knee amputations [29].These techniques may be particularly be more useful in oncological patients who are pre-treated with opioids for pre-operative pain management and in patients who are chronic drug addicts as opioid sparing strategy.

Q7

Describe multimodal analgesia options for a patient with osteosarcoma posted for amputation.

Multimodal analgesia is important for these patients as involvement of various sources and pathways for acute and chronic pain makes the pain management in these patients particularly challenging. Multiple sources are involved in pain process such as pain due to tumour involvement of the limb, co-existing musculoskeletal pain, phantom limb sensation and phantom limb pain. Various strategies that can be applied for multimodal analgesia are pharmacological, interventional and others. Pharmacological agents such as acetaminophen, non-steroidal anti-inflammatory agents, opioids and non-opioid systemic (gabapentinoids, *N*-methyl D-aspartate (NMDA) receptor antagonists, alpha-2 adrenergic agents, glucocorticoids, antidepressants, cannabinoids, etc.) analgesics are frequently used. Interventional techniques such as neuraxial and regional nerve blocks with or without catheters can be considered. Other techniques such as the use of walker, splints and gait training to avoid weight bearing on the affected limb may prevent pain during walking as well as pain due to possible pathological fracture which might also affect the disease prognosis.

These patients are on many occasions on opioids and so are prone to tolerance and dependence. This entails detailed planning in order to escalate the opioid drug dosing regimen.

Multimodal analgesia options		
Opioid analgesics	Morphine Fentanyl Hydromorphone Oxycodone	
Non-opioid systemic analgesics	Acetaminophen Non-steroidal anti-inflammatory drugs (NSAIDs) Aceclofenac, diclofenac, ketorolac, etc.	
Interventional pain procedures	Local infiltration analgesia Lumbar plexus + sacral plexus blockade Femoral/saphenous + sciatic nerve block Subarachnoid block Epidural blockade Combined spinal epidural block	±Continuous catheter
Gabapentinoids	Gabapentin Pregabalin	
N-methyl D-aspartate (NMDA) receptor antagonists	Ketamine Memantine	
Alpha-2 adrenergic agents	Clonidine	
Glucocorticoids	Dexamethasone	
Others	Antidepressants Calcitonin Nicotine Capsaicin Cannabinoids Dextromethorphan Magnesium Lidocaine	

Q8

How do you manage nausea and vomiting in these patients?

The postoperative nausea and vomiting (PONV) has multifactorial aetiology. The use of regional anaesthesia techniques decreases the PONV incidences significantly. Patients undergoing surgical resection under general anaesthesia need to be evaluated for risk of nausea and vomiting, and accordingly anti-emetic medications should be given. The use of opioids intraoperatively and postoperatively is a risk factor for PONV together with other causes such as type of procedure, length of inhalational anaesthetic agent exposure, use of nitrous oxide and patient risk factors. The postoperative nausea and vomiting prophylaxis and management may be done as per latest consensus guidelines [30].

Q9

Explain in brief wound care post amputation.

The amputation wound needs to be examined daily for the signs of infection (discharge from wound, warmth, erythema and wound dehiscence). The patients with unexplained fever or excessive stump pain have to be kept in vigilance. The wound drains are monitored daily, and when the volume of fluid collected in the drain is minimal, drain can be removed.

Q10

Describe postoperative recovery and rehabilitation for these patients.

After the surgery, the patient has to be shifted to either recovery ward, high dependency unit or intensive care unit as per the patient's pre- and intra-operative status. Postoperative pain control is paramount for recovery and rehabilitation. Pain management can be best dealt with pre-emptive preventive analgesia approaches. Though these analgesic approaches have favouring results, conflicting evidence is also eminent such as a meta-analysis comparing non-steroidal anti-inflammatory agents (NSAIDs), pre-surgical incision opioids, N-methyl-D-aspartic acid (NMDA) receptor antagonists and regional analgesia [31]. Postoperative local anaesthetic with opioid patient control epidural analgesia has been found to be better analgesic strategy compared to intravenous patient control analgesia in orthopaedic malignancy patients [18].

A team-based and patient centric approach is needed for early recovery and regaining functionality. Team members include orthopaedic surgeon, anaesthesiologist, pain physician, psychiatrist and physical therapist. The team must devise a plan for the patient to maximise patient's participation in therapy with minimum discomfort.

Q11

Give a brief account on stump pain.

Acute pain in the amputation stump gradually reduced in 1–3 weeks. Phantom limb pain can be reduced by optimum pain control in whole perioperative period [32]. Multimodal pain management with the help of modalities described above is paramount for optimal rehabilitation post amputation [32, 33]. Despite adequate counselling and pain management, few patients land up in depression. Majority of amputation patients report developing chronic pain. Pain may initially persist due to stump ischaemia, neuroma formation, stump infection and manifestation of phantom limb syndrome. Depression may complicate the treatment of pain in many amputees. Stump pain due to ischaemia may be difficult to diagnose. A transcutaneous oxygen tension below 20 mmHg at the level of the stump signifies stump ischaemia. Neuroma is frequently developed at the level of nerve transaction [34, 35]. Neuroma pain is usually localised and can be blocked by nerve blockade by anaesthetic agent. Symptomatic neuromas show heterogeneity on T2-weighted magnetic resonance imaging [36]. Bony spurs at the stump may also cause stump pain. Chronic postoperative pain can be a manifestation of stump infection and must be evaluated. Phantom pain syndrome is a diagnosis of exclusion and is diagnosed when all possible causes of stump pain are ruled out.

Q12

What is phantom limb pain? What are the strategies to manage this?

Phantom limb pain is a phenomenon where the patient feels that pain is coming from a part of body that is non-existent. The incidence has been reported to around 64% in a recent meta-nalysis [37]. The mechanism is complex and not clearly understood. It is due to complex interplay of the peripheral mechanism and maladaptive rearrangement of the somatosensory and motor areas in the brain. It is considered a neuropathic character and usually episodic. The treatment options include mirror therapy, visual feedback, transcranial magnetic stimulation and motor imagery [38]. Some drugs like gabapentin, ketamine and morphine have shown limited effectiveness [39].

Q13

Explain the considerations for postoperative physical therapy in these patients.

Weight bearing depends on various issues such as level of amputation, healing issues in the stump, etc. Patients not being mobilised and are non-ambulatory should receive thromboprophylaxis for deep vein thrombosis until activities are restricted.

After adequate wound healing, a 'shrinker' is applied on the stump to decrease oedema and to mould the stump for future prosthetic fitting. Ambulation in prosthetic is carried out gradually after complete wound healing and with the assistance of interdisciplinary rehabilitation team.

Range of motion can be regained with the help of continuous passive motion (CPM) machines and passive and active physiotherapy. These patients are also prone to develop lack in self-esteem and body image apprehension. It might be useful to take help from psychologist and join support group therapy session.

At discharge from the hospital, patient should be educated about identifying the red flags and contacting medical facility, the further course of chemotherapy and structured planning for prosthetic use and rehabilitation. Early physiotherapy and mobilisation prevent complications (depressed psychological state, joint contracture, etc.). The scheduled physiotherapy is gradually increased to improve on weight bearing, gait and physical therapy to achieve acceptable range of motion with full extension and 90° flexion. The patient's rehabilitation therapy sessions may be clubbed with the chemotherapy sessions together with outpatient sessions. Adequacy of prosthesis use and leg length discrepancies can be assessed with the help of timely follow-up.

The process of rehabilitation aims at obtaining maximum independence for the patient. Efforts are directed towards prevention of oedema, controlling pain, achieving and maintaining joint range of motion, preventing muscle atrophy and muscle weakness, preventing pressure sores, addressing sensory reduction and supporting the patient psychologically throughout the rehabilitation process.

These aims are achieved with the help of various modalities such as active and passive range of motion, desensitising techniques, resistance exercises, mobilisation, stump management, pain management and patient counselling/education.

References

1. Anderson MR, Jeng CL, Wittig JC, Rosenblatt MA. Anesthesia for patients undergoing orthopedic oncologic surgeries. J Clin Anesth. 2010;22(7):565–72. https://doi.org/10.1016/j.jclinane.2010.02.011.
2. Vijayanarasimha D, Nayanar SK, Vikram S, Patil VM, Babu S, Satheesan B. Clinico-pathological study of limb salvage surgery for osteosarcoma: experience in a rural cancer center. Indian J Surg Oncol. 2017;8(2):136–41. https://doi.org/10.1007/s13193-016-0547-8. Epub 2016 Aug 30.
3. Kundu ZS. Classification, imaging, biopsy and staging of osteosarcoma. Indian J Orthop. 2014;48(3):238–46.
4. Ottaviani G, Jaffe N. The epidemiology of osteosarcoma. In: Jaffe N, et al., editors. Pediatric and adolescent osteosarcoma. Cancer treatment and research, vol. 152. New York: Springer; 2009. p. 3–13.
5. Saghieh S, et al. Seven-year experience of using Repiphysis expandable prosthesis in children with bone tumors. Pediatr Blood Cancer. 2010;55:457–63.
6. Lee RKL, et al. Pathological fracture as the presenting feature in pediatric osteosarcoma. Pediatr Blood Cancer. 2013;60:1118–21.
7. Zhang L, Gong Q, Xiao H, Tu C, Liu J. Control of blood loss during sacral surgery by aortic balloon occlusion. Anesth Analg. 2007;105:700–3.
8. Hansen TB, Bredtoft HK, Larsen K. Preoperative physical optimization in fast-track hip and knee arthroplasty. Dan Med J. 2012;59(2):A4381.
9. Bhuvaneswar CG, Epstein LA, Stern TA. Reactions to amputation: recognition and treatment. Prim Care Companion J Clin Psychiatry. 2007;9:303.
10. Kashani JH, Frank RG, Kashani SR, et al. Depression among amputees. J Clin Psychiatry. 1983;44:256.
11. Bratzler DW, Houck PM, Surgical Infection Prevention Guidelines Writers Workgroup, et al. Antimicrobial prophylaxis for surgery: an advisory statement from the National Surgical Infection Prevention Project. Clin Infect Dis. 2004;38:1706.
12. Antimicrobial prophylaxis for surgery. Treat Guidel Med Lett. 2009;7:47.
13. McIntosh J, Earnshaw JJ. Antibiotic prophylaxis for the prevention of infection after major limb amputation. Eur J Vasc Endovasc Surg. 2009;37:696.
14. Souroullas P, Barnes R, Carradice D, Smith G, Huang C, Chetter I. Extended-course antibiotic prophylaxis in lower limb amputation: randomized clinical trial. Br J Surg. 2022;109(5):426–32. https://doi.org/10.1093/bjs/znac053.

15. Raichle KA, Osborne TL, Jensen MP, Ehde DM, Smith DG, Robinson LR. Preoperative state anxiety, acute postoperative pain, and analgesic use in persons undergoing lower limb amputation. Clin J Pain. 2015;31(8):699–706. https://doi.org/10.1097/AJP.0000000000000150.
16. Malek F, et al. Does limb-salvage surgery offer patients better quality of life and functional capacity than amputation? Clin Orthop Relat Res. 2012;470:2000–6.
17. Von Plato H, Kontinen V, Hamunen K. Efficacy and safety of epidural, continuous perineural infusion and adjuvant analgesics for acute postoperative pain after major limb amputation—a systematic review. Scand J Pain. 2018;18(1):3–17. https://doi.org/10.1515/sjpain-2017-0170.
18. Weinbroum AA. Superiority of postoperative epidural over intravenous patient-controlled analgesia in orthopedic oncologic patients. Surgery. 2005;138:869–76.
19. Scarlet S, Isaak RS, McGinigle KL. Design and implementation of an enhanced recovery after surgery (ERAS) pathway for major limb amputation in vascular surgery. Am Surg. 2018;84(4):e147–9.
20. Bosanquet DC, Glasbey JC, Stimpson A, Williams IM, Twine CP. Systematic review and meta-analysis of the efficacy of perineural local anaesthetic catheters after major lower limb amputation. Eur J Vasc Endovasc Surg. 2015;50(2):241–9. https://doi.org/10.1016/j.ejvs.2015.04.030. Epub 2015 Jun 9.
21. Horlocker TT. Complications of regional anesthesia and acute pain management. Anesthesiol Clin. 2011;29(2):257–78.
22. Kehlet H. General vs. regional anesthesia. In: Rogers MC, Tinker JH, Covino BG, Longnecker DE, editors. Principles and practice of anesthesiology, vol. 2. St Louis, MO: Mosby; 1933. p. 1218–34.
23. Baron JF, Coriat P, Mundler O, Fauchet M, Bousseau D, Viars P. Left ventricular global and regional function during lumbar epidural anesthesia in patients with and without angina pectoris. Influence of volume loading. Anesthesiology. 1987;66:621–7.
24. Moreira CC, Farber A, Kalish JA, et al. The effect of anesthesia type on major lower extremity amputation in functionally impaired elderly patients. J Vasc Surg. 2016;63:696–701.
25. O'Brien PJ, Cox MW, Shortell CK, Scarborough JE. Risk factors for early failure of surgical amputations: an analysis of 8,878 isolated lower extremity amputation procedures. J Am Coll Surg. 2013;216:836–42; discussion 842–844.
26. Siracuse JJ, Gill HL, Schneider DB, et al. Assessing the perioperative safety of common femoral endarterectomy in the endovascular era. Vasc Endovasc Surg. 2014;48:27–33.
27. Bode RH Jr, Lewis KP. Con. Regional anesthesia is not better than general anesthesia for lower extremity revascularization. J Cardiothorac Vasc Anesth. 1994;8:118–21.
28. Rodgers A, Walker N, Schug S, McKee A, Kehlet H, van Zundert A, Sage D, Futter M, Saville G, Clark T, MacMahon S. Reduction of postoperative mortality and morbidity with epidural or spinal anaesthesia: results from overview of randomised trials. BMJ. 2000;321(7275):1493. https://doi.org/10.1136/bmj.321.7275.1493.
29. Arjun BK, Prijith RS, Sreeraghu GM, Narendrababu MC. Ultrasound-guided popliteal sciatic and adductor canal block for below-knee surgeries in high-risk patients. Indian J Anaesth. 2019;63(8):635–9. https://doi.org/10.4103/ija.IJA_296_19.
30. Gan TJ, Belani KG, Bergese S, Chung F, Diemunsch P, Habib AS, Jin Z, Kovac AL, Meyer TA, Urman RD, Apfel CC, Ayad S, Beagley L, Candiotti K, Englesakis M, Hedrick TL, Kranke P, Lee S, Lipman D, Minkowitz HS, Morton J, Philip BK. Fourth consensus guidelines for the management of postoperative nausea and vomiting. Anesth Analg. 2020;131(2):411–48. https://doi.org/10.1213/ANE.0000000000004833. Erratum in: Anesth Analg 2020;131(5):e241.
31. Møiniche S, Kehlet H, Dahl JB. A qualitative and quantitative systematic review of preemptive analgesia for postoperative pain relief: the role of timing of analgesia. Anesthesiology. 2002;96:725–41.
32. Karanikolas M, Aretha D, Tsolakis I, et al. Optimized perioperative analgesia reduces chronic phantom limb pain intensity, prevalence, and frequency: a prospective, randomized, clinical trial. Anesthesiology. 2011;114:1144.
33. Ephraim PL, Wegener ST, MacKenzie EJ, et al. Phantom pain, residual limb pain, and back pain in amputees: results of a national survey. Arch Phys Med Rehabil. 2005;86:1910.
34. Huang YJ, Assi PE, Drolet BC, et al. A systematic review and meta-analysis on the incidence of patients with lower-limb amputations who developed symptomatic neuromata in the residual limb. Ann Plast Surg. 2022;88:574.
35. List EB, Krijgh DD, Martin E, Coert JH. Prevalence of residual limb pain and symptomatic neuromas after lower extremity amputation: a systematic review and meta-analysis. Pain. 2021;162:1906.
36. Chung BM, Lee GY, Kim WT, et al. MRI features of symptomatic amputation neuromas. Eur Radiol. 2021;31:7684.
37. Limakatso K, Bedwell GJ, Madden VJ, Parker R. The prevalence and risk factors for phantom limb pain in people with amputations: a systematic review and meta-analysis. PLoS One. 2020;15(10):e0240431.
38. Herrador Colmenero L, Perez Marmol JM, Martí-García C, et al. Effectiveness of mirror therapy, motor imagery, and virtual feedback on phantom limb pain following amputation: a systematic review. Prosthetics Orthot Int. 2018;42:288.
39. Richardson C, Kulkarni J. A review of the management of phantom limb pain: challenges and solutions. J Pain Res. 2017;10:1861.

18 Anaesthesia for Bone Marrow Aspiration and Biopsy

Mahima Gupta

18.1 Case

A 5 year old male child admitted with fever and anaemia, with WBC—33,000, Hb-7 g/dL, and platelet count of 40,000. Now is being posted for bone marrow aspiration (BMA) and biopsy (BMB)?

18.2 What Is BMA and BMB?

These procedures are usually performed to diagnose and for the follow-up of haematological disorders.

18.3 What Are the Indications of Bone Marrow Aspiration (BMA) [1]?

1. Investigation in children with abnormal peripheral blood findings (e.g. atypical cells [or blasts], pancytopenia, unexplained anaemia, leukopenia or thrombocytopenia)
2. Diagnosis of malignant haematological disorders, hypoplastic anaemias, congenital bone marrow failure syndromes and metastatic spread of tumours
3. Obtaining microbiological cultures in paediatrics for pyrexia of unknown origin (PUO)
4. Investigating hypersplenism, lymphadenopathy, mediastinal or abdominal masses
5. For follow-up after chemotherapy or haematopoietic stem cell transplant

18.4 What Are the Indications of Bone Marrow Biopsy (BMB)?

1. Investigation and staging of Hodgkin's and non-Hodgkin's lymphoma, and small blue round cell tumours of childhood (neuroblastoma, rhabdomyosarcoma and Ewing's sarcoma)
2. Diagnosis of aplastic anaemia, myelodysplastic syndromes and acute megakaryoblastic leukaemia (AML-M7) [2]

M. Gupta (✉)
Department of Anaesthesia and Pain, Hamdard Institute of Medical Sciences and Associated HAHC Centenary Hospital, New Delhi, India

N. Gupta et al. (eds.), *Problem Based Learning Discussions in Onco-Anesthesia and Onco-Critical Care*, https://doi.org/10.1007/978-981-99-6339-3_18

18.5 What Are the Contraindications for BMA and BMB?

1. Acquired or congenital coagulation factor deficiencies—factor replacement prior to bone marrow procedure and hospital observation for 24 h after the procedure may be indicated.
2. Patients on anticoagulants having PT or aPTT more than the therapeutic range [3].
3. Isolated thrombocytopenia is not a contraindication if performed properly and no technical difficulties are encountered. Platelets to be transfused to increase the count above 15,000 cells/microlitre [4].
4. Sternal bone marrow aspiration is contraindicated in patients with diseases associated with bone resorption (like multiple myeloma).
5. Skin infections at the site.
6. Recent radiation therapy at the site.

18.6 How It Is Performed?

At birth, numerous sites of haematopoiesis exist; however, by adolescence haematopoiesis becomes restricted to the axial skeleton. Posterior iliac crest is the most preferred site for sampling due to patient comfort and safety reasons. In obese patients having huge amount of adipose tissue or in patients with wound overlying the posterior iliac crest, sampling can be done from the anterior iliac crest. Sometimes both of the sites may be unfit for sampling, where aspiration can be done from the proximal sternum or tibia (in neonates).

Position—right or left lateral decubitus position with the thigh and knee flexed for aspiration from posterior the iliac crest. Jamshidi needle is commonly used. It is radially tapered towards the cutting edge that allows marrow tissue to freely enter the needle without clogging the tip [5]. The biopsy needle is held with the handle in the palm and the index fingertip on the shaft to control needle penetration. The needle is inserted and advanced with steady pressure to reach periosteum and by twisting motion into the bony cortex. Obturator is removed from the needle and the needle is pushed back and forth into the bony cortex and bone marrow to obtain biopsy core. Trephine core is collected on a glass microscopic slide or piece of sterile gauze and the adequacy of the core is inspected.

18.7 What Are the Complications?

It is a safe procedure with low risk of morbidity. Mortality is extremely rare with bone marrow aspiration and biopsy of iliac crest and unusual with sternal marrow aspiration. However, complications of the procedure include the following:

1. Haemorrhage at biopsy site, intra-abdominal and retroperitoneal haemorrhage [6]
2. Cardiac tamponade—due to laceration of right ventricle or root of aorta—causing death [7]
3. Sternal-manubrial separation [7]
4. Pulmonary bone marrow emboli [8]
5. Needle breakage or separation of the handle during insertion into the bone

18.8 Need for Anaesthesia during BMA and BMB

Invasive procedures are an essential part of cancer treatment. For instance, a child with standard risk B-cell ALL without central nervous system involvement may undergo somewhere 17–22 lumbar punctures over the entire treatment course [9]. Factors like previous experiences, fear, anxiety or other behavioural components have direct effects on individual's pain perception. Efficacy of modalities to reduce pain during invasive procedure is reduced in children who has received inadequate analgesia for their initial procedures during cancer diagnosis/treatment. The ASA advocates the use of sedation for painful procedures to relieve anxiety, discomfort and pain. They also describe sedation as a continuum that can be classified as mild, moderate and deep sedation/general anaesthesia [10].

18.9 How Will You Do the Pre-anesthetic Evaluation?

The pre-anaesthetic evaluation of a paediatric patient is essentially similar as for other procedures in addition to specific evaluation which needs to be considered in these cases. The child should be evaluated for any congenital diseases and syndromes. During preoperative assessment, it is important to know the underlying diagnosis and ongoing active treatment if any. Mediastinal mass is commonly seen in children with Hodgkin's, non-Hodgkin's lymphoma and acute lymphoblastic leukaemia of T-cell variety. Respiratory and cardiovascular symptoms are mainly due to compression of the heart, major vessels and airway by mediastinal mass. However, severity of symptoms does not always correlate with the degree of compression. Any history of difficulty in sleeping in supine position or any preferential position of the child should be elicited from the caregiver. Children with more than 50% tracheal compression are at high risk of anaesthetic complications. Respiratory symptoms become more evident in supine position whereas cardiovascular symptoms may manifest during Valsalva manoeuvre.

In child presenting with severe cardiovascular/respiratory symptoms or adverse radiological features, consideration should be given to obtain a diagnosis without recourse to general anaesthesia. This may be possible from peripheral blood film analyses or obtaining a tissue sample using local anaesthesia. Alternatively, tumour shrinkage therapy can also be commenced before anaesthesia but that may compromise obtaining a complete histological diagnosis. However, limiting the period of pre-diagnostic treatment will usually limit the extent of this problem [11].

Diagnostic imaging like chest X-ray for confirmation of the diagnosis can be done, while advanced imaging modalities like computerised tomography (CT) is done echocardiography or pulmonary function tests (in older children) are sought to look for dynamic airway compression. Flexible fibreoptic bronchoscopy under local anaesthesia may be required to detect tracheomalacia as a result of long-standing airway compression [11].

Children with Wilm's tumour with abdominal distension maybe at risk of aspiration and airway should be secured as needed. Post steroid therapy, the mask ventilation may be difficult, and there is a risk of airway obstruction, so all emergency airway equipment should be kept handy.

Evaluate for any active or recent upper or lower respiratory tract infection as neutropenic children are very prone for this. But the severity of the infection and risks associated with anaesthetising such patients have to weighed against the benefit and need of this important diagnostic procedure. IV should be sited as securing an intravenous line in emergency can be a little challenging in these patients since they can be undergone post chemotherapy.

Complete blood count has to be obtained to determine their neutrophil count and rule out significant anaemia or thrombocytopenia and PT/INR to rule out coagulopathic state.

Standard NPO should be followed as elucidated in the guidelines for monitoring and management of paediatric patients before, during and after sedation for diagnostic and therapeutic rocedures [10].

For adults, BMA and BMB are usually done under local anaesthesia (LA) but are administered general anaesthesia or additional analgesia if required.

18.10 Care of Immunocompromised Child

With increasing incidence of leukaemia and improving a five-year survival, anaesthetists are more likely to encounter these children, providing care during diagnostic procedures, chemoradiotherapy and surgical treatment and in intensive care. Children with a haematological malignancy are frequently immunocompromised due to disease per se or neutropenia secondary to chemotherapy.

18.10.1 Strict Aseptic Measures

Strict adherence to standard infection control measures like proper hand hygiene and minimise patient contact with known infective cases or healthcare providers. Such patients to have be taken preferably before any known infective cases.

18.10.2 Care of Central Venous Lines

Common source of infection in children with haematological malignancy is an indwelling central venous catheter (CVC) which is inserted for administration of chemotherapy and frequent blood sampling. Four possible sources of infection of these lines could be due to skin, direct contact of catheter hub by an infected source (hand/fluid), seeding from another source through blood or infected IV fluid/drug administration. While accessing CVC, sterile gloves should be worn, and catheter hubs should be disinfected using chlorhexidine skin preparation. All the preloaded drugs have to be kept in a sterile tray with hubs of the syringe covered. Post-procedure before transfer to the recovery room, the line has to be flushed with sufficient volume of normal saline to ensure there is no residual drug in the cannula. Alternatively inhalational induction can be done to avoid contact with CVC altogether.

18.11 What Are the Goals of Anaesthesia?

The main of anaesthesia is to reduce patient's discomfort and anxiety, provide amnesia, and minimise movements and safe return to the preanaesthetic state for ready to discharge and prompt management of complications.

Table 18.1 shows the minimal requirements at non-operating room locations as per guidelines by ASA [10].

Parental presence should be acknowledged to reduce the anxiety of the paediatric patient. Consent should be obtained from the caregiver and from the patient in case of adults. The identity of the patient should be confirmed along with NBM status. Any evidence of anticipated difficult airway (Cushingoid facies), kissing tonsils, history of snoring and symptomatic mediastinal mass should be identified, and appropriate equipment should be kept ready.

Table 18.1 Minimal requirements at non-operating room locations [10]

Reliable source of oxygen with backup
Suction apparatus
Waste gas scavenging
Electrical outlet
Adequate illumination of patient and anaesthesia workstation
Staff trained to support the anaesthesiologist
Emergency cart—self-inflating bag, emergency drugs, anaesthesia drugs and defibrillator
Reliable source of communication to call for help
All applicable building and safety codes
Post-anaesthesia care unit

A commonly used acronym for paediatric preparation is SOAPME. This acronym stands for the following:

S—suction catheters, appropriate size
O—oxygen supply
A—airway equipment
P—pharmacy, essential drugs
M—monitors
E—equipment (special—defibrillator)

What monitoring will you do?

The ASA guidelines for sedation in paediatrics recommend pulse oximetry, electrocardiogram, heart rate, non-invasive blood pressure, respiration and gas monitoring for deep sedation [10].

18.12 What Anaesthesia Is Used for BMA and BMB?

18.12.1 Adults

For adults, LA is usually used. Lignocaine is used to infiltrate the intended site of BMA and BMB. EMLA cream can be locally applied at least 60–90 min before infiltrating skin with

LA. Proper time should be given after local infiltration before puncturing. To reduce anxiety, intravenous sedation such as midazolam can be given; analgesia can be managed with intravenous fentanyl 0.5–1 mcg/kg and IV paracetamol 15 mg/kg, but these patients then need to be monitored in the post-anaesthesia care unit before discharge to home. If no contraindication, ketamine can be used in a dose of 0.5–1 mg/kg.

In children having IV cannula in situ, IV induction with propofol (3 mg/kg) can be done followed by maintenance with either remifentanyl (1 mcg/kg) and propofol (0.5–1 mg/kg) or sevoflurane and nitrous oxide with spontaneous respiration. Fentanyl can also be used instead of remifentanyl. Paediatric patients are initially supine and then turned lateral as soon as they are asleep. Propofol dose requirement for maintenance of anaesthesia significantly reduces when remifentanyl is used along with it, and it is an ideal analgesic for short painful procedures as it allows quick recovery because of its rapid metabolism.

In children without IV line, inhalational induction is preferred with sevoflurane and nitrous oxide in parental presence to reduce the child's anxiety and fear until the child becomes unconscious. General anaesthesia can be supplemented by local infiltration at the skin and periosteum that will reduce the dose of propofol and prevent movement during painful stimulus.

Strategies to reduce the risk of airway compromise include the use of anti-sialagogue agents, inhalational induction in head-up or lateral position and maintenance of spontaneous ventilation. Positive pressure ventilation in such patients can cause cardiorespiratory collapse due to the loss of negative intrapleural pressure, resulting in drastic reduction in venous return. Any airway compromise or decrease in cardiac output can be managed by immediately shifting the child to lateral or prone position to relieve the compression. For distal airway compression, the use of rigid bronchoscope may be considered [12].

Non-pharmacological methods to reduce pain during BMA and BMB. The first biopsy experience is the most frightening; it should be made less painful as far as possible. An experienced person should conduct the procedure.

18.13 Post Procedure Care

Patient should be monitored in well-equipped post-anaesthesia initial recording of vital signs for at least five-minute intervals; when the patient awakens, it can be extended to 5–10 min. Respiratory depression can occur with opioid administration; respiration should be supported with oxygen as required, till patient fully awake. Memories of inadequate pain control during initial procedures may lead to anticipatory anxiety for subsequent procedures [13].

References

1. Riley RS, Hogan TF, Pavot DR, Forysthe R, Massey D, Smith E, Wright L Jr, Ben-Ezra JM. A pathologist's perspective on bone marrow aspiration and biopsy: I. Performing a bone marrow examination. J Clin Lab Anal. 2004;18(2):70–90. https://doi.org/10.1002/jcla.20008.
2. Bain BJ. Bone marrow trephine biopsy. J Clin Pathol. 2001;54:737–42.
3. Knowles S, Hoffbrand AV. Bone-marrow aspiration and trephine biopsy (1). Br Med J. 1980;281:204–5.
4. Williamson PJ, Smith AG. Bone marrow aspiration and biopsy. Br J Hosp Med. 1991;46:328–30.
5. Hyun BH, Gulati GL, Ashton JK. Bone marrow examination: techniques and interpretation. Hematol Oncol Clin N Am. 1988;2:513–23.
6. Steinke B. Complications after bone marrow biopsy. Dtsch Med Wochenschr. 1992;117:1003–4.
7. Bakir F. Fatal sternal puncture. Report of a case. Dis Chest. 1963;44:435.
8. Yoell JH. Bone marrow embolism to lung following sternal puncture. Arch Pathol Lab Med. 1959;67:373.
9. Matloub Y, Bostrom BC, Hunger SP, et al. Escalating intravenous methotrexate improves event-free survival in children with standard-risk acute lymphoblastic leukemia: a report from the Children's Oncology Group. Blood. 2011;118(2):243–51.
10. Cote JC, Wilson S. Guidelines for monitoring and management of pediatric patients before, during and

after sedation for diagnostic and therapeutic procedures. Pediatr Dent. 2019;41(4):E26–52.
11. Hack HA, Wright NB, Wynn RF. The anaesthetic management of children with anterior mediastinal masses. Anaesthesia. 2008;63:837.
12. Oduro-Dominah L, Brennan LJ. Anaesthetic management of the child with haematological malignancy. Continu Educ Anaesth Crit Care Pain. 2013;13(5):158–64.
13. Iannalfi A, Bernini G, Caprilli S, Lippi A, Tucci F, Messeri A. Painful procedures in children with cancer: comparison of moderate sedation with general anesthesia for lumbar puncture and bone marrow aspiration. Pediatr Blood Cancer. 2005;45:933–8.

19 Paediatric Case of Medulloblastoma for Whole Brain Radiotherapy

Snigdha Bellapukonda and Praneeth Suvvari

19.1 Case Vignette

A five-year-old male child presented with complaints of headache, vomiting and gait abnormalities. The computed tomography (CT) scan and magnetic resonance imaging (MRI) scan of the child revealed paramedian mass involving the right medulla very close to the fourth ventricle, depicting medulloblastoma. Surgical decompression has been done but there is residual tumour and he has been posted for radiotherapy.

1. What is the incidence and survival rate of medulloblastoma in children?

   Medulloblastoma is the most common type of malignant brain tumour in children. The incidence of medulloblastoma in children is approximately 0.5–1 in 100,000. However, long-term survival of low- and moderate-risk patients is >80% [1, 2].
2. What is the role of MRI scans in the treatment course of medulloblastoma after surgical decompression? When is it performed?

   MRI scan needs to be performed within 24–48 h of the immediate postoperative period for precise assessment of the residual tumour. However, when this is not possible, it can done 2–3 weeks (but not more than 4 weeks) after the surgery. This allows the resolution of postoperative changes and thus accurately delineates the residual tumour. MRI spine needs to be performed preoperatively to assess the spread of tumour, but if this is not done, it is recommended to wait for 2–3 weeks postoperatively. The risk stratification will then be done and radiotherapy will be initiated [3, 4].

   Apart from this cerebrospinal fluid (CSF), analysis should be done 2–3 weeks post-surgery for risk stratification.
3. How will you risk stratify medulloblastoma based on MRI and CSF analysis findings?

   Children with medulloblastoma are risk stratified as the following:

   Average risk/standard risk: Children >3 years with no or small residual tumour (<1.5 × 1.5 cm^2) and no leptomeningeal metastases (M0 status) both on neuraxial imaging as well as CSF cytology are classified as having disease with >80% long-term survival with standard therapy.

   High risk: Age <3 years, residual tumour >1.5 × 1.5 cm^2, or metastases (M1–M4 status), any one or more of these features makes it a high-risk disease with the long-term survival ranging from 40% to 60% even with intensified therapy. Patients with incomplete neuraxial staging should also be classified as high risk [5, 6].

S. Bellapukonda · P. Suvvari (✉)
Department of Onco-anaesthesia, Pain and Palliative Medicine, Basavatarakam Indo American Cancer Hospital and Research Institute (BIACH&RI), Hyderabad, Telangana, India

N. Gupta et al. (eds.), *Problem Based Learning Discussions in Onco-Anesthesia and Onco-Critical Care*, https://doi.org/10.1007/978-981-99-6339-3_19

4. What is the most acceptable radiation treatment regimen for average-risk medulloblastoma?

   The current standard for treatment of average-risk medulloblastoma in childhood involves reduced dose CSI (23.4 Gy in 13 fractions) followed by tumour-bed boost (30.6 Gy in 17 fractions) amounting to a total tumour-bed dose of 54 Gy in 30 fractions over 6 weeks. This is followed by adjuvant chemotherapy (Packer's regimen)with lomustine (CCNU), cisplatin and vincristine chemotherapy [7]. The treatment for high risk medulloblastomas is not established. However, Hyper-fractionated radiotherapy with craniospinal irradiation (CSI) followed by chemotherapy is being evaluated for its treatment.
5. What is the modified medulloblastoma staging system according to Chang?

   Modified medulloblastoma staging system according to Chang [8]:

T-stage	Tumour extent
T1	Tumour <3 cm in diameter
T2	Tumour >3 cm in diameter
T3a	Tumour >3 cm in diameter with extension into the aqueduct of Sylvius and/or the foramen of Luschka
T3b	Tumour >3 cm in diameter with unequivocal extension into the brainstem
T4	Tumour >3 cm in diameter with extension up past the aqueduct of Sylvius and/or down past the foramen magnum
M-stage	**Degree of metastasis**
M0	No evidence of gross subarachnoid or hematogenous metastasis
M1	Microscopic tumour cells found in the cerebrospinal fluid
M2	Gross nodular seeding demonstrated in the cerebellar/cerebral subarachnoid space or in the third or lateral ventricles
M3	Gross nodular seeding in the spinal subarachnoid space
M4	Metastasis outside the cerebrospinal axis

6. What are most common type of cancers in paediatric population?

   The most common paediatric malignancies worldwide are leukaemia, central nervous system cancers and lymphoma [9].
7. What is the different type of radiations used in paediatric population?

   Broadly speaking, there are three different types of radiotherapy used for paediatric patients. Two are external-beam therapies: photon beam radiotherapy and proton beam radiotherapy. A third type is brachytherapy which is a short-distance method.
8. What is photon beam radiotherapy?

   It is a composed of high-energy electromagnetic waves of photons. As these photons travel through the body, they interact with electrons of both diseased and healthy tissue and deposit energy [10]. This deposited energy leads to cellular death by two distinct mechanisms: (1) direct DNA damage, which results in single- and double-stranded DNA breakage, leading to cell death, and (2) generation of cellular free radicals causing single- and double-strand DNA breakage and subsequent cell death indirectly [11].
9. What are the recent modalities in photon beam radiotherapy?

   Three-dimensional conformal radiation therapy (3D conformal RT) and intensity-modulated radiation therapy (IMRT) are now the treatment standards in most hospitals for photon beam therapy [12]. Images from computed tomography (CT), magnetic resonance imaging (MRI) and positron emission tomography scans are used to plan a treatment area through a process called 'simulation' or 'planning' for three-dimensional conformal RT. This information allows precise irradiation of the tumour whilst minimising damage to nondiseased tissue. IMRT is a subtype of three-dimensional-conformal RT and enables radiation beams to be aimed at the tumour from a number of different angles. This allows manipulation of the radiation dose, concentrating it in certain areas of the tumour (Fig. 19.1) [13].

10. What are the limitations of photon beam radiotherapy?

    A photon's peak dose deposition occurs shortly after entering the body and decreases exponentially until it exits. With target tumours located at a depth greater than 3 cm, each photon delivers more radiation to healthy tissue than to the target tumour [14].

11. What is the principle behind proton beam radiotherapy?

    In proton beam radiotherapy, charged hydrogen particles or protons are accelerated at a target tissue. With a similar mechanism of cell death to photon therapy, proton radiation possesses physical properties that make it superior in minimising side effects [10]. Protons travel in a straight line and deposit their energy consistently as they travel towards a target tissue. Due to a unique physical characteristic called the Bragg peak, there is a steep fall-off of energy when the beam stops. The resulting outcome is concentrated radiation in the tumour, which does not travel any farther through the body (Fig. 19.2) [15].

12. What are the side effects of radiotherapy?

    Short-term side effects [16]: Emotional upset (patient and family), altered taste, fatigue, nausea and vomiting, diarrhoea, hair loss, headache, blurry vision and skin changes, including radiation burns and mucositis.

    Long-term side effects: Tissue scarring, abnormal growth, regression in behaviour, claustrophobia, hormonal dysfunction, fertility impairment, neurocognitive deficit, urinary and bladder changes, induction of secondary malignancy and risk of vascular complications such as stroke and heart disease.

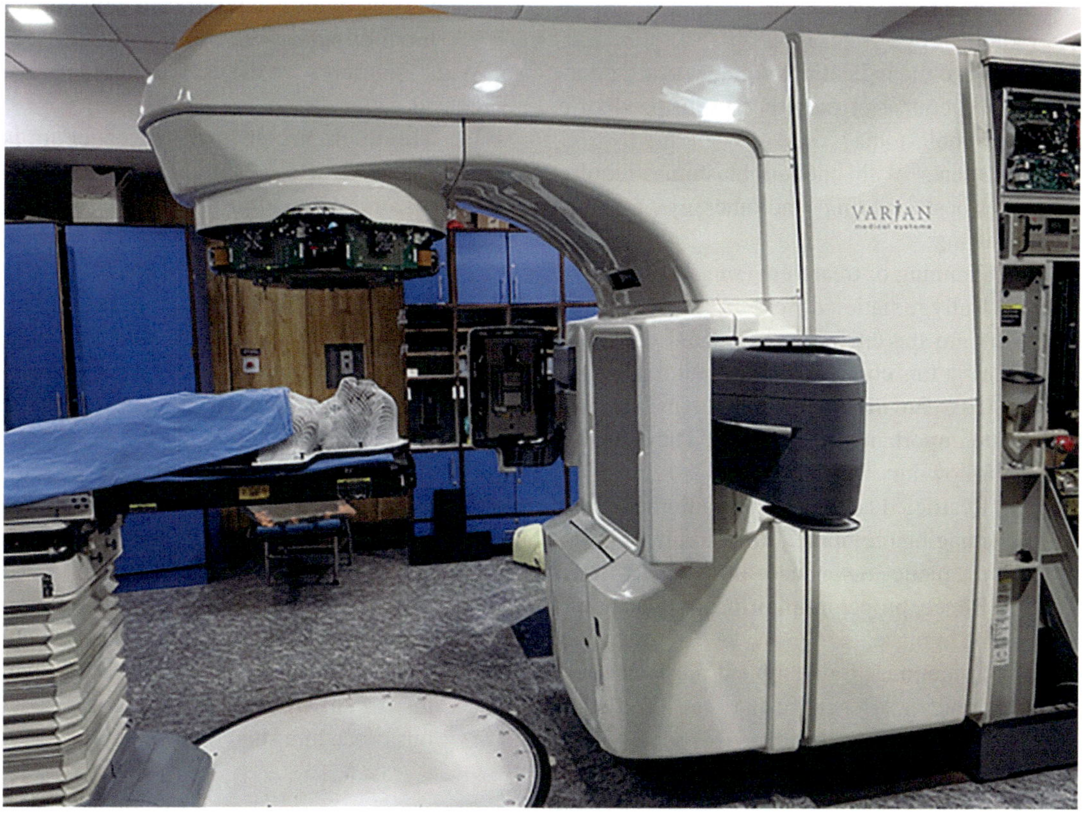

Fig. 19.1 Patient with the mould in situ for proton beam radiotherapy in radiotherapy suite

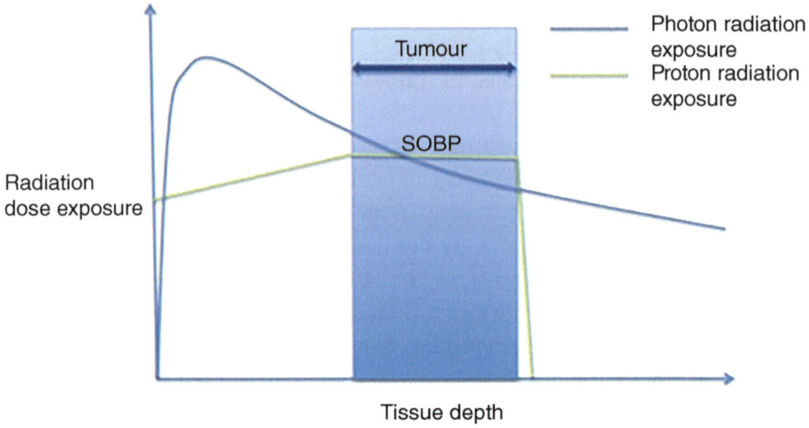

Fig. 19.2 Comparison of ionising radiation exposure in 10-MeV photon versus proton therapy. SOBP, spread-out Bragg Peak and the therapeutic radiation distribution. Adapted from Rombi et al. (2014) [14]

13. What is the duration of radiotherapy in paediatric patients with medulloblastoma?

    The duration of radiotherapy in these children varies with the grade of medulloblastoma. It ranges from 5 to 9 weeks [17]. The presence of residual tumour can increase the duration of radiotherapy. Hence, the investigations need to be repeated accordingly if the patient is in chemotherapy in addition to radiotherapy.

14. What are the indications for anaesthesia during the course of radiotherapy in paediatric medulloblastoma?

    Patients with medulloblastoma require anaesthesia during radiotherapy for the following:

    (a) Planning of treatment (*simulation*).
    (b) Daily radiation doses.

15. What are the environment-related considerations in this child posted for radiotherapy?

    Ans: Environmental concerns are of prime importance in this child. They involve the following:

    (a) Restricted access during radiotherapy or imaging (computed tomography (CT) or magnetic resonance imaging (MRI)). Hence, proper monitoring system should be in place.
    (b) Sometimes, loud ambient noise can be a concern. Hence, using ear protection should be mandated.
    (c) Radiation safety of the staff needs to be ensured with radiation monitoring badges.
    (d) Reduced access to mobile phones or Internet services as a consequence of the design of the building. This structural design of the building reduces the escape of electro-magnetic radiation and conversely reduces interference with patient monitoring as well.

16. What are the patient-specific considerations?

    (a) Thorough pre-anaesthetic checkup is required which should include birth history, evaluation for the presence of congenital diseases, bronchial asthma, seizures, previous episodes of any allergies to medicine, snoring/upper airway obstruction and feeding difficulties; recent history of upper respiratory and lower respiratory tract should be noted.
    (b) Tumour involving the brainstem or prior craniotomies can affect the lower cranial nerves and swallowing/gag reflex increasing the risk for regurgitation and aspiration. Review of any previous procedures or surgeries and anaesthesia with complications should be noted. Any history of airway compromise during previous procedure should be documented.

(c) Good communication between treatment centres is a vital part of patient safety. Hence, when patients are referred from one centre to another, previous records need to be examined for details of treatment, any complications and adverse effects of treatment. Patients requiring sedation or general anaesthesia should be cared for by paediatric-trained anaesthesia and recovery staff.
(d) These children have increased risk of aspiration as a result of delayed gastric emptying from stress, chemotherapy and opioid use and post-surgery as for medulloblastoma. Hence, adequate fasting (at least 6 h for solids and formula feeds, 4 h for breast milk and 2 h for clear liquids) needs to be ensured.
(e) These children may have UTI due to their immunosuppressed state. Risk/benefit assessment needs to be considered before delaying or proceeding with treatment. The choice of airway management (endotracheal tube placement or supraglottic airway or allowing the patient to breath spontaneously on venturi mask) depends on the condition of the patient, choice of the anaesthesiologist and the local resources.
(f) Physical examination should focus on general examination—weight and airway examination for any tonsillar hypertrophy, mandibular hypoplasia or craniofacial abnormality.
(g) Look for the presence of raised ICP like feeding difficulties, irritability, sunset sign and bulging fontanelle in children with supra-tentorial tumours. Ketamine should be avoided in such patients.
(h) Large Wilms' tumour may impair respiration.
(i) Children with mediastinal masses may have trachea-bronchial compression, SVC compression which must be thoroughly evaluated due to risk of airway collapse, hypotension and cardiorespiratory arrest following anaesthesia. History of orthopnoea should be elicited.
(j) Preoperative investigations include chest X-ray, computed tomographic scan and flow volume loops in sitting and supine position.

17. What are the other anaesthetic concerns in the preoperative period?
    (a) Answer: Long-term intravenous access (IV) is preferred in these children to avoid repeated venipuncture for chemotherapy. Chemotherapy per se causes thrombosis of veins making venous cannulation difficult. Strict asepsis needs to be maintained while assessing the line as these children are immunosuppressed. The IV access should be flushed after every use to ensure that there is residual drug and thus avoid inappropriate drug administration.
    (b) Usually, radiotherapy is administered 5 days a week for 4–5 weeks. Thus, the child is exposed to repeated airway manipulation and soft tissue damage. It is more pronounced when the patient has head and neck cancer like in this child with medulloblastoma. Complications like laryngospasm and bronchospasm need to be considered especially in these children due to soiling as a result of respiratory tract infections or due to chemotherapy and radiotherapy induced mucositis. Supraglottic airway (SGA) placement is a better choice in these patients as repeated endotracheal intubations may cause subglottic stenosis.
    (c) Although radiotherapy sittings and scanning take <1 h duration, maintenance of normothermia needs to be emphasised as the child may be partially undressed to facilitate positioning by aligning markings (on mould or the skin) with lasers. Blankets or warming devices

should not be allowed at the target site as this can cause deflection, scattering or dampening of electromagnetic waves. However, increasing the ambient temperature or using warming devices outside the treatment field can help.

(d) These children are on multiple medications. Therefore, careful review of drugs and dosing (especially analgesics and antiemetics) should be done on every day of treatment to prevent double dosing of medication.

(e) Regular monitoring of complete blood count, renal function test and liver function test should be done. Optimal level of haemoglobin and platelets should be maintained for both effective treatment and safety.

(f) The face moulds applied over the face or neck may obstruct the airway, interfere with access to airway or obstruct the movement of the chest during ventilation or may disturb the already placed airway device.

(g) Nutrition remains another concern in this patient population due to repeated fasting. Care should be taken to ensure consumption of regular diet after every anaesthesia exposure and complete awakening.

18. What are the specific considerations during simulation process?

(a) The treatment planning session prior to the actual radiotherapy is called "simulation". This session helps the radiation oncologist to decide the plan of treatment by identification and marking the location of anatomical sites which will be included in the radiation field.

(b) The expected position during the actual procedure is determined during simulation which remains a major anaesthetic concern in view of anaesthetic management.

(c) The plaster immobilisation casts for the head and body are made during simulation session which requires the child to be motionless during the procedure to ensure exact fitting cast as ill-fitting or tight cast may lead to airway compromise.

(d) GA/MAC depending upon the underlying disease site and extent of the tumour. Duration of simulation is usually longer than the actual procedure of RT and hence GA may be preferred. For example, GA is preferred during simulation for retinoblastoma wherein quite eye is required, similarly during simulation for medulloblastomas which is done in prone position.

19. Is premedication necessary in children posted for radiotherapy in medulloblastoma?

Answer: The children undergoing radiotherapy for medulloblastoma are above 2 years (after the development of central nervous system). Separation anxiety persists from 7 months to 7 years of age. Hence, premedication is necessary in this patient population.

20. What are the methods of premedication in these children?

Answer: The methods of premedication can be pharmacological and non-pharmacological [18].

Pharmacological methods: Various drugs used for premedication are the following:

Drug	Route and dose	Onset of action	Side effects
1. Benzodiazepines (BDZ) Most commonly used (BDZ) midazolam If there is an intravenous (IV) line in situ, IV midazolam can be used just before wheeling in the child for radiotherapy.	Oral: 0.5–0.75 mg/kg, up to a maximum of 20 mg Intranasal (0.3 mg/kg) Rectal (0.5 mg/kg) Sublingual (0.3 mg/kg) routes Intravenous (0.05–0.2 mg/kg)	20–25 min 10–15 min 10–15 min 10–15 min 30–60 s	Nausea, vomiting, headache and rarely respiratory depression
2. Alpha agonists [19] Clonidine Dexmedetomidine	Per oral: 3–4 μg/kg Intranasal: 2–4 μg/kg Intranasal: 1–4 μg/kg	60–90 min 30–60 min	Emergence delirium, postoperative nausea and vomiting and shivering
3. NMDA Antagonists [20] Ketamine Intramuscular use of ketamine is indicated in uncooperative older children with developmental delay.	Per oral (5–8 mg/kg) Intramuscular (4–6 mg/kg) Intravenous (0.5–1 mg/kg) Intranasal (3–5 mg/kg) routes	10 min 3–5 min 1 min	Emergence reactions and increased secretions
Chloral hydrate	Per oral dose: 20–75 mg/kg up to maximum of 2gm	30 min	Long half -lives of metabolites can lead to respiratory depression.
Melatonin	Per oral: 0.5 mg/kg	30 min	

Non-pharmacological approaches include family-centred approach and parental presence at induction of anaesthesia. Apart from these techniques, hypnosis, music therapy and videos may help the child cope with anxiety.

21. What are various methods of induction and maintenance of anaesthesia?

Induction can be by either inhalational or intravenous agents depending on the age of the patient and presence/absence of intravenous (IV) access. EMLA cream can be applied to secure IV access if time permits. Being immunosuppressed, recurrent UTI is common. Hence, IV induction is better tolerated with least risk of respiratory complications [21]. Moreover, IV induction is rapid and smooth. IV propofol (2–3 mg/kg) with or without ketamine (2–3 mg/kg) can be given. The child can be allowed to maintain spontaneous breathing, and oxygen supplementation can be given by venturi mask or SGA can be placed. Sevoflurane with oxygen and air can be used as maintenance. Duration of a single session of whole brain radiation therapy is between 10 and 15 min. A survey of anaesthesia, sedation and non-sedation practices for children undergoing repetitive cranial or craniospinal radiotherapy reported propofol-based total intravenous anaesthesia without intubation as the preferred anaesthetic technique during radiotherapy both in supine and prone positions.

Inhalational induction is preferred when there is no IV access. It has the advantage of maintaining spontaneous breathing till IV access is achieved. It also has the advantage in cases of difficult airway as the induction is slow, easy and reversible. Various techniques used for inhalational induction include single breath vital capacity technique, incremental induction technique and high initial concentration sevoflurane technique [22]. However, inhalational induction is a better choice in them if obtaining a venous access is difficult.

22. What parameters should be monitored during the procedure?

The American Academy of Pediatrics and American Academy of Pediatric Dentistry in collaboration have provided guidelines for monitoring and management of paediatric patients during and after sedation for diagnostic and therapeutic procedures which can be extrapolated for monitoring and management of patients in the radiotherapy suite.

The monitors include electrocardiogram (ECG), pulse oximeter (SpO_2), non-invasive blood pressure (NIBP) and capnography (end-tidal carbon dioxide, $EtCO_2$).

Two monitors are used in the radiology suite with one focused on the patient while the other one focused on the monitor connected to the anaesthesia machine. A slave monitor is also attached to monitor vitals outside the radiology suite. A microphone can be connected to the loudspeaker of the monitor, so that the pulse oximetry and ECG sounds are heard distinctly. The circuit and the monitoring equipment should have extension lines so that the desired length can be achieved avoiding entanglement during the movement of the operating table.

23. What are the complications associated with radiotherapy?

Respiratory	Cardiovascular	Others
Bronchospasm [23] Laryngospasm Airway obstruction Stridor Desaturation Apnoea	Tachycardia [23] Bradycardia Arrhythmias Hypotension Cardiac arrest	Nausea and vomiting [23] Sepsis-neutropenic and catheter related Excessive secretions Long-term neurocognitive effects of anaesthetic agents yet to be defined clearly

24. What are the risk factors for anaesthesia-related complications?

Answer: Propofol as a single drug has been reported to have least rate of adverse effects during sedation when used as a single drug. A study on the incidence and nature of adverse events during paediatric sedation/anaesthesia with propofol for procedures outside the operating room that included 49,836 propofol encounters at 37 locations reported that propofol sedation/anaesthesia is unlikely to yield serious adverse outcomes in a collection of institutions with highly motivated and organised sedation/anaesthesia services [24]. The study reported no deaths during sedation while cardiopulmonary resuscitation was required twice. Aspiration during sedation/anaesthesia occurred four times. Desaturation <90% for more than 30 were seen in 154 times per 10,000 sedation/anaesthesia administrations while central apnoea or airway obstruction occurred 575 times per 10,000 sedation/anaesthesia administrations. Stridor, laryngospasm, excessive secretions and vomiting had frequencies of 50, 96, 341 and 49 per 10,000 encounters, respectively. Unexpected admissions occurred at a rate of 7.1 per 10,000 encounters. On the other hand, the use of adjuvants (benzodiazepines, opioids or ketamine to propofol), duration of the procedure, total propofol dose (mg/kg) and simulation treatment have been reported to be risk factors for high complication rate [25]. Higher total propofol dose (mg/kg) and longer procedural times (minutes) have been associated with more complication rates. The probability of complications associated with propofol and adjuvants together was found to be 2.21 times as with propofol alone, and the probability of complications during simulation procedure was 2.78 times than during radiation treatment.

25. What are the newer modalities used for preoperative preparation and anaesthetic management in paediatric patients undergoing radiotherapy?

Various non-pharmacological techniques that have been tried include the following:

(a) A tour of radiotherapy suite, simulation of radiotherapy, educational material and virtual simulation. Radiation-specific activity-related colouring books, iPad/I phone apps (e.g. Rads4kids, ProtonU) and YouTube videos (e.g. One of a kind! A guide to radiotherapy). Practising lying still is another way of preparing the child [26, 27].
(b) Tolerance to masks can be improved by cutting holes near the eyes and mouth and decorating the mask with child's favourite character. Making mask on hand or stuffed toys can be tried.
(c) Caregiver may be allowed into the radiotherapy suite with lead apron.

(d) Distraction method by allowing to watch videos on radiation-compatible screen that are positioned above the patient's face with projector placed on the floor (e.g. Avatar, 14 developed at Stanford University, and RadFlix, developed at the University of Colorado) [26].

(e) Return gifts after each radiotherapy can act as an incentive.

26. What are ASA (American Society of Anesthesiology) recommendations for non-operating room anaesthesia?

(a) Oxygen supply: A primary oxygen source with backup is mandatory for the procedure. Central oxygen pipeline supply as primary oxygen source is strongly recommended. At least an E-type cylinder is encouraged.

(b) Suction apparatus should be available.

(c) Scavenging system should be available when inhalational agents are used.

(d) Anaesthesia drugs and supply, self-inflating resuscitation bag which can supply 90% oxygen, anaesthesia machine, equipment to perform the procedure and ASA standard monitoring equipment should be available.

(e) Appropriate electric outlets with adequate grounding should be available for anaesthesia machine and monitor should be available.

(f) Adequate illumination for anaesthesia machine, monitor and patient should be present.

(g) The suite should be spacious and resuscitation cart with emergency drugs and equipment should be available.

(h) Trained staff and means to communicate for assistance during emergency need to be available.

(i) Appropriate standards should be maintained in constructing the suite.

(j) Well-equipped post anaesthesia care unit (PACU) with adequate staff should be available. Transportation to PACU should be done with trained staff and adequate monitoring [28].

27. What are the post-procedure concerns in this child after radiotherapy?

Answer: The post-operative care unit should be equipped with ASA standard monitors, suction apparatus and oxygen supply. After the procedure, the child should be monitored for any upper airway obstruction (tongue fall or laryngospasm) and bronchospasm. As the child becomes completely awake, responds to commands and hemodynamically stable he can be shifted to ward.

References

1. Smoll NR, Drummond KJ. The incidence of medulloblastomas and primitive neurectodermal tumours in adults and children. J Clin Neurosci. 2012;19:1541–4.
2. Michalski JM, Janss AJ, Vezina LG, Smith KS, Billups CA, Burger PC, Embry LM, Cullen PL, Hardy KK, Pomeroy SL, et al. Children's oncology group phase III trial of reduced-dose and reduced-volume radiotherapy with chemotherapy for newly diagnosed average-risk medulloblastoma. J Clin Oncol. 2021;39:2685–97.
3. Meyers SP, Wildenhain SL, Chang JK, Bourekas EC, Beattie PF, Korones DN, et al. Postoperative evaluation for disseminated medulloblastoma involving the spine: contrast-enhanced MRI findings, CSF cytologic analysis, timing of disease occurrence, and patient outcomes. AJNR Am J Neuroradiol. 2000;21:1757–65.
4. Harreld JH, Mohammed N, Goldsberry G, Li X, Li Y, Boop F, Patay Z. Postoperative intraspinal subdural collections after pediatric posterior fossa tumor resection: incidence, imaging, and clinical features. AJNR Am J Neuroradiol. 2015;36:993–9.
5. Min HS, Lee YJ, Park K, Cho BK, Park SH. Medulloblastoma: histopathologic and molecular markers of anaplasia and biologic behavior. Acta Neuropathol. 2006;112:13–20.
6. von Hoff K, Hartmann W, von Bueren AO, Gerber NU, Grotzer MA, Pietsch T. Large cell/anaplastic medulloblastoma: outcome according to myc status, histopathological, and clinical risk factors. Pediatr Blood Cancer. 2010;54:369–76.
7. Seidel C, Heider S, Hau P, Glasow A, Dietzsch S, Kortmann RD. Radiotherapy in medulloblastoma—evolution of treatment, current concepts and future perspectives. Cancers. 2021;13(23):5945.
8. Dufour C, Beaugrand A, Pizer B, Micheli J, Aubelle MS, Fourcade A, Couanet D, Laplanche A, Kalifa C, Grill J. Metastatic medulloblastoma in childhood: Chang's classification revisited. Int J Surg Oncol. 2012;2012:1.

9. Irvine L, Stiller C. Childhood cancer statistics, England annual report; 2018. www.ncin.org.uk. Accessed 14 Nov 2019.
10. Steinmeier T, Schleithoff S, Timmermann B. Evolving radiotherapy techniques in paediatric oncology. Clin Oncol. 2019;31(3):142–50.
11. Rajamanickam B, Dai J, Wenlong N, et al. Biological response of cancer cells to radiation treatment. Front Mol Biosci. 2014;1:24.
12. Taylor A, Powell ME. Intensity-modulated radiotherapy what is it? Cancer Imaging. 2004;4(2):68–73.
13. National Cancer Institute. Radiation therapy to treat cancer. https://www.cancer.gov/about-cancer/treatment/types/radiation-therapy/external-beam. Accessed 8 July 2019.
14. Rombi B, MacDonald S, Maurizio A, et al. Proton radiotherapy for childhood tumours: an overview of early clinical results. Ital J Pediatr. 2014;40:74.
15. Newhauser WD, Zhang R. The physics of proton therapy. Phys Med Biol. 2015;60(8):155–209.
16. Good practice guide for paediatric radiotherapy. 2nd ed. https://www.rcr.ac.uk/system/files/publication/field_publication_files/bfco182_good_pract_paed_rt_second_ed.pdf. Accessed 5 July 2019.
17. Liu Y, Zhu Y, Gao L, Guozhen X, Yi J, Liu X, Li Y. Radiation treatment for medulloblastoma: a review of 64 cases at a single institute. Jpn J Clin Oncol. 2005;35(3):111–5. https://doi.org/10.1093/jjco/hyi038.
18. Dave NM. Premedication and induction of anaesthesia in paediatric patients. Indian J Anaesth. 2019;63:713–20.
19. Suvvari P, Mishra S, Bhatnagar S, Garg R, Bharati SJ, Gupta N, Kumar V, Khan MA. Comparison of intranasal dexmedetomidine versus intranasal ketamine as premedication for level of sedation in children undergoing radiation therapy: a prospective, randomised, double-blind study. Turkish J Anaesthesiol Reanimation. 2020;48(3):215.
20. Tanaka M, Sato M, Saito A, Nishikawa T. Reevaluation of rectal ketamine premedication in children: comparison with rectal midazolam. J Am Soc Anesthesiol. 2000;93(5):1217–24.
21. Von Ungern-Sternberg BS, Boda K, Chambers NA, Rebmann C, Johnson C, Sly PD, Habre W. Risk assessment for respiratory complications in paediatric anaesthesia: a prospective cohort study. Lancet. 2010;376:773–83.
22. Smith RM. Methods of induction in pediatric anesthesia. NEJM. 1949;240:761–5.
23. Verma V, Beethe AB, LeRiger M, Kulkarni RR, Zhang M, Lin C. Anesthesia complications of pediatric radiation therapy. Pract Radiat Oncol. 2016;6(3):143–54. https://doi.org/10.1016/j.prro.2015.10.018. Epub 2015 Oct 31.
24. Cravero JP, Beach ML, Blike GT, Gallagher SM, Hertzog JH, Pediatric Sedation Research Consortium. The incidence and nature of adverse events during pediatric sedation/anesthesia with propofol for procedures outside the operating room: a report from the Pediatric Sedation Research Consortium. Anesth Analg. 2009;108(3):795–804. https://doi.org/10.1213/ane.0b013e31818fc334.
25. Anghelescu DL, Burgoyne LL, Liu W, et al. Safe anesthesia for radiotherapy in pediatric oncology: St. Jude Children's Research Hospital Experience, 2004-2006. Int J Radiat Oncol Biol Phys. 2008;71(2):491–7. https://doi.org/10.1016/j.ijrobp.2007.09.044.
26. Holt DE, Hiniker SM, Kalapurakal JA, Breneman JC, Shiao JC, Boik N, Cooper BT, Dorn PL, Hall MD, Logie N, Lucas JT Jr. Improving the pediatric patient experience during radiation therapy-a children's oncology group study. Int J Radiat Oncol Biol Phys. 2021;109(2):505–14.
27. Tennant M, Anderson N, Youssef GJ, McMillan L, Thorson R, Wheeler G, McCarthy MC. Effects of immersive virtual reality exposure in preparing pediatric oncology patients for radiation therapy. Techn Innov Patient Support Radiat Oncol. 2021;19:18–25.
28. ASo A. Statement on Nonoperating Room Anesthetizing Locations. 2013. Accessed 15 July 2022. Reference Source.

Anaesthetic Considerations for a Patient with Carcinoma Prostate Planned for Brachytherapy

20

Shayak Roy, Satyaki Sarkar, and Vinod Kumar

20.1 Case Vignette

A 65-year-old male with history of low back pain for 4 months increased in severity since 1 month and obstructive urinary symptoms for 1 month. On evaluation, prostate-specific antigen was 20 ng/mL; transrectal ultrasound-guided biopsy revealed presence of adenocarcinoma of the prostate. Gleason score was 7 and clinical stage T2b. He had history of uncontrolled diabetes mellitus and CVA (cerebrovascular accident). He had a known case of ischaemic heart disease and had undergone PTCA with placement of drug-eluting stent 3 years back. Effort tolerance was poor. Echo-cardiography was suggestive of severe LV dysfunction with an ejection fraction of 45%. He was posted for prostate brachytherapy.

S. Roy
Onco-anaesthesiology and Palliative Medicine, Dr BRA IRCH AIIMS Delhi, New Delhi, India

Department of Anaesthesiology, Lady Hardinge Medical College and Associated Hospitals, New Delhi, India

S. Sarkar
Onco-anaesthesiology and Palliative Medicine, Dr BRA IRCH AIIMS Delhi, New Delhi, India

V. Kumar (✉)
Onco-anaesthesiology and Palliative Medicine, Dr BRA IRCH AIIMS Delhi, New Delhi, India

Department of Anesthesiology, University of Minnesota, Minneapolis, MN, USA
e-mail: kuma0351@umn.edu

20.2 Introduction

Q1

Describe briefly the epidemiology of carcinoma prostate. What are the treatment options available for carcinoma prostate?

Answer:

Carcinoma prostate is the second most common cancer in males across the world (after carcinoma lungs) with an annual incidence of nearly 1.4 million and mortality of approximately 375,000 per year, as per GLOBOCAN 2020 data. The high incidence of prostate cancer is thought to be partly due to the aggressive screening programmes employing PSA (prostate-specific antigen) levels.

Prostate carcinomas are a disease of the elderly male—mostly in the fifth and sixth decades of life, and unlike most other malignancies, the low-risk cases have an indolent course, spanning over 15–20 years. This makes it possible to have "watchful waiting" or "active surveillance" as one of the management modes for low-stage, low-risk prostate cancers. Among the interventions available for localised (non-metastatic) disease are external beam radiation therapy (EBRT), brachytherapy, radical prostatectomy by surgery and hormonal therapy (anti-androgens) [1, 2].

N. Gupta et al. (eds.), *Problem Based Learning Discussions in Onco-Anesthesia and Onco-Critical Care*, https://doi.org/10.1007/978-981-99-6339-3_20

Q2

What is TNM staging for prostate carcinoma? (Tables 20.1 and 20.2)

Q3

What is Gleason grading?

Table 20.1 TNM staging of prostate carcinoma

Prostate	
T1	**Not palpable**
T1a	Tumour incident histological finding in 5% or less of tissue resected
T1b	Tumour incident histological finding in more than 5% of tissue resected
T1c	Tumour identified by needle biopsy (e.g. because of elevated PSA)
T2	**Confined within prostate**
T2a	Tumour involves <half one lobe
T2b	Tumour involves >half one lobe
T2c	Tumour involves both the lobes
T3	**Tumour extends through prostatic capsule**
T3a	Extracapsular
T3b	Seminal vesicle(s)
T4	**Fixed or invades adjacent structures: bladder neck, external sphincter, rectum, levator, muscles and pelvic wall**
N1	**Regional lymph node(s)**
M1a	**Non-regional lymph node(s)**
M1b	**Bone(s)**
M1c	**Other site(s)**

Donald Gleason devised a grading system consisting of 1–5 grades based on histological tumour architecture. The International Society of Urological Pathology (ISUP) modified Gleason score (GS) in 2014 in which Gleason grades 1 and 2 were eliminated. As prostate carcinoma often has areas with different grades, modified GS of biopsy-detected PCa comprises the Gleason grade of the most extensive (primary) pattern, plus the second most common (secondary) pattern, if two are present. If one pattern is present, it needs to be doubled to yield the GS. These two grades are added to yield the Gleason score. The highest a score can be is 10. For three grades, the biopsy GS comprises the most common grade plus the highest grade, irrespective of its extent. The lowest score found on a biopsy is 6. These types of cancers are typically called low-grade and are likely to be less aggressive. Cancers that score 8–10 are considered high grade [2].

International Society of Urological Pathology 2014 group system

Grade group 1: GS 6 or under
Grade group 2: GS 3 + 4 = 7
Grade group 3: GS 4 + 3 = 7
Grade group 4: GS 4 + 4 or 3 + 5 or 5 + 3 = 8
Grade group 5: GS 9–10

Q4

Describe the risk stratification of prostate cancer.

Table 20.2 Stage grouping of carcinoma prostate

Stage	Tumour	Lymph nodes	Metastases	PSA	Gleason grade group
I	cT1, cT2a or pT2	N0	M0	<10	1
IIA	cT1, cT2a or pT2 cT2b or cT2c	N0 N0	M0 M0	≥10 but <20 <20	1 1
II B	T1T2	N0	M0	<20	2
IIC	T1T2	N0	M0	<20	3 or 4
IIIA	T1T2	N0	M0	≥20	1–4
IIIB	T3T4	N0	M0	Any PSA	1–4
IIIC	Any T	N0	M0	Any PSA	5
IVA	Any T	N1	M0	Any PSA	Any grade
IVB	Any T	Any N	M1	Any PSA	Any grade

cT—clinical estimate of extent of disease (determined by physical exam, prostate biopsy and imaging
pT—extent of disease that is based on pathologic examination of the prostate

Low risk	Intermediate risk	High risk	
PSA <10 ng/mL GS <7 (ISUP grade 1) cT1-2a	PSA 10–20 ng/mL or GS 7 (ISUP grade 2/3) or cT2b	PSA >20 ng/mL or GS >7 (ISUP grade 4/5) or cT2c	Any PSA any GS (any ISUP grade) cT3–4 or cN+
Localised			Locally advanced

Q5

What is the role of brachytherapy in carcinoma prostate?

Answer:

Brachytherapy is a form of radiation therapy in which radioactive isotopes are placed in close proximity to the tumour site, resulting in better conformal and concentrated dosing to the tumour with reduced impact on the surrounding normal tissues.

According to the current recommendations, patients of prostate cancer with clinical staging T1-T2a, a Gleason's score of ≤6 and a serum PSA level ≤10 ng/mL are considered candidates for monotherapy with brachytherapy. For patients with large prostate size (>60 g), usually brachytherapy is combined with subsequent to androgen ablative therapy to reduce the gland size, while for higher-risk patients with suspicion of extracapsular spread, it is usually combined with EBRT [3].

Q6

What are the various types of brachytherapy modalities used for carcinoma prostate?

Answer:

Brachytherapy for prostate cancer is generally of two major subtypes [2]:

- Low-dose rate (LDR) therapy:

  With low energy, short half-life isotopes in the form of permanent implants—either as needles or seeds. In the 1920s, radium needles were first used, to be replaced by iodine-125 and palladium-103 isotopes in the form of gold seeds around 1960–1980. In the early 2003, cesium-137 was introduced with the shortest half-life among the above. The radiation dose is delivered continually over months till the decay of the isotopes in the permanent implants.
- High dose rate (HDR) therapy:

  With higher energy radio-isotope—iridium-192—after-loaded for short periods through trans-perineal hollow catheters, fixed to a template. This allows for very high doses, almost comparable to linear accelerators (EBRT), to be delivered over a few fractions—typically 3–4 fractions. The trans-perineal applicators are inserted under trans-rectal ultrasonographic (TRUS) guidance in the lithotomy position [4].

Q7

What are the advantages and disadvantages of brachytherapy as compared to other treatment modalities in carcinoma prostate?

Answer:

Advantages

1. Definitive treatment for low- or intermediate-risk patients.
2. May be combined with external beam radiation therapy if needed.
3. Major side effects of surgery (urinary incontinence, rectal injury, wound infection, DVT) can be avoided.
4. Side effects of chemotherapy like gonadotropin-releasing hormone (GnRH) agonists (leuprolide, goserelin acetate, buserelin, triptorelin), GnRH antagonists (Degarelix), nonsteroidal antiandrogens [flutamide (hepatotoxicity), enzalutamide (gynecomastia)], adrenal suppression (ketoconazole), 5α-reductase inhibitors (finasteride, dutasteride) and CYP17A1 inhibitor (abiraterone) can be minimised by combining with brachytherapy.

Disadvantages

1. Pronounced acute lower urinary tract symptoms (LUTS).
2. Potential late effects include urinary retention, cystitis, erectile dysfunction and second malignancy

Q8

What is the need of anaesthesia/analgesia for carcinoma prostate brachytherapy?

Answer: To provide the following:

1. Immobility—It is crucial for ultrasound (U/S) probe placement within the rectum using a U/S stabilisation device. The U/S stabilisation device helps to ensure reproducibility from the time of initial U/S image acquisition and treatment planning to final seed insertion. So it is of paramount importance to minimise readjustment of the U/S stabilisation device after a treatment plan has been finalised, as this could lead to a geometric miss during seed insertion [5].
2. Analgesia—Placement of needle causes severe pain. So adequate analgesia is required for the precise needle placement under U/S guidance.
3. Position—During the entire procedure of 2–3 h, extended dorsal lithotomy position is required to minimise pubic bone interference during seed placement. The pelvis must be flexed so that pubic arch is elevated.

Q9

Describe the nerve supply of the prostate and the perineal region.

Answer: The prostate is innervated by parasympathetic fibres of the pelvic splanchnic nerves by way of the prostatic plexus, which receives its fibres from the inferior hypogastric plexus (for erection and secretomotor of acini). The inferior hypogastric plexus also receives preganglionic sympathetic fibres from the superior hypogastric plexus to provide motor innervation to the smooth muscles of the stroma of the prostate (for ejaculation and smooth muscle contraction)

Q10

What are the anaesthetic modalities that have been described for brachytherapy in prostatic carcinoma?

Answer: Many different anaesthetic techniques including sedation with systemic analgesia, general anesthesia, local anesthesia and regional anesthesia have been used in patients requiring administration of brachytherapy for carcinoma prostate, but combined spinal epidural techniques have been found closest to the ideal technique, as it can fulfil almost all the requirements of procedure [6].

20.3 Pre-procedural Concerns: Patient-Related Factors

Q11

Apart from routine preoperative assessment that we do for all patients preoperatively, what different evaluations are required for patients requiring administration of brachytherapy for carcinoma prostate?

Answer [7]:

- Determining which patients are good candidates for prostate brachytherapy is highly operator/institutional dependent and relies on the skill and experience of the treating physician.
- Volume study with U/S or CT may be needed. Ideal volume is <60 cc as per American Brachytherapy Society's recommendations; but larger glands are also implanted successfully at selected centres.
- If prostate volume is too large or pubic arch interference exists, hormone therapy can be initiated 2–3 months prior to implantation for gland size reduction if needed—that is why

the detailed knowledge of the drugs and its side effects are to be evaluated preoperatively.

- EBRT is an appropriate option for all patients with intermediate- and high-risk prostate cancer. EBRT with brachytherapy boost can be considered in high-intermediate and high-risk patients.
- Selected intermediate-risk patients may be candidates for short-term androgen deprivation therapy (ADT) (4–6 months) in combination with EBRT.
- High-risk patients are candidates for pelvic lymph node irradiation and the addition of neoadjuvant and adjuvant ADT for a total of 2–3 years.
- From the above discussions, we can conclude that although brachytherapy is not a major invasive procedure, the stage and previous treatment history of the prostate cancer and associated comorbidities of the patient is of utmost importance in the preoperative phase.

Q12

What are the specific anaesthetic considerations in these patients?

Answer [8]:

- The patient is required to be in extended dorsal lithotomy position for easy insertion of TRUS probe and subsequent placement of applicators. The patient then receives HDR in the radiotherapy suite.
- The placement of applicators for administration of intracavitary and interstitial brachytherapy in lithotomy position is extremely painful, and hence sensory level of blockade till T10 dermatomal level is required for successful outcomes.
- Patients will require analgesia till the applicators are in situ.
- Most of these patients are elderly with concurrent comorbidities as well as physiological changes due to ageing that put them at higher risk of occurrence of perioperative complications.
- The duration of brachytherapy procedure is variable and treatment session can take place at multiple locations.
- The whole treatment session may involve operation theatre for ultrasound-guided insertion of applicator under anaesthesia, mobilising the patient to radiology suite for computerised tomography (CT)/magnetic resonance imaging (MRI) for confirming correct placement of applicators, computer-based planning of brachytherapy with applicator in situ and finally radiotherapy room for administration of brachytherapy.

20.4 Intra-procedural Concerns: Procedure-Related, Positioning, Anaesthetic Options

Q13

Discuss the special monitoring that may be essential for these patients.

Answer: When patient receives HDR in radiotherapy suit, all the operating room staff including anaesthesiologist, radiation oncologist and nursing and technical staff are away from the patient. The patient is usually monitored through two monitors in the radiology suite. One is focused on the patient while the other one is focused on the monitor connected to the anaesthesia machine. A slave monitor is attached that helps in monitoring of patient from outside the radiology suite. Thus, the ideal anaesthetic technique administered should be safe and effective under such dynamic conditions.

Q14

Enumerate the different anaesthetic plans available and discuss their main pros and cons.

Answer: Different techniques have been selected from the anaesthesiologists armamentarium to provide adequate anaesthesia and analgesia to the patients requiring administration of brachytherapy for carcinoma prostate.

- Local anaesthesia—Wallner et al. [1] demonstrated the technique and feasibility of prostate brachytherapy under local anaesthesia only. Pros—The technique did not require allocation of significant operating room time. Cons—The patients experienced discomfort due to lithotomy position and needle insertion and moved under effect of local anaesthesia, which required adjustments in positioning of TRUS probe.
- Saddle block—Clarke et al. [9] favoured the use of saddle block for HDR brachytherapy in carcinoma prostate. Pros—Less haemodynamic fluctuations and motor involvement. Cons—T10 sensory level may not be attained. This may cause patient discomfort during positioning and hinder the procedure. Also, it is not ideal for post-op analgesia.
- Spinal catheter vs. CSE—Benrath et al. [10] use spinal anaesthesia, spinal catheter and combined spinal epidural (CSE) anaesthesia for prostate brachytherapy. Cons—Hypotension and bradycardia were observed in 10% of patients who received regional anaesthesia (more with spinal catheters). The shorter duration of anaesthesia obtained after administration of spinal block may not be sufficient for successful completion of procedure and also in the post procedure.
- Pudendal nerve block vs. CSE [11] —Schenck et al. compared pudendal nerve block (PNB) and CSE anaesthesia for performing pain-free HDR brachytherapy. Pros—PNB has been found be satisfactory to provide analgesia during the entire procedure. But sometimes the duration of entire procedure can be prolonged and PNB was associated with multiple injections, patient discomfort and shorter duration of analgesia. Patients who received CSE anaesthesia reported better subjective well-being score.
- General anaesthesia: The administration of general anaesthesia in elderly patients with comorbidities can be associated with multiple complications in perioperative period. As the procedure may be performed at multiple locations, the conduct of general anaesthesia is not always feasible.
- Among all the techniques, CSE anaesthesia is closest to the ideal technique, as it can fulfil almost all the requirements of procedure.

Pros

1. Rapid and reliable onset of sensory and motor blockade attributed to spinal block and extension of dermatomal level with prolongation of duration of analgesia due to epidural catheter.
2. As lower doses of local anaesthetic can be given intrathecally, it results in fewer incidences of cardiorespiratory complications in elderly patients. The patient's safety is not compromised, even if the procedure is performed at multiple locations.

Cons

1. It cannot be used where regional anaesthesia is contraindicated.
2. The common side effects of central neuraxial blockade will also be there.

Q15

Discuss the anaesthesia considerations in extended lithotomy position.

Answer: Extended lithotomy position (the patient's hips are flexed until the angle between the posterior surface of the patient's thighs and the OR bed surface are approximately 130°–150° and propped upward on a pillow or pad [12, 13]. The patient's lower legs are almost vertical) leads to following changes:

- CVS—Increased preload leading to transient increase in cardiac output, cerebral venous and intracranial pressure, increased BP.
- Respiratory—Increased airway pressure, decreased lung compliance and tidal volume due to cephalad shift of the diaphragm by abdominal viscera.
- Nerve injury—Common peroneal nerve, sciatic nerve, lateral femoral cutaneous nerve and obturator nerve—risk factors are low body mass index, recent cigarette smoking and prolonged duration of procedure (>2 h).

- Backache—Normal lordotic curvature of the lumbar spine is lost due to the lithotomy position and prolonged pelvic flexion might aggravate any previous lower back pain.
- Lower extremity compartment syndrome—Local arterial pressure decreases 0.78 mmHg for each centimetre the leg is raised above the right atrium. In extended lithotomy position, this decreased perfusion pressure can cause a vicious cycle of ischaemia, oedema, further ischaemia and rhabdomyolysis.
- Genitalia—The genitalia are carefully taped anteriorly out of the field.

Q16

How will you minimise the deleterious effects of lithotomy?

Answer:

- Initiation of lithotomy should be gradual and coordinated (especially in geriatric population to minimise the physiologic effects of increased venous return).
- Both legs should be simultaneously raised together and flexed at the hips and knees.
- Legs should be properly supported and wrapped to protect the nerves mentioned above.
- When raising the foot end of the table at the end of surgery, strict attention to the position of the hands must be paid to avoid crush injury to the fingers.
- The duration of the lithotomy should be kept minimum. If the procedure time crosses 2 h, then the legs should be periodically lowered to the level of the body to prevent nerve injury and compartment syndrome.

Q17

What are the pros and cons of administering general anaesthesia in this patient population?

Ans: Most of the patient in this population are geriatric with multiple comorbidities like DM, HTN, COPD and CAD along with the prostate cancer and its treatment-related side effects. The effects of general anaesthesia might augment or mask the intraoperative fluctuations of these comorbidities which might be easier to detect in an awake patient under regional anaesthesia. So general anaesthesia should be reserved for those patients in whom regional anaesthesia is contraindicated or has failed.

Other than the comorbidities, all other considerations for geriatric patients will apply to these patients:

- **CVS**—Decreased beta response to hypotension, preload dependent cardiac output, less sensitive baroreceptor reflexes, decreased cardiac contractility, increased calcification, stenosis and rigidity of arteries, increased systemic vascular resistance, wider pulse pressure and disproportionately large changes in blood pressure from small changes in preload and contractility—labile hypertension, marked hypotension upon induction with intravenous anaesthetic agents and difficulty controlling postoperative hypertension, higher prevalence of coronary artery disease and perioperative coronary ischaemia and age-related arrhythmias due to fibrotic changes, inhibiting conduction pathways and promoting re-entry.
- **Pulmonary**—Increased work of breathing, chest wall stiffens, flattened diaphragm and intercostal muscles weakness—decreased inspiratory capacity, alveolar airspace and physiologic dead space increase while surface area decreases—ventilation-perfusion mismatch; decreased forced expiratory volume (FEV1), decreased diffusion capacity of the lung (DLCO) and increased A-a gradient; blunting of central responses to hypoxia and hypercarbia.
- **Neurologic**—Increase susceptibility to medications such as diphenhydramine, scopolamine, benzodiazepines, metoclopramide, meperidine and non-steroidal anti-inflammatory drugs (NSAIDs); decreased brain volume, cerebrospinal fluid and dendrite synapses causing memory loss, cognitive

decline, sleep disorders, delirium, depression and decreased neuroplasticity and decreased cerebral autoregulation.

- **Renal**—Decreased glomerular filtration rate (1 mL per minute per metre squared each year after the age of 40), decreased response to renin, angiotensin, aldosterone and vasopressin, difficulty with volume status, electrolyte abnormalities and acid-base derangements, decreased clearing capacity of aging renal and hepatic systems—reduced doses of many medications.
- **Endocrine and metabolism**—Malnutrition—Heat production, insulation and the ability to thermoregulate commonly decline with age, type 2 diabetes mellitus is an increasingly common and particularly complicating comorbidity in the ageing population.

Therefore, from the above discussion, we can conclude that regional anaesthesia is a relatively safer option in this patient population.

Q18

Discuss the fluid management for this patient.

Answer: The perioperative fluid management should be according to ERAS protocol keeping in mind the elderly population, post-regional hemodynamic fluctuations, extended lithotomy position and preoperative bowel preparations.

Q19

Enumerate the possible intraoperative complications that may arise and discuss the management options for complications specific to these patients.

Answer:

- Haematuria—Drops of haematuria is considered normal through urethral meatus during the procedure. If frank blood comes continually, procedure should be stopped and further imaging/urology consultation should be sought to rule out bladder/vessel injury. If patient goes into shock, appropriate resuscitation protocol should be followed.
- Bowel injury—Inadvertent bowel injury may happen during the procedure due to the needles. It rarely causes any significant haemodynamic fluctuations intraoperatively.

20.5 Post-procedural Concerns: Analgesia, Resuming Normal Activities and Discharge

Q20

Why is it essential to control postoperative pain in these patients? Enumerate the postoperative pain relief options available and discuss their pros and cons.

Answer: It is important to control postoperative pain due to the applicator as it requires patient immobility in multiple sessions. Increased pain negatively impacts patient outcome and the quality of hospital stay. CSE is an excellent choice in this regard to continue analgesia up to 48–72 h postop along with round-the-clock paracetamol. NSAIDs can be used as adjuvants and opioids for rescue analgesia.

References

1. Wallner K, Simpson C, Roof J, Arthrus S, Korssjoen T, Sutlief S. Local anesthesia for prostate brachytherapy. Int J Radiat Oncol Biol Phys. 1999;45:401–6.
2. Sarah S, et al. Essentials of clinical radiation oncology. 2nd ed. Demos Medical; 2021.
3. Videtic GMM, et al. Handbook of treatment planning in radiation oncology—an updated pocket-sized guide on delivering radiation treatment. 3rd ed. Demos Medical; 2020.
4. Tselis N, Hoskin P, Baltas D, Strnad V, Zamboglou N, Rödel C, et al. High dose rate brachytherapy as monotherapy for localised prostate cancer: review of the current status. Clin Oncol (R Coll Radiol). 2017;29:401–11.
5. Lam ST, Cho PS, Marks RJ 2nd, Narayanan S. Detection and correction of patient movement in prostate brachytherapy seed reconstruction. Phys Med Biol. 2005;50:2071–87.

6. Wallner K. Prostate brachytherapy under local anesthesia; lessons from the first 600 patients. Brachytherapy. 2002;1:145–8.
7. Roessler B, Six LM, Gustorff B. Anesthesia for brachytherapy. Curr Opin Anaesthesiol. 2008;21:514–8.
8. Yildirim I. Anesthesia techniques in brachytherapy. Turk J Oncol. 2019;34(Supp 1):99–101.
9. Clarke HA, Tarshis J, Lam-McCulloch J, Kay J. Saddle block analgesia for high-dose-rate brachytherapy: a prospective study. Brachytherapy. 2009;8:335–8.
10. Benrath J, Kozek-Langenecker S, Hupfl M, Lierz P, Gustorff B. Anesthesia for brachytherapy 51/2 yr of experience in 1622 procedures. Br J Anaesth. 2006;96:195–200.
11. Schenck M, Schenck C, Rübben H, Stuschke M, Schneider T, Eisenhardt A, et al. Pudendal nerve block in HDR-brachytherapy patients: do we really need general or regional anesthesia? World J Urol. 2013;31:417–21.
12. Kumar V, Ahuja D, Gupta N, Bharati SJ, Garg R, Mishra S, Haresh KP, Gupta S, Bhatnagar S. Anesthesia concerns in prostate brachytherapy: an institutional experience. Indian J Cancer. 2020;57(4):411–5. https://doi.org/10.4103/ijc.IJC_666_18.
13. Podder T, Song D, Showalter T, Beaulieu L. Advances in radiotherapy for prostate cancer treatment. Prostate Cancer. 2016;2016:3079684.

21 Wilms Tumour

Anju Gupta and Stuti Gupta

21.1 Case Scenario

A three-year-old child presented with right-sided abdominal swelling with fever. On further evaluation, the abdominal mass was found to be a Wilms tumour originating from the upper lobe of the right kidney. How will you plan anaesthesia management for this patient?

Q1

What is the incidence and origin of Wilms tumour?

Answer: The name is based on German anatomist and surgeon Max Wilms who described his seven cases of nephroblastoma in 1899.

Wilms tumour also known as nephroblastoma accounts for the most common childhood renal tumour (85%). It accounts for 6% of childhood malignant tumours. The incidence of Wilms tumour is 1:10,000 in the USA and European populations. Its incidence is 2.5 times higher in an African population [1]. Wilms tumour originates from embryonic pluripotent renal precursor cells, found mainly in kidneys and some extrarenal places like the retroperitoneum, testis, sacrococcygeal region, inguinal ligament and mediastinum.

Q2

How is Wilms tumour distributed in different age groups?

Most commonly this tumour arises in children between 1 and 3 years of age with a peak age of presentation of 3 years. It is very rare in children older than 15, though adult cases of Wilms tumour are also reported. Females present 6 months later than males.

There is no sex preponderance in this tumour but in Asian countries M:F ratio is 1:4 [2, 3].

Q3

Explain the genetic association and congenital anomalies associated with it.

Answer: Wilms tumour can arise in three manners [3]:

1. Sporadic (M/C)
2. Familial (1.5%)
3. Genetic syndromes (10%)

Two-hit model is proposed for Wilms tumour, similar to retinoblastoma leading to recessive mutation causing a tumour.

A. Gupta · S. Gupta (✉)
Department of Anaesthesia, Pain Medicine and Critical Care, All India Institute of Medical Sciences, New Delhi, India

N. Gupta et al. (eds.), *Problem Based Learning Discussions in Onco-Anesthesia and Onco-Critical Care*, https://doi.org/10.1007/978-981-99-6339-3_21

Sporadic and familial tumours arise most commonly with two gene deletions WT1 and WT2, tumour suppressor genes.

WT1 is present on chromosome 11p13. Its expression is necessary for the maturation of blastemal cell absence which leads to stromal predominant WT, deleted in WAGR and Denys–Drash syndromes.

WT2 is present on chromosome 11p15. It is related to IGF2 and deleted in Beckwith-Weidemann syndrome.

Congenital syndromes associated with Wilms tumour are the following:

1. Overgrowth syndromes
    (a) Beckwith–Wiedemann (10–20% incidence of Wilms tumour)
    (b) Isolated hemihypertrophy (3–5% incidence of Wilms tumour)
    (c) Soto's cerebral gigantism
    (d) Perlman's gigantism with renal dysplasia
    (e) Simpson–Golabi–Behemel (phenotypically similar to Beckwith–Wiedemann)
2. Non-overgrowth syndromes
    (a) Congenital aniridia
    (b) Denys–Drash (pseudohermaphroditism, glomerulopathy; 95% incidence of Wilms tumour)
    (c) WAGR (2% incidence: Wilms' tumour, aniridia, genitourinary malformations and mental retardation) [4]
    (d) Trisomy 18

Q4

What are the manifestations of Wilms tumour?

Answer: The tumour arises from embryonal renal precursor cells; it can double within 11–13 days. So most of the symptoms arise when it crosses its pseudomembranous capsule, disrupts renal physiology and compresses other organs and vessels. The most common presentation is abdominal mass (40%) with various symptoms like haematuria (25%), nausea, vomiting, malaise, fever, abdominal pain and anorexia. About 10% are associated with familial syndromes such as aniridia, hemihypertrophy and genitourinary abnormalities. Tumours may be associated with von Willebrand's disease (<10%). It can be associated with paraneoplastic syndromes such as anaemia, renin and ACTH secretion [1, 2].

Hypertension is associated with 50% of cases which is an important anaesthesia concern. The presumed mechanism of hypertension is the following:

1. Renal ischaemia due to growing mass
2. Release of renin from tumour
3. Release of pressor substances from tumour

Hypertension can be severe and can lead to encephalopathy and cardiovascular compromise.

Q5

Enumerate congenital syndromes associated with Wilms tumour?

Answer: Following are congenital syndromes associated with Wilms tumour [1, 5]:

1. **Beckwith Weidemann syndrome**: Macroglossia, visceromegaly, omphalocele and gigantism. Hence it can be associated with a difficult airway.
2. **WAGR syndrome**: Wilms tumour, aniridia, genitourinary abnormalities and mental retardation are found in this syndrome. Cardiopulmonary problems, head anomalies, neurobehavioral disorders, musculoskeletal defects and metabolic problems can also be present.
3. **Denys–Drash syndrome**: Male pseudohermaphroditism, glomerulonephritis and Wilms tumour are found in this syndrome.
4. **Perlman syndrome:** This syndrome can be associated with WT and includes macrosomia, islet cell hyperplasia, renal hamartomas and an atypical face shape.

Other associations with trisomy 13 and 18 can be present.

Q6

What are the methods to diagnose Wilms tumour?

Answer: Initial diagnoses are made by ultrasound (USG) and computed tomography (CT) scan. Ultrasound can be used to rule out renal or extra-renal mass that moves with respiration. It is seen as an echogenic mass with areas of hypoechogenicity, signs of necrosis with coccygeal distortion causing renal displacement called as "claw sign". USG can be used to diagnose WT antenatally and inferior vena cava (IVC) doppler for infiltration of IVC.

Contrast-enhanced CT scans and magnetic resonance imaging (MRI) are more effective techniques for diagnosing and staging tumours. Cross-sectional imaging with CT or MRI is useful to detect other organ metastases, IVC and renal vein involvement, bilateral disease and ruling out neuroblastoma.

Chest CT is required for identifying lung nodules as the lungs are the most common site for metastasis.

Renal biopsy is rarely needed for Wilms tumour diagnosis.

Q7

Write down the surgical staging of Wilms's tumour.

Answer: Wilms tumour staging is done by National Wilms tumour staging 5 as mentioned in Table 21.1 [1].

Extrarenal intravascular extension of renal tumours is classified by Novick classification of cavoatrial tumour extension with RCC as mentioned in Table 21.2 [6].

Another terminology associated with Wilms tumour is a synchronous and metachronous disease when another tumour is detected in addition to the primary disease. Synchronous cancers were defined as those occurring within 6 months of the first primary cancer, while metachronous cancers were defined as those occurring more than 6 months later on [7].

Synchronous disease: Tumour in the bilateral kidney (6%) has more chances of renal failure than other cases of Wilms tumour. So after biopsy and staging of a tumour independently, pre-nephrectomy 6–8 weeks of chemotherapy shrinks the tumour size. If the one-sided tumour is remitted completely, the persistent affected kidney can undergo delayed unilateral radical nephrectomy. If the both-sided lesion is present even after chemotherapy, then bilateral partial nephrectomy can be done.

Metachronous disease: It is generally a second Wilms tumour arising in the leftover kidney after treatment of first Wilms tumour (1–3%). Prognosis is poor when the resected kidney contains nephrogenic rests; the age of presentation of the first tumour was less than 12 months of age [7].

Table 21.1 National Wilms tumour staging 5

Stage 1	Tumour confined to kidney capsule and complete resection is possible. No tumour spillage No renal sinus extension
Stage 2	Extracapsular extension Renal sinus extension Local spillage during resection No lymph node involvement Complete resection possible
Stage 3	Non-haematogenous spread beyond the kidney to abdominal lymph nodes, renal vein and IVC thrombus. Macroscopic or microscopic residual tumour Peritoneal surface spillage during resection
Stage 4	Haematogenous spread or extra-abdominal lymph node spread
Stage 5	Bilateral synchronous tumour: Biopsy and staging done separately

Table 21.2 Novick classification for extrarenal intravascular extension of renal tumours

Level 1	IVC extension but less than 2 cm above the renal vein
Level 2	Thrombus below the intrahepatic vena cava
Level 3	Thrombus in infrahepatic vena cava until the level of the diaphragm
Level 4	Thrombus extending to the right atrium

Q8

Apart from surgical evaluation what routine investigations should be performed for nephroureterectomy?

1. Answer: Following investigations can be useful in a case of Wilms tumour depending on individual case: Haemoglobin levels: patients can be anaemic due to protein loss, anorexia, coagulopathy and chemotherapy-related immunosuppression. The patient can be polycythaemic due to erythropoietin secretion by the tumour itself.
2. Total leukocyte count: to rule out infections (poor nutrition, malignancy obstructive nephropathy chemotherapy-related immunosuppression).
3. Platelet count: WT can be associated with Von Willebrand's disease and coagulopathies.
4. Blood group for cross-matching.
5. Kidney function tests: malignancy can disrupt renal physiology.
6. Hepatic function tests: IVC extension can cause hepatic dysfunction and ascites.
7. Coagulation tests: To rule out coagulopathies.
8. Two-dimensional echocardiograph: To rule out congenital heart syndrome as associated with congenital syndromes or chemotherapy involves doxorubicin.
9. Electrolytes: Disruption of renal physiology and hypertension.
10. Urine routine microscopy: Protein loss and infection.
11. Chest x-ray: To rule out chest metastasis and pleural effusions.
12. Genetic evaluation: To rule out congenital and familial syndromes associated with WT.

Q9

Enumerate the anaesthetic concerns in a case of Wilms tumour.

Answer: The anaesthetic concerns include various syndromic associations, anaemia, poor nutrition, renal dysfunction, chemotherapy-related side effects and complications, optimisation of hypertension, maintenance of intraoperative thermoregulation, surgical interference with intraoperative ventilation due to raised intraabdominal pressure, fluid management, vascular extension of tumour with possibility of tumour embolism, intermittent IVC compression, thromboembolism, potential for intraoperative haemorrhage and perioperative analgesia management.

Q10

How will you optimize the patient of Wilms tumour posted for nephroureterectomy?

Answer: A patient with Wilms tumour should be evaluated and optimised preoperatively on following lines:

1. Most Wilms tumour cases present in childhood, and since there is a potential for intraoperative haemorrhage, so adequate blood arrangement is a prerequisite.
2. Building up nutrition in the Wilms tumour patients is important because protein loss during malignancy, anorexia and chemotherapy causes anaemia. Haematinics and protein diet should be considered for adequate muscle mass and wound healing.
3. Preoperative transfusion should be carried out if necessary to maintain Hb at least more than 8 to manage intraoperative blood loss and postoperative care.
4. Antibiotic prophylaxis or treatment if any signs of infection.
5. Evaluation of genetic overgrowth syndromes to look for any airway difficulty such as micrognathia macroglossia and hypotonia. So appropriate airway equipment should be available.
6. Hyperinsulinism (Soto syndrome), congenital heart syndrome (Simpson syndrome) electrolyte disturbances due to Renin secretion and hyperaldosteronism and hypertension to be managed preoperatively.

7. Preoperative evaluation of IVC and another renal vein extension should be carried out to estimate intraoperative blood loss and risk of thromboembolism.
8. Preoperative management of chemotherapy side effects and complications beforehand.
9. Intraoperative arterial blood pressure fluctuation can happen due to renin release from tumours and IVC compression.
10. Intraoperative risk of thromboembolisation so central line placement may be mandatory in case of intravascular extension. But surgical venous access device is already placed for chemotherapy, so the percutaneous approach should always be ultrasound-guided.
11. IVC obstruction can cause retroperitoneal collaterals to dilate to conduct lower body venous return. These collaterals can communicate with epidural venous plexuses.
12. Postoperative analgesia, nausea and vomiting and pulmonary complications should be managed appropriately.
13. Postoperatively ERAS protocol should be followed for early recovery and discharge.

Q11

What are the chemotherapy agents used in Wilms tumour treatment and what are the side effects involved?

Answer: The most common chemotherapy agents used are the following [1]:

1. Vincristine—most possible side effects are reversible peripheral neuropathy, myelosuppression, SIADH, liver impairment, CNS depression and convulsions.
2. Actinomycin D—severe diarrhoea (max at 2–3 days), myelosuppression (max at 2–3 weeks), liver impairment, nausea and vomiting.
3. Doxorubicin:
   (a) Acute toxicity—myelosuppression, thrombocytopenia and cardiac dysrhythmias
   (b) Chronic toxicity—decreased cardiac contractility progressing to cardiac failure over a cumulative dose of more than 200 mg/m2. So serial Echo and EKG and Holter monitoring with increasing stress
4. Cyclophosphamide—myelosuppression, haemorrhagic cystitis, nausea and vomiting, SIADH, pulmonary fibrosis, myocardial necrosis, dysrhythmias and renal toxicity
5. MESNA—nausea and vomiting
6. Etoposide—myelosuppression and nausea and vomiting and anaphylaxis
7. Carboplatin—myelosuppression especially thrombocytopenia, nausea and vomiting, reversible nephrotoxicity, peripheral neuropathy and hepatotoxicity

Q12

What are the paraneoplastic phenomena associated with Wilms tumour and its anesthetic considerations?

Answer: Wilms tumour can be associated with a paraneoplastic syndrome which is characterised by the local hormones and substances [1, 2, 5]:

1. **Hypertension**: Association between hypertension and Wilms tumour is found to be 50% [8–10]:
   (a) Renin secretion: Renin is produced from the renal cortex and perivascular spaces enclosed in the cortex. Renin converts from angiotensinogen to angiotensin 1 and to angiotensin 2 which are potent arteriolar vasoconstrictors. Angiotensin 2 and aldosterone-induced renal wasting can be associated with polydipsia and electrolyte disturbances. Hypertension can be labile and severe. It can cause encephalopathy, intravascular volume constriction and left ventricular hypertrophy. So the use of invasive blood pressure monitoring is justified in this setting. Treatment of this hypertension is ACE inhibitors and Saralasin (angiotensin 2 analogs). Beta-adrenergic and adrenergic

blockade cannot be used perioperatively to control hypertension. Intraoperatively nitroglycerin and sodium nitroprusside can be used to control labile hypertension.
   (b) Renal ischaemia due to mechanical compression and the hyperactive renin-angiotensin system.
   (c) Release of vasopressor substances: release of angiotensin 2 and aldosterone.

   Renin levels can become normal after resection within hours but left ventricular hypertrophy and hypertension may take months to be controlled. Hence, antihypertensives should be continued postoperatively for a month.
2. **Coagulopathy:** Wilms tumour can be associated with acquired von Willebrand disease. It is characterised by abnormal Ristocetin aggregation test and bleeding time. It might be a concern for epidural placements. Fresh frozen plasma and cryoprecipitates should be kept ready preoperatively.
3. **Polycythaemia:** It is a rare association with Wilms tumour but can be the only presenting feature. Polycythaemia can be present with normal erythropoietin levels as the following:
   (a) Wide physiological range that is 5–30mIu/mL.
   (b) Episodic secretion, so testing time may miss peak serum level.
   (c) Shorter half-life that is only 1.5–3 h.
   (d) Others: The tumours may secrete ACTH, VIP-like substances, insulin, etc. and may manifest accordingly.

Q13

What is the preoperative operation theatre (OT) preparation and intraoperative monitoring required for this case?

Answer: The following preparation should be ensured in the OT for this case apart from routine OT preparation for a paediatric case:

1. Emergency drugs should be prepared (these include atropine, adrenaline, noradrenaline, dopamine, dobutamine, vasopressin, adenosine, amiodarone, amrinone, etc.).
2. Back-up ventilation equipment and defibrillator should be checked and functional.
3. Thermoregulation is an important and valuable parameter. So warming the operation theatre up till 27°, warm fluids, warm gamgee rolls, radiant warmer and warm sheets to be kept.
4. Standard ASA monitoring is required like pulse oximetry, NIBP, ECG, EtCo2, temperature and urine output.
5. Ventilatory parameters such as peak airway pressures or a precordial stethoscope to look for chest sounds and pulmonary embolism.
6. Invasive BP monitoring or CVP monitoring may be required in case of a large tumour or IVC or renal extension is present for fluid management and blood loss management.
7. A transesophageal echo probe can also help in the early diagnosis of pulmonary embolism and fluid management.

Q14

What is the plan of anesthesia management for this case?

Answer: After OT preparation and attaching ASA levels of monitoring.

Premedication: Premedication with midazolam 0.01 mg/kg or short-acting opioids such as fentanyl can be done if IV is available. If IV is not available, oral midazolam or nasal midazolam or dexmedetomidine can be given.

Anaesthesia induction: In an otherwise healthy child with Wilms tumour, depending on venous access available inhalational or intravenous induction with sevoflurane or thiopentone 3–5 mg/kg, fentanyl 2–3 mcg/kg and atracurium 0.5 mg/kg, respectively

Rapid sequence induction if the tumour is large and splinting diaphragm or ascites due to venous obstruction with thiopentone and succinylcholine 1 mg/kg if renal functions are normal

Regional anaesthesia: Epidural or caudal 19G catheter placement with a bolus of 1.25 mL/

kg of levobupivacaine with 30–50 μg/kg of morphine

Incision and positioning: Careful positioning, padding of pressure areas and eye protection are standard practices. For unilateral nephrectomy, an ipsilateral subcostal incision is enough, but for a bilateral tumour or inspection of both the kidneys, a single supraumbilical transverse incision is to be given. A chevron or rooftop incision is required if cavoatrial extension is present. Analgesia is provided according to incision (question 13) to cover the dermatomes.

Antibiotic prophylaxis is not recommended routinely. It is recommended in case of high-risk cases, renal dysfunction or urinary tract infection.

Thromboprophylaxis is recommended in such surgeries due to the high risk of thromboembolism thus graduated elastic stockings perioperatively or calf compression devices or low molecular weight heparin.

Maintenance of anaesthesia with isoflurane with MAC of 1.0 and top up with fentanyl boluses of 0.5mcg/kg and atracurium with 0.5 mg/kg. Maintenance of thermoregulation and urine output of more than 1 mL/kg/h

A fluid according to holidays Segar formula and replacement of blood loss after more than 20% blood loss

Most of our patients are extubated on the table as the surgeries are usually uneventful.

Postoperative mechanical ventilation may be required depending on the following:

1. Major blood loss and major fluid shifts
2. Large abdominal mass
3. Preoperative cardiac dysfunction
4. Difficult airway situations (syndromes)
5. For pain management
6. Coagulopathies associated with
7. Haemodynamic instability
8. Cavoatrial extension.

Q15

What are the methods to provide analgesia to this patient?

Answer: Multimodal analgesia is the key to providing opioid-sparing analgesia in any kind of abdominal surgery. General practice is to use both loco-regional techniques.

Adequate analgesia must be provided perioperatively because incision can be large depending upon the tumour size and excessive manipulation, development of chronic pain and post-traumatic stress disorder. These patients can be undertreated for pain as the estimation of pain scores can be difficult in paediatric patients. Following techniques can be used in providing adequate pain relief:

1. **Caudal or epidural analgesia**: This has been the most common mode of analgesia in abdominal surgeries. 19G epidural catheter can be inserted into caudal space or lower thoracic space for continuous infusion. Local infusion or bolus can be given. 1.25 mL/kg of 0.25% of levobupivacaine, bupivacaine or ropivacaine can be given according to the modified Armitage formula after calculating the toxic dose for a patient. Continuous infusion with local anaesthetics can be the most effective way to control perioperative pain.

   Effective dermatomes to be blocked according to incision are mentioned in Table 21.3.

   Disadvantage of continuous catheter technique is that in cases of major blood loss and repeated transfusion, placement of catheter can pose a risk of epidural haematoma due to potential coagulation disturbances. There is a risk of an impediment to respiratory efforts with the thoracic epidural technique. It can cause hypotension and haemodynamic instability.
2. Other regional techniques: Paravertebral block, erector spinal block, quadratus lumbo-

Table 21.3 Dermatomal levels required for various surgical incisions in Wilms tumour surgery

Incision	Dermatomes
Flank	T9–T11
Thoracoabdominal	T7–T12
Transabdominal	T6–T12

rum and transversus abdominis plane block can be used. These techniques are as effective as a thoracic epidural in providing analgesia during the intraoperative period. Advantages of these techniques over thoracic epidural technique are the following:

(a) It can be used even in case of major blood loss and transfusions.
(b) Decreased risk of hypotension.
(c) No blockade of respiratory efforts.

3. Local infiltration: Local infiltration with 2% lignocaine with a wound catheter can be one of the options.

   Disadvantage: Surgical site infection can occur with local catheters.

4. Intravenous drugs: Intravenous paracetamol 15 mg/kg TDS can supplement analgesia with intermittent fentanyl boluses. Intravenous fentanyl infusion and patient-controlled analgesia pumps with fentanyl or morphine can be used. Ketamine or lignocaine infusion can also be used to decrease the need for opioids in the perioperative period. NSAIDs should always be avoided.

Q16

What are the postoperative concerns of this surgery?

Answer: Major complications after nephrectomy can be divided into immediate, early and late complications [2, 3].

The immediate complications include vascular injury, injury to the spleen and injury to the bowel and pneumothorax. The early complications include bowel obstruction, peritonitis, acute renal failure and deep vein thrombosis. Chronic renal failure, wound infection and incisional hernia are late complications. All these complications depend preoperatively on respiratory function and cardiovascular functions, type and size of the tumour, histological type of tumour stage of disease or metastasis at presentation.

Long-term complications of Wilms tumour are the following [11]:

(a) Renal function—Proteinuria and hypertension may occur after nephrectomy due to compensatory hypertrophy. The risk of renal failure in unilateral Wilms tumour is only 0.25%. The most common causes of renal failure are an unrecognised renal disease in Denys–Drash syndrome and renal injury followed by radiation therapy followed by surgical complications. Close monitoring of renal function in long-term follow-up is required for routine monitoring of renal function for tumour recurrence.
(b) Lung damage: Chemotherapy and lung irradiation in case of pulmonary metastasis can cause severe lung fibrosis. Prophylaxis against pneumocystis carinii is advisable in case of lung radiotherapy
(c) Infertility: Chemotherapy and radiation can cause severe damage to prepubertal cells and hormonal dysfunction. Vincristine can cause azoospermia.
(d) Secondary neoplasms: Risk is 1.5–5.6%. It is mainly secondary in the irradiated field such as hepatocellular, bone, breast and thyroid malignancies.
(e) Liver damage: Irradiation and chemotherapy with actinomycin D and vincristine can cause hepatotoxicity and veno-occlusive disease characterised by hyperbilirubinemia, elevated liver enzymes and ascites.
(f) Congestive heart failure: It is a well-known complication after anthracyclines such as doxorubicin cause dose-related cardiomyopathy and myocyte necrosis and fibrosis. The incidence is 5% after a cumulative dose of 400–500 mg/m^2. So regular follow-up of cardiac function should be done for timely discontinuation of doxorubicin.
(g) Musculoskeletal function: Flank and abdominal radiation therapy >20–30 grey can cause a decrease in height according to age. A decrease in sitting height is found in certain patients followed by abdominal radiation. Other defects are rib hypoplasia and limb length inequality.

Table 21.4 Special anaesthetic considerations in the case of vascular extension of tumour and thrombus

Consideration	Remarks
The extent of intravascular extension	Hepatic venous congestion, hepatic dysfunction and ascites if venous drainage is impaired Pleural effusions may affect respiratory reserve.
Tricuspid obstruction on right atrial extension	Cardiopulmonary bypass may be needed. Surgical plan to be decided in close communication with the team.
Intravenous access (large-bore cannula in upper limbs or central venous access)	Potential for excessive haemorrhage and need to intermittently clamp of IVC.
CVP monitoring	Desirable because of the potential for intraoperative embolisation. But the risk of tumour dislodgements is always there. Any percutaneous approach should be ultrasound-guided. The surgical venous access device may also be there for preoperative chemotherapy and can be used intraoperatively.
Epidural placement	IVC obstruction may lead to retroperitoneal venous collaterals to conduct lower venous return. Such collaterals can communicate with epidural venous plexus so risk of inserting epidural catheters should be anticipated especially in case of full heparinisation is needed for CPB.
Transesophageal echocardiography	In case of right atrial extension of thrombus, tricuspid obstruction. To look for residual tumour or thromboembolus.

Q17

What is the special consideration in the case of vascular extension of tumour and thrombus?

Answer: A multispeciality approach including radiologists, anaesthesiologists, cardiovascular surgeons, urologists and hepatobiliary specialists is essential. The special anaesthetic considerations in such cases are mentioned in Table 21.4.

References

1. Whyte SD, Mark AJ. Anesthetic considerations in the management of Wilms' tumour. Ped Anaesth. 2006;16:504–13.
2. Chapman E, Pichel AC. Anaesthesia for nephrectomy. BJA Educ. 2016;16(3):98–101.
3. Bhutani N, Kajal P, Sharma U. Many faces of Wilms tumour: recent advances and future directions. Ann Med Surg. 2021;64:102202.
4. Fischbach BV, Trout KL, Lewis J, Luis CA, Sika M. WAGR syndrome: a clinical review of 54 cases. Pediatrics. 2005;116:984–8.
5. Goodrich M, Keatley V, Norwood B. Anesthetic management of an infant undergoing radical nephrectomy for Wilms tumour: a case report. AANA J. 2008;76:199–201.
6. Novick AC, Kaye MC, Cosgrove DM, Angermeier K, Pontes JE, Montie JE, Streem SB, Klein E, Stewart R, et al. Experience with cardiopulmonary bypass and deep hypothermic circulatory arrest in the management of retroperitoneal tumors with large vena caval thrombi. Ann Surg. 1990;212:472–6.
7. Moertel CG. Multiple primary malignant neoplasms: historical perspectives. Cancer. 1977;40(Suppl 4):1786–92.
8. Cobb ML, Vaughan RW, Louis S. Severe hypertension in a child Wilms tumour; a case report. Anesth Analg. 1976;55:519–21.
9. Ganguly A, Gribble J, Tune B, Kempson RL, Luetscher JA. Renin-secreting Wilms' tumour with severe hypertension. Ann Intern Med. 1973;79:835.
10. Matsui A, Ono K, Nakagawa M. Hyperreninemia, hypertension, and congestive heart failure in focal interstitial nephritis. Nephron. 1996;74:405.
11. Egeler RM, Wolff JE, Anderson RA, Coppes MJ. Long-term complications and post-treatment follow-up of patients with Wilms tumour. Semin Urol Oncol. 1999;17:55–61.

22 Paediatric Case of Mediastinal Mass for USG-/CT-Guided Biopsy

Sachidanand Jee Bharti and Wasimul Hoda

22.1 Case Scenario

A one-year-old child weighing 10 kg presented to paediatric emergency with history of fever, subcostal retraction and excessive crying in supine position. On examination, child was febrile, tachypnoeic with oxygen saturation of 92–94% on oxygen support through nasal prongs. On auscultation, air entry was almost absent in the right hemithorax with normal audible heart sounds. Initial chest radiograph (AP view) showed huge mass in anterior mediastinum. Suspecting as a case of mediastinal mass, child was shifted to paediatric oncology for further management, hereby discussing the various anaesthetic implications, challenges and management of child with mediastinal mass posted for diagnostic tissue biopsy under computed tomography (CT) guidance.

22.2 Give an Overview of Mediastinal Masses

- Mediastinal masses in paediatric population can be benign or malignant and may require anaesthesia for diagnostic procedures such as CT- or USG-guided biopsy or mediastinoscopy and biopsy.
- Commonly present as anterior mediastinal masses (AMM) and include T-acute lymphoblastic leukaemia, T-non-Hodgkin lymphoma (T-NHL) and Hodgkin lymphoma, neuroblastoma and germ cell tumours [1]. Lymphomas account for majority of these cases while reminder is due to teratomas, vascular malformations, bronchial cysts and neurogenic tumours [1].
- Most of the lymphomas have mediastinal involvement at presentation, and nearly half of the patients with lymphomas have respiratory symptoms at the time of presentation [2].
- A common misconception is that children are symptomatic during presentation which is not true always [3]. In fact, children are less symptomatic as compared to adults. In addition, the severity of symptoms may not correlate with the degree of trachea-bronchial obstruction [4, 5].
- Orthopnoea is suggestive of significant tracheal narrowing and should alert the anaesthesiologist for possible airway collapse following induction of anaesthesia [6]. The degree of orthopnoea should be assessed although it is difficult to assess in infants and small child. Asymptomatic infant is comfortable in supine position while symptomatic child will appear distressed or upset in supine position. But categorising as moderate or severe is challenging as in either case the

The original version of the chapter has been revised. A correction to this chapter can be found at https://doi.org/10.1007/978-981-99-6339-3_37

S. J. Bharti (✉) · W. Hoda
Onco-Anaesthesiology and Palliative Medicine, DRBRAIRCH, AIIMS, New Delhi, India

N. Gupta et al. (eds.), *Problem Based Learning Discussions in Onco-Anesthesia and Onco-Critical Care*, https://doi.org/10.1007/978-981-99-6339-3_22

infant would be severe distressed with gasping or even cyanosed.

- Life-threatening complications have been reported even in asymptomatic infants and children [7].
- Anaesthetic management in these cases for diagnostic and therapeutic purposes is extremely challenging in nature [8].
- They may present with pre-existing major airway (superior mediastinal syndrome) and vascular compression (compression of the superior vena cava), which may be exacerbated during anaesthesia causing perioperative morbidity and mortality [9].
- Deaths related to anaesthesia have been reported [7] which has been attributed to the causes such as more compressible cartilaginous airway structure, poor correlation between tumour size and presenting symptoms, difficulty in obtaining reliable history and more chances of receiving general anaesthesia (GA) even for tissue biopsy.
- Also, the diagnostic procedures are carried in remote areas as non-operating room anaesthesia (NORA), which add up the stress and difficulty to an anaesthesiologist [10].
- Therefore, a multidisciplinary diagnostic team approach with clear understanding of nature of mediastinal mass, its pathophysiology, relation to its surrounding structures and meticulous preoperative assessment and preparation to manage any life-threatening respiratory and cardiovascular complication is the key to its successful management.

22.3 What Are the Clinical Presentation of Children with Mediastinal Mass?

A thorough preoperative assessment and planning of anaesthesia with multidisciplinary team involving surgical and paediatric oncologist, anaesthesiologist and interventional radiologist is required.

- The initial presentation can be asymptomatic with mild non-specific respiratory symptoms.
- Asymptomatic patients may be overlooked where even a lymph node biopsy under sedation may turn to be catastrophic. In such cases, mediastinal masses can be an incidental finding after a chest X-ray [9]. In few cases, it may present as an emergency which can be fatal due to impending airway obstruction and cardiorespiratory collapse [11]. As symptoms may be acute and life-threatening, it is recommended to manage these patients only in centres having paediatric intensive care unit (PICU) and availability of paediatric oncologist.
- Respiratory signs and symptoms may be due to the tracheobronchial obstruction. The obstruction can be at single or multiple levels along the tracheal length. The common symptoms may be dyspnoea, wheezing, cough, stridor and chest retraction [12, 13]. These symptoms may be variable depending upon patient position. For example, orthopnoea is worse in supine position. It is due to the combined effects of gravity on lying down and increased intrapleural pressure at the end of expiration [9]. Cardiovascular sign and symptoms may be due to compression of superior vena cava (SVC) leading to superior vena cava syndrome [12]. Patient may present with dyspnoea, dilated collateral veins in the upper body and oedema in the face, neck and arms [2]. Some may have features of the right heart and pulmonary vascular compression [14]. They may have dyspnoea, arrhythmias and cardiac murmurs. Occasionally, mass may obstruct venous return leading to decreased venous return and cardiac output. Some may present with cardiac tamponade due to malignant pericardial effusions.
- Severe cardiopulmonary collapse may occur in few patients with critical mediastinal mass syndrome (CMMS) [15]. The result may be fatal even after the use of all appropriate resuscitative measures. CMMS is seen in patients with anterior mediastinal mass associated with sign and symptoms of respiratory compromise with radiological evidences of compression and deviation of airway and/or great vessels, SVC syndrome and pleural and pericardial effusion [11].

- Since the symptoms of cardiac and respiratory systems are so overlapping, it is advised to have preprocedural radiological scans in order to look for compression on tracheobronchial tree, right heart and major pulmonary vessels. It helps in better planning and management of anaesthesia. Orthopnoea is the most common presentation and may be considered as the most significant predictor of anaesthetic complications [16].
- As clinical presentation of childhood mediastinal masses is often nonspecific or incidental, patients can be asymptomatic and can go undetected. In such cases, ambulatory anaesthesia for even a lymph node biopsy may prove fatal [17]. Severe cardiovascular and/or respiratory collapse may occur following induction of anaesthesia in a patient with critical mediastinal mass syndrome (CMMS). The outcome may be fatal despite expeditious use of all appropriate resuscitative manoeuvres [18].
- CMMS in infants are identified by factors such as anterior mass, lymphoma, superior vena cava syndrome, vessel compression or displacement and pericardial and pleural effusion. Cardiac tamponade and superior vena caval syndrome are known complications of anterior mediastinal mass when it involves great vessels [19].

22.4 What Are the Predictors of Acute Perioperative Cardiorespiratory Complications in Patients with Anterior Mediastinal Mass? (Table 22.1)

Table 22.1 Risk factors for perioperative cardiorespiratory complications [20]

Clinical signs and symptoms	Diagnostic imaging findings
Orthopnoea Wheeze Stridor Upper body oedema (signs of SVC syndrome)	Tracheal, bronchial or carinal compression Great vessel compression and SVC obstruction Pulmonary artery outflow obstruction Ventricular dysfunction Pericardial effusion

Table 22.2 Possible anaesthetic mediastinal mass syndrome – risk classification

Category	Clinical/CT findings
Safe	Asymptomatic or minimal symptoms Tracheobronchial diameter >50% on CT scan
Unsafe	Moderate to severe orthopnoea Presence of pericardial effusion or SVC obstruction Children with trachea-bronchial narrowing <50% irrespective of symptoms
Uncertain	Inability to provide history in case of older children Children with mild orthopnoea whose tracheobronchial diameter is not known

Table 22.3 Grading of severity of symptoms

Grade	Symptoms
Asymptomatic	Children without symptoms
Mild	Can lie supine with mild cough and/or pressure symptoms
Moderate	Can lie supine albeit for short duration due to the increase in severity of symptoms
Severe	Inability to tolerate supine position

22.5 How Do You Risk Stratify These Patients?

The risk stratification is based on clinical symptoms and diagnostic results. It can be classified as [21] follows (Table 22.2):

The severity of the symptoms is graded based on how it affects lying down in supine position. For anterior and superior mediastinal tumours, the symptoms can be graded as the following (Table 22.3):

22.6 Describe the Pre-operative Management of Mediastinal Mass

- The main objective of evaluation is to estimate the size of mediastinal mass and its relations to the major airway and vascular structures. The localisation and extent of compression and mass effect help in assessing the anaesthetic risk and formulating an optimal anaesthetic plan. This can be done on the basis of clinical symptoms, chest X-ray, dynamic CT scan, three-dimensional CT scan, virtual bronchoscopy and two-dimensional echo. Two-dimensional echo is indicated in the presence of pericardial effusion and SVC syndrome or if CT scan shows evidence of major cardiovascular compression. It should also be borne in mind that absence of radiological evidence and or clinical findings does not exclude the probability of perioperative risk.

- Routine investigations including biochemistry, haematology and coagulation profiles must be done beforehand. Any correction or need for transfusion should be done preprocedural. In oncological patients, care should be taken to prevent risk of tumour lysis syndrome. Adequate hydration and optimal fluid management is the key to prevent its development. The use of dexamethasone can trigger tumour lysis syndrome. Therefore, it should be used judiciously.
- Based on the clinical and radiological findings, risk stratification should be done which helps to standardise the perioperative management.
- Patients with tracheal compression and SVC syndrome can be pre-treated with steroid, radiotherapy and chemotherapy [22] which may help in shrinkage of tumour and alleviating the obstructive symptoms [23]. However, there is considerable controversy regarding the use of pre-treatment steroid and radiotherapy based on the fact that it may affect the histology leading to diagnostic confusion. Therefore, its use before tissue biopsy should be discussed with the multidisciplinary team. Its use should be guided based on the risk benefit ratio.
- Avoid sedative pre-medication in patients with mediastinal mass syndrome.
- Patients must be transported in Fowler's position in presence of positional symptoms accompanied by an anaesthesiologist.
- In patients with SVC syndrome, intravenous access must be secured in lower extremity due to altered pharmacokinetics of the drugs which may lead to uncertain efficacy of the drugs.
- An alternate airway management plan should be in place. Endotracheal tubes of different sizes, spiral reinforced tubes, rigid bronchoscopes and flexible bronchoscopes should be available. An experienced bronchoscopist should be available in cases with mediastinal mass syndrome.
- How do you manage these children posted for CT-/USG-guided biopsy?
- Discussion with the multidisciplinary team especially the personnel involved during the biopsy is most important. Detailed discussion regarding the symptoms of patients, nature of tumour, presence and degree of airway or vascular compression, type of anaesthesia, backup for general anaesthesia, arrangement for resuscitation, management of catastrophic events, postprocedural management and other options to save child's life should be planned.
- It is highly recommended to avoid general anaesthesia for biopsy under ultrasonography or CT guidance [24]. Local anaesthesia is ideal in symptomatic large mediastinal masses. Alternative tissues from extramediastinal sites such as pleural effusion, peripheral lymph node or bone marrow can be done safely under local anaesthesia in order to establish oncological diagnosis. If at all, procedure cannot be done under local anaesthesia, sedation can be given. Mild sedation can be given to reduce the depth of anaesthesia in order to maintain spontaneous respiration. Maintaining spontaneous respiration is of prime importance to prevent complication [9].
- Sedation with maintenance of spontaneous respiration and avoidance of muscle paralysis should be the goal of anaesthesia [25]. Positioning can affect the severity of obstruction. Therefore, history regarding the most comfortable breathing position should be noted. This position may be helpful before and after the procedure. However, lateral, semi-erect, sitting or prone positioning can also be used for induction. Biopsy under ultrasonography (USG) and computed tomography (CT) guidance can be done in monitored anaesthesia care (MAC). Informed high-risk consent with parent and care giver is paramount. For

any catastrophic event, cardiothoracic and perfusion team should be informed prior to the procedure. Difficult airway cart and resuscitation medications should be kept in hand.

- American Society of Anaesthesiologists (ASA) fasting guidelines should be followed. After shifting to the radiological suite, patient should be nursed in the most comfortable or sitting position. A good peripheral intravenous cannula is established. Routine American Society of Anaesthesiologists monitor including echocardiograph (ECG), pulse oximetry, end-tidal carbon dioxide ($ETCO_2$) and non-invasive blood pressure (NIBP) should be attached, and a baseline reading of pulse, blood pressure, respiratory rate and oxygen saturation (SPO_2) should be noted. $ETCO_2$ can be measured through a nasal cannula having sensing capability. It helps to provide a continuous positive airway pressure (CPAP) and oxygen delivery at 3–4 L/min. In asymptomatic and stable patients, injection midazolam (0.05–0.1 mg/kg) and fentanyl (1 mcg/kg) can be given. This allows to attach monitors and oxygen supplementation via mask or nasal cannula. If patient is agitated, injection of ketamine (1 mg/kg) can be given intravenously. After sterile preparation and draping, the biopsy site is infiltrated with 2% local anaesthetic like lignocaine with adrenaline.
- Ketamine (1 mg/kg) can be used as boluses so as to reach a desired level of sedation with maintenance of spontaneous respiration. Ketamine is considered to be an ideal intravenous agent which has been used previously with good outcome. It helps in reducing negative inotropic and chronotropic effects and maintaining spontaneous respiration. It also contributes to haemodynamic stability during the whole diagnostic procedure.
- Some authors have advocated the use of dexmedetomidine in combination with ketamine [26]. As the use of dexmedetomidine as a sole agent fails to provide adequate analgesia in painful procedures like biopsy, combined use of both drugs provides optimal level of sedation and analgesia with least effect on cardiopulmonary function [27, 28]. A loading dose of dexmedetomidine (1 mcg/kg) and ketamine (1 mg/kg) over 5 min can used to induce the anaesthesia. Dexmedetomidine infusion can be continued at 0.5 mcg/kg per hour. According to patient's response, ketamine boluses at a dose of 0.3–0.5 mg/kg can be supplemented [29].
- Propofol is considered to be the drug of choice for procedural sedation. However, in cases of mediastinal biopsy, it is better avoided. It is deleterious side effects on cardiopulmonary function can lead to apnoea, airway obstruction and haemodynamic instability.
- Continuous monitoring is needed throughout the procedure. It can be easily done if biopsy is under USG. However, if it is done under CT guidance, both prevention from harmful radiation and continuous monitoring remain the goal. The monitor which is attached to the patient should be ideally visualised through the transparent glass window from operator's console side. In order to prevent any fall, patients can be wrapped well with a piece of cloth. Sedation is given just before the topogram is acquired by the radiologist. It can be repeated if needed to prevent any movement by the patient. Vital signs should be recorded before and after the procedure, after every 5 min if the procedure is prolonged in a time-based chart. Drugs administered, doses, routes and any unwanted event should be documented for future assessment and planning. This information can be used in future if the patient is planned for surgical removal under GA.
- Some patient many require general anaesthesia (GA) with controlled ventilation which has its own disadvantages.
- A backup plan for GA both in low and high risk should be planned and discussed. Additional precaution should be taken in case of asymptomatic or minimally symptomatic patients, as they may experience severe complications during the anaesthesia [30]. For GA, standard monitors and good intravenous access preferably in lower limb are needed. Awake fibreoptic intubation, inhalational induction with maintenance of spontaneous ventilation, avoidance or use of short-acting muscle relaxant, intubation distal to obstruc-

tion, proper positioning, standby rigid bronchoscopy and elective cardiopulmonary bypass for extreme cases should be considered in case of GA [31].

22.7 What Are the Mechanisms by Which General Anaesthesia Causes Cardiorespiratory Collapse in a Patient with Anterior Mediastinal Mass?

Changes in physiological pressure conditions in airway due to positioning and induction of general anaesthesia with positive pressure ventilation cause an increase in critical airway pressure leading to difficulty in ventilation and consequent hypoxia. Various factors which contribute to these changes include the following:

- A decrease in transverse diameter of thorax occurs in supine position along with cephalad displacement of the diaphragm. The increase in central blood volume increases the size of well-vascularised tumours. This increases the extrinsic compression on airways. These effects are further accentuated under anaesthesia.
- Anaesthesia causes decrease in transverse diameter of the thorax, increase in abdominal muscle tone and decrease inspiratory muscle tone which reduces the thoracic volume by 500–1000 ml [32]. Relaxation of the tracheobronchial smooth muscles enhances extrinsic compressibility of the airways.
- There is elimination of normal trans-pleural gradient due to loss of spontaneous diaphragmatic movement with the use of muscle relaxants.
- During controlled ventilation, poorly perfused anterior lung segments are preferentially ventilated with dorsal atelectasis and the increase in shunt and ventilation perfusion mismatch. There is occurrence of post-stenotic turbulent flow due to reduction in cross-sectional area and acceleration of gas molecules which may be insufficient to ventilate the distal bronchi.
- Positive pressure ventilation reduces the preload with cardiovascular instability. The effect can be severe in patients with pre-existing cardiac tamponade and compromised cardiac function.
- Increased intra-thoracic pressure during mechanical ventilation causes the tumour to compress adjacent organs that further worsens the negative airway changes [33].

22.8 What Is the Post Procedural Management of These Cases?

- The patient should be shifted and monitored carefully in post anaesthesia care unit (PACU).
- Trained paediatric nursing staff and anaesthesiologist should be vigilant enough to detect and intervene at the earliest.
- Patient should be in propped-up position, and oxygen should be supplemented via oxygen mask until the patient is fully awake with stable haemodynamics.
- Pulse-oximetry should be continued throughout the procedure till complete emergence and recovery from anaesthesia in PACU.
- A post-operative X-ray chest should be done in order to rule out pneumothorax or haemothorax due to inadvertent biopsy needle.

22.9 What Are the Complications of This Procedure?

(a) Airway obstruction.
(b) Glottic oedema and stridor in the presence of SVC. Hack et al. have found stridor to be the only predictor of post anaesthetic complication [34].
(c) Hypoxemia and hypotension are the common complications that can occur unexpectedly at any time of anaesthesia from induction to recovery in PACU [35].
(d) Complete airway obstruction and cardiovascular collapse are the most dreaded complications, when there is significant airway and vascular compression [36].

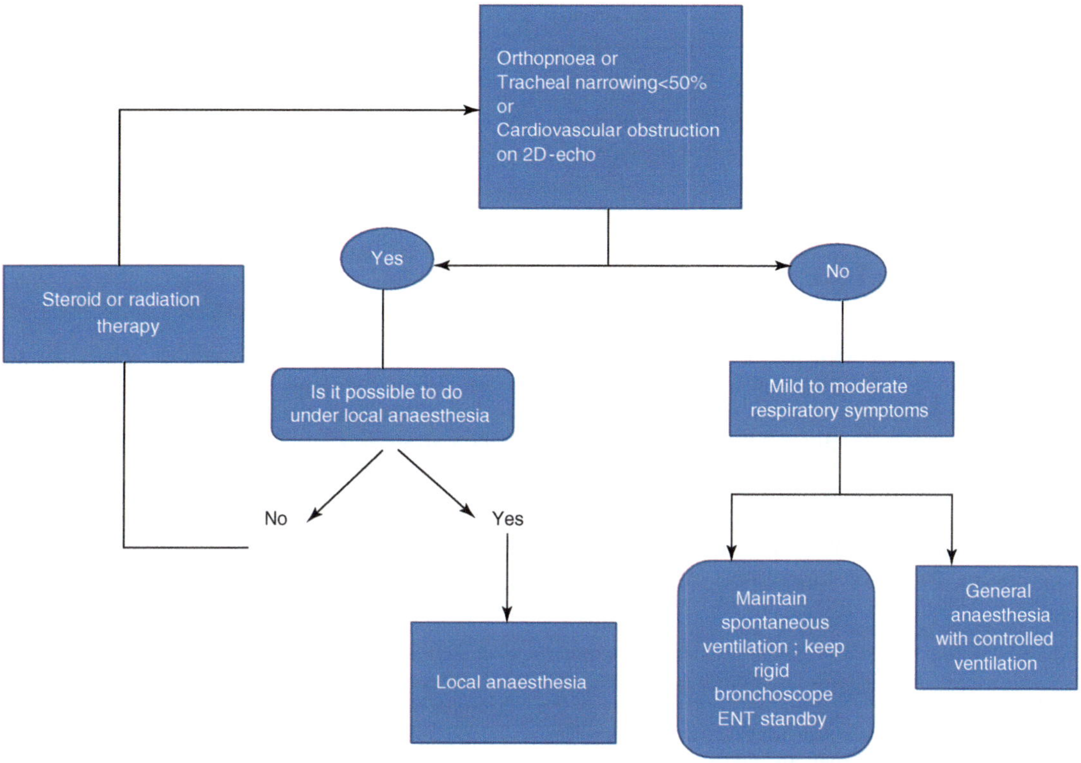

Flow chart depicting anaesthetic management in mediastinal mass

References

1. Wright CD. Mediastinal tumours and cysts in pediatric population. Thoracic Surg Clin. 2009;19:47–61.
2. King DR, Patrick LE, Genn Piasse ME. Pulmonary function is compromised in patient with mediastinal lymphoma. J Pediatr Surg. 2007;32:294–9.
3. Narang S, Harte BH, Body SC. Anesthesia for patients with a mediastinal mass. Anesthesiol Clin N Am. 2001;19:559–79.
4. Takeda SI, Miyoshi S, Akashi A, Ohta M, Minami M, Okumura M, et al. Clinical spectrum of primary mediastinal tumors: a comparison of adult and pediatric populations at a single Japanese institution. J Surg Oncol. 2003;83:24–30.
5. Azarow KS, Pearl RH, Zurcher R, Edwards FH, Cohen AJ. Primary mediastinal masses: a comparison of adult and pediatric populations. J Thorac Cardiovasc Surg. 1993;106:67–72.
6. Shamberger RC, Holzman RS, Griscom NT, Tarbell NJ, Wein Stein HJ. CT quantification of tracheal cross-sectional area as a guide to the surgical and anesthetic management of children with anterior mediastinal mass. J Pediatr Surg. 1991;26:138–42.
7. Victory RA, Casey W, Doherty P, Breatnach F. Cardiac and respiratory complications of mediastinal lymphomas. Anaesth Intensive Care. 1993;21:366–9.
8. Perger L, Lee EY, Shamberger RC. Management of children and adolescents with a critical airway due to compression by an anterior mediastinal mass. J Pediatr Surg. 2008;43(11):1990–7.
9. Karnik PP, Dave NM, Rawlani SS, Dhabe VV. Discretion is the better part of valour: non-operating room anaesthesia for tissue diagnosis of a mediastinal mass. Airway. 2022;5(2):92.
10. Lerman J. Anterior mediastinal masses in children. Semin Anesth Perioper Med Pain. 2007;26(3):133–40. WB Saunders.
11. Viswanathan S, Campbell CE, Cork RC. Asymptomatic undetected mediastinal mass: a death during ambulatory anesthesia. J Clin Anesth. 1995;7(2):151–5.
12. Vas L, Naregal F, Naik V. Anaesthetic management of an infant with anterior mediastinal mass. Pediatr Anesth. 1999;9(5):439–43.
13. FRCPC P. Principles and practice of anesthesia for thoracic surgery. Slinger P, editor. New York: Springer; 2011.
14. Kawaguchi Y, Saito T, Mitsunaga T, Terui K, Nakata M, Matsuura G, Kouchi K, Yoshida H. Prediction of

respiratory collapse among pediatric patients with mediastinal tumors during induction of general anesthesia. J Pediatr Surg. 2018;53(7):1365–8.
15. Graeber GM, Shriver CD, Albus RA, Burton NA, Collins GJ, Lough FC, Zajtchuk R. The use of computed tomography in the evaluation of mediastinal masses. J Thorac Cardiovasc Surg. 1986;91(5):662–6.
16. Blank RS, de Souza DG. Anesthetic management of patients with an anterior mediastinal mass: continuing professional development. Can J Anesth/J Can Anesth. 2011;58(9):853–67.
17. Scrace B, McGregor K. Anterior mediastinal masses in paediatric anaesthesia. ATOTW. 2015;320:1–7.
18. Robie DK, Gursoy MH, Pokorny WJ. Mediastinal tumors—airway obstruction and management. Semin Pediatr Surg. 1994;3(4):259–66.
19. Sibert KS, Biondi JW, Hirsch NP. Spontaneous respiration during thoracotomy in a patient with a mediastinal mass. Anesth Analg. 1987;66(9):904–7.
20. Anghelescu DL, Burgoyne LL, Liu T, Li CS, Pui CH, Hudson MM, Furman WL, Sandlund JT. Clinical and diagnostic imaging findings predict anesthetic complications in children presenting with malignant mediastinal masses. Pediatr Anesth. 2007;17(11):1090–8.
21. Hensley FA. A practical guide to cardiac anaesthesia. 3rd ed. Philadelphia: Lippincott Williams and Wilkins; 2003.
22. Garey CL, Laituri CA, Valusek PA, Peter SS, Snyder CL. Management of anterior mediastinal masses in children. Eur J Pediatr Surg. 2011;21(05):310–3.
23. Bray RJ, Fernandes FJ. Mediastinal tumour causing airway obstruction in anaesthetised children. Anaesthesia. 1982;37(5):571–5.
24. Malik R, Mullassery D, Kleine-Brueggeney M, Atra A, Gour A, Sunderland R, Okoye B. Anterior mediastinal masses—a multidisciplinary pathway for safe diagnostic procedures. J Pediatr Surg. 2019;54(2):251–4.
25. Frawley G, Low J, Brown TC. Anaesthesia for an anterior mediastinal mass with ketamine and midazolam infusion. Anaesth Intensive Care. 1995;23(5):610–2.
26. Corridore M, Phillips A, Rabe AJ, Tobias JD. Dexmedetomidine-ketamine sedation in a child with a mediastinal mass. World J Pediatr Congen Heart Surg. 2012;3(1):142–6.
27. Tobias JD. Dexmedetomidine and ketamine: an effective alternative for procedural sedation? Pediatr Crit Care Med. 2012;13(4):423–7.
28. Goyal R, Singh S, Bangi A, Singh SK. Case series: Dexmedetomidine and ketamine for anesthesia in patients with uncorrected congenital cyanotic heart disease presenting for non-cardiac surgery. J Anaesthesiol Clin Pharmacol. 2013;29(4):543.
29. Tinker TD, Crane DL. Safety of anesthesia for patients with anterior mediastinal masses: I. J Am Society Anesthesiol. 1990;73(5):1060–4.
30. Piro AJ, Weiss DR, Hellman S. Mediastinal Hodgkin's disease: a possible danger for intubation anesthesia: intubation danger in Hodgkin's disease. Int J Radiat Oncol Biol Phys. 1976;1(5–6):415–9.
31. Stewart AS, Smythe WR, Aukburg S, Kaiser LR, Fox KR, Bavaria JE. Severe acute extrinsic airway compression by mediastinal tumor successfully managed with extracorporeal membrane oxygenation. ASAIO J. 1998;44(3):219–21.
32. Goh MS, Liu XY, Gou YS, Case report. Anterior mediastinal masses.An anaesthetic challenge. Anaesthesia. 1999;54:674–82.
33. Luckhaupt Koch K, Jantzen JP, Dick W. Anaesthesiological aspects of mediastinal mass syndrome. Anasth Intensivmed. 1990;31:363–8.
34. Hack HA, Wright NB, Wynn RF. The anaesthetic management of children with anterior mediastinal masses. Anaesthesia. 2008;63(8):837–46.
35. Keon TP. Death on induction of anesthesia for cervical node biopsy. Anesthesiology. 1981;55:471–3.
36. Levin H, Bursztein S, Heifetz M. Cardiac arrest in a child with an anterior mediastinal mass. Anesth Analg. 1985;64(11):1129–30.

23 Unresectable Carcinoma Gall Bladder for Percutaneous Transhepatic Biliary Drainage

Aditi Suri and Gaurav Sindwani

23.1 Case Study

A 72-year-old female patient presented with gradually progressive obstructive jaundice and loss of weight for 2 months. An abdominal CT scan confirmed metastatic gall bladder cancer involving extensive metastases to the liver and hilar bile duct. She complained of dull aching pain in the abdomen and generalised pruritis, both of which were gradually progressive and described as distressing, especially at night. The patient, along with her family, was well aware of the diagnosis and wanted doctors to take all measures for her to have the best possible quality of life.

23.2 What Is the Worldwide Incidence of Carcinoma Gall Bladder [1]?

Gall bladder cancer (CAGB) is an uncommon malignancy with an incidence of 0.8–1.2%. Despite this, it accounts for almost half of the biliary tract malignancies. CAGB ranked 14th among all cancers as per GLOBOCAN data of 2018 [2]. It is the sixth most common malignancy [1]. Owing to the advanced nature of the illness due to delayed presentation, its prognosis is usually poor, with a five-year survival rate of 5%. Females are more prone to develop cancers of the liver and GI tract.

Anatomical features like an absent serosa and the perimuscular connective tissue in continuity with the connective tissue of the liver enable metastasis to the liver [3].

23.3 Discuss Epidemiology of CAGB in India

The incidence of CAGB in India carries a strong geographic and ethnic influence. Northern, Eastern and Central India are known to have a higher incidence of the disease. There has been a rise in cases of CAGB in both males and females in India. The age-adjusted incidence among women was 10.4/100,000 from 2012 to 2014 as per ICMR. Neighbouring countries like Pakistan, Bangladesh, Bhutan and Nepal too report a high incidence. Certain ethnic groups like Asian Indians, Mexican Indians and Hispanics demonstrate increased likelihood of the disease. There has been an increasing trend in prevalence and mortality due to GB diseases in India over the years possible due to environmental pollutants and lifestyle [4–6].

A. Suri (✉)
Department of Anesthesia, Pain Medicine and Critical Care, All India Institute of Medical Sciences, New Delhi, India

G. Sindwani
Department of Transplant Anesthesia, Institute of Liver and Biliary Sciences, New Delhi, India

N. Gupta et al. (eds.), *Problem Based Learning Discussions in Onco-Anesthesia and Onco-Critical Care*, https://doi.org/10.1007/978-981-99-6339-3_23

23.4 Describe in Brief the Pathophysiology and Risk Factors for CAGB [3, 7, 8]

The pathogenesis if CAGB is poorly understood. Both environmental and genetic factors play a contributory role in a susceptible host.

23.4.1 Anatomical Factors

- Being a dependent part of the GB, the fundus is an area of high mucosal contact, thus the commonest site of CAGB.
- It is an excretory organ that aids the liver to flush out toxins into the biliary system.
- Its own musculature is weak and it depends upon a functional digestive system for its emptying.
- Bacteria easily colonise it causing chronic inflammation and release of toxins. Once colonised, bacteria are difficult to eradicate.
- **Structural anomalies**: Porcelain gall bladder, gall bladder polyps, anomalous pancreatico-biliary junction and sclerosing cholangitis.

23.4.2 Geographic or Environmental Factors

- Regions with high incidence of CAGB in India lie along major rivers of Sutlej, Ganges, Yamuna and Brahmaputra. This is because these rivers gather industrial pollutants, agricultural effluents and human waste along their course. This causes faecal coliform count like *Salmonella typhi* and *H. pylori* to exponentially increase as the river flows downstream.
- The presence of heavy metals, nitrates and pesticides has been identified in the Ganges.

23.4.3 Dietary Factors

- Use of adult-rated mustard oil as cooking oil in North India is an important factor. Mustard oil is an irritant to the gut. Carcinogenic adulterants like diethyl nitrosamine, sanguinarine, etc. are implicated.

23.4.4 Others

- **Age and gender**: The average age of presentation is around 71 ± 12.5 years in the West while it is 51 ± 11 years in India. The early age at disease presentation in India is possibly due to multitude of environmental and lifestyle factors. Women are 2–6 times more prone because women have higher oestrogen and progesterone levels. GB mucosa has receptors for oestrogen and progesterone which favours stasis and gallstone formation.
  - Lack of education and access to healthcare resources.
  - Prevalence of malnutrition among Indian females thus poor immune status that promotes carcinogenesis [9].
- **Obesity**: The higher the BMI (>30), the more the incidence of CAGB.
- **High parity**: Increased risk of CAGB exists with higher parity.
- **Family history** of CAGB.
- **Genetic factors: The** presence of KRAS, TP53 and c-ERB-B2 genetic alterations is known to be associated with adverse outcome in CAGB.

23.5 Discuss Clinical Presentation and Staging of CAGB [3, 8]

In early stages of CAGB, patients are often asymptomatic and often incidentally diagnosed after cholecystectomy for GSD, cholecystitis or routine imaging. Some patients may complain of non-specific symptoms like dyspepsia or pain in the abdomen.

The disease is usually advanced for most patients at the time of presentation. Symptoms are epigastric or right hypochondrial pain (54–83%), vomiting (15–43%), jaundice (10–46%), weight loss (10–39%), anorexia (4–41%) and mass per abdomen (3–8%). Weight loss and jaundice often indicate advanced disease [7, 10, 11]. Disease spread towards celiac plexus can precipitate abdominal pain. Intestinal obstruction, severe pruritis and cholangitis are other complications that may cause significant deterioration in patients' quality of life.

Histopathology: Most common histological type of CAGB remains the adenocarcinoma (AC) (80–90%). Two-thirds of these are poorly differentiated. The rest 10% may either be squamous cell, papillary, adeno-squamous, small cell or undifferentiated.

Pattern of spread: CAGB may metastasise by the following:

- Local invasion to the liver (segments IV and V)
- Lymphatic route
- Peritoneal seeding
- Hematogenous spread

Based on TNM staging system of the American Joint Committee on Cancer (AJCC) [12, 13], it can be categorised as the following:

Stages I and II are potentially resectable and thus approached with curative intent.
Stage III is a locally unresectable disease.
Stage IV indicated unresectable due to distant metastasis.

23.6 What Are Presenting Symptoms of CAGB [4, 14]?

Patients usually present with non-specific features like vague abdominal pain which may mimic cholecystitis, loss of appetite and weight loss. Early stages of the disease are largely asymptomatic. A large proportion of patients are in fact diagnosed incidentally either during a laparoscopic or postoperatively as histopathological finding after an uneventful laparoscopic cholecystectomy [15]. An elderly patient presenting with right upper quadrant pain, anorexia and weight loss and jaundice should raise suspicion of an advanced malignancy. The presence of jaundice in particular indicates adverse outcome.

23.7 What Are the Diagnostic Modalities for Diagnosis of CAGB [8, 16, 17]?

Ultrasonography (USG) is an inexpensive, readily available modality which may reveal cholelithiasis, gall bladder calcification, gall bladder mass or even invasion of adjoining structures. The presence of a GB thickness >3 mm, GB calcification, mass in the lumen and GB polyp >10 mm with enhanced vascularity should raise suspicion of malignancy. But USG has limited use in establishing a diagnosis and disease extent.

Endoscopic ultrasonography (EUS): Endoscopic ultrasonography allows USG probe to be placed much closer to biliary tree for precise imaging of GB. Moreover, it makes simultaneous FNAC (fine needle aspiration cytology) also possible.

Computed tomography (CT) scan: It is used to assess extent of involvement of adjacent structures like lymph node spread, spread to liver or distant structures.

Magnetic resonance imaging (MRI) has limited utility for evaluation of CAGB. MR angiography on the other hand is a valuable tool to detect vascular invasion with a sensitivity of 100% and specificity of 87% [15].

FDG-PET is an indispensable tool for not only preoperative disease staging but also for differentiating benign from malignant disease and detecting postoperative residual disease.

23.8 Common Symptoms Associated with Advanced CAGB [18, 19]

Since a large proportion of CAGB patients cannot undergo curative treatment, palliation of symptoms remains the only effective approach. In patients suffering from progressive jaundice with associated symptoms of cholestasis and cholangitis, providing biliary drainage is the foremost goal. This has significant impact by alleviating cholestatic symptoms and improves quality of life of the patients. Selected patients awaiting curative surgery but with total bilirubin levels >20 mg/dl may benefit from biliary drainage prior to surgery. The presence of cholangitis, jaundice with pain in the abdomen and incoercible pruritis are other indications for biliary drainage.

Endoscopic and percutaneous or surgical bypass are available options for biliary drainage. Being less invasive, percutaneous transhepatic biliary drainage (PTBD) and endoscopic procedures are preferred over surgical bypass.

23.9 What Are Current Treatment Options Available for CAGB [20]

Surgery: The only curative approach remains surgical resection. This is often coupled with hepatectomy and lymphadenectomy in advanced stages. The primary tumor invasion (T) as per the AJCC staging is the sole determinant of surgical approach to follow.

Stage T_{Ia}: Simple cholecystectomy is the recommended approach.

Stages T1b-T2: Radical cholecystectomy with resection of adjacent liver parenchyma (segments IVb and V) may be feasible. Resection of common bile duct (CBD)/common hepatic duct is performed in case of gross or microscopic involvement of margin of cystic duct intraoperatively.

Stages T3–T4: These may involve direct invasion of adjacent structures like the liver, duodenum or colon. In such cases, radical resections are debatable and may be considered only in medically fit patients after consensus of a multidisciplinary team. However, radical resections have not shown to prolong overall or disease-free survival. T4 disease is mostly deemed unresectable and palliation is the recommended route to follow.

Port site recurrence: This needs attention in incidentally diagnosed CAGB after laparoscopic cholecystectomy. It may occur by the following:

- Contamination
  - Direct: during retrieval of tissue or by contaminated instruments
  - Indirect (chimney effect): tumor seeding on post sites secondary to gas leakage
- As a result of immune response of the individual
- Haematogenous spread

It is advocated by some authors to excise port sites or drain sites during the second radical surgery. But others advise against the same because port site excision offers no survival advantage and rather increased risk of generalised peritoneal disease [21].

23.9.1 Adjuvant Treatments

Chemotherapy: gemcitabine, fluoropyrimidines and platinum compounds are the agents of choice. These are used in combination for better results. It is a combination of gemcitabine with cisplatin as shown to confer a significant survival advantage [22].

Radiotherapy: External beam radiotherapy (EBRT) is utilised only as an adjuvant treatment which may provide a survival advantage at 1 year but not at 5 years (70 hundal). Some retrospective studies demonstrated a better survival with adjuvant RT with 5-FU chemotherapy when compared to surgery alone [23–26].

Other: Targeted therapy against epidermal growth factor receptor (EGFR) is a promising modality under research [24].

Palliation: Palliative chemotherapy administered using a combination of gemcitabine and 5-FU is usually well tolerated with mild toxicity. Gemcitabine may also be combined with capecitabine or cisplatin [7, 27].

23.10 What Are Modalities of Palliation for Obstructive Jaundice in Advanced or Unresectable CAGB [19]

Owing to its late diagnosis and poor five-year survival rate of just 5–10%, palliation of distressing symptoms goes a long way in preserving quality of life of patients. Obstructive jaundice is the most distressing symptom that is seen in almost **33–56%** patients and is managed primarily using either endoscopic retrograde cholangiopancreatography (ERCP) or PTBD [18].

The selection of either of the above procedures depends upon the level of obstruction to bile tract, expertise to perform either procedure and postprocedural care available.

In the presence of a blocked hepatic confluence along with blocked segmental ducts, a PTBD is the preferred method of drainage. It is also indicated in the event of a failed endoscopic approach which otherwise is the gold standard approach.

PTBD catheters allow bile to drain externally using a pigtail catheters or there may be a combined external-internal drainage using a ring biliary catheter [28].

23.11 What Is the Procedure of PTBD and Its Benefits and Uses. Describe the Procedure of PTBD [29]

Fluoroscopic PTBD was first described in the year 1962.

It is indicated in 1. Either before surgery to relieve biliary obstruction, 2. To allow biliary drainage and its associated side effects or 3. Facilitate palliative chemotherapy.

Although both fluoroscopic and USG-guided techniques described in literature, yet no standardised techniques or guidelines exist. Most clinicians prefer to use both fluoroscopy and USG while others prefer USG only.

Investigations including complete blood count, serum electrolytes and renal and liver function tests are done. Platelet transfusion is done if platelet count is <50,000/cumm and FFP transfusion to correct an INR if >1.5.

Prophylactic antibiotics are administered 30–60 min prior to the procedure. After sufficient administration of local anaesthesia, a convex (3–5 MHz) USG probe is used to puncture a peripheral bile duct with an 18G or 20 G needle. The biliary anatomy and level of obstruction are identified using injection of contrast dye (50% Omnipaque) under fluoroscopy.

An 8F or 10F biliary drainage catheter is then inserted using Seldinger technique after dilating the track satisfactorily. A drainage catheter with multiple side holes may also be placed which allows bile to be drained both internally and externally. Internal drainage aids enterohepatic circulation. Left-sided biliary duct system is preferred to the right. A post procedure observation period of 24 hours is recommended.

23.12 What Are the Types of PTBD?

There are three types of PTBD:

1. External
2. Internal-external
3. Percutaneous SEMS placement

   PTBD is preferred on the right side in the presence of high obstruction. The presence of ascites deems a superior benefit from a left-sided PTBD.

23.13 What Are the Available Approaches for PTBD?

The procedure to perform PTBD can be guided using fluoroscopy or combined USG and fluoroscopy. A USG-guided combined approach boasts of a reduced exposure to ionising radiation, shorter procedure time, lesser punctures and in all lesser procedure-related complications.

23.14 What Is Percutaneous SEMS?

Percutaneous SEMS is an approach of PTBD. It can be a one-step (primary stenting) or two-step procedure (secondary stenting). A two-step technique allows time margin in the instance of procedural bleeding.

23.15 What Are the Possible Complications During PTBD?

Stent occlusion, dislodgement of catheter, cholangitis, bleeding, leakage of bile around the catheter, pain and infection are common side effects that may accompany a PTBD. Unlike PTBD, endoscopic drainage (EBD) is devoid of such complications and has a shorter duration of hospital stay [30]. Mahjoub and colleagues reported a much lower morbidity rate in EBD group as compared to PYBD group (3.8% vs 21%) [31].

23.16 What Are Other Alternatives to Achieve Biliary Drainage Apart from PTBD [18, 32, 33]?

ERCP-guided biliary drainage may involve endoscopic nasobiliary drainage (ENBD) or insertion of a self-expanding metallic or plastic stent (SEMS).

1. **Endoscopic nasobiliary drainage**: ENBD involved insertion of a 5–7 Fr tube inside the biliary tree and then exteriorising it through the nose to allow biliary drainage. Studies have reported a lower incidence of cholangitis, pancreatic fistula and stent dysfunction with this approach. Nevertheless, this approach carries risk of catheter dislodgment and is thus used as a temporary measure preoperatively.
2. **Endoscopic retrograde cholangiopancreatography (ERCP):** Internal drainage of bile is achieved using ERCP-guided insertion of either plastic stents (PS) or metallic stents (self-expanding metallic stents (SEMS)). Plastic stents are made of Teflon, polyethylene or polyurethane. Their diameter ranges from 5F to 12F and light ranges between 1 and 18 cm. SEMS are made of metal alloys like nickel or titanium. They may be 4–12 cm in length while their diameter may be 6–10 mm. Both types of stents are radiopaque Table 23.1 [18].

   Of the three types of SEMS, U-SEMS is the choice for palliative drainage because of ingrowth of tumor and resultant adhesion of the stent has to be inserted permanently. PC stent has a metallic proximal and distal end while the centre is made of plastic. The ends prevent migration of stent and the plastic centre allows easy removal if needed. FC sent and PC stent are thus preferred when curative surgery is planned in future. Procedural complications include pneumoperitoneum, bleeding and stent migration.
3. **Endoscopic Ultrasound-Guided Biliary Drainage (EUS-BD):** EUS-BD has recently gained popularity in management of malignant biliary obstruction owing to its multiple advantages. It finds its utility in cases where ERCP has failed, there is altered anatomy post surgery or when repeated interventions have failed.

Table 23.1 Advantages and disadvantages of plastic stents and metallic stents (SEMS)

Stent type	Advantage	Disadvantage
Plastic stent	• Mouldable: can adapt to the shape of biliary tree • Removable • Inexpensive	• Risk of stent migration (5–10%) • Stent occlusion due to biliary sludge, clots and biofilm (30%) • Need to be changed every 3–6 months
SEMS **Fully covered (FC SEMS)** **Partially covered (PC SEMS)** **Uncovered (U SEMS)**	• Gold standard for palliative biliary drainage • Low risk of stent occlusion, cholangitis and procedural failure • Better nutrition absorption • No loss of electrolytes	• Technically difficult • Steep learning curve • Difficult to remove eventually

Though uncommon, it is not free of risk of bleeding, peritonitis, bile leak, cholangitis, migration of stent or pneumoperitoneum. Moreover, it requires technical expertise of a sonographer which may be available in a tertiary centre only. Thus limited experience and insufficient availability limit its use.

4. **Palliative chemotherapy** is considered in patients with good performance status. Gemcitabine in combination with cisplatin is used to provide symptom palliation.

23.17 What Is the Evidence for Utility of EUS-BD [34]?

An international multicentre study evaluated the preference of EUS over PTBD and found that almost 80% patients preferred EUS over PTBD ($p < 0.001$) because it was associated with internal drainage better success rate and much lower morbidity. It allowed a significantly improved quality of life due to the absence of an external drain tube and its associated problems.

References

1. Singh BP, Khan WF, Rathore YS, et al. Incidental carcinoma gallbladder: incidence, risk factors, and factors affecting survival—5-year experience from a tertiary care institute. J Gastrointest Canc. 2020;51:980–7. https://doi.org/10.1007/s12029-019-00347-1.
2. Sung H, Ferlay J, Siegel RL, Laversanne M, Soerjomataram I, Jemal A, et al. Global cancer statistics 2020: GLOBOCAN estimates of incidence and mortality worldwide for 36 cancers in 185 countries. CA A Cancer J Clin. 2021;71(3):209–49.
3. Hundal R, Shaffer EA. Gallbladder cancer: epidemiology and outcome. Clin Epidemiol. 2014;6:99–109. https://doi.org/10.2147/CLEP.S37357.
4. Dutta U, Bush N, Kalsi D, Popli P, Kapoor VK. Epidemiology of gallbladder cancer in India. Chin Clin Oncol. 2019;8(4):33. https://doi.org/10.21037/cco.2019.08.03.
5. Malhotra RK, Manoharan N, N.K. Shukla G.K. Rath: gallbladder cancer incidence in Delhi urban: a 25-year trend analysis. Indian J Cancer. 2017;54:673.
6. Krishnatreya M. Gall bladder cancer in Delhi-some thoughts. Indian J Cancer. 2019;56:182.
7. Lai EC, Lau WY. Aggressive surgical resection for carcinoma of gallbladder. A N Z J Surg. 2005;75:441–4.
8. Okumura K, Gogna S, Gachabayov M, Felsenreich DM, McGuirk M, Rojas A, Quintero L, Seshadri R, Gu K, Dong XD. Gallbladder cancer: historical treatment and new management options. World J Gastrointest Oncol. 2021;13(10):1317–35.
9. Baskaran V, Vij U, Sahni P, et al. Do the progesterone receptors have a role to play in gallbladder cancer? Int J Gastrointest Cancer. 2005;35:61–8.
10. Dixon E, Vollmer CM Jr, Sahajpal A, et al. An aggressive surgical approach leads to improved survival in patients with gallbladder cancer: a 12-year study at a North American Center. Ann Surg. 2005;241:385–94.
11. Taner CB, Nagorney DM, Donohue JH. Surgical treatment of gallbladder cancer. J Gastrointest Surg. 2004;8:83–9.
12. Greene FL, Page PL, Fleming IP, et al. American Joint Committee on cancer: AJCC cancer staging manual. 6th ed. New York: Springer; 2002. p. 139–44.
13. Sobin LH, Wittekind CH, editors. Digestive system: gallbladder. In TNM classification of malignant tumors. 6th ed. New York: Wiley-Liss; 2002. p. 84–6.
14. Misra S, Chaturvedi A, Misra NC. Gallbladder cancer. Curr Treat Options Gastro. 2006;9:95–106. https://doi.org/10.1007/s11938-006-0028-1.
15. Reid KM, Ramos-De la Medina A, Donohue JH. Diagnosis and surgi- cal management of gallbladder cancer: a review. J Gastrointest Surg. 2007;11(5):671–81.
16. Kim HJ, Lee SK, Jang JW, et al. Diagnostic role of endoscopic ultrasonography-guided fine needle aspiration of gallbladder lesions. Hepato-Gastroenterology. 2012;59(118):1691–5.
17. Joo I, Lee JY, Kim JH, Kim SJ, Kim MA, Han JK, Choi BI. Differentiation of adenomyomatosis of the gallbladder from early-stage, wall-thickening-type gallbladder cancer using high-resolution ultrasound. Eur Radiol. 2012;23(3):730–8.
18. Schepis T, Boškoski I, Tringali A, Bove V, Costamagna G. Palliation in gallbladder cancer: the role of gastrointestinal endoscopy. Cancers. 2022;14(7):1686.
19. Gupta A, Gupta S, Chauhan U, Kumar U, Sharma N, Ahuja R, Rajput D, Gupta M. Symptom palliation in advanced GallBladder cancer: an institutional experience. Indian J Palliat Care. 2019;25(4):514–6. https://doi.org/10.4103/IJPC.IJPC_94_19.
20. Aloia TA, Járufe N, Javle M, Maithel SK, Roa JC, Adsay V, et al. Gallbladder Cancer: expert consensus statement. HPB. 2015;17(8):681–90.
21. Fuks D, Regimbeau JM, Le Treut YP, Bachellier P, Raventos A, Pruvot FR, et al. Incidental gallbladder cancer by the AFC-GBC-2009 Study Group. World J Surg. 2011;35:1887–97.
22. Valle J, Wasan H, Palmer DH, et al. Cisplatin plus gemcitabine versus gemcitabine for biliary tract cancer. N Engl J Med. 2010;362(14):1273–81.
23. Houry S, Barrier A, Huguier M. Irradiation therapy for gallbladder carcinoma: recent advances. J Hepato-Biliary-Pancreat Surg. 2001;8:518–24.

24. Kresl JJ, Schild SE, Henning GT, et al. Adjuvant external beam radiation therapy with concurrent chemotherapy in the management of gallbladder carcinoma. Int J Radiat Oncol Biol Phys. 2002;52:167–75.
25. Itoh H, Nishijima K, Kurosaka Y, et al. Magnitude of combination therapy of radical resection and external beam radiotherapy for patients with carcinomas of the extrahepatic bile duct and gallbladder. Dig Dis Sci. 2005;50:2231–42.
26. de Aretxabala X, Roa I, Berrios M, et al. Chemoradiotherapy in gallbladder cancer. J Surg Oncol. 2006;93:699–704.
27. Uno T, Itami J, Aruga M, et al. Primary carcinoma of the gallbladder: role of external beam radiation therapy in patients with locally advanced tumor. Strahlenther Onkol. 1996;172:496–500.
28. Ramachandran K, Kannan S. Laryngeal mask airway and the difficult airway. Curr Opin Anaesthesiol. 2004;17(6):491–3. https://doi.org/10.1097/00001503-200412000-00007.
29. Italian College of Interventional Radiology (ICIR) Rising Stars Group, Giurazza F, Corvino F, Contegiacomo A, Marra P, Lucarelli NM, et al. Safety and effectiveness of ultrasound-guided percutaneous transhepatic biliary drainage: a multicenter experience. J Ultrasound. 2019;22(4):437–45.
30. Hameed A, Pang T, Chiou J, Pleass H, Lam V, Hollands M, Johnston E, Richardson A, Yuen L. Percutaneous vs. endoscopic pre-operative biliary drainage in hilar cholangiocarcinoma—a systematic review and meta-analysis. HPB. 2016;18:400–10.
31. Al Mahjoub A, Menahem B, Fohlen A, Dupont B, Alves A, Launoy G, Lubrano J. Preoperative biliary drainage in patients with resectable perihilar cholangiocarcinoma: is percutaneous transhepatic biliary drainage safer and more effective than endoscopic biliary drainage? A meta-analysis. J Vasc Interv Radiol. 2017;28:576–82.
32. Kawashima H, Itoh A, Ohno E, Itoh Y, Ebata T, Nagino M, Goto H, Hirooka Y. Preoperative endoscopic nasobiliary drainage in 164 consecutive patients with suspected perihilar cholangiocarcinoma: a retrospective study of efficacy and risk factors related to complications. Ann Surg. 2013;257:121–7.
33. Lin H, Li S, Liu X. The safety and efficacy of nasobiliary drainage versus biliary stenting in malignant biliary obstruction: a systematic review and meta-analysis. Medicine. 2016;95:e5253.
34. Nam K, Kim D, Lee T, Iwashita T, Nakai Y, Bolkhir A, et al. Patient perception and preference of EUS-guided drainage over percutaneous drainage when endoscopic transpapillary biliary drainage fails: an international multicenter survey. Endosc Ultrasound. 2018;7(1):48.

24 Case of Liver Metastasis for RFA

Manoj Kamal and Priyanka Sethi

24.1 Case History

An 80-year-old male patient, with a history of diabetes, hypertension and coronary artery disease, presented to OPD (outpatient department) with pain in right hypochondrium. He was a known case of carcinoma colon for which hemicolectomy was done 2 years back. Post-surgery he received seven cycles of capecitabine and oxaliplatin. Preliminary ultrasound showed multiple liver nodules. CT scan was done to confirm the findings which showed three liver metastasis nodules of 2–3 cm in size. They were 2 cm inside the liver tissue without any proximity to the vascular structure. A PET scan was done to rule out any extrahepatic metastasis. The patient is now posted for RFA ablation of liver metastasis.

24.2 Introduction

The liver is the most common site for metastases from gastric and colorectal cancer. Various treatment options available for these includes surgical resection, non-surgical ablation techniques and systemic chemotherapy. Treatment option is decided as per the condition of patient, type and location of tumor. Percutaneous radiofrequency ablation (PRFA) of solid tumours is a minimally invasive procedure intended to treat primary and/or metastatic solid tumours with thermal tissue destruction and coagulative necrosis. It has got wider acceptability due to its safety profile [1].

The lung, kidney, thyroid, pancreatic, soft tissue and bone tumors are also treated by RFA. The RFA for liver metastasis are usually performed outside operating room under ultrasound and CT guidance.

With ultrasound guidance, RFA needle is inserted into the tumor, penetrating through the liver. This needle will deliver high-frequency electrical current at the site of tumor. Many times, RFA is reserved for patients who are not suitable for surgical resection, secondary to poor hepatic reserve, severe comorbidities, advanced age or cancer stage.

24.3 What Are the Different Modalities of Treatment for Liver Metastasis?

The treatment modality treatment depends on size, site, number of tumors, vascularity or extrahepatic involvement of the tumor [2, 3].

(a) Surgery: It is a standard treatment modality in resectable tumors. The surgery is not a feasible option for small, multiple tumors and patients with poor liver functions.

M. Kamal · P. Sethi (✉)
Department of Anaesthesiology and Critical Care, AIIMS, Jodhpur, India

N. Gupta et al. (eds.), *Problem Based Learning Discussions in Onco-Anesthesia and Onco-Critical Care*, https://doi.org/10.1007/978-981-99-6339-3_24

(b) Chemotherapy/radiotherapy: Various treatments such as systemic chemotherapy, hepatic arterial infusion (HAI) of chemotherapy and radiotherapy are also proposed for better outcomes in patients with advanced tumor not amenable for resection or sometimes before surgical treatment.
(c) Local ablation: It is a less invasive technique usually used for the treatment of unresectable hepatic tumors. It can be achieved with percutaneous ethanol injection, microwave coagulation therapy and radiofrequency ablation (RFA). This resulted in local necrosis of lesion. RFA claims to provide good local control with a smaller number of treatment sessions in unresectable tumors.

24.4 What Is RFA?

Radiofrequency ablation is a minimal invasive technique for ablating solid tumors (primary or secondary). Alternating current of radiofrequency waves are delivered through uninsulated tip of needle into tissue. These waves increase the local temperature >60 °C which causes thermal tissue destruction and coagulative necrosis [4].

24.5 What Are the Advantages of RFA?

It is a minimal invasive technique with low morbidity, fewer complications and repeatability for recurrent lesions. The RFA can be done either percutaneously, laparoscopically or open surgical method. In some cases, superficial tumors can be wedged out (excised), while deeper lesions can be destroyed by RFA, thereby preserving most of the liver tissue [5].

24.6 How RFA Performed?

The RF is delivered by 14–21 G partially insulated electrodes placed percutaneously on the desired site, which is connected with radiofrequency generator. The electrode is usually expandable and multi-tined so that, when deployed and extended, it can treat lesions up to 5 cm in diameter. The number of electrode placement depends on size of tumor to be ablated. Tissue temperature achieved and duration of heat determines area of necrosis. Usually, tissue necrosis is achieved at a temperature of 60–100 °C for 4–6 min, but in cases where thermal conduction into the lesion is slow, the duration of current needs to increase up to 20–30 min [2, 4].

24.7 Indication of Liver RFA?

1. Primary and metastatic liver tumors with a maximum diameter of 3–5 cm are the most frequent indications for RFA.
2. It can also be used as bridge therapy for liver transplantation.
3. If surgical resection of tumor is not possible due to poor hepatic reserve, severe comorbidities, advanced cancer stage or advanced age.
4. Recurrent Hepato Cellular Carcinoma.

24.8 Limitations of RFA

1. Multiple lesions in the liver is a relative contraindication for RFA.
2. If maximum diameter of target tumor is more than 3 cm, then results of RFA become unpredictable.

24.9 What Are the Goals of Anaesthesia in a Patient Posted for Liver RFA?

Anaesthesia for radiofrequency ablation involves, the titrated use of short-acting opioids and sedatives to enable intervention radiologist to perform procedures effectively, while monitoring the patient closely for potential adverse effects [4, 6]. Goals to be achieved for anesthesia during RFA include the following:

1. Immobile.
2. Analgesia: These patients have considerable pain, due to the initial skin puncture along with the deeper pain associated with thermal tissue necrosis.
3. Minimise procedural discomfort during the performance of the procedure. With monitored anaesthesia care (MAC) or with regional anaesthesia, patient cooperation is very important to localise tumor and needle. In case if patient is not cooperative, general anaesthesia needs to be given.

24.10 What Are the Anaesthesia Concerns in RFA?

1. Anaesthetic consideration of non-operating room anesthesia (NORA) includes lack of familiar working environment, trained manpower, specialised monitoring, equipment and workstations.
2. Proper preoperative evaluation along with informed consent and adequate on-site preparations is mandatory for safe conduct of procedure. These patients are usually high risk with multiple comorbidities, so a thorough preoperative cardiac and respiratory assessment should be done.
3. Patient positioning should be confirmed. Complete airway examination should be done prior to sedation or induction of general anesthesia. All airway equipment for managing difficult airway should be ready. There should be an alternative plan in place to deal with periprocedural crisis.
4. The patients with liver malignancy often have associated cirrhosis and other haemostatic disorders which may lead to increased risk of bleeding. These patients may be on various anticoagulant medications.
5. Anaesthesia plan must be clearly discussed with intervention radiologist. There may be need for deep breaths and apnoeic pause along with pain management during the procedure.
6. Post procedure, patients must be monitored at least for 30 min in properly equipped recovery area. If needed, the patient must be transferred to the post-anaesthesia care unit (PACU) or the intensive care unit (ICU).

24.11 What Are Different Anaesthesia Techniques Used for Liver RFA?

The choice of anaesthetic technique depends on site, size of tumor and practitioner experience. The liver RFA can be performed under MAC, regional anaesthesia, general anaesthesia and sometimes under local anesthesia.

The anaesthesia plan for radiofrequency ablation of the liver is dependent on planned RFA technique. The percutaneous approach can be performed with local infiltration and MAC and is preferred anaesthetic technique. The optimum sedation can be achieved by administering one or more of the following drugs: propofol, dexmedetomidine, midazolam, fentanyl and remifentanil.

Doses of various anaesthetic agents to be used are the following:

1. Propofol: Loading dose of 0.5–1 mg/kg, followed by maintenance dose of 1–3 mg/kg/h. Effect site dose concentration of 2–4 mcg/mL to be achieved by Target Controlled Infusion pump.
2. Midazolam: Bolus dose of 0.1 mg/kg.
3. Dexmedetomidine: Loading dose of 1 μg/kg, followed by maintenance dose of 0.5–0.7 μg/kg/h.
4. Fentanyl: Bolus dose of 1–2 μg/kg followed by boluses as per the need.
5. Remifentanil: Infusion dose of 0.05–0.15 μg/kg/min.

Higher doses of analgesics as fentanyl at the rate of 1–2 μg/kg need to be administered sometimes as severity of pain is more in RFA due to combined effect of Glisson's capsule puncture and heat produced during the procedure. Adequate perioperative monitoring is needed to assess patency of airway and sedation levels.

RFA is sometimes performed under general anaesthesia, if even slight movement is not allowed during the procedure. It also controls severe pain and procedural discomfort.

If RFA is planned by laparoscopic approach, than general anesthesia is required. In general, laparoscopic approaches are typically indicated for the treatment of lesions that may be difficult to target via percutaneous puncture. During laparoscopy, apnoeic pauses may be needed in between to reduce the interference of respiratory movements.

Regional anaesthesia techniques as thoracic epidurals and thoracic paravertebral block are also an option for providing anaesthesia to patients posted for RFA. Coagulation abnormalities need to be ruled out before finalising the anaesthesia plan.

24.12 The Minimum Monitoring Required for RFA?

1. Pulse oximetry
2. ECG
3. Non-invasive blood pressure
4. Capnography
5. Temperature
6. Invasive blood pressure monitoring: In known case of significant coronary artery disease or other cardiac diseases.

24.13 Minimum Anaesthesia Equipment for PRFA Procedures

1. Difficult airway cart
2. Anaesthesia drugs (depending on type of anaesthesia chosen for the procedure)
3. Emergency crash cart
4. Anaesthesia workstation
5. Suction machine and catheters
6. Gas scavenging system (if inhaled general anaesthesia is planned)
7. Automated infusion pump
8. Defibrillator with paddles

24.14 Enumerate the Complications of RFA

Being a minimally invasive procedure, complications rate is very less. The associated complications are the following:

1. Bleeding
2. Pneumothorax
3. Biliary fistula and biliary perforation
4. Intestinal fistula
5. Liver abscess
6. Needle track seeding
7. Portal vein thrombosis

24.14.1 Prognosis

RFA is an effective method to treat liver metastases especially if it is a solitary lesion. Its survival is comparable to survival after surgical resection [6].

24.15 Perioperative Antibiotic Prophylaxis

The prevention of peri procedure infection is very important especially if procedure is done outside operating room. There is always a risk contamination of the surgical field. Periprocedural IV antibiotic prophylaxis is recommended for liver tumour ablation as chances of infection are high in comparison to other RFAs. The Society of Interventional Radiology in 2018 recommended routine prophylaxis for liver tumour ablation in guidelines on antibiotic prophylaxis during vascular and interventional radiology procedures. In low-risk patients, the guidelines recommend the administration of IV cefazolin 1–2 g. In patients at high risk for postoperative infection as, patients with cirrhosis, diabetes and history of biliary-enteric anastomosis, various regimens are proposed: levofloxacin combined with metronidazole, neomycin and erythromycin, ampicillin/sulbactam and vancomycin or clindamycin with gentamicin. There is no such recommendation of routine antibiotic prophylaxis for patients posted for renal, lung, adrenal or bone tumour RFA.

Adequate level of asepsis and antiseptic handling of equipment along with sterile dressing of the surgical field are recommended to further minimise risk of infection.

To conclude, there is no ideal technique of anaesthesia for liver RFA. It depends on multiple factors including type, site of lesion, patient profile, cooperation and expertise of intervention radiologist. Overall aim should be to provide ideal operating conditions for intervention, minimise perioperative complications and enhance recovery with reduced need of postprocedural care.

References

1. Lee JW, Choi MH, Lee YJ, Ali B, Yoo HM, Song KY, Park CH. Radiofrequency ablation for liver metastases in patients with gastric cancer as an alternative to hepatic resection. BMC Cancer. 2017;17:185.
2. Bai YH, Chen G, Xu Y, Cui L, Li XH, Wang XQ, Wang MQ, Duan F. General versus local anesthesia for percutaneous radiofrequency ablation of hepatocellular carcinoma at unusual regions. J Cancer Res Ther. 2020;16:1686–90.
3. Giustiniano E, Nisi F, Rocchi L, Zito PC, Ruggieri N, Cimino MM, Torzilli G, Cecconi M. Perioperative management of complex hepatectomy for colorectal liver metastases: the alliance between the surgeon and the anesthetist. Cancers (Basel). 2021;13:2203.
4. Piccioni F, Poli A, Templeton LC, Templeton TW, Rispoli M, Vetrugno L, Santonastaso D, Valenza F. Anesthesia for percutaneous radiofrequency tumor ablation (PRFA): a review of current practice and techniques. Local Reg Anesth. 2019;12:127–37.
5. Shamim F, Asghar A, Tauheed S, Yahya M. Radiofrequency ablation of hepatocellular carcinomas: a new spectrum of anesthetic experience at a tertiary care hospital in Pakistan. Saudi J Anaesth. 2017;11:21–5.
6. Wong J, Lee KF, Lee PS, et al. Radiofrequency ablation for 110 malignant liver tumours: preliminary results on percutaneous and surgical approaches. Asian J Surg. 2009;32:13–20.

Tumour Lysis Syndrome

25

Shagun Bhatia Shah and Rajiv Chawla

25.1 Case History

A 62-year-old 54 kg male diagnosed as B-cell non-Hodgkin's lymphoma was administered a chemotherapy regimen (R-CHOP) comprising cyclophosphamide, doxorubicin, vincristine, prednisone and rituximab (monoclonal antibody). He presented to the emergency department 72 h after initiation of chemotherapy with complaints of sudden onset nausea, vomiting, flank pain, dark-coloured urine, generalised seizures and circumoral numbness. On examination his vitals were BP 90/64 mmHg, HR 107/min. General physical examination revealed bilaterally palpable cervical and supraclavicular lymph nodes. When the tourniquet of the BP cuff was inflated, he developed carpal spasm in the right hand. Investigations revealed haemoglobin, 8.2 g%; blood urea, 84 g%; serum creatinine, 1.5 mg%; serum potassium, 6.6 meq/L; serum calcium, 6.9 mg%; serum phosphate, 6.1 mg%; and uric acid, 8.2 mg%. ECG showed tall, peaked T-waves, broad QRS complex and prolonged QT interval. Positron emission tomography (FDG-18 PET-CT) for staging revealed multiple supradiaphragmatic and infradiaphragmatic lymph nodes with conglomerated mass appearance.

S. B. Shah · R. Chawla (✉)
Department of Anesthesiology, Rajiv Gandhi Cancer Hospital, New Delhi, India

Q1

What Is the Clinical Diagnosis Based Upon the Signs and Symptoms Presented Above?

The provisional clinical diagnosis is tumour lysis syndrome (TLS), which is an oncologic emergency.

Q2

Define TLS and Describe in Detail the Etiopathogenesis of TLS.

Chemotherapy-induced or spontaneous cancer cell lysis/death releases the intracellular material into the bloodstream precipitating a constellation of haematological, metabolic and electrolyte derangements, collectively called TLS (Fig. 25.1).

Since the intracellular cation with highest concentration is potassium, and the predominant intracellular anion is phosphate, tumour cell lysis produces hyperkalaemia (6–72 h after chemotherapy initiation) and hyperphosphataemia (24–48 h) [1–6]. Hypocalcaemia occurs secondary to hyperphosphataemia (calcium phosphorus multiple exceeding 70 leading to precipitation of calcium phosphate crystals in the renal tubules and extra-renal tissue) [1, 2, 4, 7]. Hyperphosphataemia mops up the ionised serum calcium. To distinguish true hypocalcaemia from pseudohypocalcaemia in presence of

N. Gupta et al. (eds.), *Problem Based Learning Discussions in Onco-Anesthesia and Onco-Critical Care*, https://doi.org/10.1007/978-981-99-6339-3_25

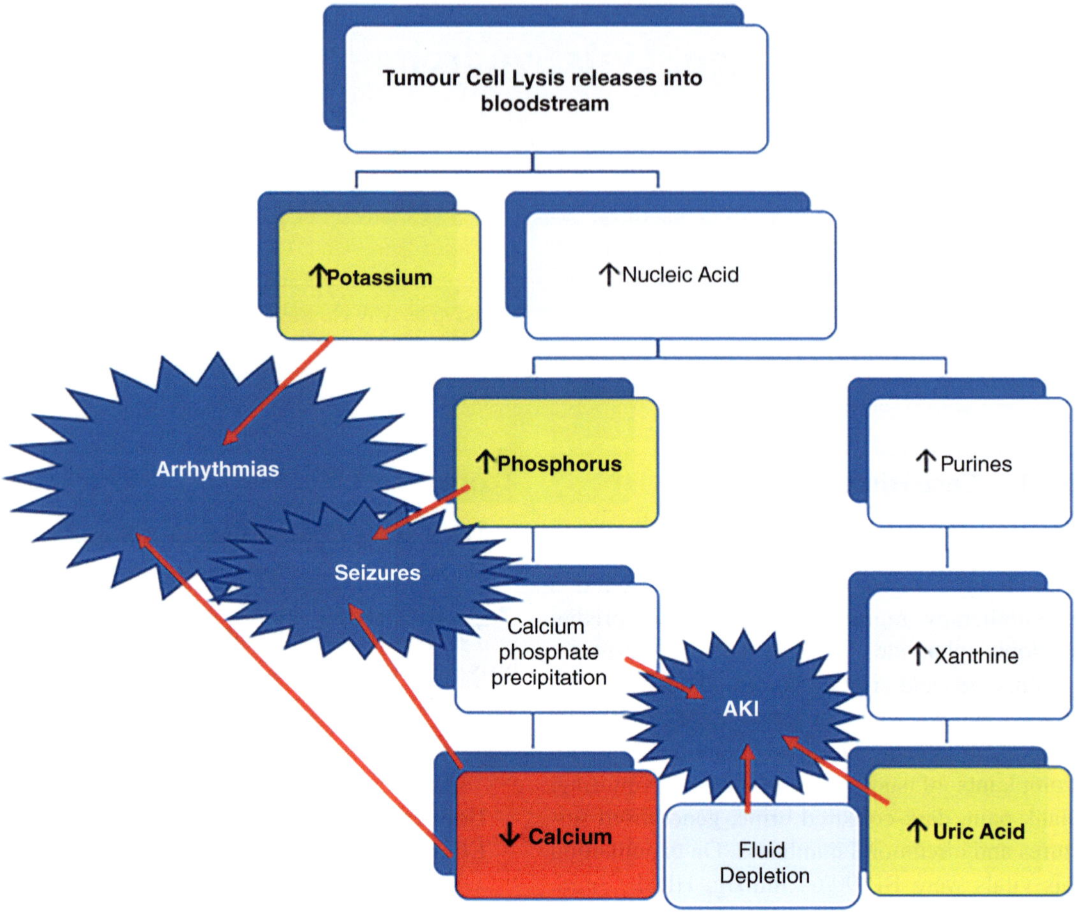

Fig. 25.1 Etiopathogenesis of tumour lysis syndrome

hypoalbuminaemia, an ionised calcium level is ordered. Tumour cell lysis releases nucleic acids that are degraded to purines (adenine and guanine), whose further breakdown produces hyperuricaemia (48–72 h later). This produces uric acid crystal deposition within the renal tubules causing uraemia [2, 3]. Uraemia may be produced by additional mechanisms during TLS (calcium phosphate/xanthine precipitation, renal parenchymal infiltration by tumour cells, tumour-related obstructive uropathy, acute onset sepsis, nephrotoxic drugs) which should also be investigated when a patient with haematologic malignancy on chemotherapy develops uraemia [7].

As laboratory tests become progressively abnormal, the threshold for clinical symptoms is breached, potentially resulting in multi-organ dysfunction and death.

A high tumour burden/load calculated by number and diameter of metastasis, presence of rapidly dividing cells and mitotic figures (acute leukaemia or high-grade lymphoma) and paradoxically highly chemosensitive tumours display maximum risk of TLS development. Although TLS can occur spontaneously [2] (before cancer treatment), it more commonly presents 3–7 days after initiation of chemotherapy. In addition to traditional chemotherapy patients, TLS may be observed in association with steroid [3], hormonal [2] and targeted therapy, after radiotherapy [2, 3] and in conjunction with invasive techniques (tumour biopsy, embolisation of feeding vessels, surgical treatment) [5].

Q3

What Is the Incidence of TLS in NHL Patients?

Bedrna and Polcák are credited with the earliest description of TLS in 1929 [5]. Hande et al. retrospectively studied 102 patients with high-grade non-Hodgkin's lymphoma (NHL) and reported a 42% incidence of laboratory TLS versus a mere 6% incidence of clinical TLS [6]. Incidence of clinical TLS varies between 3 and 27% in patients with haematological malignancy [5].

Q4

What Is the Risk Stratification of Tumour Lysis Syndrome?

Risk prediction for development of TLS entails a thorough knowledge of the type and growth rate of cancer, the nature of chemotherapy and the degree of responsiveness to treatment being administered. The known TLS-associated risk factors can be clubbed into three distinct categories [1, 3] (Table 25.1, Fig. 25.2):

(a) Patient specific
(b) Treatment specific
(c) Malignancy specific

The development of TLS is not limited to the systemic route of chemotherapeutic drug administration. Intrathecal administration and chemo-embolisation are also implicated.

Malignancies can be categorised as having high/moderate/low risk for TLS. Solid-organ tumours traditionally exhibit a comparatively lower risk for TLS versus haematological malignancy, but with advent of novel cancer-treatment modalities, there is expanding literature with case reports citing TLS in solid tumours (testicular cancer, breast cancer and pulmonary microcytoma) [7]. In addition to the type of malignancy, size of the tumour/burden of cancer cells, rate of proliferation of tumour cells and their chemosensitivity are other factors that are directly proportional to the risk of TLS development.

Table 25.1 Risk stratification of tumour lysis syndrome into patient, treatment and malignancy specific categories [1, 3]

Patient specific	Treatment specific	Malignancy specific
Male gender	Cytotoxic drugs • Paclitaxel • Fludarabine • Etoposide • Thalidomide • Bortezomib • Hydroxyurea • Carfilzomib	High risk • Non-Hodgkin's lymphoma • Burkitt lymphoma • Lymphoblastic lymphoma • B-cell acute lymphoblastic leukaemia (ALL) • ALL with white blood cell count (WBC) >100,000/μL • Acute myelogenous leukaemia (AML) + WBC count >50,000/μL, monoblastic cell type
Increased age	Immunotherapy • Sorafenib	
Pre-existing ↑uric acid	Radiation therapy	Intermediate risk • Diffuse large B-cell lymphoma • ALL with WBC 50,000–100,000/μL • AML with WBC 10,000–50,000/μL • Chronic lymphocytic lymphoma (CLL) with WBC 10,000–100,000 after treatment with fludarabine • Haematological malignancy with rapid proliferation after initiation of therapy
	Biphosphonate (zoledronic acid)	
Acidic urine	Corticosteroids	
↓ Urine output	Hormonal agents	
Dehydration	Biologic response modifiers • Abatacept • Adalimumab • Etanercept • Tocilizumab	
Pretreatment AKI CKD	Monoclonal antibodies First-generation anti-CD20 monoclonal antibody rituximab has a lower risk than Obinutuzumab (4.6%)	Low risk • Indolent non-Hodgkin's lymphoma • ALL with WBC <50,000/μL • AML with WBC <10,000/μL • CLL with WBC <10,000/μL

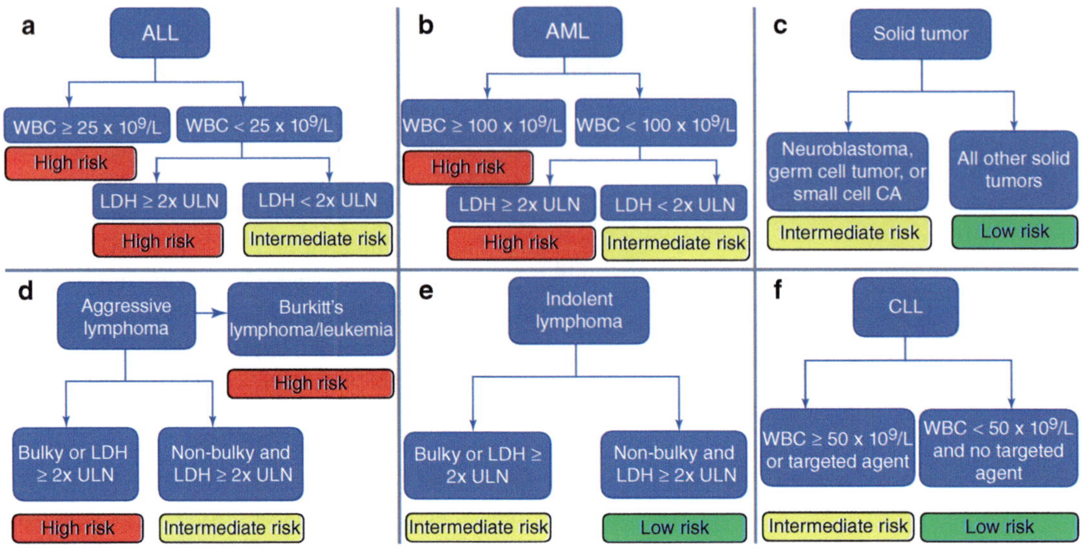

Fig. 25.2 Risk stratification of TLS corresponding with Acute Lymphoblastic Leukemia (ALL), Acute Myelogenous Leukemia (AML), Solid Tumors, Agressive Lymphomas, Indolent Lymphomas, and Chronic Lymphocytic Leukemia (CLL)

It was postulated that surgical debulking of the tumour/cytoreductive surgery prior to chemotherapy administration may reduce the probability of developing TLS. Current literature suggests that surgical debulking is an ineffective approach, owing to deferring of return to intended oncotherapy (induction chemotherapy), risk of complications (TLS during surgery) and prompt reappearance of resected tumour [2].

Q5

Describe the Cairo and Bishop Criteria for Diagnosis of TLS? What Are the Limitations of These Criteria?

Cairo-Bishop criteria [8, 9] for laboratory TLS entail presence of ≥2 of the criteria listed below in the time period ranging from 3 days pre-chemotherapy until 7 days post-chemotherapy.

- Uric acid: ≥8 mg/dL (alternatively 25% rise from baseline values)
- Potassium: ≥6 mEq/L (alternatively 25% rise from baseline values)
- Phosphorous: ≥6.5 mg/dL (paediatric patients) or ≥4.5 mg/dL in adults (alternatively 25% rise from baseline values)
- Calcium: ≤7 mg/dL (alternatively 25% fall in baseline values)

Clinical TLS appears when laboratory TLS is accompanied by at least one criterion listed below:

- Serum creatinine >1.5 times the upper border of reference range for that age group
- Sudden cardiac death/arrhythmias
- Convulsions

Howard et al. [10] proposed some modifications to cater to the limitations of Cairo-Bishop criteria:

1. Concomitant presence of ≥2 metabolic derangements.
2. The 25% rise/fall clause should be removed.
3. The definition of clinical TLS should be expanded to cover symptomatic hypocalcaemia.

Wilson and Berns proposed further modifications:

1. Chemotherapy as a prerequisite should be removed to accommodate patients with spontaneously occurring TLS.

Table 25.2 Cairo-Bishop grading classification of TLS

	Grade 0[a]	Grade I	Grade II	Grade III	Grade IV	Grade V
LTLS	–	+	+	+	+	+
Creatinine[b,c]	≤1.5 × ULN	1.5 × ULN	>1.5–3.0 × ULN	>3.0–6.0 × ULN	>6.0 ULN	Death[d]
Cardiac arrhythmia[c]	None	Intervention not indicated	Non-urgent medical intervention indicated	Symptomatic + incompletely controlled medically or controlled with device (defibrillator)	Life-threatening (arrhythmia CHF, hypotension, syncope, shock)	Death[d]
Seizure[c]	None	–	One brief generalised seizure; seizure(s) well-controlled by anti-convulsants; infrequent focal motor seizures not interfering with ADL	Altered consciousness during seizure poorly controlled with breakthrough generalized seizures despite medical intervention	Seizure of any kind which are prolonged, repetitive or difficult to control (status epilepticus, intractable epilepsy)	Death[d]

[a]No laboratory tumour lysis syndrome (LTLS)
[b]Creatinine levels: patients will be considered to have elevated creatinine if their serum creatinine is 1.5 times greater than the institutional upper limit of normal (ULN) below age-/gender-defined ULN. If not specified by an institution, age/sex ULN creatinine may be defined as 1–12 years (all genders), 61.6 μmol/L; 12–16 years (all genders), 88 μmol/L; ≥16 years, female, 105.6 μmol/L; ≥16 years, male 114.4 μmol/L
[c]Not directly or probably attributable to a therapeutic agent (e.g. rise in creatinine after amphotericin administration)
[d]Attributive probably or definitely to CTLS

2. To accommodate CKD patients, the requirement of creatinine >1.5 times upper limit for clinical TLS should be replaced by absolute creatinine increase of 0.3 mg% or 50% increase in creatinine levels above baseline.

The most severe manifestation of TLS (renal, cardiac, neuro) delineates the grade of clinical TLS as per the Cairo-Bishop grading classification (Table 25.2) [9, 10].

Q6

What Is the Clinical Presentation of TLS?

Although TLS may develop spontaneously, the signs and symptoms of TLS typically develop 3–7 days post chemotherapy initiation. The focus of history-taking and physical examination of TLS patients should be elicitation of the primary causes of tumour lysis. Constitutional symptoms like anorexia and weight loss herald the onset of malignancy in time. Dyspnoea, orthopnoea or tachypnoea may signify primary tumour-induced airway compression.

25.2 Physical Examination

Focal point of the physical examination should be the associated tetrad of electrolyte dysfunction.

(a) Hyperkalaemia

Primary hyperkalaemia may result in muscle cramps or weakness, paresthesia, fatigue, nausea, vomiting, diarrhoea, cardiac arrhythmias (tachycardia or ventricular fibrillation), electrocardiographic changes (wide flat P-wave, broad QRS complex, tall-peaked T-waves in Gothic fashion), syncope and sudden death [5, 7, 11, 12].

(b) Hyperphosphataemia

Primary hyperphosphataemia may result in malaise, nausea, vomiting, diarrhoea and convulsions [5].

(c) Hypocalcaemia

Secondary hypocalcaemia can result in neuromuscular irritability, tetany, carpopedal spasm, Chvostek sign, Trousseau's sign, lengthening of ST segment and prolonged QT interval on ECG, cardiac arrhythmias, seizures and bronchospasm (wheezing) [4, 5].

(d) Hyperuricaemia

Primary hyperuricaemia may result in acute kidney injury, oliguria/anuria, lethargy, dysuria, flank pain and haematuria [1, 13, 14].

(e) Uraemia [7]

Hyperuricaemia and obstructive uropathy can lead to manifestations of uraemia including malaise, asthenia, nausea, vomiting, dysgeusia, agitation, pruritus, crackles (uremic heart failure), muffled heart sounds (uremic pericarditis), joint ache, kidney calculi and renal colic, dermal deposition of calcium phosphate crystals and even gangrene.

Other clinical manifestations of TLS include syncopal attack, palpitations, dependent pedal pitting oedema, periorbital oedema and ascites (fluid overload).

Q7

When Would a Patient with TLS Require ICU Admission?

Severe TLS may manifest as life-threatening cardiac arrhythmias, acute renal failure, lethargy requiring intervention for airway protection (endotracheal intubation), seizures and multiple organ dysfunction syndrome. Any of the above critical presentations requires ICU admission.

Q8

What Haematological Investigations Would You Order for a Laboratory Diagnosis of TLS?

Serum potassium, calcium, uric acid, phosphate and creatinine levels are essential. Laboratory diagnosis of TLS requires ≥ 2 of the criteria listed below, observed in the same 24-h interval.

1. Hyperuricaemia (uric acid >8.0 mg/dL or 25% rise above baseline levels)
2. Hyperkalaemia (potassium >6.0 mmol/L or 25% rise above baseline levels)
3. Hyperphosphataemia (phosphorus >4.5 mg/dL in adults, >6.5 mg/dL in children or 25% rise above baseline levels)
4. Hypocalcaemia (corrected serum calcium <7.0 mg/dL or ionised calcium <1.12 mmol/L or 25% fall below baseline)

Corrected calcium = serum calcium + [0.8 × (normal albumin − serum albumin)].

Acute kidney injury is defined as elevated serum creatinine (increased by ≥ 0.3 mg/dL) or oliguria (urine output <0.5 mL/kg/h).

Q9

Describe the Importance of Imaging Modalities in TLS Patients.

Chest radiograph and computed tomography (CT) scan for diagnosis and further assessment of a mediastinal mass or an associated pleural effusion. Abdominal and retroperitoneal CT-scan and ultrasound to evaluate mass lesions located in the abdomen/retroperitoneum. Cautious use of intravenous (IV) contrast is warranted in view of any associated AKI. Fluorodeoxyglucose positron emission tomography (PET)/CT has emerged as the latest benchmark imaging technique for staging fluorodeoxyglucose-avid histology since it evaluates organ involvement (liver, spleen) in addition to lymph node involvement.

Q10

Describe the Clinical Management of a TLS Patient.

The primary aim in patients with an intact renal function is to flush out tumour lysis products like uric acid by aggressive intravenous fluid therapy to prevent acute kidney injury and also correct the electrolyte imbalance.

25.3 Renoprotective Measures

25.3.1 Rapid Expansion of Intravascular Volume

TLS management commences with rapid volume expansion with crystalloids (NS, RL, avoid high potassium solutions) to increase the glomerular filtration rate (GFR) and hasten excretion of solutes liberated by tumour lysis. Intravenous fluid therapy should commence 48 h prior to chemotherapy initiation continued until 48 h post chemotherapy. Hydration with 3 L/m^2/day or 200 mL/kg/day if ≤10 kg (4–5 L/day) is considered adequate to maintain a urine output of ≥100 mL/m^2/h or 3 mL/kg/h if ≤10 kg (3 L/day) [13–17].

25.3.2 Diuresis

Diuretics (mannitol (0.5 mg/kg) and furosemide (0.5–1.0 mg/kg) are administered if urine output is inadequate despite the absence of acute obstructive uropathy and/or hypovolaemia. Severe oliguria/anuria may necessitate furosemide (2–4 mg/kg) bolus to increase urinary output and maintain a urinary specific gravity of ≤1.010. Hydration fluids should initially be free of potassium, calcium and phosphate so as to avert hyperkalaemia, hyperphosphataemia and calcium phosphate crystal deposition. Avoid thiazides that interact with allopurinol or elevate uric acid levels (hydrochlorothiazide) by inhibiting renal reabsorption [1, 13–15].

25.4 Correction of Electrolyte Imbalance

25.4.1 Hypocalcaemia

Intravenous calcium gluconate, 1 g, repeated if required, should be administered for symptomatic hypocalcaemia (seizures, tetany, cardiac dysrhythmias). Acute iatrogenic obstructive uropathy may be triggered by treating asymptomatic hypocalcaemia, owing to precipitation of additional calcium as calcium phosphate crystals resulting in exacerbation of AKI (nephrocalcinosis is promoted by calcium phosphate product >60 mg^2/dL^2) requiring haemodialysis. Therefore, hyperphosphataemia correction is prioritised over asymptomatic hypocalcaemia rectification [11].

25.4.2 Hyperkalaemia

Correction of hyperkalaemia secondary to TLS should assume precedence. Calcium gluconate, β-adrenergic agonists and glucose in insulin infusions are indicated whenever serum potassium levels surpass 6 meq/L [1, 7].

25.4.3 Hyperphosphataemia

Treat hyperphosphataemia >4.5 mg/dL or 25% rise above baseline as follows [7, 15–17]:

- IV furosemide 20–40 mg
- Phosphate binders such as aluminium hydroxide 50–150 mg/kg/day in four divided doses.
- Renal replacement therapy may be indicated for severe/symptomatic hyperphosphataemia.

25.4.4 Hyperuricaemia

25.4.4.1 Allopurinol

First-line treatment of hyperuricaemia comprises allopurinol initiated 2–3 days prior to chemotherapy and continued for 10–14 days [11]. Being a structural isomer of hypoxanthine, allopurinol acts like a competitive inhibitor of xanthine oxidase, hampering the conversion of xanthine to uric acid, thereby preventing hyperuricaemia in TLS. Allopurinol is ineffective once hyperuricaemia is already established [11, 12].

Xanthine oxidase enzymatically promotes conversion of allopurinol to oxypurinol (active metabolite), whose renal excretion is impaired in CKD or AKI. Elevated serum and urinary xanthine levels accompany allopurinol administration. Owing to poor solubility, xanthine may form crystals in the kidney tubules worsening any TLS-associated obstructive uropathy.

Vigilance for 'allopurinol hypersensitivity syndrome' (skin rash, eosinophilia, acute hepatitis), an adverse effect and potential drug-interaction with azathioprine (immunosuppressant used in solid-organ transplant and autoimmune disorder patients) is required. Dose: oral 600–800 mg/day in 2–3 divided doses and IV 200–400 mg/m^2/day in 1–4 divided doses.

25.4.4.2 Recombinant Urate Oxidase (Rasburicase) [5, 18–20]

Rasburicase is obtained from *Aspergillus* using recombinant technology and causes catalytic breakdown of uric acid producing allantoin, carbon dioxide and hydrogen peroxide. Hydrogen peroxide, a powerful oxidiser, may trigger severe methemoglobinemia or haemolytic anaemia in glucose-6-phosphate dehydrogenase (G6PD)-deficient individuals.

Approved by FDA in 2009, rasburicase has become the drug of choice for treating hyperuricaemia in leukaemia, lymphoma and solid tumour patients on chemotherapy intramuscularly or intravenously in dose range of 50–100 U/kg/day (IV 0.2 mg/kg once, infused over 30 min). Humans lack urate oxidase that catalyses metabolism of uric acid to the more soluble allantoin, for renal excretion. Compared with allopurinol, rasburicase has better efficacy in serum uric acid reduction in TLS and is better tolerated by TLS patients, and dose adjustment for alterations in serum creatinine is not necessary.

Four important caveats regarding rasburicase use are as follows: administration in catalase and G6PD deficient patients may cause life-threatening rasburicase-induced methemoglobinemia, concurrent alkalinisation of urine is avoided owing to correlation with acute renal failure, an antibody response to rasburicase may reduce effectiveness of subsequent doses and lastly since rasburicase remains active ex vivo, any blood samples drawn must promptly be laid on ice during transfer for laboratory evaluation of UA levels for monitoring [3].

25.4.4.3 Febuxostat

Unlike allopurinol, febuxostat (a newer xanthine oxidase inhibitor) does not cause the hypersensitivity reactions but is more expensive. As reported by the Febuxostat for Tumour Lysis Syndrome Prevention in Hematologic Malignancies (FLORENCE) clinical trial, febuxostat is more efficacious in regulating hyperuricaemia in TLS, with fewer safety concerns and conservation of kidney function [3, 21].

25.4.4.4 Sodium Bicarbonate (Alkalisation of Urine) [1, 14–18]

Although alkalinisation of urine (pH ≥6.5) promotes renal urate elimination, the existing concept of using sodium bicarbonate for alkalinisation of urine is contentious. A urinary pH of 7.5 is essential for solubility of urate while at urine pH ≥6.5 the solubility of xanthine and hypoxanthine is reduced substantially, leading to deposition of renal tubular xanthine crystals throughout and following allopurinol treatment. Metabolic alkalosis and xanthine-induced obstructive nephropathy may stem from overenthusiastic blood and urinary alkalinisation. Normal urinary pH is acidic (pH 5). Alkalinisation of urine by adding 40–50 mEq/L of sodium bicarbonate to the hydrating intravenous fluid produces a tenfold rise in urinary uric acid solubility. The flipside is reduced ionised calcium levels because of reduced bonding of calcium to albumin, worsening the TLS-associated hypocalcaemia precipitating arrhythmia or tetany. Alkalinisation of urine also favours the deposition of calcium and phosphate salts in the renal tubules worsening any TLS-associated AKI. Hence the importance of monitoring serial serum calcium levels cannot be overemphasised, and alkalinisation of urine is only advisable in event of non-availability of rasburicase is not readily available. Three ampoules of 7.5% sodium bicarbonate (135 mEq total) are added to 1 L of D5W and infused at twice the maintenance rate titrated to a urinary pH of 7.1–7.5.

25.4.4.5 Haemodialysis

In life-threatening or refractory hyperkalaemia, hyperphosphataemia or hyperuricaemia accompanying TLS-associated AKI, early haemodialysis is an attractive option and probably the best treatment modality. Continuous renal replacement therapy with a high dialysate/replacement fluid flow rate is the soundest technique for solute removal, in face of a continuous release of intracellular ions. If intermittent haemodialysis is utilized for extracorporeal clearance, rebound hyperkalaemia/hyperphosphataemia might develop [7, 11].

Q11

Sudden Deterioration Is Occasionally Seen in Patients with TLS Despite Above Measures. What Is the Emergency Management Approach in Such Cases?

Worsening electrolyte imbalance is the commonest reason behind decompensation in TLS patients. Interventions should target both the symptoms (cardiac arrhythmia, seizure) and the underlying root cause (electrolyte abnormality).

Immediately obtain a 12-lead ECG to rule out a life-threatening arrhythmia.

Cardiac arrhythmias may result from either hypocalcaemia or hyperkalaemia.

- **Hypocalcaemia:**
  - Calcium gluconate 1–3 ampoules (1 g [4.5 mEq] per 10-mL ampoule); 100–200 mg/kg for paediatric patients
  - Calcium chloride 1 ampoule (1 g [13.5 mEq] per 10-mL amp) through central line

Calcium supplementation in TLS may cause precipitation of calcium phosphate but can also antagonize the cardiac arrhythmias of hyperkalaemia.

- **Hyperkalaemia** [3, 11]
  - Calcium gluconate
  - Salbutamol/albuterol 10–20 mg nebulized
  - Insulin 10 units IV bolus with 1–2 ampules of D50W IV; insulin 0.1 units/kg IV with 2 mL/kg of D25W IV in pediatric patients
  - Sodium polystyrene sulfonate (Kayexalate) 30 g PO or PR; 0.5–1 g/kg per dose in paediatric patients
- **Acute Kidney Injury:**

Dialysis is indicated in following situations [7]:

- Fluid overload and pulmonary oedema refractory to intravenous medication
- Unrelenting hyperkalaemia despite medical therapy
- Metabolic acidosis despite medical therapy
- Blood urea nitrogen (BUN) >100 mg/dL
- Rapidly rising BUN
- Symptomatic uraemia or electrolyte imbalance

- **Seizures:**

Severe hypocalcaemia or hyperphosphataemia may culminate in seizures managed with the following:

- IV lorazepam 2–4 mg
- IV diazepam 5–10 mg

No particular vasopressor is preferred over the others.

Q12

What Is the Role of a Multidisciplinary Team in Management of TLS?

Multidisciplinary approach involving the services of an oncologist, nephrologist, internist, intensivist and ICU nurses is required for TLS management. TLS entails coordination with the medical oncologist, frequent laboratory investigations and intensive nursing care, often necessitating an ICU admission.

Q13

What Is the Prognosis of a Patient Who Develops TLS?

Although clinical TLS is rare, it produces a deadly metabolic crisis (mortality of 29–79%) [15]. With early and aggressive therapy, the mortality rate in TLS can be greatly improved.

Q14

Is TLS Preventable? Elaborate Upon the Preventive Measures Available.

Serum electrolyte balance is maintained by urinary excretion. Hence, adequate renal function is paramount for recovery from TLS. Prophylactic and initial therapeutic measures focus on renoprotection and enhancing flow rate through the renal tubules to boost renal excretion of excess potassium, phosphate and urate.

Patients receiving chemotherapy should be well hydrated since IV fluids aid renal flushing out of toxins in the urine. High urine flow rates inhibit uric acid crystal deposition in renal tubules. Close monitoring of urine output is essential to assess optimal fluid balance and for any signs of oliguric renal failure. Laboratory monitoring of serum potassium, calcium, phosphorus and uric acid levels during chemotherapy is recommended. Uric acid-lowering medication (allopurinol and rasburicase) may be prescribed prophylactically for laboratory-diagnosed hyperuricaemia.

Q15

What Is the Differential Diagnosis of TLS?

Clinical conditions that may produce hyperkalaemia, hyperphosphatemia, hyperuricaemia and hypocalcaemia need to be distinguished from TLS (Table 25.3).

Q16

What Are the Implications of TLS in a Pregnant Lady with NHL?

The fourth most common malignancy diagnosed during pregnancy (1:6000 deliveries) is lymphoma [22]. Two major contributary factors for the rising incidence are current trend to postpone pregnancy to later years and the high incidence of AIDS-related non-Hodgkin's lymphoma

Table 25.3 Differential diagnosis of tumour lysis syndrome

Hyperkalaemia	Hyperphosphatemia	Hyperuricaemia	Hypocalcaemia
Hypocalcaemia	Waldenstrom macroglobulinaemia	Hyperparathyroidism	Hypoalbuminaemia • Cirrhosis • Nephrosis • Malnutrition • Burns • Sepsis
Metabolic acidosis	Monoclonal gammopathy	Hypothyroidism	Hypoparathyroidism
Congenital adrenal hyperplasia	Multiple myeloma	Nephrolithiasis	Hypomagnesemia
Digitalis toxicity	Pseudohypoparathyroidism	Ketoacidosis (diabetic, alcoholic)	Pseudohypoparathyroidism
Acute tubular necrosis	Rhabdomyolysis	Uric acid nephropathy	Kidney dysfunction
Electrical burn	Hypervitaminosis D	Gout/pseudogout	Vitamin D deficiency
Head trauma	Oral saline laxative (phospho-soda) abuse	Type 1 a glycogen storage disease	Calcium deficiency
Rhabdomyolysis	Pseudohyperphosphatemia	Haemolytic anaemia	Pancreatitis
Thermal burns		Hodgkin's lymphoma	

(NHL) in developing countries [22]. Acute spontaneous TLS in a pregnant woman with non-Hodgkin's lymphoma has been reported [23]. A 27-week pregnant lady developed epistaxis, malaise, vomiting and dehydration and had developed TLS secondary to undiagnosed NHL. Although she delivered a healthy baby at 28 weeks, unfortunately he expired after a few days. The ethical dilemma encountered is that although chemotherapy can induce remission, potential foetotoxicity is a major concern.

If the mother is diagnosed with high-grade NHL (Burkitt or lymphoblastic lymphoma) during the first trimester of pregnancy, urgent chemotherapy administration is essential, to avoid potential maternal fatality. Medical termination of pregnancy is advisable to avoid chemotherapy-induced major foetal congenital malformations and spontaneous abortion. For mothers diagnosed with NHL during the second/third trimester of pregnancy, literature review revealed that chemotherapy may be instituted minus teratogenicity and with minimal foetotoxicity. IUGR and microalbuminuria may occur. Alkylating agents should be avoided. In the third trimester, it is preferable to withhold CT till after delivery. Cancer chemotherapy is incompatible with breast feeding [22].

Q17

What Are the Different Types of NHL?

The World Health Organization (WHO) classification is the most frequently used classification for NHL (Table 25.4) [24].

First introduced in 2001, as an elaboration upon the REAL approach, the latest update of the WHO classification was in 2016. Based on morphology and cell lineage, it broadly describes two categories/groups of NHL: B-cell origin and T-cell/natural killer (NK)-cell origin. Two subdivisions are recognized in each group: precursor neoplasms (earliest stages of differentiation) and more mature differentiated neoplasms.

The WHO classification subtypes for NHL precursors are listed below:

- Precursor B-lymphoblastic leukaemia/lymphoma
- Precursor T-lymphoblastic lymphoma/leukaemia

Table 25.4 WHO classification subtypes for differentiated NHL

	Peripheral B-cell neoplasms	Peripheral T-cell and NK-cell neoplasms
1	B-cell chronic lymphocytic leukaemia/small lymphocytic lymphoma	T-cell chronic lymphocytic leukaemia/prolymphocytic leukaemia
2	B-cell prolymphocytic leukaemia	T-cell granular lymphocytic leukaemia
3	Lymphoplasmacytic lymphoma/immunocytoma	Mycosis fungoides/Sézary syndrome
4	Mantle cell lymphoma	Peripheral T-cell lymphoma, not otherwise characterised
5	Follicular lymphoma	Hepatosplenic gamma/delta T-cell lymphoma
6	Extranodal marginal zone B-cell lymphoma of mucosa-associated lymphatic tissue (MALT) type	Subcutaneous panniculitis-like T-cell lymphoma
7	Nodal marginal zone B-cell lymphoma (± monocytoid B-cells)	Angioimmunoblastic T-cell lymphoma
8	Splenic marginal zone lymphoma (± villous lymphocytes)	Extranodal T-/NK-cell lymphoma and nasal type
9	Hairy cell leukaemia	Enteropathy-type intestinal T-cell lymphoma
10	Plasmacytoma/plasma cell myeloma	Adult T-cell lymphoma/leukaemia (human T-lymphotropic virus [HTLV] 1+)
11	Diffuse large B-cell lymphoma (DLBCL)	Anaplastic large cell lymphoma, primary systemic type
12	Burkitt lymphoma	Anaplastic large cell lymphoma, primary cutaneous type
13		Aggressive NK-cell leukaemia

Table 25.5 Non-Hodgkin's lymphoma staging

Stage	Area of involvement	Extranodal (E) status
I	Single node or adjacent group of nodes	Single extranodal lesions without nodal involvement
II	Multiple lymph node groups on same side of the diaphragm	Stage I or II by nodal extent with limited contiguous extranodal involvement
II Bulky[a]	Multiple lymph node groups on same side of diaphragm with 'bulky disease'	N/A
III	Multiple lymph node groups on both sides of diaphragm; nodes above the diaphragm with spleen involvement	N/A
IV	Multiple noncontiguous extranodal sites	N/A

Suffixes A and B are not required. X for bulky disease replaced with documenting of largest tumor diameter
[a]Stage II bulky disease is considered limited or advanced; this distinction is made on the basis of histology and a number of prognostic factors

Q18

Describe the Staging of Non-Hodgkin's Lymphoma (NHL)

The Lugano Modification (2014) of the Ann Arbor staging system [25, 26] for NHL was promptly adopted by the National Comprehensive Cancer Network and provides the following revised recommendations (Table 25.5):

- Positron emission tomography-computed tomography (PET-CT) is preferred for fluorodeoxyglucose (FDG)-avid lymphomas; CT is indicated for non-avid lymphomas.
- PET-CT is preferred for pretreatment assessment and routine staging.
- Contrast-enhanced CT is more accurate for lymph node size assessment and for radiation planning.
- PET-CT is the preferred modality for ascertaining splenic involvement (cut-off value being splenomegaly >13 cm).
- In case of PET-CT scans negative for bone/marrow infiltration, a bone marrow biopsy is indicated to identify involvement by discordant histology, with clinical correlation.
- Since hepatic size is not conclusive, liver involvement is suggested by diffusely increased or focal uptake, with or without focal or disseminated nodules.
- Prior Ann Arbor staging categorised patients according to absence (A) or presence (B) of disease-related symptoms (weight loss >10%, fever, drenching night sweats); these are non-essential in NHL staging since they have no prognostic value.

References

1. Belay Y, Yirdaw K, Enawgaw B. Tumor lysis syndrome in patients with hematological malignancies. J Oncol. 2017;1:968–86.
2. Friedman M, Patel PR, Rondelli D. A focused review of the pathogenesis, diagnosis, and management of tumor lysis syndrome for the interventional radiologist. Semin Intervent Radiol. 2015;32(2):231–6.
3. Sury K. Update on the prevention and treatment of tumor lysis syndrome. J Onco-Nephrol. 2019;3(1):19–30.
4. Davidson MB, Thakkar S, Hix JK, Bhandarkar ND, Wong A, Schreiber MJ. Pathophysiology, clinical consequences, and treatment of tumor lysis syndrome. Am J Med. 2004;116:546–54.
5. Alakel N, Middeke JM, Schetelig J, Bornhäuser M. Prevention and treatment of tumor lysis syndrome, and the efficacy and role of rasburicase. Onco Targets Ther. 2017;10:597–605.
6. Hande KR, Garrow GC. Acute tumor lysis syndrome in patients with high-grade non-Hodgkin's lymphoma. Am J Med. 1993;94(2):133–9.
7. Attinà G, Tepedino R, Ruggiero A. Acute tumor lysis syndrome: a metabolic emergency in cancer patients. Biomed Pharmacol J. 2021;14(5):1721.
8. Cairo MS, Bishop M. Tumour lysis syndrome: new therapeutic strategies and classification. Br J Haematol. 2004;127(1):3–11.
9. Cairo MS, Coiffier B, Reiter A, Younes A, TLS Expert Panel. Recommendations for the evaluation of risk and prophylaxis of tumour lysis syndrome (TLS) in adults and children with malignant diseases: an expert TLS panel consensus. Br J Haematol. 2010;149(4):578–86.

10. Howard SC, Jones DP, Pui CH. The tumor lysis syndrome. N Engl J Med. 2011;364(19):1844–54.
11. Puri I, Sharma D, Gunturu KS, Ahmed AA. Diagnosis and management of tumor lysis syndrome. J Community Hosp Intern Med Perspect. 2020;10(3):269–72.
12. Jones GL, Will A, Jackson GH, British Committee for Standards in Haematology. Guidelines for the management of tumour lysis syndrome in adults and children with haematological malignancies on behalf of the British committee for standards in haematology. Br J Haematol. 2015;169(5):661–71.
13. Abu-Alfa AK, Younes A. Tumor lysis syndrome and acute kidney injury: evaluation, prevention, and management. Am J Kidney Dis. 2010;55(5):1–19.
14. Ostermann M, Liu K, Kashani K. Fluid management in acute kidney injury. Chest. 2019;156(3):594–603.
15. Klemencic S, Perkins J. Diagnosis and management of oncologic emergencies. West J Emerg Med. 2019;20(2):316–22.
16. Darmon M, Vincent F, Camous L. Tumour lysis syndrome and acute kidney injury in high-risk haematology patients in the rasburicase era. A prospective multicentre study from the Groupe de Recherche en Réanimation Respiratoire et Onco-Hématologique. Br J Haematol. 2013;162(4):489–97.
17. Criscuolo M, Fianchi L, Dragonetti G, Pagano L. Tumor lysis syndrome: review of pathogenesis, risk factors and management of a medical emergency. Expert Rev Hematol. 2016;9(2):197–208.
18. Spring J, Munshi L. Oncologic emergencies. Crit Care Clin. 2021;37:85–103.
19. Kassem N, Ghazy AA, Abu-Tineh M, Omar NE, Nashwan AJ, Prem CP. Tumor lysis syndrome in chronic lymphocytic leukemia: conventional treatment versus novel agents. Medicine. 2020;99(51):e23632.
20. Lopez-Olivo MA, Pratt G, Palla SL. Rasburicase in tumor lysis syndrome of the adult: a systematic review and meta-analysis. Am J Kidney Dis. 2013;62(3):481–92.
21. Spina M, Nagy Z, Ribera JM. FLORENCE: a randomized, double-blind, phase III pivotal study of febuxostat versus allopurinol for the prevention of tumor lysis syndrome (TLS) in patients with hematologic malignancies at intermediate to high TLS risk. Ann Oncol. 2015;26(10):2155–61.
22. El-Sonbaty MR, Bitar Z, Abdulrazak A. Acute spontaneous tumor-lysis syndrome in a pregnant woman with non-Hodgkin's lymphoma. Int J Hematol. 2001;73(3):386–9.
23. Pereg D, Koren G, Lishner M. The treatment of Hodgkin's and non-Hodgkin's lymphoma in pregnancy. Haematologica. 2007;92(9):1230–7.
24. Swerdlow SH, Campo E, Pileri SA, Harris NL, Stein H, Siebert R, Advani R, Ghielmini M, Salles GA, Zelenetz AD, Jaffe ES. The 2016 revision of the World Health Organization classification of lymphoid neoplasms. Blood. 2016;127(20):2375–90.
25. Cheson BD, Fisher RI, Barrington SF, Cavalli F, Schwartz LH, Zucca E. Recommendations for initial evaluation, staging, and response assessment of Hodgkin and non-Hodgkin lymphoma: the Lugano classification. J Clin Oncol. 2014;32(27):3059.
26. Munakata W, Terauchi T, Maruyama D, Nagai H. Revised staging system for malignant lymphoma based on the Lugano classification. Jpn J Clin Oncol. 2019;49(10):895–900.

Carcinoma Base of the Tongue with Acute Stridor

26

Swapna Charie, Akhilesh Gupta, and Anshu Gupta

26.1 Case

A 50-year-old male has a mass in base of tongue. The patient had difficulty in swallowing and breathing. The mouth opening was 2 cm and Mallampati was IV. He was posted for resection of mass.

26.2 Cancer of the Base of the Tongue

Q1

What is the surgical anatomy of carcinoma base of the tongue and relevant anaesthesia considerations?

Answer: Tongue is a muscular organ divided into oral tongue and pharyngeal or base of the tongue (BOT).

The genioglossus muscle forms the main bulk of the tongue. Tumors can easily extend towards the anterior floor of the mouth owing to the anatomic characteristic of the muscle. The prognosis and the treatment options depend on the depth of invasion. The management changes if the tumor crosses the midline and/or extends to the posterior into the base of the tongue. Innervated by the hypoglossal nerve, and supplied by the lingual artery, pathway of tumor spread in the tongue can occur into the floor of the mouth mandible and/or base of the tongue via local extension. The lingual septum acts as the barrier for spread of tumor.

Anatomy of the tongue is a crucial factor while considering the options for strategising definitive surgery as well as subsequent airway management. The oral tongue or the two-thirds is treated like lip cancer whereas the posterior one-third of the tongue is treated like oropharyngeal cancer.

Lesions less than 4 cm are called local cancers and >4 cm are referred to as locally advanced cancers. Treatment of the tongue and floor of the mouth is performed by factoring a balance between achieving tumor-free margin and functional rehabilitation as well as aesthetic preservation.

Small T1 lesions are typically treated with glossectomy. However, medial lesions crossing midline require total/near-total glossectomy with a myocutaneous flap to fill the defect. Such lesions may also require a marginal or a segmental mandibular resection or a cervical pull through of the tongue to allow access and achieve tumor-free margin. Reconstruction of the surgical defects depends on their size and the location. For patients with mandibular involvement, reconstruction depends on the location of defect.

S. Charie · A. Gupta (✉) · A. Gupta
Department of Anesthesiology, ABVIMS and RMLH Hospital, New Delhi, India

N. Gupta et al. (eds.), *Problem Based Learning Discussions in Onco-Anesthesia and Onco-Critical Care*, https://doi.org/10.1007/978-981-99-6339-3_26

Segmental mandibular defects require composite-free flaps like fibular flaps whereas larger defects may require radial forearm flaps or anterolateral thigh flaps.

MRI modality for imaging the tongue as it has superior soft tissue characterisation.

26.3 Anaesthesia Considerations

26.3.1 Pre-op Considerations

Q2

What are the pre-operative airway-related concerns?

History of snoring or OSA is important as the presence of either gives a clue of difficult mask ventilation. Patency of the external nares and condition of the nasal turbinates has to be examined to facilitate nasal intubation or for passing of fibrescope.

The difficulty can be both difficult mask ventilation and intubation and laryngoscopy or both. The feasibility of rescue plans in achieving oxygenation should be planned out.

The patient must be primed about the possibility of requirement of awake intubation. The need for tracheostomy and the aspect of not being able to resume verbal communication after the procedure should also be explained about. However, change in voice, dysphagia, hoarseness and orthopnoea should be quickly obtained as they point towards airway compromise. Prior receipt of radiation therapy or co-existence of conditions like submucosal fibrosis should be ruled out.

Q3

What are pre-operative non-airway-related concerns?

Answer: These patients can be candidates with severe cardiorespiratory disease like coronary artery disease, COPD, peripheral arterial disease, cerebrovascular disease and poor nutritional status linked with their smoking and excessive alcohol consumption. The perioperative risks associated with a major surgery and the risk of anaesthesia increase exponentially in patients with increasing age and co-morbidities. These conditions also predispose the patients to develop both major adverse cardiac events and grave post-operative pulmonary complications.

The role of anaesthetists here is not only to optimise the pre-operative status of the patient, but they also form a crucial part of the multidisciplinary team that decides the available treatment options for the cancer weighing the potential benefit obtainable from undergoing the anaesthesia and the surgery and the risks entailed.

Q4

What pre-operative investigations are required?

Answer: Pre-anaesthetic evaluation should include CBC, biochemistry, coagulation profile, renal and liver function tests and electrocardiogram. Further investigations like chest X-ray, arterial blood gas analyses, echocardiography and pulmonary function tests are requested on a case-to-case basis based on the risk factors and the symptomatology.

Chest X-ray may reveal a hyper-inflated chest with flattened diaphragm and emphysematous changes in chronic smokers with COPD.

ABG may reveal a baseline respiratory acidosis with a compensated metabolic alkalosis and the pO_2 value on room air can give a snapshot of the phenotype.

Pink puffers have a $PaCO_2$ which is near normal and a PaO_2 >60 mmHg are more likely to have emphysematous changes in the lung with associated lung destruction and bullae formation. Hence ventilating with lower airway pressures intra-operatively becomes paramount in order to avoid inadvertent rupture of bullae and subsequent pneumothorax.

Blue bloaters on the other hand have a $PaCO_2$ >45 mmHg and PaO_2 <60 mmHg and suffer from subclinical or clinical hypoxia and have pulmonary hypertension secondary to chronic hypoxic pulmonary vasoconstriction. These patients are at increased risk of acute cor pulmonale in the event of intraoperative or post-operative hypoxia.

Flow volume loops from PFT can help to differentiate respiratory distress from airway disease or the upper airway obstruction due to the malignant disease process. Any reversible component of obstruction should be optimised before surgery.

Cardio-pulmonary exercise testing can be done if available and patients with a metabolic equivalent <11–13 mL/kg/min are considered as increased risk for cardiac complications.

Pre-operative malnutrition due to the oral lesion, prior radiotherapy and trismus predisposes these patients to dyselectrolytemia, poor wound healing and development of acute refeeding syndrome. Cases where patients developed acute Wernicke's encephalopathy due to prolonged poor oral intake and concomitant alcohol consumption have also been reported which manifested as immediate post-operative delirium.

Hence pre-operative assessment should also include nutritional screening to identify patients at high risk for these complications like those with BMI <18.5 or with loss of >10% of body weight in the recent period, and these patients have to be subjected to nutritional rehabilitation prior to listing for elective surgery. Rehabilitation can be achieved by oral/oro-gastric/percutaneous gastrostomy feeding.

Patients with ongoing alcohol/consumption and addiction to smoking or tobacco should be carefully identified by history and examination and appropriate measures to facilitate withdrawal has to be instituted at least 72–48 h before surgery to allow optimisation of hydration, nutritional status and electrolytes.

Q5

Describe the intraoperative management of a patient with carcinoma base of the tongue.

Securing IV cannula: A 18G/16 G peripheral cannula with attached multiple ports may be needed in face of blood loss and the possibility of requirement of transfusion of blood products as well as infusion of vasopressors.

Pre-operative discussion with the surgical counterparts on the preferred limb/site for the flap will allow planning for the site for intravenous access.

Regional anaesthesia with ropivacaine or bupivacaine can be performed prior to anaesthesia to facilitate harvest of the graft and thereby minimise intraoperative anaesthesia and surgical time.

Q6

How airway is managed in these patients?

Special attention should be given for airway management. The foremost step in management is to analyse the pre-op imaging along with the surgeon [1]. The rapidly progressive nature of the disease and the tell-tale effects of the treatment received during the medieval period can warrant a revision of an airway plan already made during the pre-anaesthetic checkup.

An algorithm or a strategy than one particular plan is to be adopted as recommended by the NAP4 in the face of difficult intubation or ventilation which may include but not limited to awake fibreoptic intubation, video laryngoscopy and crico-thyroidotomy/jet ventilation [2]. The plan should be chalked out and discussed in detail with the surgical team, patient and the family. In cases involving the posterior one-third of the tongue, the tumour may also extend to the oropharynx or lingual epiglottis virtually making access to visualisation of the cords difficult. In such cases, pre-op CT/MRI can give important information regarding need for elective tracheostomy. The need for elective tracheostomy can also stem from obtaining adequate surgical access to ensure achieving disease-free margins. Hence, the need for post-operative tracheostomy in more radical procedures should also be factored in and the patient and the family need to be counselled about.

Nasal intubation/oral intubation depends on the site and depth of tumour. In lesions of the base of the tongue where tongue protrusion is not possible, and for lesions fixated to the floor of the mouth, awake fibreoptic intubation/video-laryngoscopy intubation is adopted.

In contrast to the recommended difficult airway algorithm where supraglottic airway device remains Plan B after failed direct laryngoscopy, malignant lesions of the tongue preclude placement of SADs and awake fibreoptic intubation with total intravenous anaesthesia and/or combined with airway blocks are the choice of interventions for securing the airway.

Pre-operative planning should answer important questions like the following:

- Is face mask ventilation feasible?
- Is direct laryngoscopy and intubation likely to be difficult?
- Is an awake technique preferable, and if yes, is it feasible from aspects of nature of the growth, bleeding tendency, expertise, equipment availability, patient co-operation and consent.
- Is elective tracheostomy a more safer option?
- Is emergency FONA feasible and is expertise available for consistent execution of the same?

A team of anaesthetists should be deployed for the case on the day of surgery, and they should be able to be anticipate errors and maintain situational awareness and be able to maintain closed communication and execute the primary and rescue plans.

26.3.2 Awake Fibreoptic Technique

The first step is to determine the ability to secure airway after induction of GA or resort to an awake technique. The awake technique has advantages of preserving airway patency, ventilation and aspiration prevention. However, the risk of bleeding and lack of patient co-operation can be the limiting factors.

Fibrescope intubation after induction of GA may cause worsening of airway obstruction [3] and loss of landmarks. Hence with failed awake fibreoptic technique, there may be a need to consider awake elective tracheostomy under airway blocks or local anaesthesia.

Q7

Which mode of induction is preferred in these patients?

26.3.3 Inhalational Induction

Earlier inhalational induction was thought of as a safe technique as patient's spontaneous ventilation is preserved and reversal of anaesthesia is possible in the event of a failed intubation. However, NAP4 guidelines cautiously warn that preferring inhalational induction as the primary plan although offers theoretical advantages and is associated with high rates of failure and the dangerous complication of cork in bottle type of airway obstruction due to instrumentation where the exhalation of anaesthetic gases is severely limited triggering the downward spiral of rapid hypoxia. Hence, the rescue plan should be in place before inhalational induction.

Q8

What are the concerns if direct laryngoscopy is chosen as primary plan?

If direct laryngoscopy is chosen as the primary plan, then the attempt is to be done under optimal positioning, using optimal laryngoscope and alternative blades as backup with adequate neuromuscular blockade. Repeated attempts should be taken by a second intubator with a higher success rate as subsequent attempts may bring in additional caveats of airway oedema, bleeding, trauma to the friable and necrosed tumours.

Q9

What are the intraoperative non-airway-related concerns?

- Majority of the tongue surgeries are carried out in supine position with 15°–30° head-up. This position facilitates venous drainage adequately and helps in decreasing surgical site congestion.

- Temperature monitoring using core temperature probe is essential in prolonged procedures with major blood loss.
- Goal-directed fluid therapy can be accomplished by invasive arterial monitoring for extensive resections where pulse pressure variation PPV and area under the curve of the arterial trace can give us a guide regarding the stroke volume and volume responsiveness. This helps to avoid both flap vascular compromise due to hypo-perfusion or volume loading.
- Placement of central venous catheters is not routinely warranted in minor resections. However, in extensive surgeries, cancer patients with poor venous access, and in the event of major blood loss, the insertion of a femoral central line may be needed for vasopressor and blood product administration.
- Anaesthesia can be maintained with a combination of inhalational and intravenous anaesthesia with opioids. Remifentanil enables rapid blunting of haemodynamic response with surgical stimulation and can avoid mishaps like inadvertent mal-positioning or dislodgement of endo-tracheal tubes/ tracheostomy tubes.
- In patients with chronic hypertension evidence suggests targeting a higher MAP of around 70–75 mmHg and avoid induced hypotension as it can precipitate compromise of the flap vascularity as well. Induced hypotension should be avoided to prevent adverse consequences like type II myocardial infarction or embolic events.

Q10

What are the post-operative concerns in these patients?

Post-operative analgesia is usually accomplished by longer acting opioids like morphine.

Tongue surgeries are notorious to have high incidence of post-operative nausea and vomiting. Hence dexamethasone 0.15 mg/kg can be given as it also helps to decrease airway oedema.

26.3.4 Anaesthesia for a Patient with Acute Stridor

Q11

What is stridor and its types?

Stridor is a harsh, high-pitched noise created by turbulent airflow through a partially obstructed airway. It implies a reduction in airway diameter of at least 50% [4]. In the inspiratory phase, stridor points to obstruction at a supraglottic or glottic level, whereas biphasic inspiratory expiratory stridor implies subglottic compromise [5]. Expiratory stridor or wheeze suggests tracheal or tracheobronchial obstruction.

Obstruction of the airway at its most extreme is an anaesthetic emergency requiring immediate intervention. Two important aspects to be quickly identified are the site of obstruction and the cause of stridor.

Q12

What is the cause of stridor in a case of carcinoma base of the tongue?

In a case of Ca tongue, the obstruction is usually supraglottic. However, the glottic or subglottic extension of the disease and the external compression of the airway due to involvement of neck nodes and consequent radiation therapy to the neck can also be possible. The patient should also be quickly evaluated for the cause of the stridor, namely, proliferative or ulcero-proliferative nature of the growth, bleeding from the tumor, superimposed infection of the lesion or inflammation.

Management of the obstructed airway is particularly challenging and accounted for 40% of all cases (72 out of 184 patients) reported to the fourth UK National audit project of major airway complications (NAP 4) [6].

Q13

What are the specific findings in history and examination of these patients?

26.3.5 History

The patient should be quickly enquired for other pertinent symptoms like change of voice, difficulty in lying down, hoarseness of voice, drooling due to inability swallow secretions and sitting forward to maintain airway patency as these are ominous signs of sudden deterioration.

26.3.5.1 Examination

- The posture adopted by the patient should be noted. They may be dyspnoeic, using accessory muscles of respiration and require supplementary oxygen.
- Assessment of the airway should include mouth opening, dentition, tongue protrusion, Mallampati classification, jaw subluxation and neck movement.
- The neck should also be examined for masses, mobility of the trachea, airway distortion and any potential difficulties for front of neck access (e.g. previous radiotherapy).
- A quick fibreoptic nasal endoscopy can be performed in the theatre depending upon the oxygenation of the patient and the urgency of the situation. It gives a fair idea about the nature of the mass: friable, ulcerative/ulceroproliferative/verrucous, the extent and attachment to surrounding structures and the degree of obstruction.
- A quick ultrasound examination of the neck can give an idea about the degree of airway distortion especially if landmarks are not palpable and also helps in precisely marking the cricothyroid membrane and identifying an overlying vascular structure like innominate artery or big veins in case front of neck access is contemplated.

Q14

Describe the management of acute airway obstruction secondary to carcinoma base of the tongue?

The underlying bottom line of the management algorithm is that recognition and management of acute airway obstruction require a multidisciplinary approach involving the surgical counterparts as well.

A multidisciplinary approach which actively incorporates inputs from the surgical team, senior anaesthetists who have expertise in handling acute airway obstruction and ICU team should be urgently sought.

Management demands answering few important questions prior to devising the plan to secure the airway:

- What is the level, extent and nature of obstruction?
- Is the patient able to lie down flat?
- Is there a possibility of failed mask ventilation?
- Is awake tracheostomy possible or required?
- Feasibility to mobilise ECMO or institute cardiopulmonary bypass in case of a cannot-intubate cannot-oxygenate CICO scenario?

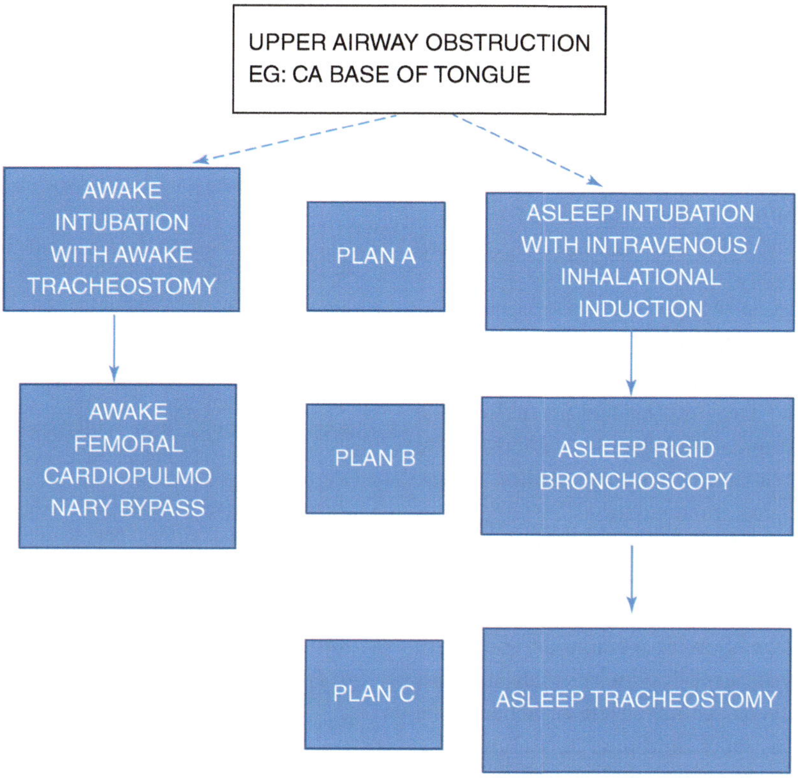

- The theatre personnel should be promptly intimated and prepared with the equipment and the required manpower.
- Careful consideration of the relative risks and the benefits of the proposed airway management strategy and the need for the surgical and anaesthesia team to concur with the proposed strategy is mandatory.
- Clear assignment of the leader with expertise, role assignment, preparation of equipments for primary plan and rescue plan, contingency management, clear communication between team members and most importantly anticipation of possible errors and considering human factors are crucial in the management of an acutely stridorous patient.
- The technique of transnasal humidified rapid-insufflation ventilator exchange (THRIVE) or NO-DESAT where high flow oxygen is delivered via nasal cannula may be considered in isolation or to complement oxygenation prior to intubation. However, one should always remember that achieving oxygenation in an obstructed airway can be tricky and should remain cautious about the false sense of security it offers.
- Techniques like administration of Heliox and administration of intravenous corticosteroids can be considered to decrease the airway oedema.

Q15

What is the role of awake tracheostomy in such patients with acute stridor?

The decision to perform awake tracheostomy depends on available expertise, location and availability of other contingency plans.

The indications are the following:

- Severe stridor.
- Grossly distorted anatomy.
- Inability to visualise glottis with fibrescope inserted nasally.
- The possibility of the surgical intervention decreasing the airway calibre post-operatively.

This procedure has been deemed to be safe and effective in securing the airway in acutely stridor patients. The limiting factors include the demand for technical expertise to tracheostomise in a distorted anatomy and the ability of the patient to tolerate supine position.

Where awake tracheostomy is not deemed necessary, elective narrow-bore needle crico-thyroidotomy may be considered as an option prior to induction allowing a cannula to be left in situ. This may be used for jet ventilation in the event of failure to secure an endotracheal tube and conversion via a Seldinger technique to a wide-bore crico-thyroidotomy if necessary.

In the CICO situation, NAP-4 warns of a significant failure rate with cannula cricothyroidotomy, and the DAS guidelines also recommend a surgical approach when emergency front-of-neck access is required.

References

1. Nikhar SA, Sharma A, Ramdaspally M, Gopinath R. Airway management of patients undergoing oral cancer surgery: a retrospective analysis of 156 patients. Turk J Anaesthesiol Reanim. 2017;45(2):108–11.
2. Frerk C, Mitchell VS, McNarry AF, Mendonca C, Bhagrath R, Patel A, Difficult Airway Society Intubation Guidelines Working Group, et al. Difficult Airway Society 2015 guidelines for management of unanticipated difficult intubation in adults. Br J Anaesth. 2015;115(6):827–48.
3. Wong P, Wong J, Mok MU. Anaesthetic management of acute airway obstruction. Singap Med J. 2016;57(3):110–7.
4. Mason RA, Fielder CP. The obstructed airway in head and neck surgery. Anaesthesia. 1999;54(7):625–8.
5. Zheng G, Feng L, Lewis CM. A data review of airway management in patients with oral cavity or oropharyngeal cancer: a single-institution experience. BMC Anesthesiol. 2019;19:92.
6. Royal College of Anaesthetists. 4th National Audit Project: major complications of airway management in the UK. London: Royal College of Anaesthetists; 2011.

A Case of Carcinoma Colon with Febrile Neutropenia

27

Jitendra Mahajan, Rohini Dattatri, and Nishkarsh Gupta

A 63-year-old male with Sigmoid colon cancer, metastatic to the liver and lungs, was treated for past 3 years with oxaliplatin, irinotecan, bevacizumab and panitumumab (RAS and BRAF wild type). Most recently, he received regorafenib but progressed after 4 months with 80% of tumour burden in the liver. He has ECOG PS 1/2, MSI-high disease, no family history of hereditary non-polyposis colorectal cancer (CRC) and negative germline testing for Lynch syndrome.

1. **Among all cancers, where does colorectal cancer rank in terms of incidence and death?**
   - Second most common cause of cancer-related deaths is CRC, which accounts for 8.4% of all cancer deaths.
   - Lifetime incidence of CRC is about 5%.
2. **What is the median overall survival of CRC?**
   - Overall, one-third of patients diagnosed with colon cancer will die from the disease.
   - Median survival: 48 months.
   - Five-year survival for all CRC patients (all stages and sites) is 61%.

J. Mahajan · R. Dattatri · N. Gupta (✉)
Department of Onco-Anaesthesiology and Palliative Medicine, Dr. BRAIRCH, AIIMS, New Delhi, New Delhi, India

27.1 Aetiology and Risk Factors

1. What is the typical cytopathological pattern of colon cancer development?
   - The majority of colon cancers develop through an orderly sequence of histologic stages beginning with the normal colonic epithelium, which advances to the adenoma, and culminates in the carcinoma driven by the development of progressive genetic mutations. This process evolves over 10 years in patients without inherited genetic defects.
2. What are the major molecular pathways of CRC development, and what molecular alterations do they involve? There are three major pathways described:
   - Chromosomal instability pathway is present in 75–80% of sporadic colon cancers. It contributes to the development of a number of inherited CRCs such as familial adenomatous polyposis (FAP) (adenomatous polyposis coli [APC]). It is characterised by the sequential accumulation of mutations in the APC, KRAS, SMAD and p53 genes, among others.
   - CpG island methylator phenotype (CIMP) pathway is present in 15% of sporadic colon cancer. It involves the methylation and, therefore, the inactivation of the promoter regions of various tumour suppressor genes such as CDKN2A and THBS1.

N. Gupta et al. (eds.), *Problem Based Learning Discussions in Onco-Anesthesia and Onco-Critical Care*, https://doi.org/10.1007/978-981-99-6339-3_27

- Microsatellite instability (MSI) high pathway is inherited mutations in DNA repair enzymes (MLH1, MSH2, MSH6, PMS2 and EPCAM). These genetic defects cause Lynch syndrome, which is commonly referred to as hereditary nonpolyposis colorectal cancer (HNPCC).

1. **What are the major risk factors associated with CRC?**

Factors that impact CRC screening recommendations are the following:

- Personal history of colon cancer or adenomas with size >1 cm and tubulovillous or villous histology and high-grade dysplasia.
- IBD (inflammatory bowel disease), particularly in patients with pancolitis. Risk increases with the degree of extent, duration and inflammatory activity. Proctitis or proctosigmoiditis alone does not increase the risk of CRC.
- First-degree relative(s) with colon cancer or advanced adenoma.
- Hereditary CRC syndromes: HNPCC: About 3% of CRC, autosomal dominant mutation in DNA mismatch repair genes (hMLH1, hMSH2, hMSH6, PMS2). Lynch syndrome is reserved for the classification of families with germline mutation in mismatch repair genes. FAP: About 1% of CRC. Germline mutation in APC gene.

MUTYH-associated polyposis (MAP): This is an autosomal recessive condition that occurs secondary to biallelic germline mutation in a gene involved in base excision repair mutY homolog (MUTYH) and presents with differing clinical presentations. It can be associated with polyposis phenotype, usually <500 adenomas, and has a high incidence of somatic APC mutations. Cowden syndrome, Bannayan–Riley–Ruvalcaba syndrome (PTEN hamartoma syndrome): autosomal dominant inheritance, usually from mutations in the PTEN gene, but also can result from mutations in the SDHB, SDHD or KLLN gene.

- Abdominal and pelvic radiation: higher risk of CRC 10 years after treatment with at least 30 Gy to the abdomen.
- Increased age. Over 90% of CRCs occur after age 50 years.

Factors that do not impact CRC screening recommendations are the following:

- Excessive alcohol use, cigarette smoking, obesity, race, although incidence and mortality are higher in African Americans
- Gender, although CRC is more common in men than women

27.2 Screening

1. Screening for CRC is recommended to begin at what age?
    - For the average-risk patient: Start screening at age 50 years.
    - Family history of CRC or advanced adenoma: Colonoscopy 10 years before the age of earliest occurrence or beginning at age 40 years (whichever comes first), if an affected first-degree relative is <60 years old at diagnosis or if CRC or advanced adenomas are present in more than two first-degree relatives.
2. For patients who develop CRC before age 50, what clinical workup is recommended?
    - Clinical genetic consultation with testing for MSI (microsatellite instability), with germline mutational assessment of DNA mismatch repair genes (MLH1, MSH2, MSH6 and PMS2) if their tumour is MSI high. Additional germline mutational assessment, for example, of the APC or MYH genes if the family history or patient's clinical presentation is suggestive for these mutations.
3. Until what age is screening recommended?
    - Screening is recommended to be continued up to 10 years before a patient's life expectancy.
4. **What are the acceptable tests for screening and at what intervals should they be performed?**
    - Colonoscopy every 10 years
    - Flexible sigmoidoscopy every 5 years

- CT scan of the colon (virtual colonoscopy) every 5 years
- Double-contrast barium enema every 5 years
- Faecal occult blood testing each year
- Faecal immunochemical testing each year
- Faecal DNA testing every 1–2 years

27.3 Prevention

1. What lifestyle modifications and interventions reduce the risk of CRC?
   - Daily use of aspirin and nonsteroidal anti-inflammatory medications
   - Postmenopausal oestrogen and progesterone hormone replacement therapy
   - Reduced intake of fat and meat
   - Diets rich in folate, fibre, calcium, vitamin D, magnesium, garlic and omega-3 fatty acids
   - Polypectomy with adenoma removal
   - Increased physical activity

27.3.1 Pathology

1. What are the major subtypes of CRC?
   - Majority are carcinomas, with >90% adenocarcinomas CK20 (cytokeratin 20) and CDX2 (caudal-type homeobox 2) positivity which are sensitive and specific markers of adenocarcinoma of colorectal origin (with exception of medullary carcinomas due to high microsatellite instability).
   - Mucinous carcinomas produce extracellular mucin that comprises ≥50% of tumour mass and dissects through tumour wall, increasing risk of local spread. Associated with one or more mismatch repair gene deficiencies.
   - Non-gland-forming carcinomas: Signet ring cell carcinoma: ≥50% of tumour made up of cells with intracellular mucin that displaces the nucleus. They are aggressive tumours with high risk of intramural spread and peritoneal carcinomatosis.
   - Medullary carcinoma: large eosinophilic, polygonal cells growing in solid sheets with heavy infiltration of small lymphocytes. These tumours are characterised by high degree of microsatellite instability.
   - Other non-adenocarcinoma CRC are adenosquamous carcinoma, squamous cell carcinoma, spindle cell, undifferentiated carcinomas and non-Hodgkin lymphomas, particularly mantle cell lymphoma and neuroendocrine tumours (NETs).
2. **How is CRC graded?**
   - Based on the degree of well-formed glands. Tumours are low grade (grade 1 or 2) if >50% of the tumour has well-formed glands and high grade (grade 3) if less.
3. **How are appendiceal tumours classified?**
   - About 50% of appendiceal tumours will be low-grade NETs.
   - "Goblet cell carcinoids" are adenocarcinomas with some neuroendocrine differentiation. Considerable disagreement exists about this histologic type, but in general they should be treated like adenocarcinomas.
   - Adenocarcinoma.
   - Signet ring carcinomas.
   - Appendiceal mucinous neoplasms are rare and do not have an agreed upon classification.

27.4 Signs and Symptoms

1. **What are some of the most common clinical presentations of CRC?**
   - Gross or occult blood in stool
   - Alterations in bowel habits, including constipation, cramping or diarrhoea
   - Abdominal pain or discomfort
   - Bowel obstruction
   - Decreased appetite, early satiety, weight loss and fatigue
   - Iron-deficiency anaemia secondary to blood loss

27.5 Diagnostic Workup

1. **What is the most accurate mode of diagnosis of CRC?**
   - Colonoscopy is the most accurate mode of diagnosis since it permits direct visualisation and biopsy of a suspected lesion.

27.6 Prognostic and Risk Factors

1. **What are the poor prognostic factors related to CRC?**
   - Depth of tumour invasion through the colorectal wall
   - Presence of one or more lymph node metastases
   - Degree of tumour regression after preoperative treatment for rectal carcinomas
   - Presence of distant metastases
   - Positive surgical margins (i.e. circumferential/radial margin)
   - Less than 12 lymph nodes resected with surgical removal of CRC
   - Irregular tumour border
   - Elevated carcinoembryonic antigen (CEA)
   - Absence of microsatellite instability
   - Poor histologic differentiation
   - Lymphovascular invasion and perineural invasion
   - Bowel perforation or obstruction
   - The presence of KRAS or BRAF mutations

27.6.1 Medical Therapeutic Modalities

What are the frequently employed chemotherapy agents and regimens for the treatment of CRC?

- 5-Fluorouracil (5-FU)/leucovorin (folinic acid)
- Capecitabine
- Oxaliplatin
- Irinotecan
- Trifluridine-tipiracil (TAS-102). Tipiracil is an inhibitor of thymidine phosphorylase, preventing the degradation of trifluridine, a nucleoside analog that inhibits thymidylate synthase. Approved for third- or fourth-line metastatic CRC
- FOLFOX (combination 5-fluorouracil/leucovorin/oxaliplatin)
- FOLFIRI (combination 5-flurouracil/leucovorin/irinotecan)
- FOLFOXIRI (combination 5-flurouracil/leucovorin/oxaliplatin/irinotecan)
- CapeOX (combination capecitabine/oxaliplatin)

What targeted agents have been currently employed in the treatment of CRC?

- Bevacizumab: a humanised monoclonal antibody that targets vascular endothelial growth factor A (VEGF-A). VEGF-A is the ligand for vascular endothelial growth factor receptors A and B (VEGFR-1, VEGFR-2)
- Ramucirumab: It is a vascular endothelial growth factor receptor 2 (VEGFR-2) antagonist and is a monoclonal antibody(human).
- Cetuximab: a chimeric mouse/human antibody that targets the epidermal growth factor receptor (EGFR)
- Panitumumab: a human monoclonal antibody that targets the EGFR
- Aflibercept: an intravenous fusion protein with binding portions of VEGF-1 and VEGF-2 receptors linked to the Fc portion of human IgG1, preventing VEGF-A and VEGF-B and placenta growth factor (PGF) from binding to their respective receptors
- Regorafenib: an oral inhibitor of angiogenic tyrosine kinases

Before beginning the treatment with cetuximab or panitumumab in any regimen, what testing must be performed?

- Mutations in exons 2 (codons 12 and 13), 3 (codons 59 and 61) and 4 (codons 117 and 146) in KRAS and NRAS must be looked for in the tumour as these can contribute to the failure of anti-EGFR therapy due to development of resistance. Mutations in KRAS and NRAS are usually mutually exclusive.

27.7 The Febrile, Neutropenic Patient

1. **How do you define febrile neutropenia?**
   - **Definition.** "1. Fever in a neutropenic patient is a single oral temperature of 38.3 °C (101 °F) or a temperature of 38.0 °C (100.4 °F) for 1 h". An absolute neutrophil count (ANC) of <500 cells/µL or an ANC between 500 and 1000 cells/µL that is falling can be referred to as neutropenia. Severe neutropenia is an ANC of 100 cells/µL". Serious infections occur when the duration and severity of neutropenia are more than 7 days.
2. **How do you stratify the risk in neutropenic patients?**

Neutropenic patients can be categorised as low-risk and high-risk.

1. **Low-risk patients** are those in whom the anticipated duration of neutropenia is 7 days, and the risk of complications from chemotherapy-induced neutropenia is relatively less. In addition, no significant medical comorbidities should be present to be classified as a low-risk patient. Such patients can be managed on a day-care basis.
   - Criteria for exclusion: Presence of diabetes mellitus, low blood pressure, neurological changes, bleeding episodes, pneumonia, dehydration and history of fungal infection in the last 6 months.
2. **High-risk patients** (requiring hospitalisation for the initial management)—patients are considered as high risk
   - When the ANC count is 100 cells/µL (severe neutropenia) or the expected period of neutropenia of >7 days
   - The presence of medical comorbidities (i.e. elderly patients with >60 years of age, low blood pressure, altered neurological status, unremitted cancer and pneumonia) or alemtuzumab treatment in the recent past
   - Those with an increased risk of complications due to reduced neutrophil count
   - Stem cell transplant recipients
   - Patients with acute leukaemia with ongoing chemotherapy
3. **Describe the epidemiology of febrile neutropenia**
   - 20–30% of patients with neutropenia-associated fever can have an infectious pathology found in 20–30% of patients having neutropenic fever with bacteraemia demonstrable in 10–25%. In 80% of the cases, the isolated organisms are mostly from the patient's flora (chiefly gut percolation of bacteria).
   - *Pseudomonas aeruginosa*, a gram-negative organism, is the most common organism causing infections in this population. Infections with gram-negative organisms require empirical antibiotic therapy as they cause significant morbidity and mortality.
   - The use of fluoroquinolones as prophylactic agents at the onset of neutropenia has led to an increased prevalence of gram-positive organisms especially methicillin-resistant *Staphylococcus aureus* [MRSA] and vancomycin-resistant enterococci [VRE]).
4. **Explain the aetiology and pathophysiology of febrile neutropenia**
   - The duration of neutropenia determines the risk and timing of infection. Lungs (25%) and oropharynx (25%), central venous catheter (CVC) sites (15%) and skin, sinuses (5%), gastrointestinal (GI), perineum (5%) and genitourinary sites (5%) are the commonly affected sites.

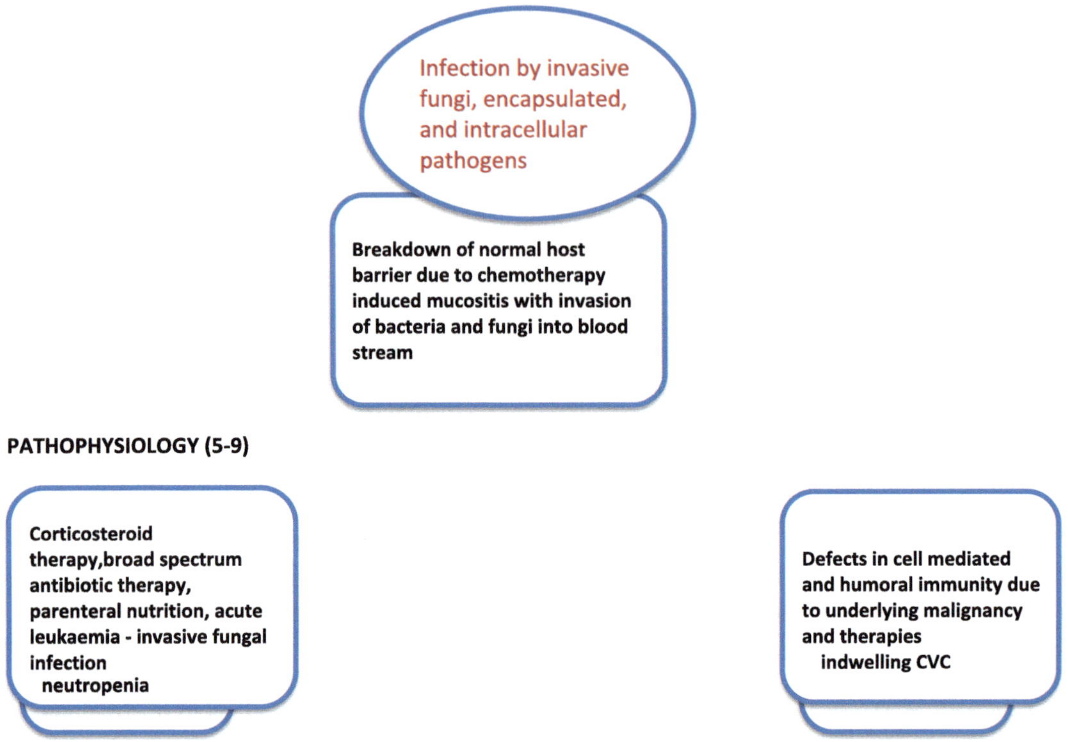

27.8 Pathophysiology [1–5]

5. **How do you do risk assessment in a patient with febrile neutropenia?**

   The Multinational Association for Supportive Care in Cancer (MASCC) risk index score has been commonly used to identify patients with febrile neutropenia who are at a low risk and high risk of serious complications and mortality. This helps in guiding the empiric antibiotic therapy based on the risk (Table 27.1). The maximum score is 26 and an MASCC score >21 in a patient with febrile neutropenia is suggestive of a low risk for complications and may be considered for treatment in an ambulatory setting if he/she stays within an hour of the hospital facility and can return to the medical facility quickly for emergency and follow-up. A caregiver should also be present at home.

Table 27.1 MASCC Index

Characteristics	Weight
Febrile neutropenia burden • Asymptomatic or only mild symptoms • Moderate symptoms	 5 3
Absence of hypotension (SBP >90 mmHg)	5
Active COPD not present	4
Solid tumour or no history of fungal infection	4
No dehydration which requires parenteral fluids	3
Outpatient status	3
Age <60 years	2

6. **Explain the management of febrile neutropenia**

   (A) **Clinical presentation.** 1. Neutropenic patients may present with fever, which could be the only sign of an underlying serious infection in the absence of other signs of inflammation, and sepsis should be considered in any patient who presents with tachypnoea, hypotension, hypoxemia and altered mental status.

(B) **Differential diagnosis.** In a patient presenting with febrile neutropenia, assume that it is due to infection and start empiric broad-spectrum antibiotic therapy until fever and neutropenia resolve. Other non-infectious causes should also be considered.

(C) **History**: A thorough history and physical examination are a must in the evaluation of a patient presenting with febrile neutropenia. The presence of any new complaints must be noted with a detailed review of the respiratory, gastrointestinal, neurological systems, ENT, skin and eye.

(D) **Physical Examination**

- Physical examination should be performed as a part of the initial work-up and daily. Head-to-toe examination including the skin, vascular catheter sites, fundus and recent surgical wounds should be performed. Inflammatory signs may be minimal or absent in neutropenic patients.
- Head and neck examination may reveal that the presence of vesicles in the ear canal may be suggestive of herpes infection. Attention should be paid to telltale signs of invasive fungal infection of orbits and sinuses such as discharge from the eyes, pain in the eyes, difficulty in eye movement, redness and eschar or scar in the nasopharynx.
- Examination of the skin: One should look at the CVC entry sites for the presence of redness, induration and tenderness suggesting the presence of a catheter-related infection. Systemic bacterial, viral and fungal infections can be suspected by the presence of necrotic ulcers, vesicles and nodules, respectively, in the skin.
- The presence of rales or rhonchi may be due to community-acquired or nosocomial bacterial, fungal and viral pathogens. However, exacerbation of airway or interstitial lung diseases may mimic respiratory infections.
- Abdomen—Neutropenic patients may not present with overt abdominal pain or distension. Diarrhoea from infective aetiology should be differentiated from the ones due to mucositis or chemotherapy-induced. The presence of abdominal pain and tenderness may be due to liver abscess, neutropenic enterocolitis or *Clostridium difficile* colitis.

d. Sepsis due to *P. aeruginosa* and *Clostridium perfringens* or *Clostridium septicum* not commonly seen in healthy patients must be considered in neutropenic patients [6, 7].

(E) **Laboratory Evaluation**

See Table 27.2.

Table 27.2 Shows initial and definitive diagnostic tests

	Initial diagnostic tests	Definitive diagnostic tests
1	Complete blood count including platelet count and differential count	Specimens obtained by biopsy, bronchoalveolar lavage (BAL), GI endoscopy or invasive means—subjected to histological examination and special culture techniques
2	Liver function tests	Fungal antigen testing—serum galactomannan assay, galactomannan testing of BAL fluid and beta-D-glucan assay
3	Renal function tests and electrolytes	
4	Peripheral blood cultures (2 sets)	
5	Urinalysis and urine culture	
6	Sputum culture Stool culture, assay for *C. difficile*—diarrhoea history	
7	Swabs, smears, aspiration, cultures or biopsy of suspicious skin or mucous membrane lesions	

27.9 Radiologic Studies

1. Chest radiograph (CXR) or computed tomography (CT) scan of the chest.
   - The characteristics of infiltrates on the CXR/CT chest can provide a clue for the diagnosis, for example, focal or multifocal infiltrates—bacterial or invasive fungal pneumonia.
   - Diffuse interstitial infiltrates—viral pneumonia, *P. jirovecii* or noninfectious processes.
   - Cavitary and nodular pattern—bacterial/fungal aetiology (e.g. mycobacteria, *P. aeruginosa*, *Staphylococcus aureus,* anaerobes), Nocardia species, *Legionella* and noninfectious processes.
2. Imaging of the abdomen may be obtained if indicated.

27.10 Treatment [2, 4, 5, 8–12]

(A) Principles

1. Life-threatening infections can occur in patients with neutropenia and require prompt treatment with broad-spectrum IV antibiotics after obtaining appropriate cultures.
2. Empiric antibiotics should be administered preferably within 60 min of presentation to the medical facility while continuing diagnostic tests. Gram-negative coverage for pseudomonas should be included in empiric therapy while gram-positive cover can be added in the presence of a specific indication.
3. Local antibiogram should be considered in initiating empirical antibiotic therapy for high-risk patients which should cover *P. aeruginosa* but could include one of the following options mentioned in Table 27.3:
4. In case of suspicion of bacteraemia due to *Staphylococcus* or other gram-positive organisms, severe mucositis, cellulitis, tunnel or entry site infection, vancomycin should be added to any of the above empiric regimens which can be discontinued after 3 days of empiric treatment, if no causative agent requiring vancomycin for treatment is isolated. However, it can be continued if used in a patient with penicillin allergy in combination with aztreonam. Beta-lactams should be administered before vancomycin to prevent delay in coverage of gram-negative organisms as vancomycin infusion requires at least 1 h for administration.
5. Administration of an aminoglycoside is only for targeting specific organisms in the presence of documented infection [13].
6. If mucocutaneous lesions are suspicious of herpes simplex virus (HSY) or varicella-zoster virus (VZV) infection, antiviral agents should be added.
7. In patients with evidence of sepsis, persistent fever for 4–7 days or the presence of risk factors for invasive fungal infection, empiric anti-fungal therapy should be considered [14].
   (a) Empiric anti-fungal agents of different classes should be considered in patients who have received prophylactic antifungal agents.

Table 27.3 Empiric antibiotic therapy

	Dose	Frequency	Indication
Ceftazidime/cefepime	2 g IV	q 8th h	No localising symptoms or signs
Piperacillin/tazobactum	3.375 g IV	q 6th h	Suspected dental, oral, intra-abdominal, anaerobic or polymicrobial infection
Aztreonam + vancomycin	2 g IV 1 g IV	q 6th h Q12th h	Penicillin allergy
Imipenem	500 mg	q 6th h	Infection with extended spectrum beta-lactamase-producing organism

(b) Fluconazole can be started empirically in neutropenic patients with persistent fever with no risk factors for fungal infection and not received prophylaxis with fluconazole. In case, fluconazole prophylaxis has been given, antifungal to target resistant candida species should be started.

(c) In patients who satisfy the following six criteria, an antifungal agent that covers *Aspergillus* species or other filamentous fungi should be considered:
- Colonisation by fungi with filaments.
- Treatment with corticosteroids >1 mg/kg/day dose.
- Neutropenia lasting >20 days.
- Presence of lung infiltrates suspicious for fungal invasion.
- AML patients.
- Stem cell transplant recipients.

8. The dose and route of administration of antifungals depends on various factors such as the presence of mucositis and kidney and liver function. Commonly followed regimens include the following have been mentioned in Table 27.4:
9. Removal of indwelling CVCs is recommended in the following conditions:
   (a) Candida species, bacillus species, pseudomonas and vancomycin-resistant enterococci-related bacteraemia.
   (b) The presence of septic thrombophlebitis.
   (c) Evidence of tunnel or exit site infection.
   (d) Irrespective of the organism isolated, if the bacteraemia persists or recurs.
10. If no infection is documented, along with resolution of fever and recovery of ANC >500 cells/μL, empirical antibiotic therapy may be discontinued.

(B) Supportive care

Inotropic—vasopressors should be started based on ICU protocols and guided by haemodynamic monitoring. Ventilatory support should be provided as and when required.

(C) Guidelines for the dosing of antibiotics
1. Renal and hepatic dysfunction should be considered and the appropriate dose modifications should be done.
2. The antibiotic dose used for gram-negative sepsis should be appropriate to target *P. aeruginosa*.
3. Institutional and published guidelines for the management of febrile neutropenia should be followed for appropriate dosing of the antibiotics.
4. Discontinuation of antibiotic therapy.
   (a) Following the resolution of fever and neutropenia, empiric antibiotic therapy may be discontinued.
   (b) Although antimicrobial therapy targeting specific organisms may be started after isolation of the causative organism, gram-negative coverage (including *P. aeruginosa*) should be continued until the resolution of neutropenia.

(D) The treatment should always be based on published guidelines [7].

(E) Prognosis
1. High mortality rate is seen in neutropenic patients with gram-negative sepsis when untreated or inadequately treated and

Table 27.4 Commonly used antifungal agents

Drug	Loading dose	Maintenance dose
Fluconazole	800 mg IV or PO-day 1	400 mg IV or PO
Voriconazole	6 mg/kg IV or PO q 12 h–day 1	4 mg/kg IV or PO q 12 h
Amphotericin B/liposomal amphotericin B	3–5 mg/kg IV once a day	
Caspofungin	70 mg IV—Day 1	50 mg IV once a day
Micafungin	100 mg once a day—candidemia	

also in patients suffering from multiple co-morbidities.
2. The use of empiric therapy in febrile, neutropenic patients has significantly reduced mortality rates to <15%; however, it is also dependent on other factors such as the presence of comorbidities and time to initiation of empiric antibiotic therapy and the patient profile.
3. High mortality in patients with multiple comorbidities [6–10].

References

1. Bodey GP, Jadeja L, Elting L. *Pseudomonas bacteremia*. Retrospective analysis of 410 episodes. Arch Intern Med. 1985;145(9):1621.
2. Mikulska M, Viscoli C, Orasch C, Livermore DM, Averbuch D, Cordonnier C, Akova M. Aetiology and resistance in bacteraemias among adult and paediatric haematology and cancer patients; fourth European conference on Infections in Leukemia Group (ECIL-4), a joint venture of EBMT, EORTC, ICHS, ELN and ESGICH/ESCMID. J Infect. 2014;68(4):321. Epub 2013 Dec 24.
3. Holland T, Fowler VG Jr, Shelburne SA 3rd. Invasive gram-positive bacterial infection in cancer patients. Clin Infect Dis. 2014;59:S331.
4. Freifeld AG, Bow EJ, Sepkowitz KA, et al. Clinical practice guideline for the use of antimicrobial agents in neutropenic patients with cancer: 2010 update by the Infectious Diseases Society of America. Clin Infect Dis. 2011;52:e56.
5. National Comprehensive Cancer Network (NCCN) Clinical Practice Guidelines in Oncology. Prevention and treatment of cancer-related infections. Version 1.2018. http://www.nccn.org. Accessed 1 Aug 2018.
6. Fishman JA. Infection in solid-organ transplant recipients. N Engl J Med. 2007;357(25):2601–14.
7. Koo S, Marty FM, Baden LR. Infectious complications associated with immunomodulating biologic agents. Infect Dis Clin N Am. 2010;24(2):285–306.
8. Taplitz RA, Kennedy EB, Bow EJ, et al. Outpatient management of fever and neutropenia in adults treated for malignancy: American Society of Clinical Oncology and Infectious Diseases Society of America clinical practice guideline update. J Clin Oncol. 2018;36:1443.
9. de Naurois J, Novitzky-Basso I, Gill MJ, Marti FM, Cullen MH, Roila F. Management of febrile neutropenia: ESMO clinical practice guidelines; ESMO guidelines working group. Ann Oncol. 2010;21(Suppl 5):v252.
10. Averbuch D, Cordonnier C, Livermore DM, Mikulska M, Orasch C, Viscoli C, Gyssens IC, Kern WV, Klyasova G, Marchetti O, Engelhard D, Akova M. Targeted therapy against multi-resistant bacteria in leukemic and hematopoietic stem cell transplant recipients: guidelines of the 4th European conference on infections in leukemia (ECIL-4, 2011), ECIL4, a joint venture of EBMT, EORTC, ICHS, ESGICH/ESCMID and ELN. Haematologica. 2013;98(12):1836.
11. Rolston KV. Challenges in the treatment of infections caused by gram-positive and gram-negative bacteria in patients with cancer and neutropenia. Clin Infect Dis. 2005;40(Suppl. 4):S246.
12. Sipsas NV, Bodey GP, Kontoyiannis DP. Perspectives for the management of febrile neutropenic patients with cancer in the 21st century. Cancer. 2005;103(6):1103.
13. Freifeld AG, Bow EJ, Sepkowitz KA, et al. Clinical practice guideline for the use of antimicrobial agents in neutropenic patients with cancer: 2010 update by the Infectious Diseases Society of America. Clin Infect Dis. 2011;52(4):e56.
14. Koo S, Bryar JM, Page JH, et al. Diagnostic performance of the (1–3)-beta-D-glucan assay for invasive fungal disease. Clin Infect Dis. 2009;49(11):1650.

CA Breast with Spinal Cord Compression

28

Jyotsna Goswami, Angshuman Rudra Pal, and Suparna Mitra

28.1 Case Scenario

A 45-year female with triple-negative locally advanced breast cancer has undergone modified radical mastectomy after 4 months of neoadjuvant chemotherapy. The surgical specimen biopsy report was ypT2N2M0. She was scheduled for radiotherapy (RT) to the chest wall and supraclavicular fossa. However, just before the planned RT date, the patient presented to emergency with symptoms of severe back pain and weakness in both lower limbs. MRI lumbosacral spine has shown multiple skeletal metastases in L3, L4, L5 and S1 with cord compression.

28.2 What Is the Incidence and Common Symptoms of Presentation of Metastatic Spinal Cord Compression (MSCC) from Various Carcinoma?

Although rare, MSCC is a dreaded complication of carcinoma, which is associated with severe pain and progressive impairment of neurologic function [1]. Due to this danger of permanent motor loss and paralysis, MSCC is considered as an oncological emergency that requires urgent intervention in terms of prompt diagnosis and treatment.

The true incidence is difficult to get as it depends on the hospital admission and correct diagnosis [2, 3]. The reported incidence is approximately 3–5%, although it varies with the type of the primary tumour. It is more (19%) in case of lung, prostate or breast cancers, which comprises of more than 50% of all MSCC patients requiring hospitalisation [4–6].

Approximately 20–34% of cancer patients present with symptoms of MSCC. In case of multiple myeloma and lymphoma, when it is diagnosed, often it has already spread extensively. A cancer patient presenting with back pain has a high possibility of having MSCC. They should be diagnosed and treated without any delay to prevent further neurologic damage and control of pain and thus provide a reasonable quality of life. Simultaneous palliative care, particularly for non-ambulatory patients, is helpful [5].

In 95% of patients, back pain, which lasts for a prolonged period, presents as the first symptom followed by limb weakness. While developing MSCC, patients are usually very sick with multiple comorbidities and poor performance status. Depending upon the presenting condition of the patient, future plan should be decided either for curative or palliative intent.

J. Goswami (✉) · A. R. Pal · S. Mitra
Department of Oncoanaesthesia, Tata Medical Center, Kolkata, India

N. Gupta et al. (eds.), *Problem Based Learning Discussions in Onco-Anesthesia and Onco-Critical Care*, https://doi.org/10.1007/978-981-99-6339-3_28

28.3 How Do Patients with MSCC Present? What Are the Key Clinical Findings That Help Us to Diagnose?

Usually, the onset of the symptoms of MSCC is slow but progressive. There may be rapid deterioration in the course of the disease. The clinical feature depends on the level of the spinal cord affected and the resulting neural compression. Detailed neurological examination must be conducted including assessment of strength, sensory function, motor reflexes and sphincter function. The area below the affected part of the spinal cord usually develops reduced sensation and upper motor neuron features with symmetrical deficit. If the part below the termination of the spinal cord is affected, patients present with cauda equina syndrome with asymmetrical lower motor neuron deficits involving distal extremity initially [7]. ASIA Impairment Scale Scoring Chart is helpful for detailed documentation [6].

Back pain is the commonest presenting symptom in 80–95% of cases [8]. It is a continuous aching pain with increased severity at night and aggravated by Valsalva manoeuvres, coughing, sneezing and lying on the back [3]. This high-intensity pain usually presents as spinal or radicular pain. In the advanced stage, the nature of pain may change to radicular burning type or referred pain. High index of suspicion and alertness for the development of symptoms is of utmost importance in malignant patients for early diagnosis of MSCC.

Red flags for MSCC are the following:

1. Weakness of limbs with difficulty in walking (35–75%)
2. Sensory loss (may not be proportional to the level of spinal lesion)
3. Bladder or bowel dysfunction (which indicates poor functional outcome after treatment)
4. Neurological signs
5. Pain at various levels of spinal cord
6. Pain precipitated by straining will be more than usual nocturnal spinal pain

28.4 Explain the Different Theories of Pathophysiology Behind the MSCC

The spinal cord compression is classified as intradural or extradural depending on the site of metastatic deposit. Intradural can again be classified into intramedullary or extramedullary. Extradural lesions can be of either epidural origin or may be migration of lesions from adjacent vertebrae, causing compression effect [9].

Among the three mechanisms, haematogenous spread is the commonest mode of spread in MSCC [10]. The other two modes are direct extension of the tumor into the vertebral column from adjoining places and as the primary site of tumor [11]. The usual sites of deposition are thoracic spine followed by the lumbosacral and cervical spine [12]. This deposited mass causes compression of the adjacent vital structures like epidural venous plexus, spinal artery, thecal sac and spinal cord [13]. This may result in neurological symptoms or venous congestion and oedema leading to neural demyelination and cell damage. Thus, chronic and untreated pressure results in vascular injury leading to spinal cord infarction with permanent damage of neuronal function [14].

28.5 What Are the Investigations Required to Diagnose the MSCC?

Clinical signs and symptoms alone are not sufficient for estimating the severity of compression. Plain radiography also has very poor sensitivity as a diagnostic tool. Magnetic resonance imaging (MRI) of the entire spine is the investigation of choice to diagnose the metastatic spinal cord compression, with a sensitivity as high as 93% and a specificity of 97% [10, 15]. Computed tomography (CT) scanning with sagittal T1 and short T1 inversion recovery (STIR) sequences can detect metastatic disease within the bone and may help in planning of the treatment. To detect the soft tissue components of mass and the degree of spinal cord compression, the sagittal T2 imaging supplemented with axial T1- or T2-weighted scans needs to be used. CT myelography and positron emission tomography scanning (PET) are used for diagnosis in patients with MRI-incompatible implant.

28.6 What Should Be Your Initial Plan of Management?

After the MRI confirms the diagnosis, the treatment should be started promptly with the aim to prevent further neurological deterioration, relieve pain and restore neurological function. In most cases, the treatment consists of early administration of corticosteroids and then either surgical decompression followed by radiation therapy or only radiation therapy. The National Institute for Health and Care Excellence (NICE) have provided guidelines on the management of spinal cord compression in 2008 [16]. Before starting treatment, the patient's performance status, neurological ability, the systemic disease burden and previous treatments should be taken into account.

28.7 How Can the Patient with Suspected MSCC Be Positioned for Care?

Patients with neurological symptoms suggestive of MSCC need to be positioned flat with the spine in neutral alignment carefully. Once the spinal shock is settled, patients can be positioned gradually from supine to 60° head-up over a period of time for further assessment and monitoring. Patients who are not immediately going for surgery or RT need to be encouraged to maintain their position by themselves and mobilise as per tolerance with the aid of braces and collars or halo jackets for the neck to stabilise the spine.

28.8 What Is the Role and Dose of Glucocorticoids?

Glucocorticoids reduce spinal cord oedema and prevent irreversible injury, thus providing analgesia and preserving neurologic function [17]. After thorough assessment, it should start as a stat dose of at least 16 mg of dexamethasone, unless contraindicated, followed by 16 mg on daily basis for a short period of time, while multidisciplinary decision is being made. Once surgery is performed or the radiotherapy has started, the dose needs to be tapered off gradually over a few days as tolerated and steroid-related side effects are monitored. The dose of steroid should be increased temporarily if there is deterioration of neurological function at any point of time. If there is fast improvement in the motor function after starting of glucocorticoid therapy, then there are high chances of neurological recovery after the final treatment [18].

28.9 Which Modalities Are Available for Pain Relief?

For pain management, patients are offered NSAID, opioid and nonopioid analgesics [19, 20]. WHO's three-step pain management ladder is helpful for escalation of doses. Adjuvant analgesics that can be prescribed are anticonvulsants like gabapentin, pregabalin and tricyclic antidepressants [21]. Caregivers should be aware of side effects like sedation, anticholinergic effects, orthostasis and cardiac arrhythmias. For invasive procedures like epidural or intrathecal analgesia, patients should be referred to pain specialists, and for intractable pain, neurosurgical interventions should be considered. Physical methods of pain relief like heat, cold, ultrasound and electrical stimulation can also be helpful in many cases.

28.10 When Will the Patient Be Considered a Candidate for Surgery?

According to NICE guidelines, surgery should be offered to patients with spinal metastases and having evidence of structural spinal failure with spinal instability to stabilise the spine and prevent cord compression and damage [16]. Spinal stabilisation can also be considered for patients suffering from mechanical pain which is resistant to conventional analgesia even if completely paralysed [22–24]. Surgery is also the first modality of treatment for MSCC in case of radio-resistant tumors. If patients have too poor prognosis, or the patient is too frail, surgery is not recommended. Cord decompression and spinal stabilisation can be done by conventional approach or by minimal access. Procedure like vertebroplasty or kyphoplasty is considered if there is vertebral body collapse [25]. Many randomised trials have shown excellent results with surgery and RT compared to only RT [14, 26].

28.11 Are There Any Objective Criteria to Decide Between Surgery and Radiotherapy?

There are various scoring systems to guide clinician to take decisions regarding surgery and RT [18, 27]. One of them is the neurologic, oncologic, mechanical and systemic disease (NOMS) decision framework which takes into account the degree of spinal cord compression by using the Spine Oncology Study Group [SOSG] scoring system, radiosensitivity of the tumor, stability of the spine, presence of myelopathy and the patient's ability to undergo the proposed treatment [28]. Ambulatory status of the patient has been the most important prognostic indicator.

28.12 When Is the Radiation Therapy Indicated?

The current practice is to give fractionated radiotherapy, rather than a single fraction, to patients with good prognosis and have radiotherapy as their primary treatment [29]. Even if paraplegia is complete, palliative radiotherapy in the form of 8 Gy single fraction is offered to patients with spinal metastases having non-mechanical spinal pain [30]. It helps in significant pain control and improvement in neurological function [6]. If the tumor is radio-resistant, radiotherapy can still be used for patients who are not suitable for surgery. Patients who have been paraplegic for more than 24 h are less likely to recover neurological function after radiotherapy. To avoid unnecessary surgical procedures and associated complications, palliative RT alone can be a good reasonable treatment of choice for patients with an expected limited survival. If surgery is planned, preoperative radiotherapy is not given. In patients who have a satisfactory surgical outcome, fractionated radiotherapy is routinely offered after surgery [14, 31].

28.13 What Is the Role of Bisphosphonates?

Bisphosphonates are helpful for patients with MSCC, if the vertebral involvement is from breast cancer or myeloma. It helps in reducing pain and the risk of vertebral collapse [32]. It can also reduce hypercalcaemia associated with osteolytic metastases from primary cancers.

28.14 What Is the Role of Rehabilitation in These Patients?

Because of the advanced nature of the disease process, patients with MSCC most commonly encounter functional disability along with the emotional pinch. So rehabilitation and supportive care are very important parts of management in order to promote independence and improve the quality of life [33–35]. The NICE guidelines regarding 'improving supportive and palliative care for adults with cancer' are very useful in implementing holistic, goal-directed and patient-centred rehabilitation programmes. The rehabilitation will aim at relief of pain and spasticity, prevention of complications and maximise functional independence and improvement of quality of life and psychological status.

28.15 What Thromboprophylaxis Measures Should Be Taken for These Patients?

Graduated compression stockings and/or intermittent pneumatic compression devices or foot impulse equipment should be offered to patients on bedrest [36, 37]. In addition to mechanical thromboprophylaxis, subcutaneous low molecular weight heparin (LMWH) is indicated in patients who are at high risk of venous thromboembolism [37, 38]. Duration of treatment will depend on mobility status, presence of risk factors and overall clinical condition.

28.16 How Will You Prevent Pressure Ulcers?

Patients suffering from MSCC are prone to develop pressure ulcers because of restricted mobility and impaired sensation [39]. To prevent this complication, they should be turned on the bed carefully using a log-roll technique once every 2–3 h. Those who are not advised bed rest should be encouraged to mobilise regularly. Air mattresses and cushions with high-grade pressure-relieving properties are comfortable for the patients [40]. While turning the patient, risk assessment and documentation for pressure ulcers should be done on daily basis.

28.17 How to Manage Bladder and Bowel Continence?

Incontinence, retention, constipation and obstruction have a huge effect on care and well-being of the patients with MSCC. Initially a urinary catheter can be used to manage bladder dysfunction. In case of long-term requirement, intermittent catheterisation or suprapubic catheters are recommended [41, 42]. Other measures such as diet modification, faecal softeners, oral or rectal laxatives, abdominal massage and irrigation techniques are helpful [43].

28.18 How Will You Ensure Adequate Circulatory and Respiratory Functioning?

Vitals like heart rate (HR), blood pressure (BP), respiration and oxygenation with pulse oximetry should be monitored and recorded on daily basis. If a patient develops postural hypotension, he/she should be positioned carefully to improve venous return. Graduated compression devices and foot pumps are also helpful [44, 45]. Overzealous hydration can lead to pulmonary oedema and should be avoided. Chest physiotherapy and non-invasive airway clearance techniques such as deep breathing exercise and postural drainage can help to remove secretions and clearing of airway [46].

28.19 What Will Be Your Rehabilitation Plan After the Patient Is Discharged?

Community-run supportive care and rehabilitation services are very helpful to maximise the quality of life. These services should be made available, when patients with MSCC are discharged to home. Family members also should be encouraged to take active participation in caregiving. Training of the families and caregivers will help in better implementation of rehabilitation programmes [47].

28.20 How to Evaluate Quality of Life (QoL) in These Patients?

A variety of outcome measures have been used to assess QoL for patients suffering from MSCC. In 1995, Sundaresan et al. used the Functional Assessment of Cancer Therapy-General (FACT-G) scale to measure QoL [48]. Then, Mannion et al. in 2007 used 36-Item Short Form Health Survey questionnaire (SF36), which includes scoring from 0 to 100, with 100 being the perfect health [49]. More recently, the disease-specific Spine Oncology Study Group—Outcomes Questionnaire (SOSG-OQ) was developed to evaluate QoL in these groups of patients [50].

References

1. Sodji Q, Kaminski J, Willey C, Kim N, Mourad W, Vender J, et al. Management of metastatic spinal cord compression. South Med J. 2017;110(9):586–93.
2. Mak KS, Lee LK, Mak RH, Wang S, Pile-Spellman J, Abrahm JL, et al. Incidence and treatment patterns

in hospitalizations for malignant spinal cord compression in the United States, 1998–2006. Int J Radiat Oncol. 2011;80(3):824–31.
3. Cole JS, Patchell RA. Metastatic epidural spinal cord compression. Lancet Neurol. 2008;7(5):459–66.
4. Epidemiology [Internet]. Metastatic spinal cord compression: diagnosis and management of patients at risk of or with metastatic spinal cord compression. National Collaborating Centre for Cancer (UK); 2008 [cited 2022 Jul 28]. https://www.ncbi.nlm.nih.gov/books/NBK55011/
5. Robson P. Metastatic spinal cord compression: a rare but important complication of cancer. Clin Med Lond Engl. 2014;14(5):542–5.
6. Roberts TT, Leonard GR, Cepela DJ. Classifications in brief: American Spinal Injury Association (ASIA) impairment scale. Clin Orthop. 2017;475(5):1499–504.
7. Sun H, Nemecek AN. Optimal management of malignant epidural spinal cord compression. Hematol Oncol Clin North Am. 2010;24(3):537–51.
8. Loblaw DA, Perry J, Chambers A, Laperriere NJ. Systematic review of the diagnosis and management of malignant extradural spinal cord compression: the Cancer Care Ontario Practice Guidelines Initiative's Neuro-Oncology Disease Site Group. J Clin Oncol Off J Am Soc Clin Oncol. 2005;23(9):2028–37.
9. Bartels RHMA, Feuth T, van der Maazen R, Verbeek ALM, Kappelle AC, André Grotenhuis J, et al. Development of a model with which to predict the life expectancy of patients with spinal epidural metastasis. Cancer. 2007;110(9):2042–9.
10. Al-Qurainy R, Collis E. Metastatic spinal cord compression: diagnosis and management. BMJ. 2016;353:i2539.
11. Bucholtz JD. Metastatic epidural spinal cord compression. Semin Oncol Nurs. 1999;15(3):150–9.
12. Loblaw DA, Laperriere NJ, Mackillop WJ. A population-based study of malignant spinal cord compression in Ontario. Clin Oncol. 2003;15(4):211–7.
13. Prasad D, Schiff D. Malignant spinal-cord compression. Lancet Oncol. 2005;6(1):15–24.
14. Patchell RA, Tibbs PA, Regine WF, Payne R, Saris S, Kryscio RJ, et al. Direct decompressive surgical resection in the treatment of spinal cord compression caused by metastatic cancer: a randomised trial. Lancet Lond Engl. 2005;366(9486):643–8.
15. Lawton AJ, Lee KA, Cheville AL, Ferrone ML, Rades D, Balboni TA, et al. Assessment and management of patients with metastatic spinal cord compression: a multidisciplinary review. J Clin Oncol Off J Am Soc Clin Oncol. 2019;37(1):61–71.
16. Metastatic spinal cord compression: diagnosis and management of patients at risk of or with metastatic spinal cord compression [Internet]. Cardiff (UK): National Collaborating Centre for Cancer (UK); 2008 [cited 2022 Jul 26]. (National Institute for Health and Care Excellence: Guidelines). http://www.ncbi.nlm.nih.gov/books/NBK55007/
17. Malignant spinal-cord compression—PubMed [Internet]. [cited 2022 Jul 6]. https://pubmed.ncbi.nlm.nih.gov/15629272/
18. Sørensen S, Helweg-Larsen S, Mouridsen H, Hansen HH. Effect of high-dose dexamethasone in carcinomatous metastatic spinal cord compression treated with radiotherapy: a randomised trial. Eur J Cancer Oxf Engl 1990. 1994;30A(1):22–7.
19. A physician's guide to pain and symptom management in cancer patients [Internet]. [cited 2022 Jul 26]. https://www.press.jhu.edu/books/title/10494/physicians-guide-pain-and-symptom-management-cancer-patients
20. Evidence-based practice of palliative medicine—9781437737967 [Internet]. US Elsevier Health. [cited 2022 Jul 26]. https://www.us.elsevierhealth.com/evidence-based-practice-of-palliative-medicine-9781437737967.html
21. Gabapentin in the treatment of neuropathic pain after spinal cord injury: a prospective, randomized, double-blind, crossover trial—PubMed [Internet]. [cited 2022 Jul 26]. https://pubmed.ncbi.nlm.nih.gov/12137213/
22. Fehlings MG, Nater A, Tetreault L, Kopjar B, Arnold P, Dekutoski M, et al. Survival and clinical outcomes in surgically treated patients with metastatic epidural spinal cord compression: results of the prospective multicenter AOSpine study. J Clin Oncol Off J Am Soc Clin Oncol. 2016;34(3):268–76.
23. Wu J, Zheng W, Xiao JR, Sun X, Liu WZ, Guo Q. Health-related quality of life in patients with spinal metastases treated with or without spinal surgery: a prospective, longitudinal study. Cancer. 2010;116(16):3875–82.
24. Ibrahim A, Crockard A, Antonietti P, Boriani S, Bünger C, Gasbarrini A, et al. Does spinal surgery improve the quality of life for those with extradural (spinal) osseous metastases? An international multicenter prospective observational study of 223 patients. Invited submission from the Joint Section Meeting on Disorders of the Spine and Peripheral Nerves, March 2007. J Neurosurg Spine. 2008;8(3):271–8.
25. Sadeghi-Naini M, Aarabi S, Shokraneh F, Janani L, Vaccaro AR, Rahimi-Movaghar V. Vertebroplasty and kyphoplasty for metastatic spinal lesions: a systematic review. Clin Spine Surg. 2018;31(5):203–10.
26. Rades D, Huttenlocher S, Dunst J, Bajrovic A, Karstens JH, Rudat V, et al. Matched pair analysis comparing surgery followed by radiotherapy and radiotherapy alone for metastatic spinal cord compression. J Clin Oncol Off J Am Soc Clin Oncol. 2010;28(22):3597–604.
27. Ropper AE, Ropper AH. Acute spinal cord compression. N Engl J Med. 2017;376(14):1358–69.
28. Laufer I, Rubin DG, Lis E, Cox BW, Stubblefield MD, Yamada Y, et al. The NOMS framework: approach to the treatment of spinal metastatic tumors. Oncologist. 2013;18(6):744–51.
29. Hoskin PJ, Hopkins K, Misra V, Holt T, McMenemin R, Dubois D, et al. Effect of single-fraction vs multifraction radiotherapy on ambulatory status among

patients with spinal canal compression from metastatic cancer: the SCORAD randomized clinical trial. JAMA. 2019;322(21):2084–94.
30. Rades D, Stalpers LJA, Veninga T, Schulte R, Hoskin PJ, Obralic N, et al. Evaluation of five radiation schedules and prognostic factors for metastatic spinal cord compression. J Clin Oncol Off J Am Soc Clin Oncol. 2005;23(15):3366–75.
31. Witham TF, Khavkin YA, Gallia GL, Wolinsky JP, Gokaslan ZL. Surgery insight: current management of epidural spinal cord compression from metastatic spine disease. Nat Clin Pract Neurol. 2006;2(2):87–94. quiz 116
32. Wong R, Wiffen PJ. Bisphosphonates for the relief of pain secondary to bone metastases. Cochrane Database Syst Rev. 2002;(2):CD002068.
33. Huang ME, Sliwa JA. Inpatient rehabilitation of patients with cancer: efficacy and treatment considerations. PM R. 2011;3(8):746–57.
34. Ruff RL, Adamson VW, Ruff SS, Wang X. Directed rehabilitation reduces pain and depression while increasing independence and satisfaction with life for patients with paraplegia due to epidural metastatic spinal cord compression. J Rehabil Res Dev. 2007;44(1):1–10.
35. Rimaud D, Calmels P, Roche F, Mongold JJ, Trudeau F, Devillard X. Effects of graduated compression stockings on cardiovascular and metabolic responses to exercise and exercise recovery in persons with spinal cord injury. Arch Phys Med Rehabil. 2007;88(6):703–9.
36. Scottish Intercollegiate Guidelines Network. Prevention and management of venous thromboembolism: a national clinical guideline. Edinburgh: SIGN; 2010.
37. Hill J, Treasure T. Reducing the risk of venous thromboembolism (deep vein thrombosis and pulmonary embolism) in inpatients having surgery: summary of NICE guidance. BMJ. 2007;334(7602):1053–4.
38. Scottish Intercollegiate Guidelines Network. Antithrombotics: indications and management. Edinburgh: Scottish Intercollegiate Guidelines Network; 2013.
39. Royal College of Nursing (UK). The management of pressure ulcers in primary and secondary care: a clinical practice guideline [Internet]. London: Royal College of Nursing (UK); 2005 [cited 2022 Jul 26]. (National Institute for Health and Clinical Excellence: Guidance). http://www.ncbi.nlm.nih.gov/books/NBK49010/
40. National Collaborating Centre for Nursing and Supportive Care (UK). The use of pressure-relieving devices (beds, mattresses and overlays) for the prevention of pressure ulcers in primary and secondary care [Internet]. London: Royal College of Nursing (UK); 2003 [cited 2022 Jul 26]. (National Institute for Health and Clinical Excellence: Guidance). http://www.ncbi.nlm.nih.gov/books/NBK48950/
41. Niël-Weise BS, van den Broek PJ. Urinary catheter policies for short-term bladder drainage in adults. Cochrane Database Syst Rev. 2005;(3):CD004203.
42. Jamison J, Maguire S, McCann J. Catheter policies for management of long term voiding problems in adults with neurogenic bladder disorders. Cochrane Database Syst Rev. 2004;(2):CD004375.
43. Norton C, Thomas L, Hill J. Management of faecal incontinence in adults: summary of NICE guidance. BMJ. 2007;334(7608):1370–1.
44. Bloomfield DM. Strategy for the management of vasovagal syncope. Drugs Aging. 2002;19(3):179–202.
45. Claydon VE, Steeves JD, Krassioukov A. Orthostatic hypotension following spinal cord injury: understanding clinical pathophysiology. Spinal Cord. 2006;44(6):341–51.
46. Cosortium for Spinal Cord Medicine. Respiratory management following spinal cord injury: a clinical practice guideline for health-care professionals. J Spinal Cord Med. 2005;28(3):259–93.
47. Supportive care and rehabilitation [Internet]. Metastatic spinal cord compression: diagnosis and management of patients at risk of or with metastatic spinal cord compression. National Collaborating Centre for Cancer (UK); 2008 [cited 2022 Aug 3]. https://www.ncbi.nlm.nih.gov/books/NBK55015/
48. Sundaresan N, Sachdev VP, Holland JF, Moore F, Sung M, Paciucci PA, et al. Surgical treatment of spinal cord compression from epidural metastasis. J Clin Oncol Off J Am Soc Clin Oncol. 1995;13(9):2330–5.
49. Mannion RJ, Wilby M, Godward S, Lyratzopoulos G, Laing RJC. The surgical management of metastatic spinal disease: prospective assessment and long-term follow-up. Br J Neurosurg. 2007;21(6):593–8.
50. Janssen SJ, Teunis T, van Dijk E, Ferrone ML, Shin JH, Hornicek F, et al. Validation of the Spine Oncology Study Group-Outcomes Questionnaire to assess quality of life in patients with metastatic spine disease. Spine J Off J North Am Spine Soc. 2017;17(6):768–76.

29 Ca Endometrium with Long-Standing Diabetes Mellitus for Radical Hysterectomy

Swapnil Y. Parab

29.1 Case Scenario

A 60-year-old female, presented with heavy post-menopausal bleeding, for 4 months. The patient is a known case of diabetes mellitus for 10 years, on oral hypoglycemic agents. The patient is obese with a body mass index of 35.5 kg/square meters. The patient underwent transvaginal sonography that revealed an endometrial thickness of 23 mm. Hysteroscopic biopsy of the endometrium showed adenocarcinoma. The patient is planned for radical hysterectomy with bilateral salpingo-oophorectomy and bilateral pelvic lymphadenectomy.

Q.1

Discuss the epidemiology and risk factors for EC.

Endometrial cancer (EC) is the most commonly seen malignancy among women in developed countries. EC occurs usually in postmenopausal women and the incidence is highest in the seventh decade of life [1]. Surgery is the treatment option for the early stages of cancer (stages I and II), and the five-year survival rates vary between 47% and 69% [1].

Estrogens, both internal and external, play an important role in the causation of EC. In addition, other risk factors for EC include old age, white race, metabolic syndrome, diabetes mellitus, early menarche, late menopause, overweight, radiation exposure, and polycystic ovarian syndrome [2].

Q.2

What is the association between diabetes mellitus, obesity, and EC?

The relationship between obesity, diabetes mellitus (DM), and cancer is complex and multifactorial. The strongest evidence is available for postmenopausal breast, endometrial and colorectal cancers. Visceral adiposity is now recognized as an endocrine organ that secretes adipokines, inflammatory cytokines, and estrogen. In a meta-analysis of 22 studies, DM was strongly associated with EC (relative risk (RR), 1.72, 95% CI, 1.48–2.01). DM-associated obesity, hyperglycemia, and hyperinsulinemia have been proposed as the mechanism of carcinogenesis in postmenopausal ladies [3]. Another meta-analysis showed that overweight (body mass index—BMI ≥25 kg/sq m) and obesity (BMI ≥30 kg/sq m) were associated with the increased risk of EC (RR for excess body weight, 1.62, 95% CI, 1.39–1.89 and RR for obesity, 2.54, 95%CI, 2.11–3.06) [4].

S. Y. Parab (✉)
Department of Anesthesiology, Critical Care and Pain, Tata Memorial Hospital, Mumbai, India

N. Gupta et al. (eds.), *Problem Based Learning Discussions in Onco-Anesthesia and Onco-Critical Care*, https://doi.org/10.1007/978-981-99-6339-3_29

Thus, there exists a definite relationship between DM, obesity, and the risk of EC.

Q.3

How is DM defined? How is it classified?

DM is a group of metabolic diseases that occurs due to defects in the secretion and/or action of insulin and is characterized by hyperglycemia. The diagnostic criteria for DM are shown in Table 29.1 [5]. According to 2017 American Diabetes Association (ADA) guidelines, DM can be classified into the following general categories:

1. Type 1 diabetes (autoimmune destruction of β-cell of the pancreas that leads to an absolute deficiency of insulin)
2. Type 2 diabetes (insulin resistance leading to progressive loss of β-cell insulin secretion)
3. Gestational DM (diabetes diagnosed in the second or third trim ester of pregnancy that was not clearly overt diabetes prior to gestation)
4. Specific types of diabetes, for example, monogenic diabetes syndromes (maturity-onset diabetes of the young, neonatal diabetes), diseases of the pancreas (e.g., cystic fibrosis), and drug-induced diabetes (e.g., glucocorticoid) [5]

Q.4

Discuss the multisystem affection due to DM.

DM affects multiple systems in the body. The mechanism of damage due to DM is vasculopathy. DM affects major vessels (macro-vasculopathy) as well as medium and small blood vessels (microangiopathy). Microvascular complications include nephropathy, neuropathy, and retinopathy, whereas macrovascular complications include myocardial infarction and stroke. Mechanisms of injury include the formation of advanced glycosylated end products, osmotic stress from sorbitol accumulation, and free radical-mediated oxidative stress [6]. Various systems of the body affected by DM are summarized below:

1. Diabetic nephropathy:
   (a) Proteinuria-microalbuminuria
   (b) Progressive decline in glomerular filtration rate
   (c) Accelerated hypertension and progression to end-stage kidney disease
2. Diabetic neuropathy:
   (a) Chronic symmetrical distal polyneuropathy—"glove-stocking" hypoesthesia/dysesthesia, sensory loss, night-time pain, and loss of spatial location of a limb

Table 29.1 Diagnostic criteria for diabetes mellitus

1	Symptoms of hyperglycemia plus random plasma glucose concentration ≥200 mg/dL (11.1 mmol/L) "Random" means any time of the day without regard to time since the last meal. Symptoms of hyperglycemia include polyurea, polydipsia, and unexplained weight loss.
OR	
2	Fasting plasma glucose ≥126 mg/dL (7.0 mmol/L) "Fasting" is defined as no calorie intake for at least 8 h.
OR	
3	Two-hour postprandial plasma glucose ≥200 mg/dL (11.1 mmol/L) during an oral glucose tolerance test. The test should be performed as described by WHO, using a glucose load containing the equivalent of 75 grams of anhydrous glucose dissolved in water.
OR	
4.	Glycosylated hemoglobin ≥6.5% The test should be performed using a method that is National Glycohaemoglobin Standardization Programme (NGSP) certified and standardized to Diabetes Control and Complication Trial (DCCT) assay.

   (b) Progressive motor dysfunction—diabetic amyotrophy
   (c) Autonomic dysfunction-orthostatic hypotension, resting tachycardia, gastroparesis, bloating, constipation/diarrhea, erectile dysfunction, neurogenic bladder and silent myocardial infarction
3. Diabetic retinopathy:
   (a) Retinal hemorrhages, exudates, proliferative retinopathy, and retinal detachment
4. Cardiovascular affection:
   (a) Accelerated atherosclerosis
   (b) Diabetic cardiomyopathy-diastolic dysfunction leading to exertional dyspnea
   (c) Endothelial dysfunction-prothrombotic state and accelerated hypertension
   (d) Congestive heart failure
5. Central nervous system affection:
   (a) Cerebral infarction and stroke
   (b) Accelerated atherosclerosis/dyslipidemia/pro-thrombotic stat → stroke
6. Gastrointestinal system:
   (a) Gastroparesis, nausea, vomiting, bloating, diarrhea and constipation

Q.5

How would you evaluate this patient in the pre-operative period? How would you optimize the patient for surgery?

The patient has a primary disease of EC along with two major comorbidities, that is, DM and obesity. Hence the aim of pre-operative evaluation would be to know the effect of disease and comorbidities on the physiology of the body. Since EC is associated with polymenorrhoea and menorrhagia, the patient often develops normocytic-normochromic or iron deficiency anemia. Hence, it is prudent to diagnose and treat the anemia accordingly. Cessation of smoking and alcohol should be followed for at least 12 weeks prior to surgery. Secondly, from a DM point of view, preoperative evaluation should aim to ensure the adequate functioning of vital organs like the heart, kidney, and central nervous system. Optimum glycemic control in the preoperative period should be achieved using oral hypoglycemic agents (OHA) and/or insulin. Although there is no cutoff value of the glycosylated hemoglobin (HbA1c) for preoperative fitness, the risk of postoperative morbidity and mortality increases with an increase in the level of HbA1c. Lastly, since the patient has morbid obesity, preoperative evaluation should look for any obesity-related modifiable complications like obstructive sleep apnea (OSA), deranged lipid profile, and poor cardiac function. Chest and limb physiotherapy strengthens the muscles and helps in conditioning the patient for major oncosurgery. A preoperative structured weight reduction program also helps in improving perioperative outcomes. In the case of OSA, the use of a continuous positive airway pressure device reduces the frequency of apnea-hypercapnia episodes and helps in normalizing the cardiovascular effects of OSA. Details of preoperative investigations and optimization are summarized in Table 29.2.

Q.6

Discuss the antidiabetic medications and their perioperative management.

Antidiabetic medications are primarily insulin and oral hypoglycemic agents (OHAs). Commonly used OHAs and their perioperative use are summarized in Table 29.3. In a diabetic patient undergoing elective surgery, it is important to adjust the doses of these drugs in the preoperative period so that preoperative blood sugar levels are well controlled and there are no major fluctuations in the glycemic control during the surgery and postoperation.

Although OHAs are used to optimize preoperative blood sugar control, it is best to avoid OHAs on the day of surgery and to resume their intake after enteral nutrition is started postoperatively. Variable absorption of OHAs, preoperative fasting period, and surgical stress are the common reasons why OHAs need to be replaced by insulin administration prior to surgery. Various types of insulin and their preoperative use are summarized in Table 29.4. The issues with exogenous administration of insulin are the following:

Table 29.2 Preoperative evaluation and optimization

Preoperative comorbidities	Endometrial cancer	Diabetes mellitus	Obesity
Preoperative investigations	(a) Complete hemogram, (b) Serum iron (c) Serum ferritin (d) Total iron binding capacity (TIBC) (e) Vitamin B12 and folic acid levels	(a) Blood sugar (fasting and postprandial) (b) Glycosylated hemoglobin (c) Test to assess end organ damages: 1. Electrocardiogram 2. Two-dimensional echocardiography 3. Renal function test 4. Urine examination to detect glycosuria and microalbuminuria 5. Tests for sensory-motor neuropathy 6. Lipid profile (in view of associated metabolic syndrome)	(a) Polysomnography test (b) Pulmonary artery pressure on the echocardiography
Preoperative optimization	(a) Replenishment of iron stores using intravenous iron supplements (b) Replenishment of vitamin B12 and folic acid by intravenous/intramuscular injections or oral supplements (c) Nutritional optimization as per proteins and energy requirement of the body (d) Smoking and alcohol cessation	1. Adjustment of OHA and insulin doses to achieve sugar control 2. Preoperative physiotherapy and muscle strengthening exercises	1. Use of CPAP machine to reduce the episodes of apnea-hypercarbia 2. A well-planned weight reduction program

Note: Although mortality increases with the increase in HbA1c levels, there is no consensus about any particular cutoff of HbA1c value for perioperative mortality

Table 29.3 Oral hypoglycemic agents and their perioperative use

Sr no.	Class	Mechanism of action	Generic name	Common side effects	Perioperative use for elective surgery
1	Sulfonylurea	Stimulation of insulin secretion by beta cells of islets of Langerhans in the pancreas	Second-generation: glimepiride, gliclazide, and glibenclamide	Hypoglycemic episodes	Stop on the morning of the surgery and restart as soon as food intake is resumed
2	Meglitinides	Stimulation of insulin secretion by the pancreas	Repaglinide and nateglinide	Hypoglycemic episodes	Stop on the morning of the surgery and restart as soon as food intake is resumed
3	Biguanides	Inhibition of mitochondrial respiratory chain and reduction in hepatic gluconeogenesis	Metformin	Lactic acidosis (in presence of renal dysfunction)	Stop on the morning of the surgery and restart after 24 h
4	Thiazolidinediones	Enhanced insulin sensitivity by activation of PPAR-gamma	Pioglitazone and rosiglitazone	Risk of myocardial infarction with rosiglitazone	To be continued perioperatively
5	Alpha-glucosidase inhibitor	Inhibits intestinal glucose absorption	Acarbose and voglibose		Stop on the morning of the surgery and restart after food intake is resumed
6	Dipeptidyl peptidase-4 inhibitor	Inhibition of GLP-1 degradation	Sitagliptin, linagliptin, and saxagliptin	Nausea, vomiting, and delayed gastric emptying	To be continued perioperatively
7	Sodium-glucose cotransporter-2 inhibitor (SGLT-2 inhibitor)	Facilitation of renal loss of glucose	Dapagliflozin and empagliflozin	Diuresis, hypovolemia, and euglycemic ketoacidosis	To be stopped for a minimum of 24 h prior to surgery and restarted after food intake is resumed
8	Glucagon-like peptide-1 agonists	Increase activity of GLP-1 and increase glucose-dependent insulin secretion	Liraglutide and semaglutide		Research ongoing

Table 29.4 Insulin types and preoperative use

Type of insulin	Name	Peak action	Duration of action	Day before surgery	Day of surgery
Rapid-acting	Lispro, Aspart	30–90 min	2–5 h	No change	Hold the dose
Short-acting	Regular insulin	2–5 h	5–8 h	No change	Hold the dose
Intermediate-acting	NPH	4–12 h	18–24 h	No change in the daytime dose, 75% of the evening dose, depending on glucose levels	50% of the morning dose
Long-acting	Glargine	6–8 h	24–42 h	75–100% of night dose depending on the glucose levels	75–100% of the morning dose

1. Exogenously administered insulin does not match the physiological variations of endogenous insulin secretion (which usually varies with feeding and starvation status).
2. Subcutaneously administered insulin has inadequate peak concentrations for the postprandial rise in blood sugar. Also, the systemic absorption of subcutaneously administered insulin is unpredictable.
3. Exogenously administered insulin enters systemic circulation, unlike endogenous insulin which is secreted into the portal circulation. Hence, the first-pass metabolism plays an important role in regulating the metabolic actions of insulin.
4. The logistic issues with the delivery of insulin (e.g., adsorption of insulin on the surfaces of the syringe and tubing) affect the consistent delivery of insulin.

Q.7

Discuss the perioperative targets for blood sugar control.

Most problems with poor glycemic control occur when blood sugar exceeds 180 mg%. A number of studies in the last two decades have tested the pros and cons of tight sugar control (blood sugar targets of 70–110 mg%) versus moderate sugar control (blood sugar targets between 140 and180 mg%). Tight sugar control has achieved better outcomes in terms of postoperative surgical site infections, cardiac complications, and overall mortality [7, 8]. However, there is a risk of hypoglycemia episodes in chasing tight sugar control targets. Instead, some studies have demonstrated the superiority of moderate sugar control over tight sugar control [9, 10]. Permissive hyperglycemia (blood sugar levels >180 mg%) is no longer acceptable.

Blood sugar should be measured on the morning of the surgery, an hour during the surgery when insulin infusions are being used, and 2 h during the postoperative period. Longer-acting insulin preparations should be switched to short-acting insulins prior to elective surgery.

Carbohydrate loading is a part of the "Enhanced Recovery After Surgery" program, as it prevents dehydration, improves insulin resistance, maintains glycogen stores, and decreases protein breakdown following surgery. However, current ADA guidelines recommend against carbohydrate loading in diabetic patients to limit the development of hyperglycemia in them [11].

Subcutaneously administered rapid-acting insulin or continuous infusion of regular insulin is used to control hyperglycemia during the surgery. Insulin infusion is the best method to control intraoperative blood sugars in patients undergoing procedures that involve hemodynamic fluctuations, significant blood loss, fluid shifts, and the need for vasopressors. Absorption of subcutaneously administered insulin becomes erratic in such scenarios and hence is not recommended [12].

There are many regimens of intraoperative sugar control that are described in literature. A detailed description is beyond the scope of this book. We prefer to use a variable dose insulin regimen depending on the blood glucose of the patient using a simple formula to adjust the rate of insulin infusion during the surgery: rate of regular insulin infusion per hour = blood glucose level/150. Increased insulin requirement is needed in case of sepsis, steroid administration, or fever. In such cases, the denominator changes to 100 [12].

Q.8

Discuss the treatment options for EC.

Surgery forms the mainstay of the treatment, especially in the clinically early stages of the disease. Total hysterectomy and bilateral salpingo-oophorectomy form the basic minimum surgery. In addition, pelvic or para-aortic lymph node dissection is done based on the stage of the disease and findings of imaging of the abdomen and pelvis. In case of the advanced stage of the disease at the time of presentation, neoadjuvant chemotherapy is given for 3–4 cycles, and then operability is decided based on the imaging [13]. The surgical approach may vary from open, laparoscopic, or robotic, depending on the comorbidities of the patient and the expertise available.

Q.9

Patient is planned for radical hysterectomy with bilateral salpingo-oophorectomy and pelvic lymphadenectomy. Describe the anesthesia management of the case.

Preoperative preparation for the surgery involves counseling of the patient, consent, evaluation of blood group and reservation of adequate blood, and bowel preparation. In the case of bowel preparation using an enema, adequate fluid replacement should be done the night before surgery. The patient should be allowed clear liquids till 2 h prior to surgery. Solid food is to be avoided after 10 pm on the night before the surgery. It is prudent to schedule these patients as first case to avoid prolonged fasting.

Thromboprophylaxis should be offered to all patients undergoing elective oncological surgery. Low molecular weight heparin should be administered 12 h prior to the surgery. Mechanical thromboprophylaxis measures like stockings or sequential compression devices should be used perioperatively.

In the operation theatre, a single wide-bore intravenous access is sufficient for the surgery. In a diabetic patient, another intravenous access is preferred for an infusion of insulin, if required during the surgery. Standard monitors for the surgery include an electrocardiogram, pulse oximeter, capnometer, temperature monitor, and noninvasive sphygmomanometer. An invasive blood pressure monitor is preferred in case of complex surgical plans, anticipated blood loss or fluid shifts, and multiple comorbidities of the patient.

The patient is positioned supine on the operation table. Obese patients should be transferred to the operation table using Hover mattresses or slide sheets. Patients should be well strapped using belts and bean bags to prevent sliding on the operation table, especially in case of a head-low lithotomy position during laparoscopic surgery.

Temperature regulation should be done with control of operation theater temperature, use of forced warm air mattresses, and fluid warming device. Limbs should be carefully padded to prevent pressure sores.

Intravenous antibiotic chemoprophylaxis should be given in the operation theater. Anxiolysis should be provided by intravenous midazolam at 0.04 mg/kg, monitoring the respiratory rate and oxygen saturation. Adequate pre-oxygenation should be done, as obese patients have the low functional residual capacity and short apnea time.

General anesthesia with lower thoracic epidural analgesia is a suitable option for open radical surgery. Epidural analgesia can be omitted in case of minimally invasive surgery.

Induction of anesthesia should be done with etomidate (0.2–0.3 mg/kg) or high-dose fentanyl (4–5 microgram per kg)-midazolam (0.04 mg/kg) combination, as both of these options prevent precipitous hypotension at the time of induction. It is especially important in cases having autonomic dysfunction due to long-standing DM. Long-standing DM affects the mobility of the atlanto-axial joint, reducing the extension of the head. Obesity and short neck also make laryngoscopy difficult. Hence, a propped-up position should be given by putting the roles under the shoulders of the patient. It helps in achieving adequate extension of the head. DM also increases the risk of aspiration due to gastroparesis. In view of all the potential difficulties, modified rapid sequence intubation (preoxygenation → induction agent → an attempt of ventilation → depolarizing muscle relaxant → intubation) can be planned.

Airway control should be secured with a cuffed endotracheal tube placed under the guidance of a direct laryngoscope or video-laryngoscope. Second-generation supraglottic device, a stylet, and a ventilating bougie should be kept ready as a backup plan of ventilation or intubation, in case of an unanticipated difficult airway. Controlled mechanical ventilation should be done using pressure control or volume control mode, with a tidal volume of 6–8 mL/kg and adequate positive end-expiratory pressure (the one at which driving pressure is measured the least). Oxygen-air combination along with a modern inhaled anesthetic agent (isoflurane/sevoflurane titrated to the minimum alveolar concentration of 0.8–1.0) should be used to maintain the depth of anesthesia. Nitrous oxide increases the risk of postoperative nausea and vomiting (PONV), distends the bowel loops, and causes postoperative atelectasis; hence it is best to avoid the use of nitrous oxide. In case of the laparoscopic surgeries, alveolar ventilation should be increased by 20–30% to tackle the hypercarbia due to the capnoperitoneum.

Intravenous strong opioids (e.g., fentanyl or morphine) should be used to titrate analgesia as per hemodynamic response. Intraoperative epidural infusion of 0.1% bupivacaine infusion reduces the requirement for analgesic and anesthetic agents. It also prevents the sympathetic response during the surgery and helps in preventing hyperglycemia during the surgery. Epidural analgesia offers good postoperative pain relief and helps in early ambulation and early return of bowel function.

Blood loss during the surgery should be carefully monitored and replaced. A nonliberal, individually tailored fluid strategy should be used to ensure adequate perfusion of the tissues (confirmed by means of stable hemodynamic parameters, urine output (0.3–0.5 mL/kg/h), or serum lactates less than 2 mg%). In case of hemodynamic instability, cardiac output monitoring devices may be used to provide goal (i.e., adequate stroke volume)-directed fluid therapy. A balanced salt solution should be used as a crystalloid. Blood products should be used as and when necessary, at the discretion of the anesthesiologist.

Antiemetic prophylaxis should be considered using either Inj ondansetron or Inj domperidone. For those with a high risk of PONV (female gender, use of opioids, nonsmoker, and past history of PONV), dual anti-emetic prophylaxis should be offered to the patient. In the case of DM, dexamethasone should not be used as an anti-emetic drug. In case of a difficult airway, the trachea should be extubated only after regaining adequate muscle power, reflexes, and consciousness.

Q.10

Discuss the postoperative analgesia plans for this patient.

Parenteral analgesic drugs like intravenous paracetamol (15–20 mg/kg 3–4 times a day) and nonsteroidal anti-inflammatory drugs (e.g., diclofenac 1 mg/kg three times a day) or selective COX-2 inhibitors (e.g., etoricoxib 1 mg/kg once or twice a day) should be administered unless contraindicated. Epidural analgesia forms the preferred method (grade A evidence) of analgesia according to "procedure-specific postoperative pain management"—PROSPECT website [14]. For the patients in whom epidural analgesia is not used, an alternate plan of analgesia should be implemented. It includes a bilateral transversus abdominis plane block or bilateral rectus sheath block or patient-controlled opioid analgesia.

Q.11

What are the postoperative concerns in this patient?

Postoperative care concerns in patients undergoing radical abdominal hysterectomy include postoperative pain, PONV, delirium, and the development of deep venous thrombosis.

Postoperative delirium is not uncommon in elderly patients. The incidence of postoperative delirium is 17.5% and is more commonly seen in patients with hypoalbuminemia, postoperative transfusion, and immobility [15].

Postoperative analgesia and thromboprophylaxis should be continued for 4–5 postoperative days. Ambulation and early enteral nutrition should resume at the earliest. Continuous positive airway pressure devices should be considered for patients with morbid obesity. Blood sugar should be monitored every 2–4 h and should be treated with a sliding scale of subcutaneously administered rapid-acting insulin. OHAs can be resumed once the enteral nutrition is resumed.

Q.12

Discuss the acute hyperglycemic complications and their management in diabetic patients in the perioperative period.

Hyperglycemic emergencies, namely, diabetic ketoacidosis (DKA) and hyperosmolar hyperglycemic state (HHS), can occur during the perioperative period. The hallmark of both conditions is acute hyperglycemia caused due to deficiency of circulating insulin and/or concomitant elevation in counter-regulatory hormones like cortisol, glucagon, catecholamines, etc.

The pathophysiology of hyperglycemic emergencies is shown in Fig. 29.1.

DKA is more commonly seen in type 1 DM patients. Any stress in the body can trigger the development of DKA. The classical presentation of DKA includes fatigue, polyuria, polydipsia, diffuse abdominal pain (reported in 46% of patients), and nausea-vomiting (reported in 66% of patients). Nearly 50% of patients present with lethargy and stupor. Physical examination reveals signs of dehydration (dryness of mouth and con-

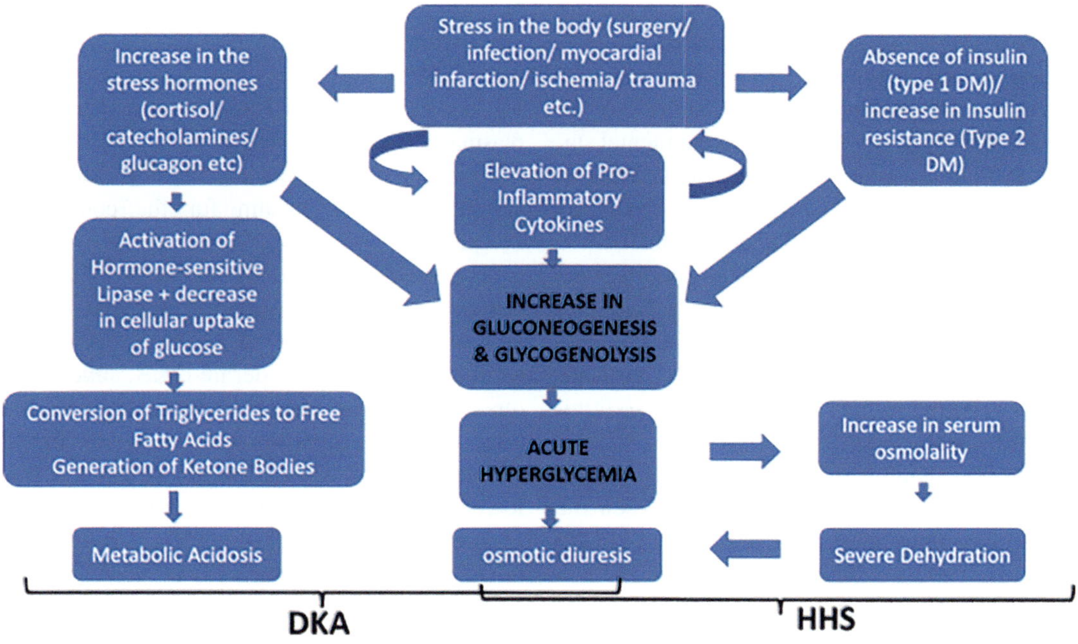

Fig. 29.1 Pathophysiology of hyperglycemic crises

Table 29.5 Diagnostic criteria for hyperglycemic crises

Parameters	Diabetic ketoacidosis (plasma glucose >250 mg%)			Hyperosmolar hyperglycemic state (plasma glucose >600 mg%)	Euglycemic DKA (plasma glucose <200 mg%)
	Mild	Moderate	Severe		
Arterial pH	7.25–7.30	7.00–7.24	<7.00	>7.30	<7.30
Serum bicarbonate (meq/L)	15–18	10–15	<10	>18	
Urine ketone	Positive	Positive	Positive	Small	Positive
Serum Ketone	Positive	Positive	Positive	Small	Positive
Effective serum osmolality	Variable	Variable	Variable	>320 mosm/kg	Variable/raised
Anion gap	>10	>12	>12	<12	
Mental status	Alert	Alert/ drowsy	Stupor/ coma	Stupor/coma	Alert
Water deficit	5%	5–7%	7–10%	>10%	5–7%
Type of DM	Type 1 DM	Type 1 DM	Type 1 DM	Type 2 DM	Type 1 or 2 DM, patients on SGLT-2 inhibitors

junctiva, poor skin turgor, hypotension, and tachycardia). Patients are often tachypneic and exhibit a classic fruity (acetone) breath odor. On investigation, patients show the classic triad of hyperglycemia, ketonemia, and high anion gap metabolic acidosis.

HHS is more commonly seen in elderly patients with type 2 DM. Relative deficiency of insulin leads to a hyperglycemic state; however, the insulin levels are adequate enough to prevent lipolysis and ketogenesis. As compared to DKA, hyperglycemia and volume deficit are more severe in HHS. HHS presents insidiously over days to weeks, with progressive decline in the mental status, leading to delirium, coma, and seizures. Hyperviscosity-associated complications like thrombosis may be seen in patients with HHS.

Euglycemic DKA is another condition in which blood glucose levels are not too high, but ketonemia and metabolic acidosis exist. It occurs in type 1 as well as type 2 DM. It is more commonly reported in patients consuming "sodium-glucose transporter-2 inhibitor" (SGLT-2 inhibitor—dapagliflozin).

Salient differentiating features between the three conditions are discussed in Table 29.5 [16, 17].

Treatment of hyperglycemic emergencies involves fluid resuscitation, insulin administration, correction of electrolytes, and vigilant monitoring.

Initial fluid therapy is administered to expand the intravascular, interstitial, and intracellular volumes. In the absence of cardiac disease, isotonic saline (0.9% NaCl) should be infused at a rate of 15–20 mL per kg per hour (nearly 1–1.5 L during the first hour). Subsequently 0.45% saline is continued at 250–500 mL/h and should be used if the corrected serum sodium is normal or high. If corrected serum sodium is low, then 0.9% NaCl is continued at a similar rate. In DKA, the mean duration in which plasma glucose drops below 250 mg% is 6 h while the mean duration for ketosis to get corrected is 12 h. Once the plasma glucose drops to 200 mg%, 5% dextrose is added to the replacement fluids to allow the administration of insulin for the control of ketonemia.

The mainstay of the treatment is the administration of intravenous insulin. Regular insulin is preferred over intermediate or long-acting insulin. For mild to moderate DKA, subcutaneous rapid-acting insulin is equally safe and effective. For complicated DKA, an initial bolus of insulin should be 0.1 U per kg, followed by an infusion at 0.1 U/kg/h. It reduces plasma glucose at the rate of 50–75 mg/dL per hour. When the blood sugar drops below 200 mg/dL in DKA and 300 mg/dL in HHS, the insulin rate should be halved, and dextrose infusion should be added to avoid hypoglycemia.

Serum potassium should be checked prior to the administration of insulin. For values less than 3.3 meq/L, supplemental potassium is administered at the rate of 20–30 meq/L per hour. Bicarbonate administration is required in severe DKA when pH drops below 7.0. Nearly 50–100 mmol of sodium bicarbonate is administered to correct the acidosis. Phosphate supplementation is advisable only if serum phosphate concentration is less than 1.0 mg%.

Vigilant monitoring is required during the correction of hyperglycemic crises. Venous pH, plasma glucose, serum electrolytes, osmolality, and signs of dehydration should be monitored every 2–4 h. In DKA, treatment is targeted to achieve plasma glucose <200 mg%, serum bicarbonate >18 meq/L, and venous pH >7.30. In HHS, serum glucose is maintained at higher plasma levels (between 250 and 300 mg%) to avoid cerebral edema [17].

References

1. Sung H, Ferlay J, Siegel RL, Laversanne M, Soerjomataram I, Jemal A, et al. Global cancer statistics 2020: GLOBOCAN estimates of incidence and mortality worldwide for 36 cancers in 185 countries. CA Cancer J Clin. 2021;71(3):209–49. https://doi.org/10.3322/caac.21660.
2. Passarello K, Kurian S, Villanueva V. EC: An overview of pathophysiology, management, and care. Semin Oncol Nurs. 2019;35(2):157–65. https://doi.org/10.1016/j.soncn.2019.02.002.
3. Saed L, Varse F, Baradaran HR, Moradi Y, Khateri S, Friberg E, et al. The effect of diabetes on the risk of EC: an updated systematic review and meta-analysis. BMC Cancer. 2019;19(1):527. https://doi.org/10.1186/s12885-019-5748-4.
4. Zhang Y, Liu H, Yang S, Zhang J, Qian L, Chen X. Overweight, obesity and EC risk: results from a systematic review and meta-analysis. Int J Biol Markers. 2014;29(1):e21–9. https://doi.org/10.5301/jbm.5000047.
5. American Diabetes Association Professional Practice Committee. 2. Classification and diagnosis of diabetes: standards of medical care in diabetes-2022. Diabetes Care. 2022;45(Suppl 1):S17–38. https://doi.org/10.2337/dc22-S002.
6. Lotfy M, Adeghate J, Kalasz H, Singh J, Adeghate E. Chronic complications of diabetes mellitus: a mini review. Curr Diabetes Rev. 2017;13(1):3–10. https://doi.org/10.2174/1573399812666151016101622.
7. Lai J, Li Q, He Y, Zou S, Bai X, Rastogi S. Glycemic control regimens in the prevention of surgical site infections: a meta-analysis of randomized clinical trials. Front Surg. 2022;9:855409. https://doi.org/10.3389/fsurg.2022.855409.
8. Jin X, Wang J, Ma Y, Li X, An P, Wang J, et al. Association between perioperative glycemic control strategy and mortality in patients with diabetes undergoing cardiac surgery: a systematic review and meta-analysis. Front Endocrinol (Lausanne). 2020;11:513073. https://doi.org/10.3389/fendo.2020.513073.
9. Bhamidipati CM, LaPar DJ, Stukenborg GJ, Morrison CC, Kern JA, Kron IL, et al. Superiority of moderate control of hyperglycemia to tight control in patients undergoing coronary artery bypass grafting. J Thorac Cardiovasc Surg. 2011;141(2):543–51. https://doi.org/10.1016/j.jtcvs.2010.10.005.
10. Sathya B, Davis R, Taveira T, Whitlatch H, Wu WC. Intensity of peri-operative glycemic control and postoperative outcomes in patients with diabetes: a meta-analysis. Diabetes Res Clin Pract. 2013;102(1):8–15. https://doi.org/10.1016/j.diabres.2013.05.003.
11. Duggan EW, Carlson K, Umpierrez GE. Perioperative hyperglycemia management: an update. Anesthesiology. 2017;126(3):547–60.
12. Duggan E, Chen Y. Glycemic management in the operating room: screening, monitoring, oral hypoglycemics, and insulin therapy. Curr Diab Rep. 2019;19(11):134. https://doi.org/10.1007/s11892-019-1277-4.
13. Oaknin A, Bosse TJ, Creutzberg CL, Giornelli G, Harter P, Joly F, et al. ESMO Guidelines Committee. Electronic address: clinicalguidelines@esmo.org. Endometrial cancer: ESMO Clinical Practice Guideline for diagnosis, treatment, and follow-up. Ann Oncol. 2022:S0923-7534(22)01207-8. https://doi.org/10.1016/j.annonc.2022.05.009.
14. https://esraeurope.org/pain-management/. Accessed on 3 Sep 2022.
15. McAlpine JN, Hodgson EJ, Abramowitz S, Richman SM, Su Y, Kelly MG, et al. The incidence and risk factors associated with postoperative delirium in geriatric patients undergoing surgery for suspected gynecologic malignancies. Gynecol Oncol. 2008;109(2):296–302. https://doi.org/10.1016/j.ygyno.2008.02.016.
16. Fayfman M, Pasquel FJ, Umpierrez GE. Management of hyperglycemic crises: diabetic ketoacidosis and hyperglycemic hyperosmolar state. Med Clin North Am. 2017;101(3):587–606. https://doi.org/10.1016/j.mcna.2016.12.011.
17. Kitabchi AE, Umpierrez GE, Miles JM, Fisher JN. Hyperglycemic crises in adult patients with diabetes. Diabetes Care. 2009;32(7):1335–43. https://doi.org/10.2337/dc09-9032.

Anaesthetic Considerations for a Child with Retinoblastoma for Orbital Enucleation

30

Renu Sinha and Soumya Sarkar

30.1 Case History

A 10-month-old boy with unilateral retinoblastoma presented for primary enucleation. The child had not received any chemotherapy or radiotherapy earlier.

30.2 Introduction

Q.1

What is Epidemilogy of Retiniblastoma and Common Presenatation?

Retinoblastoma (RB) was reported first in 1597 by Petras Pawius, and it accounts for 6% of all malignancies in children below 5 years. The annual global incidence is around 6000–8000 and over 1400 cases are from India each year [1]. Two-thirds of cases of RB are usually diagnosed before age 2 years, and 95% of cases are diagnosed before age 5 years [2]. It usually bears an autosomal dominant inheritance pattern associated with the RB1 gene mutation. Leukocoria (60%) is the most common finding at presentation. Other common symptoms are strabismus (20%), red painful eye (5%), poor vision, orbital cellulitis, unilateral mydriasis and heterochromia iridis [3]. Neovascularization, neovascular glaucoma, hyphaema, pseudohypopyon and vitreous haemorrhage may be observed in advanced cases. Mortality rate is around 95% without treatment due to metastasis in the brain.

Investigations are done to classify the tumour, to see the extent of tumour and for planning the treatment include ultrasound (USG), computed tomography (CT), magnetic resonance imaging (MRI), bone scan, bone marrow aspiration and lumbar puncture. USG is done to assess tumour size and to detect calcification within the tumour. CT also detects calcification. MRI is superior to CT for optic nerve evaluation and detection of extraocular extension but cannot detect calcification.

Q.2

What are the treatment goals for a patient with retinoblastoma?

Treatment goals include the preservation of both life and vision. Management of RB is multidisciplinary with prognosis of 80% vision salvage, 90% eye salvage and 98% life salvage [4]. Chemotherapy is the first line of treatment and 65% will be cured with it [5]. Chemotherapy is

R. Sinha (✉)
Department of Aanesthesiology, Pain Medicine & Critical Care, RP Centre, AIIMS, New Delhi, India
e-mail: renusinha@aiims.edu

S. Sarkar (✉)
Department of Anaesthesiology, AIIMS, Kalyani, India

N. Gupta et al. (eds.), *Problem Based Learning Discussions in Onco-Anesthesia and Onco-Critical Care*, https://doi.org/10.1007/978-981-99-6339-3_30

administered via intravenous route, intraarterial in the ophthalmic artery and intravitreal or periocular (subtenon). Mostly 2–3 drugs are administered simultaneously, intravenously or orally. A standard combination used to shrink intraocular RB is carboplatin, vincristine and etoposide. Combination of two drugs such as carboplatin and vincristine may be used for very small tumour. In case RB is not responding to these drugs, other drugs have been used. Intravitreal or periocular melphalan and topotecan injections are also administered for vitreous seedlings of tumour.

External radiation brachytherapy may be required after chemotherapy to save the eye. Thirty-five percent of patients require enucleation or sometimes exenteration for advanced cases. Mortality is around 8% [5].

30.2.1 Primary Concerns

Q.3

What are the Primary Anesthesia Concerns for a Patient with Retinoblastoma Scheduled for Ennucleation?

1. Paediatric age group.
2. Separation anxiety in >6-month-old patients.
3. Majority of the children with RB underwent multiple general anaesthesia exposure for ophthalmic evaluations, chemotherapy and radiotherapy which may result in development of post-traumatic stress disorder [6].
4. Potential side effects of chemotherapy: neutropenia, secondary leukaemia, cardiotoxicity, deafness, infections and other systemic (pulmonary, renal, hepatic, gastrointestinal, neurological) involvement [7].
5. Difficult intravenous access [8].
6. **Associated syndromes:** ROHHAD syndrome (rapid-onset obesity, hypothalamic dysfunction, hypoventilation and autonomic dysfunction), Costello syndrome, Noonan syndrome, neurofibromatosis type 1, Beckwith–Wiedemann syndrome, etc. [9].
7. Oculo-cardiac reflex (OCR): Dissection of the extra-ocular muscles is required during enucleation which leads to significant risk of OCR [10].
8. Blood loss.

30.2.2 Preoperative Evaluation

Q.4

Enumerate the Specific Things you will Check During Preoperative Evaluation?

1. *Comprehensive history and physical examination:* to rule out any other existing medical problems.
2. *Complete blood count:* to look for neutropenia and haemoglobin.
3. *ECG*: Patients receiving cisplatin and anthracyclines (including epirubicin and doxorubicin) often present with QT prolongation, Torsades de Pointes, which may lead to ventricular tachycardia [11].
4. *Post chemotherapy echocardiography*: The anthracyclines, cyclophosphamide, 5-fluorouracil (5-FU), bleomycin, paclitaxel and docetaxel have serious cardiac toxicity. Apart from chemotherapy, radiotherapy also can affect cardiac valves, vessels and pericardium. The impact in terms of hypotension, hypertension, arrhythmias, myocardial infarction, congestive cardiac failure, cardiomyopathy, myocarditis and pericarditis, leading to pericardial effusion, can be immediate or delayed. The echocardiogram should focus on specific details regarding cardiac wall contractility, left ventricular ejection fraction and pericardial fluid [7, 11].
5. *Site for intravenous access:* due to difficult cannulation.
6. *Drugs used for pupillary dilatation*: pupil should be dilated for adequate retinal examination. Mydriatic drugs like timolol and phenylephrine have been used for pupillary dilatation, and their systemic effects can lead to complications. Phenylephrine can lead to

bradycardia and hypertension during anaesthesia, and intraoperative pulmonary oedema has been reported which necessitates ICU admission and ventilation.

30.2.3 Anaesthesia Management

30.2.3.1 Premedication

The decision to pre-medicate the child and the modality (oral, intravenous or intra nasal) is tailored according to the requirement of the child, the preferences of the anaesthesiologist and the availability of resources. Midazolam, ketamine, dexmedetomidine and clonidine have been used for premedication [12]. However, premedication is avoided in children with an anticipated difficult airway. Alternatively, non-pharmacological techniques like video distraction, parental presence and preoperative incentive-based game therapy have shown promising results [13].

30.2.3.2 Induction of Anaesthesia

Choice of intravenous or inhalational induction depends on the child's preference, at the discretion of the anaesthetist and comorbidities. Usually, these children do not have intravenous access preoperatively. In children with intellectual disability, seizure disorder or comorbidities, IV access can be secured in the preoperative room after the application of a eutectic mixture of local anaesthetics (EMLA). Usually, the IV induction is preferred in a child with a big orbital mass to avoid eye compression with a face mask [12, 14].

30.2.3.3 Airway Management

Goals of ophthalmic surgery include akinesia, analgesia and low intraocular pressure. During ophthalmic surgery, access to the airway is also restricted for anaesthesiologist. Thus, endotracheal intubation with paralysis and controlled ventilation is preferable in very young children. Preformed south-facing RAE tube, a reinforced flexible tracheal tube (ETT) may be beneficial in this scenario. However, second-generation supraglottic airway devices (SAD) can be a good alternative in children as it allows smoother induction and emergence from anaesthesia and has much less effect on IOP [15]. SAD can be used with controlled ventilation with muscle relaxants.

30.2.3.4 Maintenance of Anaesthesia

The choice of maintenance is under the discretion of anaesthesiologists. While isoflurane or sevoflurane is preferred inhalational agents over halothane, which bears an increased risk of dysrhythmias, total intravenous anaesthesia (TIVA) with propofol can be a better alternative in terms of reducing the risk of postoperative nausea and vomiting (PONV) [12, 15]. Adrenaline soaked gauge pieces are used to reduce bleeding during surgery especially after removal of eye ball. Anaesthesiologist should calculate the maximum dose of adrenaline which can be diluted in saline. After removal of eye ball, an implant is inserted to fill the empty intra-orbital space. Surgical duration for enucleation is around 40–80 min. Usually blood loss is minimal and blood transfusion is rarely required. Surgical duration of exenteration is around 60–100 min depending on the surgeon's experience, and blood loss is more in comparison to enucleation. Pressure bandage should be done before extubation to reduce postoperative bleeding. Coughing and bucking during extubation or SAD removal should be avoided as it can lead to postoperative bleeding. Intravenous bolus of fentanyl, propofol or lignocaine will help to blunt extubation response. Face mask should not compress the eye bandage and head should be turned towards the opposite side of the operated eye while making lateral position to avoid ocular compression.

30.2.3.5 Oculocardiac Reflex (OCR)

Q.5

What is Oculocardiac Reflex? What are the Options to Manage it?

The incidence of oculocardiac (OCR) reflex is around 60% during paediatric eye surgery. Surgical traction of extra-ocular eye muscles or compression over the globe during enucleation may result in sinus bradycardia, junctional rhythms, atrioventricular block, atrial ectopics or ventricular ectopics. Pulling of the medial rectus muscle is most commonly associated with it, in which the afferent innervation is the ophthalmic division of the trigeminal nerve, which communicates through the sensory nucleus in the fourth ventricle to the efferent vagus nerve.

It resolves immediately with the withdrawal of stimulus and weakens with repetition. Intravenous atropine 10–20 μg/kg or glycopyrrolate 10 μg/kg can be used as a therapeutic modality. However, pre-emptive prophylaxis with anticholinergic is debatable. Topical local anaesthetic agents (proparacaine 0.5%), peribulbar block, sub-tenon's block, maintenance of normocarbia and a deeper plane of anaesthesia can attenuate the OCR [10, 12].

30.2.3.6 Intraoperative Analgesia

Q.6

What are the Options aAvailable for Perioperative Analgesia in this Patient?

Apart from opioids (fentanyl, morphine), non-steroidal anti-inflammatory drugs (NSAIDs) and paracetamol and regional blocks with general anaesthesia have been attributed for a significant reduction in the opioid requirement, OCR and PONV [16].

Peribulbar block shows an excellent safety margin in children [17]. There is always risk of extraocular tumour spread in case of globe perforation during peribulbar block. Sub-tenon infiltration of local anaesthetic drugs seems to be more efficacious and devoid of needle complications [18]. Maximum dose of local anaesthetic agent should be calculated before administration of block especially in infants.

Postoperative Care

Q.7

Enumerate the Concerns in the Postoperative Period for this Patient?

Mild to moderate postoperative pain is usually well managed with paracetamol and NSAIDs. Pre-emptively, they can be started preoperatively or rectally/IV at induction. The multimodal approach by means of the administration of tramadol, fentanyl and even escalation to morphine may be needed. However, there is increased risk of PONV with opioids. In the absence of anti-emetic prophylaxis, 60% of children are prone to develop PONV after ocular surgery. Intravenous ondansetron (0.15 mg/kg) alone, or with combination of dexamethasone (0.1–0.2 mg/kg), effectively reduces the incidence to 10% [19].

References

1. Rodriguez-Galindo C, Orbach DB, VanderVeen D. Retinoblastoma. Pediatr Clin N Am. 2015;62:201–23.
2. Abramson DH. Retinoblastoma: diagnosis and management. CA Cancer J Clin. 1982;32:130–40.
3. Abramson DH, Frank CM, Susman M, et al. Presenting signs of retinoblastoma. J Pediatr. 1998;132:505–8.
4. Rao R, Hanovar S. Retinoblastoma. Indian J Pediatr. 2017;84(12):937–44.
5. Kaliki S, Patel A, Iram S, Ramappa G, Mohamed A, Palkonda VA. Retinoblastoma in India: clinical presentation and outcome in 1,457 patients (2,074 eyes). Retina. 2019;39(2):379–91.
6. Resource R, Life C, Support P. Post-traumatic stress disorder in childhood cancer—WE C Hope. WE C Hope https://wechopeorg/retinoblastoma/child-life/psychological-support/ptsd/. Published 2022. Accessed 31 July 2022.
7. Allan N, Siller C, Breen A. Anaesthetic implications of chemotherapy. Continu Educ Anaesth Crit Care Pain. 2012;12(2):52–6.
8. Bahl A, Johnson S, Alsbrooks K, Mares A, Gala S, Hoerauf K. Defining difficult intravenous access (DIVA): a systematic review. J Vasc Access. 2021:11297298211059648.
9. Kamihara J, Bourdeaut F, Foulkes WD, Molenaar JJ, Mossé YP, Nakagawara A, Parareda A, Scollon SR, Schneider KW, Skalet AH, States LJ. Retinoblastoma and neuroblastoma predisposition and surveillance. Clin Cancer Res. 2017;23(13):e98–106.
10. James I. Anaesthesia for paediatric eye surgery. Continu Educ Anaesth Crit Care Pain. 2008;8:5–10.
11. Ewer M, Benjamin R. Cardiotoxicity of chemotherapeutic drugs. In: Perry M, editor. The chemotherapy source book. London: Williams and Wilkins; 1996. p. 649–59.

12. Sinha R, Ranjan RB. Anesthesia for ophthalmic procedures. Principles and practice of pediatric anesthesia. 1st ed. New Delhi: Jaypee Brothers Medical Publisher; 2017. p. 258–69.
13. Manyande A, Cyna AM, Yip P, Chooi C, Middleton P. Non-pharmacological interventions for assisting the induction of anaesthesia in children. Cochrane Database Syst Rev. 2015;2015(7):CD006447.
14. Sinha R, Shende D, Garg R. Comparison of propofol (1%) with admixture (1:1) of thiopentone (1.25%) and propofol (0.5%) for laryngeal mask airway insertion in children undergoing elective eye surgery: double masked randomized clinical trial. Indian J Anaesth. 2010;54(2):104–8.
15. Smith SJ, Pettigrew TY. Anaesthesia for eye surgery in paediatrics. Anaesth Intensive Care Med. 2019;20(12):721–4.
16. Schaller B, Sandu N, Filis A, Buchfelder M. Peribulbar block or topical application of local anaesthesia combined for paediatric strabismus surgery. Anaesthesia. 2008;63(10):1142–3.
17. Deb K, Subramaniam R, Dehran M, Tandon R, Shende D. Safety and efficacy of peribulbar block as adjunct to general anaesthesia for paediatric ophthalmic surgery. Paediatr Anaesth. 2001;11(2):161–7.
18. Kalaiyarasan R, Shende D, Parthiban M, Lomi N. Comparison of peribulbar block and subtenon infiltration in pediatric enucleation for retinoblastoma. Indian J Ophthalmol. 2021;69(8):2106–10.
19. Tramer M, Moore A, McQuay H. Prevention of vomiting after paediatric strabismus surgery: a systematic review using numbers-needed-to-treat method. Br J Anaesth. 1995;75:556–61.

Anaesthesia for Central Airway Obstruction

31

Rohini Dattatri, Anju Gupta, and Nishkarsh Gupta

A 55-year-old male with a history of exertional breathlessness for 5 months, haemoptysis for 2 weeks and acute onset stridor for a day presented to the emergency department. He was a chronic smoker for 30 years (20 pack years). On examination, he was found to have a heart rate of 100/min and respiratory rate of 35/min along with stridor and difficulty speaking in sentences. He was in a propped-up position. Respiratory system auscultation revealed extensive rhonchi and crept with a room air saturation of 90%. There was the use of accessory muscles for respiration. ABG revealed Pa02 58 mm Hg and $PaCO_2$ 60 mm Hg, pH 7.1 Multi-slice CT scan showed the presence of a tracheal mass with 5 mm stenosis together with dynamic airway collapse. He was posted for rigid bronchoscopy and tracheal stenting.

31.1 What Are the Causes of Central Airway Obstruction (CAO)?

The trachea and the main bronchi are referred to as "central airways" (Tables 31.1 and 31.2).

R. Dattatri · A. Gupta · N. Gupta (✉)
Onco-Anaesthesiology and Palliative Medicine, Dr BRAIRCH, AIIMS, New Delhi, India

N. Gupta et al. (eds.), *Problem Based Learning Discussions in Onco-Anesthesia and Onco-Critical Care*, https://doi.org/10.1007/978-981-99-6339-3_31

Table 31.1 Classification of CAO

Classification of CAO

Based on the location	Intrinsie Extrinsic Mixed Intra-thoracic Extra-thoracie Variable
Based on the type of airflow limitation	Dynamic Fixed

Table 31.2 Indications for airway stenting [1]

• Malignant	Intra-luminal	Adenoid cystic Mucoepidermoid Carcinoid
	Extra-luminal	Esophageal Ca Mediastinal tumours Sarcomas
• Benign	Trauma	Post-intubation Blunt/penetrating injury to airway Inhalational
	Inflammatory	Wegener's granulomatosis, SLE Sarcoidosis
	Infections	TB, bacterial tracheitis, viral tracheobronchitis, rhinoscleroma
	Vascular	Rings, aneurysms
	Neoplastic	Pabillomas, neurofibroma
	Anastomotic	Lung transplant, sleeve resection
	Miscellaneous	Tracheomalacia

31.2 Describe the Airway Stents

Montgomery is the pioneer of airway stents who first used it in a patient with sub-glottic stenosis in the mid-1960s. Dumon introduced silicone stents.

- Stents can be made of metal, silicone or a combination of different materials. Metal stents can be self-expanding (SEMS) or fixed in diameter, covered (polyurethane, polytetrafluoroethylene and silicone) or uncovered. SEMS is made of nickel-titanium alloy—nitinol. Silicone stents come only in fixed diameters and polypropylene/carbon fibre may be used to reinforce the stents. Radial pressure exertion and frictional forces maintain the stents in their position. Biodegradable materials have been tried in stents although not yet available for clinical use as a result of mixed results in clinical trials. Stents of different sizes and shapes are available and can be custom-made based on the indication of stenting.
- Metal stents (specifically uncovered stents) are difficult to remove and reposition due to the epithelisation and hence preferred in malignant airway obstruction where palliation is the goal. Metallic stents also carry the risk of perforation and granuloma formation [2, 3]. However, there are reports of these stents being successfully placed in benign central airway obstruction too [4].
- On the other hand, covered metal stents are easier to remove and resistant to granuloma formation. Metallic stent usage in benign conditions should be preferred only in those who are unfit for open procedures; conservative endoscopic management has failed as the long-term data regarding the safety of these stents in benign diseases is unavailable [5].
- It has been reported in the literature that nearly 95% of symptomatic patients can benefit from airway stenting in carefully chosen cases if done by experienced personnel [6]. In patients with terminal cancer, it improves the quality of life [7]. It can facilitate early extubation in patients who have become ventilator-dependent [8]. In addition, stents have been used effectively to manage bronchial dehiscence, stenoses and bronchomalacia which can occur after lung transplantation [9].
- Silicone stents are preferred in benign diseases for the ease of removal. The advantages and disadvantages of metal and silicone stents have been summarised in Tables 31.3 and 31.4, respectively.
- Hybrid stents made of more than one material are also used but are expensive.

Table 31.3 Pros and cons of metal stents [10]

	Pros	Cons
Metallic stents	The inner diameter is larger as compared to outer diameter. Stent migration is uncommon. It does not affect the muco-ciliary function. These stents can be placed using fibreoptic bronchoscope.	Removal and re-positioning Risk of vascular perforation, granuloma formation and tumour invasion is high. Covered stents are inflammable. Laser energy can be transmitted.

Table 31.4 Pros and cons of silicone stents [10]

	Pros	Cons
Silicone stents	Both repositioning and extraction of these stents are easier. Tumour invasion and granuloma formation are less common.	Rigid bronchoscopy is required for insertion. Inner diameter of the stent is smaller compared to outer diameter. Prone for migration Can affect the muco-ciliary function leading to pooling of secretions with increased susceptibility to infections Inflammable

31.3 What Are the Complications of Airway Stenting?

The complication rate following therapeutic bronchoscopy for CAO is low (3.9%) as reported by the American College of Chest Physicians Quality Improvement Registry, Evaluation and, Education ACCS AQuIRE [11].

Complications following the insertion of stents could be acute/early or long term. Close vigilance is required to prevent/or recognise the complications early to provide suitable intervention. Early complications can occur due to rigid bronchoscopy and include trauma to the teeth, oropharynx and airways. Barotrauma is a known complication. Gas embolism, tension pneumothorax, pneumomediastinum and subcutaneous emphysema can occur with the use of jet ventilation. Hypoxaemia, hypercarbia and acidosis can be expected to occur especially in those with pre-existing pulmonary disease. Acute obstruction of the airway is a catastrophic complication that can occur during the time of induction and during the procedure or post-procedure. The presence of severe hypoxia, intolerance to the supine position and resting stridor are a few risk factors predicting the occurrence of this problem. Rigid bronchoscopy should be immediately available to relieve the obstruction and identify the cause. Few cases might require VV ECHO to tide over the emergency. Bleeding during the procedure, laryngeal oedema and stent migration can predispose to airway obstruction [12].

Stent stenosis, migration and fracture of the stent and stent erosion are some late complications. Formation of granulation tissue leading to restenosis and recurrence of obstructive symptoms is possible with metallic stents [13]. Silicone stents can affect muco-ciliary clearance resulting in the impaction of secretions. There is also an increased chance of migration of these stents. Disseminated pneumonia can occur [12]. Metallic stents can erode the airway leading to the development of broncho-vascular fistula or esophago-respiratory fistula which can result in massive haemoptysis or aspiration pneumonia, respectively [14]. In case of major haemorrhage, opening the thoracic cavity might be required and the anaesthetist should be prepared for the same.

31.4 What Are the Anaesthetic Considerations in this Procedure?

- A comprehensive history and physical examination along with appropriate investigations should address these issues. The clinical status of the patient as well as the degree of physiologic compromise determines the evaluation of these patients. Cough, haemoptysis, breathlessness and wheezing are the usual presenting symptoms. The presence of stridor usually indicates advanced stenoses (5–8 mm) [15]. Numerous factors such as pre-existing pulmonary disease, cardiac disease, strength of the respiratory muscles, metabolic demand, pain and anxiety contribute to the perception of dyspnoea despite a common myth that symptoms do not occur until the tracheal diameter has reduced to 8 mm (for exertion symptoms) and 5 mm (for symptoms at rest). Postural variation in symptoms should be specifically asked for so that the patient can be positioned accordingly during induction of anaesthesia as well as help to relieve the life-threatening airway obstruction.
- Attention should be paid to the presence of comorbidities like hypertension, COPD and diabetes as they can increase the risk of complications such as bleeding and hypoxaemia. Although optimisation of comorbidities is difficult due to the emergent nature of the procedure, due consideration must be given.
- Patients with airway obstruction are considered high-risk because of compromised airway, deranged physiology and sharing of airway which requires adequate peri-procedural planning and preparation and a good team effort for a successful outcome. The procedure of airway stenting is usually done in a bronchoscopy suite which is a remote location. Hence, an anaesthetist should be prepared for anaesthesia in remote locations with specific attention paid to the presence of emergency resuscitation equipment, drugs, trained personnel, working anaesthesia machine and suction apparatus, airway equipment, reliable oxygen source with back-up, safe electrical outlets and ASA standard anaesthesia monitoring facility. Preoperative

planning involves determining the location and severity of obstruction, the procedure to be performed, the requirement of general anaesthesia, the stent type to be used, backup plans and post-operative management [10].

- In case of airway stenting due to malignancy, the local mass effects (SVC syndrome, recurrent laryngeal nerve palsy, phrenic nerve palsy, cardiac compression, tracheoesophageal fistula), systemic effects, presence of paraneoplastic syndromes (Lambert Eaton myasthenia gravis, hypercalcemia of malignancy, SIADH) and possibility of distant metastases with end-organ dysfunction (brain, liver, adrenal, bone) should be kept in mind during preoperative planning. In non-malignant diseases (Wegener's granulomatosis, sarcoidosis, amyloidosis), one should be aware of the presence of severe extra-pulmonary disease. All these would affect the choice of anaesthetic technique.
- Central airway lesions may be fixed or variable. It can be intra-thoracic or extra-thoracic. Stenting is done for lesions below the vocal cords. These lesions act as variable intra-thoracic obstruction. As in variable intra-thoracic obstruction, airflow is mainly affected in expiration as the airway expands during inspiration. This leads to the phenomenon of "air trapping" in the distal segments resulting in hyperinflation of the lungs. This can lead to barotrauma and volutrauma as well as cardiovascular compromise. This can be prevented by providing sufficient expiratory time as well as maintaining the inspiratory pressures <30 cmH_2O.
- It is imperative to understand the nature and extent of airway obstruction in all but cases but the most emergent cases [16]. Traditionally pulmonary function tests and supine and upright flow volume loops have been used to risk stratify these patients although these tests have a questionable role in the era of dynamic C-scan which can provide information on the functional anatomy. Performing spirometry itself can provoke respiratory failure in advanced obstruction.
- Detailed information on the nature and location of airway obstruction, dynamic collapse as well and its effects on the adjacent structures can be obtained by reconstructed multislice CT scans [17, 18]. Routine investigations such as full blood count, biochemistry, chest X-ray, ECG, ABG and PFT are indicated in all patients. Thyroid function tests should be done in patients with thyroid malignancy. Patients with risk factors for cardiac disease should undergo 2D-Echo.
- Proper counselling of the patients should be done by explaining the risks and benefits of the procedure.

31.5 What Are the Local and Systemic Effects of Malignancy that Can Have Anaesthetic Implications?

31.5.1 Systemic Effects [19]

- Cachexia.
- Lambert Eaton myasthenic syndrome—increased sensitivity to neuromuscular blockers.
- Metabolic effects—SIADH, Cushing's syndrome, hypercalcaemia of malignancy.
- Adverse effects of chemotherapy and radiotherapy—haematological, cardiotoxicity, nephrotoxicity and radiotherapy-related airway changes leading to difficult airway.
- Increased risk of venous thrombosis.
- Immunosuppression.

31.5.2 Local Effects [19]

- SVC obstruction—In the presence of SVC obstruction, lower limb IV access is preferred.
- Vocal cord palsy may be present.
- If any patient has received prior radiotherapy to the head and neck region, airway distortion can predispose to difficult mask ventilation, laryngoscopy and intubation.

31.6 What Pre-Procedural Preparation Can Be Done Before the Bronchoscopy?

Preoperative optimisation should be done in all cases except emergencies.

- Selective use of anti-sialogogues facilitates airway topicalisation and fibreoptic examination [20].
- Administration of steroids is beneficial in these patients. Racemic epinephrine also helps in relieving glottic oedema.
- The use of Heliox is beneficial by reducing the turbulent airflow and improving the gas exchange, thereby temporarily reducing the work of breathing [21].
- Coughing should be avoided as it may cause total obstruction. Humidified oxygen should be administered along with maintaining an upright position.
- Insertion of an arterial line helps in obtaining frequent ABG for assessing the adequacy of oxygenation and ventilation during the procedure.

31.7 What Are the Anaesthetic Considerations for Rigid Bronchoscopy?

- Rigid bronchoscopy requires general anaesthesia together with neuromuscular blockade as it causes intense airway stimulation.
- During the procedure, the airway remains unprotected increasing the risk of aspiration. It can also lead to difficulty in ventilation together with the risk of inaccessibility to the airway.
- If jet ventilation is being used, barotrauma can occur. It can also lead to hypercapnia.
- One should be aware of the technical difficulties such as shared airway, the need for total intravenous anaesthesia and use of an open circuit.
- Lastly, complications such as airway trauma, haemorrhage, gas embolism and airway fire can happen requiring prompt management.

31.8 What Are the Anaesthetic Techniques that Can Be Used in These Procedures?

The choice of anaesthetic technique depends on whether a rigid bronchoscope or flexible bronchoscope is being used for airway stenting. The major concerns during this procedure are shared airway, the potential for critical airway compromise and obstruction to ventilation. A flexible bronchoscope procedure can be performed under adequate topicalisation of the airway using local anaesthetics. Tolerance of the procedure can be improved by the administration of conscious sedation. Short-acting opioids may be administered judiciously to reduce coughing. Another useful adjunct is transnasal humidified rapid-insufflation ventilatory exchange (THRIVE) which improves the gas exchange while providing oxygenation during bronchoscopy. In addition to ASA standard monitoring, intra-arterial monitoring and depth of anaesthesia monitoring using BIS are helpful during rigid bronchoscopy when total intravenous anaesthesia (TIVA) is used. A separate IV access is required during the administration of TIVA [22].

31.8.1 Induction of Anaesthesia

Intravenous or inhalation agents can be used for the induction of anaesthesia and can be chosen based on the anaesthetist's preference and experience in addition to the condition of the patient. However, IV induction together with neuromuscular blockade provides the most suitable operating condition during the use of a rigid bronchoscope. It is desirable to prevent coughing and movement of the patient as it can lead to total airway obstruction or worsening of SVC obstruction. Extubation should also be smooth to reduce the risk of stent migration. Caution should be exercised in patients with high-grade obstruction. Spontaneous ventilation should be maintained during induction in these cases and neuromuscular blocking agents may be administered only after assessing the degree of dynamic obstruction using a flexible bronchoscope. Maintaining an adequate depth of anaesthesia along with airway topicalisation can reduce coughing during the procedure. In addition, a rigid bronchoscope or emergency VV ECMO should be available for immediate use in case of any difficulty in ventilation as rescue measures. Patient factors and the procedure being performed determine the airway device that can be used. If the insertion of an airway stent is being carried out using a flexible bronchoscope, either an endotracheal tube or a supra-glottic airway device can be used each with its advantages and disadvantages.

31.8.2 Maintenance of Anaesthesia

Volatile or intravenous agents can be used for the maintenance of anaesthesia. The disadvantages of using inhalational agents during rigid bronchoscopy are inadequate scavenging and delivery of anaesthetic agents due to the leak of volatile agents requiring high gas flows and increased risk of postoperative nausea and vomiting. Measuring the end-tidal concentration of the agents is difficult during rigid bronchoscopy. TIVA with jet ventilation has definite advantages in these cases [23]. Traditionally in a patient with stridor, spontaneous ventilation is maintained; however, literature reports the safe use of neuromuscular blocking agents even in such cases [24, 25]. Short-acting agents such as succinyl-choline may be used on a case-to-case basis.

31.9 What Are the Anaesthetic Considerations in Patients with an Airway Stent Posted for Unrelated Procedures?

- Detailed information regarding the indication, type and location of the stent and complications that occurred during the stent insertion procedure should be obtained. It is essential to know if any symptoms of airway obstruction are present even when posted for an unrelated surgery. One should consider the possibility of stent migration or obstruction from secretions and granulation tissue formation. Obstruction of stent due to tumour recurrence and invasion is also a possibility.
- Utmost importance should be given to airway management to avoid grave complications such as stent displacement resulting in CAO, airway dissection and formation of a false lumen [26].
- Hence, careful preoperative planning is imperative which can be aided by obtaining information directly from the team which performed the procedure whenever possible or going through the patient discharge summary.
- Tracheostomy may also be impossible in these situations, requiring an innovative approach for the management [27].
- The use of neuraxial or regional techniques helps to avoid airway trauma. If the need for general anaesthesia is mandated, a laryngeal mask airway can be used to minimise the risk of stent displacement. If tracheal intubation cannot be avoided, a fibreoptic bronchoscope can be used to inspect the airway and guide the endotracheal tube within the stent lumen or just proximal (in case of a carinal stent) to it. Extubation should also be followed by fibreoptic inspection of the airway to confirm the stent position. If stent migration or stenosis is a concern, an emergency rigid bronchoscopy can be done.

31.10 What Are the Modes of Ventilation that Can Be Used During Rigid Bronchoscope Procedures?

During the procedure of rigid bronchoscopy, the ventilation can be maintained by the following methods [28]:

(a) Spontaneous ventilation.
(b) Apnoeic oxygenation method (which provides a surgical intervention time of 3 min or longer) which can be accompanied by the use of oxygen insufflation and THRIVE.
(c) Intermittent positive pressure ventilation (IPPV) with bronchoscopic ventilation.
(d) Jet ventilation (manual and high frequency).

- Apnoeic oxygenation-: In this method, the patient is pre-oxygenated with 100% FIO2. The intervention is performed during this time which is followed by capping of the proximal end to allow ventilation. Following adequate ventilation and oxygenation, further interventions can be performed, and this cycle is repeated until the case is completed. This technique is obsolete due to the availability of better techniques.
- Spontaneous assisted ventilation—This technique is similar to the previous technique concerning pre-oxygenation. In addition, supplemental oxygen is provided throughout the procedure and ventilation is assisted. TIVA is used for the maintenance of anaesthesia.
- Controlled ventilation—This is the preferred ventilation mode during rigid bronchoscopy. In this method, the rigid bronchoscope itself is used to provide positive pressure ventilation. The leaks from the ports of rigid bronchoscope can be minimised by using silastic caps on the ports and packing of the oropharynx. However, it has a few disadvantages such as the need for a high flow rate, no control over the FiO2 which is being inspired and improper delivery of volatile anaesthetic agents.
- Jet ventilation—This technique involves the use of a small catheter through which a high-pressure (0.3–3 bars) gas source is applied to the open airway intermittently. It works on Bernoulli's principle in which the application of high-pressure gas through an open airway entrains the surrounding air mixing with it with the gas jet and creating a Venturi effect. It can be manual or electrically powered devices. Air entrainment leads to delivery of lower than anticipated FiO2. Low-frequency jet ventilation is used in manual devices while electrically powered ones use high frequency.
- *Manual jet ventilation*—In this technique, a narrow bore cannula attached to the port of the bronchoscope is used to deliver compressed gas at a high pressure (0.3–3 bars). This gas source is passed through the pressure-reducing valves. It delivers a pressure of 50 pounds per square inch (psi) or less, and the respiratory rate (RR) is maintained between 8 and 30 breaths/min [29]. Bulk flow (convection) is responsible for most of the ventilations. The adequacy of ventilation can be assessed by periodic ABG or transcutaneous capnography. It is desirable to maintain a peak pressure < 35 cm of H_2O.

Automated jet ventilation—In contrast to manual jet ventilation, this technique delivers breaths at a rate of 60–300 breaths/min generating a tidal volume of 1–3 ml/kg. Here, several gas-stream mechanisms including bulk ventilation are responsible for ventilation [30, 31]. The operator can control the applied pressure, respiratory rate and inspiratory time to maintain adequate oxygenation [32]. Maintaining a high respiratory rate and low tidal volume is desirable during the procedure [26, 27]. Conditions such as broncho-pleural fistula which requires maintenance of low airway pressure benefit from the use of automated jet ventilation. Insufflation pressure is limited by alarms such as pause pressure and peak inspiratory pressure. Initial settings can be a frequency of 100 counts/min, an inspiratory time of 50% and a driving pressure of 1.5 bars. Alarms for pause pressure and peak inspiratory pressure at 25 mbar [10].

ECMO/CPB—VV ECMO can be considered in cases with critical airway obstruction where even induction of anaesthesia and positive pressure ventilation can precipitate complete airway collapse. It can be used as a final rescue measure in failed ventilation; however, outcomes are better when it is initiated electively [33]. It ensures adequate gas exchange in the absence of adequate ventilation.

References

1. Finlayson G, Brodsky J. Anesthetic considerations for airway stenting in adult patients. Anesthesiol Clin. 2008;26(281–91):vi. https://doi.org/10.1016/j.anclin.2008.01.005.
2. Grillo HC. Stents and sense. Ann Thorac Surg. 2000;70(4):1142.
3. Grewe PH, Muller KM, Lindstaedt M, et al. Reaction patterns of tracheobronchial wall to implanted noncovered metal stents. Chest. 2005;128(2):986–90.
4. Thornton RH, Gordon RL, Kerlan RK, et al. Outcomes of tracheobronchial stent placement for benign disease. Radiology. 2006;240(1):273–8.
5. Ehller RL, Livingston WJ, Morgan CE. Expandable tracheal stenting for benign disease: worth the complications? Ann Otol Rhinol Laryngol. 2006;115(4):247–52.
6. Saad CP, Murthy S, Krismanich G, et al. Self-expandable airway stents and flexible bronchoscopy: long-term outcomes analysis. Chest. 2003;124(5):1993–9.
7. Vonk-Noordegraaf A, Postmus PE, Sutedja TG. Tracheobronchial stenting in the terminal care of cancer patients with central airways obstruction. Chest. 2001;120(6):1811–4.
8. Noppen M, Stratakos G, Amjadi K, et al. Stenting allows weaning and extubation in ventilator - or tracheostomy dependency secondary to benign airway disease. Respir Med. 2007;101(1): 139–45.
9. Saad CP, Ghamande SA, Minia OA, et al. The role of self-expandable metallic stents for the treatment of airway complications after lung transplantation. Transplantation. 2003;75(9):1532–8.
10. Barnwell N, Lenihan M. Anaesthesia for airway stenting. BJA Educ. 2022;22(4):160–6. https://doi.org/10.1016/j.bjae.2021.11.010.
11. Ost DE, Ernst A, Grosu HB, et al. Complications following therapeutic bronchoscopy for malignant central airway obstruction: results of the AQuIRE registry. Chest. 2015;148:450–71.
12. Makris D, Marquette CH. Tracheobronchial stenting and central airway replacement. Curr Opin Pulm Med. 2007;13(4):278–83.
13. Zakaluzny SA, Lane JD, Mair EA. Complications of tracheobronchial airway stents. Otolaryngol Head Neck Surg. 2003;128(4):478–88.
14. Urschel JD. Delayed massive hemoptysis after expandable bronchial stent placement. J Laparoendosc Adv Surg Tech A. 1999;9(2):155.
15. Pinsonneault C, Fortier J, Donati F. Tracheal resection and reconstruction. Can J Anaesth. 1999;46(5):439–55.
16. Mason RA, Fielder CP. The obstructed airway in head and neck surgery. Anaesthesia. 1999;54(7): 625–8.
17. Lee KS, Lunn W, Feller-Kopman D, et al. Multislice CT evaluation of airway stents. J Thorac Imaging. 2005;20(2):81–8.
18. Burke AJ, Vining DJ, McGuirt WF, et al. Evaluation of upper airway obstruction using virtual endoscopy. Laryngoscope. 2000;110(1):23–9.
19. Nethercott D, Strang T, Krysiak P. Airway stents: anaesthetic implications. Continuing Education in Anaesthesia Critical Care & Pain. 2010;10(2):53–8. https://doi.org/10.1093/bjaceaccp/mkq006.
20. Conacher ID. Anaesthesia and tracheobronchial stenting for central airway obstruction in adults. Br J Anaesth. 2003;90(3):367–74.
21. Ho AM, Dion PW, Karmakar MK, et al. Use of heliox in critical upper airway obstruction. Physical and physiologic considerations in choosing the optimal helium:oxygen mix. Resuscitation. 2002;52(3):297–300.
22. Nimmo AF, Absalom AR, Bagshaw O, et al. Guidelines for the safe practice of total intravenous anaesthesia (TIVA): joint guidelines from the Association of Anaesthetists and the Society for Intravenous Anaesthesia. Anaesthesia. 2019;74:211–2.
23. Galway U, Zura A, Khanna S, Wang M, Turan A, Ruetzler K. Anesthetic considerations for bronchoscopic procedures: a narrative review based on the Cleveland Clinic experience. J Thorac Dis. 2019;11:3156–7.
24. Slinger P, Karsli C. Management of the patient with a large anterior mediastinal mass: recurring myths. Curr Opin Anaesthesiol. 2007;20(1):1–3.
25. Chadha M, Kulshrestha M, Biyani A. Anaesthesia for bronchoscopy. Indian J Anaesth. 2015;59:565–73.
26. Davis N, Madden BP, Sheth A, et al. Airway management in patients with tracheobronchial stents. Br J Anaest. 2006;96(1):132–5.
27. Madden BP, Sheth A. An approach to tracheostomy in a patient with an expandable metallic tracheal stent. J Laryngol Otol. 2005;119(9):731–2.
28. Sullivan MT, Neff WB. A modified Sanders ventilating system for rigid-wall bronchoscopy. Anesthesiology. 1979;50:473–4.
29. MacIntyre NR. High frequency ventilation. In: MacIntyre NR, Branson RD, editors. Mechanical ventilation. Philadelphia: WB Saunders; 2001.
30. Evans E, Biro P, Bedforth N. Jet ventilation. Contin Educ Anaesth Crit Care Pain. 2007;7:2–5.
31. Carlon GC, Miodownik S, Ray C Jr, Kahn RC. Te chnical aspects and clinical implications of high frequency jet ventilation with a solenoid valve. Crit Care Med. 1981;9(1):47–50.
32. Bunnell JB. High frequency hardware: implementation of the latest mode of respiratory therapy. Med Instrum. 1985;19:208.
33. Malpas G, Hung O, Gilchrist A, et al. The use of extracorporeal membrane oxygenation in the anticipated difficult airway: a case report and systematic review. Can J Anaesth. 2018;65:685–97.

Anaesthetic Management of Pheochromocytoma

32

Sujata Nambiath and Raj Tobin

32.1 Case History

A 45-year-old male with no prior medical history presented with complaints of episodic headaches, palpitations and tremors. The symptoms often occurred after exercise. He was not on any medications and not abusing any drugs. On physical examination, he had an elevated blood pressure of 178/98 mm Hg, tachycardia of 126 beats per minute and a temperature of 98 °F. His investigations were suggestive of pheochromocytoma.

32.2 What Is Pheochromocytoma?

Pheochromocytoma is a pharmacologically explosive catecholamine-secreting tumour of the chromaffin cells of the adrenal medulla. They may be bilateral, extra-adrenal or malignant. Paragangliomas are neuroendocrine tumours arising from extra-adrenal paraganglia, which may produce catecholamines and present similarly. The familial tumours may be associated with multiple endocrine neoplasia 2A and 2B, 3A, Von Hippel–Lindau disease and neurofibromatosis [1, 2].

The adrenal medulla is a large sympathetic ganglion that has lost its postganglionic fibres and hence has only secretory functions. Methylation of noradrenaline to adrenaline only occurs in the adrenal medulla and depends on cortisol. Tumour disrupts the portocapillary circulation and hence cortisol cannot reach the medulla. Thus 90% of these tumours secrete noradrenaline, unlike normal adrenal medulla that secretes mostly adrenaline. Ten percent of tumours secrete adrenaline, and rarely some secrete dopamine, opioid peptides, vasoactive intestinal eptide, adrenocorticotropic hormone, calcitonin and somatostatin. Noradrenaline-secreting tumours present with hypertension while tachycardia is the predominant symptom in adrenaline-secreting ones.

During the resting basal state, catecholamines are required in minimal quantities. However, in tumours of the adrenal medulla, the excessive catecholamine secretion leads to a myriad of signs and symptoms that are an extension of its physiological action. Noradrenaline acts predominantly on $\alpha 1$ receptors while adrenaline acts on non-specific β-receptors (Table 32.1). Table 32.2 shows the summary of the effects of adrenaline and noradrenaline.

In long standing cases, there may be loss of postural reflexes and downregulation of $\alpha 1$ and $\beta 1$ receptors. $\alpha 2$ receptors show impaired occupancy response coupling. However, $\beta 2$ receptor

S. Nambiath (✉) · R. Tobin
Max Hospital, Saket, New Delhi, India

N. Gupta et al. (eds.), *Problem Based Learning Discussions in Onco-Anesthesia and Onco-Critical Care*, https://doi.org/10.1007/978-981-99-6339-3_32

Table 32.1 Actions of various inotropes on cardiovascular system

Receptor	Noradrenaline	Adrenaline	Dopamine	Effect on neurotransmission	Peripheral vessels	Heart rate	Myocardial contractility
α1	+++	++	+	Excitatory	Vasoconstriction	Reflex bradycardia	–
α2	+++	++	–	Inhibitory	Vasodilatation	Reflex tachycardia	–
β1	++	+++	++	Excitatory	–	Tachycardia (direct)	Increases
β2	+	+++	++	Inhibitory	Vasodilatation	–	–

Table 32.2 Effects of adrenaline and noradrenaline

	Noradrenaline	Adrenaline
Heart rate	Decreased	Increased
Peripheral resistance	Increased	Decreased
Mean arterial pressure	Increased	Increased[a]
Cardiac output	Decreased[b]	Increased[a]
Nervous system	Excitatory	Excitatory
Metabolic	Increased metabolic rate Glycogenolysis (liver, muscle) Mobilisation of free fatty acids	

[a]Via beta-mediated tachycardia and increased myocardial contractility
[b]Due to increased afterload

activity remains intact [2]. The clinical features of dopamine-secreting tumours are inflammatory or hypermetabolic in nature, with normal blood pressures and sugars.

Ten percent of pheochromocytomas are malignant, with metastasis to lung, lymph nodes, muscle or liver. Hyperglycaemia is a prominent symptom and is due to catecholamine-induced glycogenolysis, lipolysis and inhibition of insulin release.

32.3 Case

A 50-year-old male presents with a supra-renal mass. He has a history of poorly controlled hypertension, easy tiredness, recurrent headaches, palpitations and sweating for the past 6 months.

32.4 What Are the Signs and Symptoms of Pheochromocytoma? [1, 2]

Headache, palpitations and sweating are the classic triad of clinical presentation. Hypertension, present in 90% of cases, may be sustained or paroxysmal in 35–50%. Paroxysms may be triggered by changing position, abdominal pressure, coitus, sneezing, voiding, defaecation, exercise, anxiety and caffeine. Orthostatic hypotension is the presenting symptom in adrenaline- and dopamine-secreting tumours. This is because these two hormones act more on the vasodilatory beta-, rather than alpha-receptors. Other symptoms are summarised in Table 32.3.

Table 32.3 Signs and symptoms of pheochromocytoma

	Symptoms	Signs
Cardiovascular	Chest pain and palpitations	Hypertension—Sustained or paroxysmal, tachyarrhythmias, orthostatic hypotension, myocardial ischaemia and cardiac failure
Respiratory	Dyspnoea and orthopnoea	Pulmonary oedema
Neurological	Headache, anxiety, visual disturbance, paraesthesia, tremor and seizures	Papilledema, hypertensive encephalopathy and focal neurological deficits
Gastrointestinal	Nausea, vomiting and abdominal pain	Bowel ischaemia
Metabolic	Weakness, lethargy and sweating	Carbohydrate intolerance, hyperglycaemia, hypercalcaemia, heat intolerance, weight loss
Haematological	Facial pallor	Polycythaemia

32.5 What Is the Mechanism of Orthostatic Hypotension?

1. Extracellular volume contraction in noradrenaline-secreting tumours.
2. Beta 2 action in adrenaline- and dopamine-secreting tumours.
3. Loss of postural reflexes in long-standing tumours.
4. With initiation of alpha-blockade for control of hypertension.

32.6 What Is Catecholamine-Induced Cardiomyopathy?

Sustained catecholamine release over a prolonged period can lead to hypertrophic cardiomyopathy. Stress or takotsubo cardiomyopathy causes left heart failure. Management is by non-specific beta-blockers like carvedilol, angiotensin-converting enzyme inhibitors and diuretics. The condition is partially reversible after treatment with alpha-blockers and tumour removal.

32.7 How Will You Confirm your Diagnosis?

Diagnosis requires biochemical testing and imaging studies.

32.7.1 Biochemical Tests

Plasma catecholamines have a very short half-life and hence is not reliable for diagnosis. Since there is a diurnal variation in catecholamine secretion, 24-h urine samples are tested for elevated catecholamines and their breakdown products like vanillylmandelic acid (dopamine), metanephrine (adrenaline) and normetanephrine (noradrenaline). Urinary assay of catecholamine metabolites by high-performance liquid chromatography with electrochemical detection (HPLC-ED) has a low chance of false positives, and hence this is the screening test of choice [3]. Also, catecholamine enzyme activity within chromaffinomas may be unpredictable, and hence both plasma catecholamines and urinary metabolites should be measured. More than four times elevation of plasma fractionated metanephrines have a high sensitivity [4].

Results may be false-positive with recent exercise, smoking, caffeine, venous sampling in the sitting position, renal impairment and intake of drugs like norepinephrine re-uptake inhibitors, adrenergic receptor blockers (atenolol, phenoxybenzamine), monoamine oxidase inhibitors, cocaine, amphetamine, caffeine, acetaminophen and sympathomimetics [1].

Pheochromocytoma may be ruled out by a clonidine suppression test if the elevated plasma normetanephrine levels are reduced to less than 40% of baseline after 3 h of administration of oral clonidine.

32.7.2 Imaging Studies

Imaging studies are required to localise the tumour. Various studies like ultrasound, CT, MRI and meta-iodobenzylguanidine (MIBG) scan are complementary and are useful for differentiating these tumours from other lesions of the adrenals. MIBG-123 is a norepinephrine analog that localises to presynaptic adrenergic nerves, sympathomedullary tissue and cytoplasmic storage vesicles. The uptake of radiotracer is proportional to the number of neurosecretory granules within the tumour [5].

32.8 How Will You Evaluate and Optimise this Patient for the Surgery?

32.8.1 Evaluation

Clinical assessment—Evaluate for hypertensive end-organ damage to kidneys, myocardium and eyes, assess for symptoms of cardiac failure and enquire for presence of familial conditions.

Blood investigations—An elevated haematocrit, hyperglycaemia, hyperparathyroidism with raised plasma calcitonin concentrations (MEN syndrome), raised creatinine and electrolyte imbalance may be found in these patients.

Chest radiograph—to exclude cardiomegaly and pulmonary oedema.

An ECG may show ventricular hypertrophy, arrhythmias and ST-T changes of myocardial ischaemia.

ECHO—chamber hypertrophy and myocardial dysfunction may be present.

A stress echo may precipitate a catecholamine crisis and hence should be avoided.

32.8.2 Optimisation

Preoperative preparation is aimed towards control of blood pressure, heart rate and arrhythmias, intravascular volume restoration, optimisation of myocardial function, control of blood sugar, correction of electrolyte imbalance and amelioration of any end-organ damage.

Table 32.4 Roizen's criteria

1. Preoperative blood pressure < 160/90 mm hg for 24 h before surgery
2. Postural hypotension >80–45 mm hg
3. No ST-T changes in the ECG for 1 week
4. Ventricular premature beats not more than 1 in 5 min

Roizen et al. recommended the following criteria for preoperative optimisation in noradrenaline-secreting tumours (Table 32.4):

However, the Endocrine Society recommended in 2007 that the goal is to achieve target blood pressure of less than 130/80 mmHg when sitting and no less than 80/45 mmHg when standing with a target heart rate of 60–70 per minute when sitting and 70–80 per minute when standing [6]. They further suggested that complete prevention of perioperative hypertension and tachycardia cannot be achieved by any doses or combinations of drugs [7]. Moreover, it is now believed that ST or T wave changes may reflect Takotsubo cardiomyopathy rather than ischaemia [1].

Hyperglycaemia occurs due to increased α1-mediated glycogenolysis, α2-mediated impaired insulin release, β1-mediated lipolysis or β2-mediated peripheral insulin resistance. Renal impairment may cause hyperkalaemia. Hypercalcaemia occurs when the tumour is associated with a parathyroid adenoma as in MEN 2A.

32.9 Why Is it Necessary to Initiate Alpha-Blockade in These Patients?

Prolonged exposure to excessive circulating catecholamines results in uncontrolled hypertension leading to myocardial ischaemia, arrhythmias or congestive cardiac failure due to cardiomyopathy. Catecholamine-induced vasoconstriction may cause increased haematocrit. These effects have to be optimised before surgical resection of the tumour. Initiation of alphablockers will lead to vasodilatation, and adequate fluid intake along with a high salt diet will restore the intravascular volume, which may be titrated using serial haematocrits. A 5–10% fall in haematocrit is seen in well-prepared patients [8]. However, this is a guide to the therapy and not an end point for adequate volume expansion. Addition of beta-blockers for control of the heart rate will help in optimisation of myocardial function.

32.10 Why Should Alpha-Blockade Be Initiated before Beta-Blockade?

Non-selective β-blockers inhibit β2-mediated vasodilatation, leading to unopposed α-mediated vasoconstriction, and can precipitate a hypertensive crisis. Additionally, the negative inotropic effect of β-blockade may worsen myocardial function resulting in cardiac failure and pulmonary oedema.

32.11 What Are the Drugs Used to Control the Blood Pressure? (Table 32.5)

1. Alpha-Blockers

   Phenoxybenzamine is a non-selective, non-competitive and long-acting α-blocker. In addition to blocking the postsynaptic α1-mediated vasoconstriction, it also prevents the presynaptic α2-mediated inhibition of catecholamine release. The latter effect leads to reflex tachycardia, requiring simultaneous beta-blockade. In severe cardiomyopathy, β blockers can precipitate cardiac failure. Since the drug is long acting, it may cause postoperative refractory catecholamine-resistant hypotension and so should be stopped 24–48 h prior to surgery.

   Doxazosin is a competitive, selective α1-blocker which does not cause tachycardia, postoperative hypotension or sedation. Other newer selective α-blockers like prazosin, urapidil and terazosin do not produce reflex tachycardia and have shorter half-lives enabling rapid dose adjustments [9–11]. However, since these are competitive in mechanism of action, they may be overwhelmed by catecholamine release during tumour manipulation.

   Some authors now believe that with the advances in anaesthetic and monitoring techniques and the availability of fast-acting drugs to correct hypo- or hypertension, preoperative arterial pressure normalisation is not required in patients not in cardiac failure and without any end-organ damage. Such patients also require less vasoactive drugs and colloids in the perioperative period [2, 12].
2. Beta-Blockers

   Selective β1 antagonists like metoprolol and atenolol are used in adrenaline- and dopamine-secreting tumours or to control the tachycardia caused by non-selective α-blockade.
3. Calcium Channel Blockers.

   They are used as the first-line drug in very mild hypertension or in those who develop severe orthostatic hypotension with α-blockers.
4. α-Methylparatyrosine or metyrosine inhibits catecholamine synthesis and is specifically indicated in metastatic pheochromocytomas, patients with LV dysfunction and tachycardia caused by α-blockade [6]. The side effects are diarrhoea, crystalluria, galactorrhoea, anxiety, depression and extra-pyramidal symptoms.

Table 32.5 Drugs used for perioperative management of a patient with pheochromocytoma

Drug	Mechanism of action	Dose
Drugs for preoperative optimisation		
Phenoxybenzamine	Non-selective irreversible α 1 and 2 adrenergic antagonists	PO 10 mg BD, increased to 60–200 mg daily; started 2 weeks preop, discontinued 2 days prior to surgery
Doxazosin	Competitive, selective α1-antagonists	1 mg OD, increased up to 16 mg OD
α-Methylparatyrosine	Inhibits tyrosine hydroxylase	PO 250 mg, increased to 2 g/day for 1–3 weeks
Drugs to attenuate stressor response		
Magnesium sulphate	Inhibits catecholamine release, reduces alpha receptor sensitivity and dilates arterioles, antiarrhythmic	IV 40 to 60 mg/kg boles at induction, followed by 1 to 2 g/h infusion
Fentanyl	Inhibiting the over-activation of HPA axis	IV 3 to 5 mcg/kg at induction
Remifentanil	Inhibiting the over-activation of HPA axis	IV 1–2 mcg/kg 1 min before intubation
Esmolol	Anti-catecholamine and membrane stabiliser	IV 0.5 mg/kg, given 2 min prior to intubation
Dexmedetomidine	Centrally acting selective α2-receptor agonist	IV 1 mcg/kg (over 10 min) followed by 0.5 mcg/kg/h infusion
Drugs to decrease blood pressure intraoperatively		
Sodium nitroprusside (arteriolar) and glyceryl trinitrate (venolar)	Nitric oxide donors	IV 1 mcg/kg/min and titrate
Nicardipine	Inhibits noradrenaline-mediated calcium influx in vascular smooth muscle	IV 3–5 mg/h. for 15 min and titrate
Diltiazem	Inhibits noradrenaline-mediated calcium influx in vascular smooth muscle	5–15 mg/h
Fenoldopam	Inhibits noradrenaline-mediated calcium influx in vascular smooth muscle	0.2 mg/kg/min
Urapidil	Competitive, selective α1-antagonists	10–15 mg/h
Esmolol	Selective β1 antagonist	IV 500 mcg/kg over 1 min, followed by 50 mcg/kg/min and titrate
Drugs to increase blood pressure intraoperatively		
Vasopressin	Systemic vasoconstriction (V1 receptor) increases renal water reabsorption (V2 receptors)	IV bolus 0.4–20 units followed by 1–3 U/h
Phenylephrine	Direct α 1-receptor agonist	IV 50–100 mcg boluses or 0.5–1 mcg/kg/min titrated infusion

32.12 How Will the Surgical Technique Affect your Anaesthesia Choices?

The surgical techniques are open retroperitoneal, open transabdominal, laparoscopic or robotic. Open surgery is required for large or invasive adrenal masses and most paragangliomas. Since tumour handling is more with the open technique, stabilising the haemodynamics can be challenging.

Laparoscopic and robotic tumour resection is performed in the lateral position with table break. Catecholamine surges may occur during patient positioning and can be very severe during initiation of pneumoperitoneum. However, minimal tissue handling diminishes the stress response. There is also reduced blood loss, less postoperative pain, significantly faster recovery and shorter hospital stay. Postoperative pain can be managed with ultrasound-guided abdominal field block, patient-controlled intravenous opioid analgesia and oral analgesics.

32.12.1 What Are your Anaesthetic Considerations?

Intraoperative complications are severe hyper- or hypotension, stroke, arrhythmias, myocardial ischaemia and left ventricular failure. The increased catecholamine secretion by the tumour can lead to increased loading of sympathetic vesicles with noradrenaline. During periods of increased nerve stimulation like laryngoscopy, intubation, surgical stimulus, pain and pneumoperitoneum, excessive secretion of postganglionic neuronal noradrenaline results in exaggerated physiological sympathetic response. Intraoperative haemodynamic instability is associated with high plasma norepinephrine levels at diagnosis, large tumour size, profound postural drop after commencement of α-blockade and a pre-induction mean arterial pressure above 100 mm Hg [13]. Severe vasoconstriction can cause malignant hypertensive crisis, cerebrovascular accident, aortic dissection, myocardial infarction, arrhythmias, heart failure, pulmonary oedema and acute renal failure.

The specific anaesthetic goals and the suggested management are as follows:

1. Minimise catecholamine release:
   (a) Avoid halothane (which sensitises the heart to catecholamines) and sympathomimetics like desflurane, ketamine, ephedrine, droperidol, parasympatholytics like atropine, metoclopramide (which promotes presynaptic release or inhibits reuptake), morphine, pethidine, atracurium (histamine release) and succinylcholine (which stimulates sympathetic ganglia and provokes tumour catecholamine release due to raised intra-abdominal pressure from muscle fasciculation).
   (b) Smooth endotracheal intubation—avoid stressor response, avoid bucking and coughing which may raise intra-abdominal pressure. Drugs like magnesium, fentanyl or remifentanil, dexmedetomidine or short-acting esmolol can be used to attenuate such catecholamine surges (Table 32.4).
   (c) Avoidance of hypothermia and shivering by using forced air warmers.
   (d) Intra-abdominal pressure during pneumoperitoneum to be kept as minimal as possible.
   (e) Minimising haemodynamic responses to tumour handling by early surgical ligation of the adrenal vein. During tumour handling, severe hypertension and bradycardia are seen in norepinephrine-secreting tumours while tachyarrhythmias is seen with epinephrine-secreting tumours.
2. Maintain stable haemodynamics:
   (a) Hypertensive crises are managed with peripheral vasodilators like glyceryl trinitrate and sodium nitroprusside, calcium channel blockers like nicardipine and fenoldopam and urapidil infusion. Beta-blockers like esmolol and labetalol are used to control the heart rate.
   (b) Hypotension seen after tumour devascularisation can be managed by infusing large volumes of fluid guided by central venous pressure. Vasopressors like phenylephrine, vasopressin or noradrenaline should be added only after volume status is restored.
3. Postoperative pain control:
   (a) Continuous local anaesthetic—opioid epidural analgesia.
   (b) Ultrasound-guided abdominal field blocks.
   (c) Patient-controlled intravenous opioid analgesia.

32.13 What Is the Aetiology of Intraoperative Hypotension?

Severe refractory catecholamine-resistant hypotension may occur following ligation of the tumour-venous supply leading to sudden reduction of circulating catecholamines. Other causes are suppression of the contralateral adrenal medulla, inadequate intravascular volume replacement, residual effects of preoperative alpha-blockade, catecholamine receptor downregulation caused by chronic elevation of catecholamine levels, catecholamine-induced cardiomyopathy, anaesthetic drugs and surgical blood loss.

32.14 How Will you Monitor the Patient Intraoperatively?

1. Monitoring of 5-lead ECG, pulse oximetry, end-tidal carbon dioxide, arterial blood gases, blood glucose, urine output and body temperature.
2. Invasive arterial monitoring to be established before induction.
3. Central venous access—for drug infusions and to assess fluid status.
4. Esophageal doppler or transesophageal echocardiography to guide fluid management and to assess myocardial function where mandated.
5. Cardiac output monitoring via pulmonary artery catheter may be used to guide intravenous fluid replacement in selected cases like large tumours, cardiomyopathy and myocardial ischaemia.

32.15 Are Arterial Pulse Contour Analysis Devices Useful in Pheochromocytoma Surgery?

Cardiac output readings from algorithm-calibrated systems like PiCCO and LiDCO are not very accurate in conditions of haemodynamic instability and significantly fluctuating vascular tone [14].

32.16 What Are the Postoperative Complications?

1. Persistent hypertension.
   (a) Pain, co-existing essential hypertension, urinary retention and fluid overload are some of the common causes of postoperative hypertension. Other specific causes are inadvertent ligation of the renal artery precipitating hyper-reninism, incomplete tumour resection and metastatic disease.
2. Persistent hypotension—management is similar to that adopted during the intraoperative period. Tumour size >60 mm, urinary noradrenaline levels >600 mcg/day and urinary adrenaline levels >200 mcg/day are predictors of prolonged hypotension [15, 16].
3. Postoperative hypoglycaemia may occur due to rebound hyper-insulinism caused by elimination of the inhibitory effect of norepinephrine on pancreatic β-cells. This may be masked by persistent β blockade.
4. Lifetime steroid replacement is indicated in bilateral adrenalectomy. 100 mg of hydrocortisone is administered at induction and continued every 8 h followed by 25 mg twice daily for 72 h. Oral prednisolone is started at discharge.

32.17 How Will you Manage a Pheochromocytoma Which has Been Incidentally Detected During Routine Surgery?

Hypertension and tachyarrhythmia are the most common presenting symptoms. If suspected, intraoperative management includes immediate cessation of tumour manipulation. Hypertension should be controlled with α-blockers or nitrates followed by heart rate control with short-acting selective β1-blockers like esmolol. Surgery should be terminated as soon as possible. Postoperatively, the patient should be continuously monitored for catecholamine surges in the intensive care unit. Other complications are myocardial or cerebral infarction, acute kidney injury or mesenteric ischaemia.

32.18 How Will You Manage a Patient Who Is Diagnosed with a Pheochromocytoma During Pregnancy?

If the gestational age at presentation is less than 24 weeks, the tumour is resected during the second trimester. If it is diagnosed after 24 weeks, the patient is stabilised on α-blockers [2].

Phenoxybenzamine and propranolol are safe in pregnancy.

Labour can precipitate a hypertensive crisis, and diagnosis may be confused with eclampsia. Magnesium sulphate infusion is the management for both. Delivery should be by elective caesarean section under regional anaesthesia.

References

1. Connor D, Boumphrey S. Perioperative care of phaeochromocytoma. BJA Education. 2016;16(5):153–8.
2. Pace N, Buttigieg M. Pheochromocytoma. Br J Anaesth CEPD Rev. 2003;3(1):20–3.
3. McHenry CR. Pheochromocytoma: a clinical enigma. Endocr Pract. 2016;
4. Eisenhofer G, Goldstein DS, Walther MM, et al. Biochemical diagnosis of pheochromocytoma: how to distinguish true-from false-positive test results. J Clin Endocrinol Metab. 2003;88:2656–66.
5. Beierwaltes WH. Endocrine imaging: parathyroid, adrenal cortex and medulla, and other endocrine tumors. Part II J Nucl Med. 1991;32:1627–39.
6. Pacak K. Preoperative Management of the Pheochromocytoma Patient. J Clin Endocrinol Metab. 2007;92:4069–79.
7. Lenders JW, Duh QY, Eisenhofer G, et al. Pheochromocytoma and paraganglioma: an endocrine society clinical practice guideline. J Clin Endocrinol Metab. 2014;99:1915–42.
8. Ramachandran R, Rewari V. Current perioperative management of pheochromocytomas. Indian J Urol. 2017;33(1):19–25.
9. Lentschener C, Gaujoux S, Tesniere A, Dousset B. Point of controversy: perioperative care of patients undergoing phaeochromocytoma removal—time for a reappraisal? Eur J Endocrinol. 2011;165:365–73.
10. Subramaniam R. Pheochromocytoma-current concepts in diagnosis and management. Trends Anaesth Crit Care. 2011;1(2):104–10.
11. Goldstein DP, Voigt MR, Ruan D. Current preoperative preparation of pheochromocytoma/paraganglioma syndrome. Clin Surg. 2017;2:1517.
12. Groeben H, Nottebaum BJ, Alesina PF, Traut A, Neumann HP, Walz MK. Perioperative α-receptor blockade in phaeochromocytoma surgery: an observational case series. Br J Anaesth. 2017 Feb;118(2):182–9.
13. Bruynzeel H, Feelders RA, Groenland THN, et al. Risk factors for hemodynamic instability during surgery for phaeochromocytoma. J Clin Endocrinol Metab. 2010;95:678–85.
14. Camporota L, Beale R. Pitfalls in haemodynamic monitoring based on the arterial pressure waveform. Crit Care. 2010;14:124.
15. Namekawa T, Utsumi T, Kawamura K, et al. Clinical predictors of prolonged post resection hypotension after laparoscopic adrenalectomy for pheochromocytoma. Surgery. 2016;159(3):763–70.
16. Subramaniam R. Complications of adrenal surgery. In: Fleisher LA, Rosenbaum SH, editors. Complications in anesthesia. third ed. Philadelphia: Elsevier; 2018.

A Case of Carcinoma Breast with Brain Metastasis for Gamma Knife Radiosurgery

33

Neha Sharma, Kanwaljeet Garg, and Gyaninder Pal Singh

33.1 Case History

A 30-year-old female with carcinoma breast presented with headache. She was previously operated and had received chemotherapy and radiotherapy. The PET CT and CT scan was suggestive of a metastatic lesion in the brain. The patient was planned for gamma knife stereotactic radiosurgery.

33.2 What Are the Various Types of Breast Cancer? What Are the Risk Factors and Its Manifestations?

In women, breast cancer is the most common cancer and also the second most common cause of cancer death in females all over the world. The type of breast cancer is determined by the specific kind of breast cells that are involved. The different types are the following:

(a) Ductal carcinoma in situ (most common).
(b) Invasive ductal carcinoma.
(c) Lobular carcinoma in situ.
(d) Invasive lobular carcinoma.
(e) Triple-negative breast cancer (ER-, PR-, HER-).
(f) Paget's disease.
(g) Phyllodes tumor.
(h) Metastatic breast carcinoma.

Risk factors [1] associated with breast cancer include the following:

- Advanced age.
- Family history of breast cancer.
- Previous history of breast cancer.
- Use of oral contraceptives pill (OCP).
- Hormone replacement therapy (HRT).
- Nulliparity.
- Child birth after 30 years of age.

Common manifestations are the following:

- Mostly diagnosed during routine screening.
- Breast lump.
- Discharge.
- Redness.
- Skin erosion.
- Swelling and pain in advanced cases.
- Axillary lymphadenopathy.

33.3 What Are the Common Sites and Symptoms of Metastasis in Patients of Breast Cancer?

Metastatic breast cancer is classified as stage 4 breast cancer where the cancer cells have spread

N. Sharma · G. P. Singh (✉)
Department of Neuro-Anaesthesiology, CN Centre, AIIMS, New Delhi, India

K. Garg
Department of Neurosurgery, CN Centre, AIIMS, New Delhi, India

N. Gupta et al. (eds.), *Problem Based Learning Discussions in Onco-Anesthesia and Onco-Critical Care*, https://doi.org/10.1007/978-981-99-6339-3_33

to other parts of the body mostly by hematogenous spread and less commonly through lymphatics. The most common sites for metastasis include the lungs, bones, brain, and liver [2, 3]. The symptoms will depend upon the site of metastasis.

Bone metastasis [4] occurs in 53% of metastatic breast cancer patients. Common sites include the ribs, pelvis, spine, and long bones of the arm and lower limbs. Presenting symptoms may include joint pains, pathological fractures, fatigue, weakness, and back pain.

Liver metastasis occurs in 50% patients with stage 4 cancer. Most patients are asymptomatic for hepatic involvement and are diagnosed mostly by deranged liver function tests or on imaging studies. Symptoms may include fatigue, weight loss, decreased appetite, epigastric discomfort, fever, pedal edema, and jaundice.

Lung metastasis [5] occurs in about 35% patients with metastatic breast cancer. It is more commonly associated with HER-positive and triple-negative type of breast cancer. Symptoms include chest discomfort, shortness of breath, cough with hemoptysis, and wheeze.

Brain metastasis occurs in about 10–25% stage 4 breast cancer patients. Patients may present with headache, altered sensorium, amnesia, mood disorder, seizures, stroke, and focal neurological deficits.

33.4 What Are the Incidence, Prognosis, and Risk Factors for Brain Metastasis in Patients of Breast Cancer?

Breast cancer is the second most common cause of brain metastasis following lung cancer. The incidence of brain metastasis in patients of breast cancer varies from 10% to 25% in various studies [6–8].

The risk factors that are found to be associated with brain metastasis in these patients are advanced stage at diagnosis, age less than 40 years, BRCA1/BRCA 2 gene mutation, luminal type of breast cancer, triple-negative breast cancer, HER-2 receptor positivity, presence of lung metastasis, African American women, presence and number of extracranial metastases, high histological grade, and elevated LDH levels prior to treatment [9–17].

Factors for poor prognosis include high-grade tumors, tumor size >5 cm, presence of extra-cranial metastasis, multiple metastases, triple-negative or HER-2 biomarker positivity, and Karnofsky Performance Status (KPS) score of ≤70. Age, race, ethnicity, lymph node status, and time between diagnosis of breast cancer and brain metastasis do not impact survival [18].

33.5 What Are the Treatment Options and Prognosis After Treatment for Brain Metastasis in Breast Cancer Patients?

The various treatment options available for brain metastasis in breast cancer patients include local and systemic treatment or a combination of both along with conventional management protocol for patients with brain tumors. Conventional treatment focuses on strategies to control peritumoral edema, control of seizures, prevention of thromboembolic complications, and management of raised intracranial pressure.

Local treatment includes surgical removal of lesions, whole brain radiotherapy, stereotactic surgery, or a combination of above. The choice of treatment will depend upon number, size, and location of brain metastases, degree of mass effect and edema, presence or absence of symptoms, functional status, extent of systemic disease, and patient's preferences with regard to invasive therapy [19].

Systemic treatment involves the use of various chemotherapeutic agents and monoclonal antibodies like trastuzumab and pertuzumab for HER+ patients.

Various studies have suggested improved survival in breast cancer patients with brain metastasis due to availability of newer drugs. The overall median survival in patients with brain metastasis is about 14 months and in those with HER positivity is around 23 months due to efficacy of trastuzumab in these patients [20–23]. However, triple-negative patients with brain metastasis have an average survival period of about 3–4 months [24, 25].

33.6 What Is Stereotactic Radiosurgery?

Stereotactic radiosurgery (SRS) is a noninvasive treatment modality for brain pathologies including metastasis, where the lesion(s) are delivered high-dose radiation while sparing the adjacent normal brain parenchyma. SRS, thus, minimizes the widespread and long-lasting neurocognitive side effects of whole brain radiation therapy. SRS can be done using a linear accelerator, gamma knife or charged particles. It is the treatment of choice for some brain pathologies where the surgical resection involves high risk. It can be used as a monotherapy or as an adjunct to surgical treatment like SRS boost to the tumor bed in cases of brain metastases.

The gamma knife [26] was invented by Leksell in Sweden in 1951. It has an array of 192 cobalt-60 sources which is surrounded by an 18,000 kg shield. The sources are oriented in a manner such that all the beams converge at a single point termed as the isocenter and provides a target accuracy between 0.1 and 1 mm (Fig. 33.1). An MRI-compatible stereotactic head frame (Leksell Model G) is used for immobilization of the head (Fig. 33.2). However, the latest model of gamma knife, the Gamma Knife ICON, allows face mask immobilization of the head (Fig. 33.3). The duration of the treatment depends on the number and size of the lesions and the age of the radioisotope. The cognitive outcome has been found to be better with SRS compared to the whole brain radiotherapy.

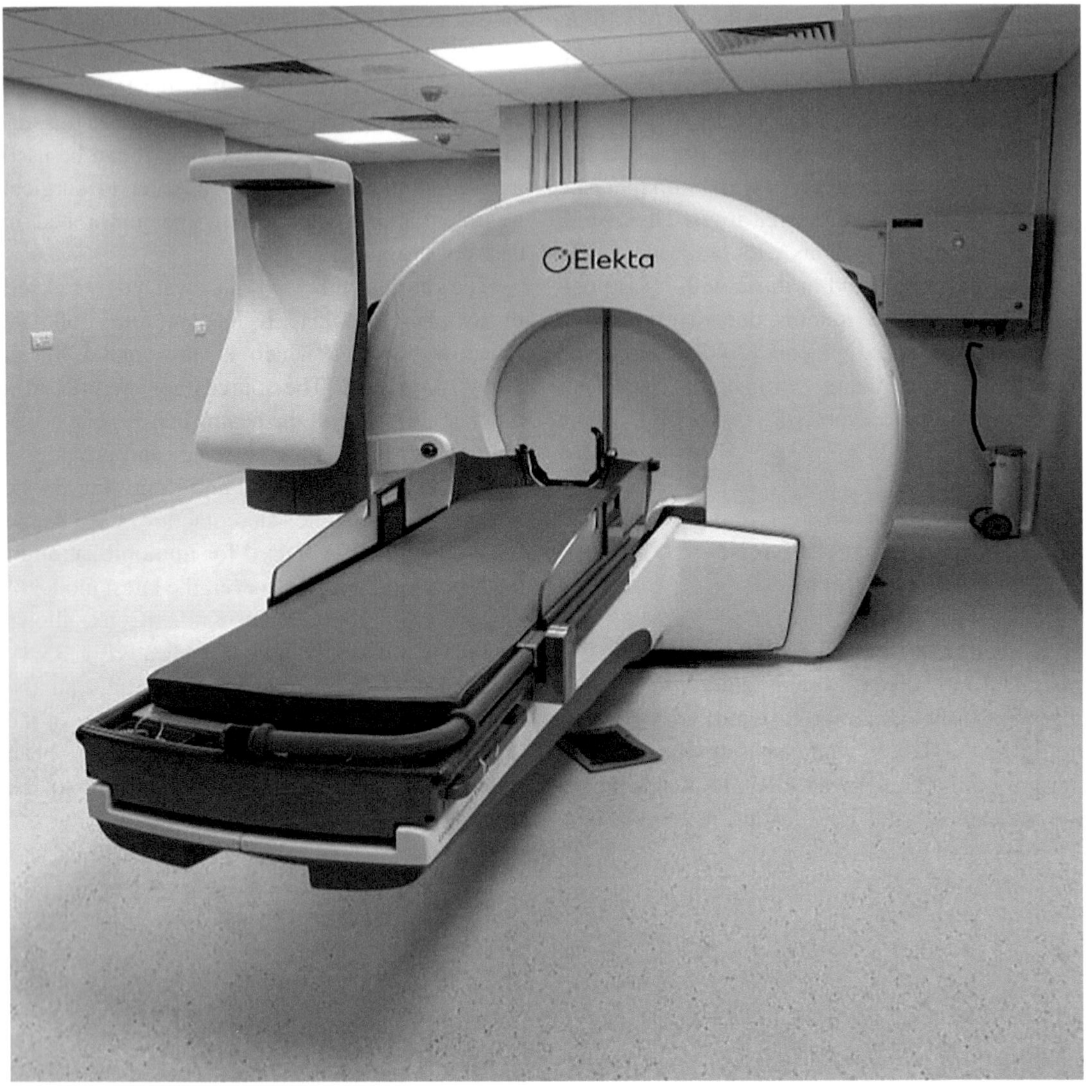

Fig. 33.1 The gamma knife radiosurgery suite

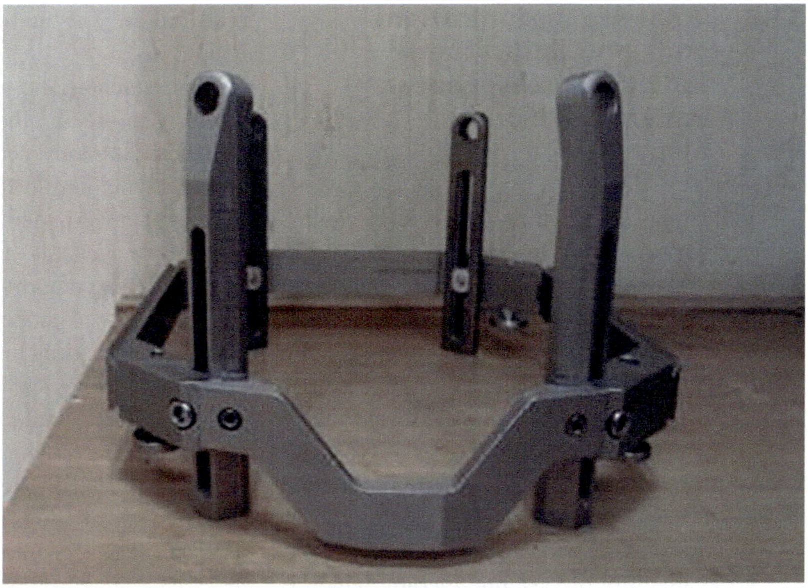

Fig. 33.2 MRI-compatible stereotactic head frame (Leksell Model G)

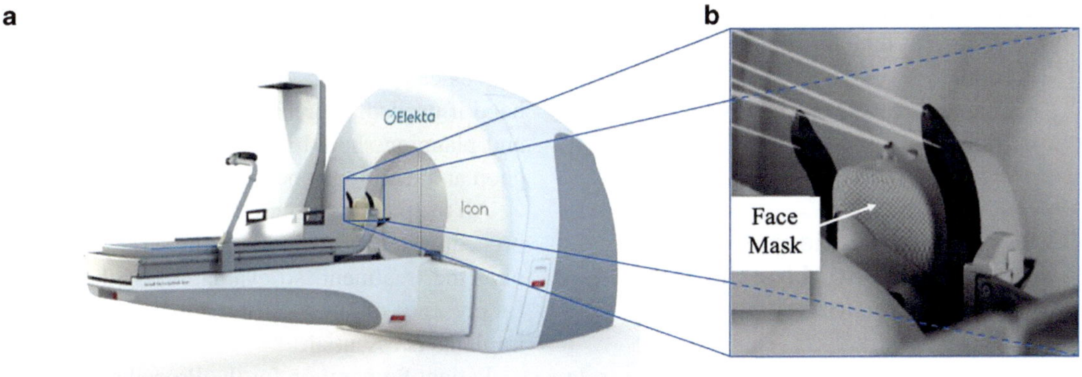

Fig. 33.3 (**a**) Gamma knife ICON and (**b**) face mask immobilization of the head

33.7 Enumerate the Advantages of SRS

The advantages of gamma knife radiosurgery are the following:

- Relatively painless procedure.
- No bleeding.
- Short treatment time.
- Less morbidity compared to surgery or whole brain radiation.
- Highly accurate.
- Less radiation exposure to the surrounding normal brain.
- Targets lesions in areas of the brain which are difficult to access surgically.
- Less damage to surrounding normal tissue.
- Day care procedure.
- Early recovery.

33.8 What Are the Indications and Contraindications for SRS in Breast Cancer Patients with Brain Metastasis?

The indications and contraindications for gamma knife surgery are the following:

(a) Indications [18].
- 3–4 small (< 10 cc) unresected brain lesions, though greater number of lesions or larger lesions can be treated using hypo-fractionated SRS
- Brain metastases post-resection (radiation to tumor bed).
- Patients with better performance status.
- Availability of systemic therapy which is known to be active in the brain.

(b) Contraindications [27].
- Multiple tumors (relative contraindication).
- Large size >10 cc (relative contraindication).

33.9 How Is a Patient Evaluated and Prepared for Gamma Knife Radiosurgery?

Gamma knife radiosurgery (GKRS) is a relatively painless procedure that does not involve any skin incision. The procedure requires an alert, cooperative patient who is comfortable and able to lie supine and remain immobile throughout the procedure. Most of the time, it is done under local anesthesia which is required only at the time of placement of head frame.

Assessment—The patient is evaluated preoperatively mostly by the neurosurgeon as general anesthesia is rarely needed for this procedure in adult patients like in this case. When the procedure is planned under monitored anesthesia care (MAC) or general anesthesia, the patient is evaluated for comorbidities, general well-being, airway, ability to cooperate and lie still, history of claustrophobia, drug history, and their side effects [28]. The neurological status and any focal neurological deficits should be documented before the procedure. The imaging and laboratory investigations are reviewed. The treatment of the patient is reviewed and all drugs are continued as per schedule. It is also very important to look for veins in these patients during preoperative visit as due to chemotherapy and multiple hospitalizations intravenous access may be difficult and a peripherally inserted central catheter (PICC) or a central venous catheter insertion can be planned beforehand if needed. Moreover, meticulous discussion and planning should be done with the neurosurgeon and radiologist before the procedure.

All the patients require MRI before the GKRS procedure for localization of the target and planning the treatment, so evaluation of the patient for presence of any MRI-incompatible devices or implants is essential.

Patient Preparation for the Procedure [29].

- Psychological preparation—Patients should be given complete information about the technique, duration, and invasive monitors, if used. It is very important to address all the queries of the patient so as to make the patient comfortable and less anxious on the day of the procedure.

- Nil per oral (NPO) orders—Patients should be kept NPO as per standard guidelines for any operative procedure if planned under general anesthesia. The patients are allowed a light breakfast if the treatment is planned under local anesthesia.
- Premedication—Alprazolam tablets can be given the night before the procedure to allay the anxiety of the patient depending on the general condition and level of sensorium.
- Steroids—Glucocorticoids are generally given to these patients before the procedure and continued for 3–5 weeks post procedure to combat the perilesional edema which may increase following the procedure.
- Consent is taken from the patient for the procedure and the patient is once again counseled. An intravenous access is secured for intravenous fluid and drug administration.

33.10 What Is the Workflow of Treatment for the Patient Posted for Gamma Knife Radiosurgery?

Gamma knife radiosurgery is usually a day care procedure. Once the patient arrives for the surgery, patient's consent, adequate preparation, and NPO status are ensured. Local anesthesia is infiltrated at the pin insertion site for the head frame application with close monitoring of vital signs. The patient undergoes a contrast MRI (alone or with CT head) after frame fixation. The MRI and CT images are transferred to the planning station and treatment planning is done. The patient is then wheeled into the gamma knife suite and positioned on the gamma knife table. Standard ASA monitors are attached and the treatment is then delivered. The workflow of standard gamma knife radiosurgery procedure is shown in Fig. 33.4.

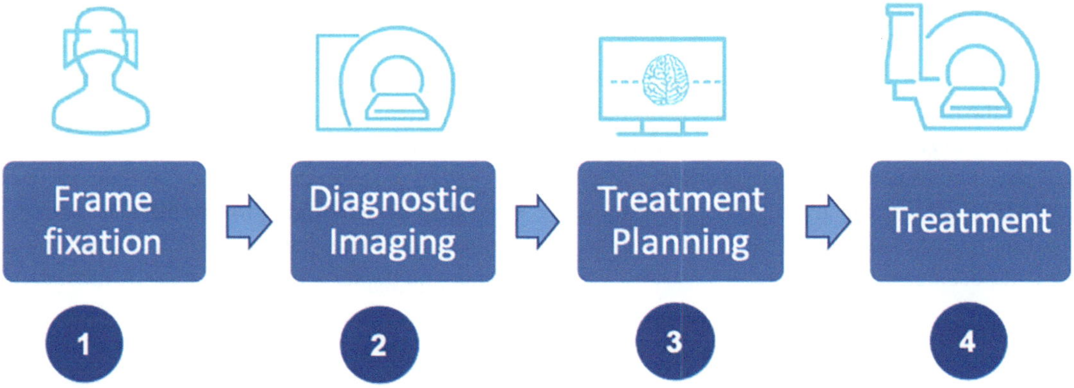

Fig. 33.4 Workflow for a gamma knife radiosurgery

33.11 What Are the Local Anesthetic Drugs that Can Be Used for Placement of the Stereotactic Frame?

Stereotactic frame placement is secured to the skull with the help of four pins. It is a painful procedure and thus requires local anesthetic infiltration before the pins are placed. The various local anesthetic drugs that can be used include lignocaine (maximum dose 5.0 mg/kg), lignocaine with epinephrine (7.0 mg/kg), bupivacaine (2.5 mg/kg), and ropivacaine (3.0 mg/kg). EMLA (eutectic mixture of local anesthetics) can also be applied to the pin site about an hour prior to pin insertion. The maximum safe dose of these drugs should be kept in mind as repeat infiltration may be needed in case of prolonged duration of procedure, thereby increasing chances of local anesthetic systemic toxicity as scalp is a highly vascular structure. Moreover, these patients are more prone to seizures due to brain metastasis, and if it occurs, it can be devastating and very difficult to manage with the head fixed in the frame.

Few patients may have a vasovagal episode during the placement of pins. One should be prepared for this and legs should be elevated immediately. It is imperative to have pulse oximeter connected during the frame placement so that one can pick the decreasing heart rate before the patient becomes unconscious.

33.12 How Is the Patient Monitored and Positioned During the Procedure?

All patients must be monitored using pulse oximetry during the application of head frame. During the radiosurgery procedure, the patients are monitored according to standard ASA (American Society of Anesthesiologists) guidelines using ECG, noninvasive blood pressure, and pulse oximetry. Oxygen should be supplemented using nasal cannula or face mask. The capnography mask (capnoxygen mask) should be used to continuously monitor end-tidal CO_2 ($EtCO_2$) to monitor patient's respiration while at the same time administering oxygen, if sedation is given.

The patient is closely watched using video cameras (focused on to the patient) and satellite monitors that will continuously display the patient's image and vital parameters on the screen outside the procedure room (Figs. 33.5 and 33.6). Also, mobile monitoring systems should be available as the patient might require transportation to the MRI suite or for CT scan. The patient should be explained that they will be able to communicate with the treating team during the procedure in case of any discomfort or query with the help of the built-in communication system.

Proper positioning of the patient is very important to ensure a comfortable and cooperative patient. The patient can be asked to lie supine and position themselves in the most com-

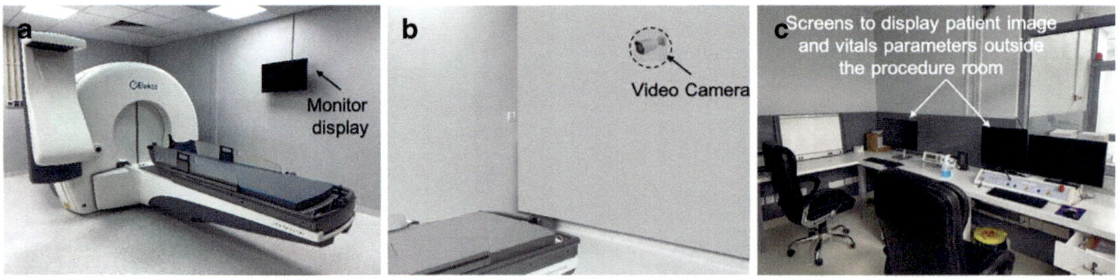

Fig. 33.5 (**a**) Gamma knife unit with monitor display, (**b**) video camera installed at the foot end of the gamma knife table focused on the patient, and (**c**) the image of the patient on the gamma knife table and vital parameters from the patient monitor are displayed on the screens outside the procedure room (remote monitoring system)

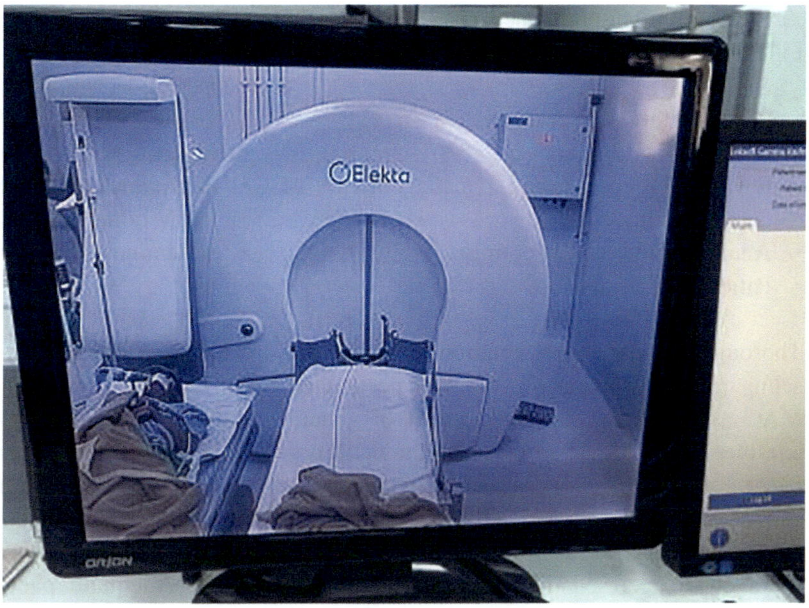

Fig. 33.6 Patient being watched on a screen outside the procedure room (patient lying on patient trolley inside the gamma knife unit)

fortable position. A pillow can be placed beneath the knees of the patient with legs flexed to prevent undue stretching of the spine especially in patients with back pain. Also, these patients are prone to have bony metastasis and so have fragile bones which are prone to fractures. Thus, utmost care should be taken during transfer of these patients to and from the procedure room. The environment of the gamma knife suite should be calm, quiet, and comfortable, and temperature should be adjusted as per comfort of the patient and blanket provided to the patient for comfort.

33.13 What Are the Anesthetic Considerations before Taking a Patient for Gamma Knife Surgery?

The most important consideration during conduct of anesthesia for this procedure involves ensuring availability of all anesthesia and resuscitation equipment along with support staff at this remote location away from the conventional operating room setup. Patients should be evaluated before the procedure and preparation should be done according to patient-specific factors. Certain factors that should be kept in mind before planning anesthesia for this procedure include the following:

- Need for complete immobility of the head after the frame is in place.
- Difficulty in accessing the airway with the head frame in situ.
- Long duration of procedure.
- Transportation of patient to multiple sites with head frame attached.
- Inability to access the patient during procedure and ensuring availability of remote monitoring systems.

33.14 How Is Monitored Anesthesia Care (MAC) Provided for Gamma Knife Surgery?

MAC is defined by the ASA as a specific anesthesia service provided by a trained anesthesiologist where the patient undergoes a diagnostic or therapeutic procedure under local anesthesia with mild sedation and/or analgesia. The patient should be cooperative to undergo the procedure under sedation [30–32].

Goals of monitored anesthesia care are the following:

- Patient safety.
- Support of vital functions.
- Early diagnosis and management of complications.
- Analgesia and patient comfort.
- Patient satisfaction.

Thorough preoperative evaluation, patient counseling, and postoperative care are needed for MAC as is needed for the conduct of general anesthesia. The anesthesiologist should be prepared for managing various complications like sudden patient movement leading to pin displacement, loss of airway, aspiration, seizures, desaturation due to deep sedation, etc. All the necessary equipment and emergency drugs should be available, and all preparation should be done for conversion to general anesthesia if need arises. Also, all the tools needed for removal of the head frame should be checked and readily available in case of emergency airway management.

Monitoring should include the following:

- Standard ASA monitors (ECG, pulse oximetry, NIBP, $EtCO_2$).
- Monitoring of response to verbal stimulation for titration of depth of sedation.

Contraindications for MAC are the following:

- Spasticity or movement disorders.
- Morbid obesity.
- History of sleep apnea.
- Patients in altered sensorium or inability to follow commands.
- Anticipated difficult airway.
- Patients with risk of airway obstruction with sedation.

Drugs (sedatives/analgesics) used for MAC are the following:

- Propofol—0.5 mg/kg bolus followed by 25–75 μg/kg/min IV as infusion.
- Opioids—Fentanyl 0.5–2 μg/kg/h infusion or 1–2 μg/kg bolus IV before stimulation.
- Dexmedetomidine—1 μg/kg loading over 10 min followed by 0.2–0.7 μg/kg/h IV infusion.
- Benzodiazepines—Midazolam 0.02–0.03 mg/kg IV bolus.
- Ketamine—0.25–1 mg /kg IV bolus.

33.14.1 Procedure

Patient planned for the procedure under MAC is sedated using either an opioid or a benzodiazepine. Continuous infusion of an appropriate sedative can be started after assessing the patient's general condition and ability to cooperate. Adequate padding is placed under the shoulders as the head frame might cause discomfort in lying supine for the duration of procedure. Warming blankets and proper padding of all pressure points is essential to make the patient comfortable. The patient is monitored throughout the procedure via remote monitoring system.

33.14.2 Discharge

After completion of the procedure, the head frame is removed, and the patient is shifted to the recovery room for observation and monitoring and later discharged after ensuring adequate recovery. Patients are given analgesics for pin site pain. Steroids, usually tablet dexamethasone, and antiepileptic drugs are continued.

33.14.3 Follow-Up

A repeat MRI of the brain, 3 months after the gamma knife radiosurgery, is done to check the response of the tumor. These patients are kept under continuous follow-up as it is not uncommon for these patients to develop new metastases over time.

33.15 What Are the Indications of General Anesthesia for Gamma Knife Radiosurgery and How Is It Accomplished?

The indications of general anesthesia are the following:

- Uncooperative patient.
- Patient with movement disorders or dystonia.
- Claustrophobic patients.
- Patients who have mental retardation.
- Pediatric patients.

After a thorough preoperative evaluation, patient preparation, ensuring adequate NPO status on the day of procedure and availability of necessary equipment and personnel, the patient is taken inside the gamma knife suite, and standard ASA monitors are attached. An intravenous line is secured beforehand, and an anxiolytic like midazolam or fentanyl can be administered depending on the general condition and comorbidities 30–45 min before the procedure.

33.15.1 Induction

Balanced anesthesia technique is used. Propofol is most widely used for induction. A short-acting opioid like fentanyl or alfentanil is given before propofol and muscle relaxation is achieved using intermediate-acting relaxants such as vecuronium, rocuronium, or atracurium/cis-atracurium (if the patient has deranged liver functions due to liver metastasis). Airway is secured using an endotracheal tube as the procedure usually takes around 4–5 h. Xylocard (preservative-free lignocaine) at a dose of 1.5 mg/kg, 90 s before the laryngoscopy, may be given intravenously to blunt the response to laryngoscopy and intubation. Alternatively, short-acting beta-blockers like esmolol or metoprolol can be used. Once the airway is secured, a stereotactic frame is applied after local infiltration at pin sites. Additional bolus of fentanyl or propofol can be given at this point to prevent sympathetic response and subsequent increase in intracranial pressure to pin insertion which is the only noxious stimulus in this procedure.

33.15.2 Maintenance

Anesthesia may be maintained either using inhalational or intravenous anesthetic. If the gamma knife suite has availability of vaporizers, inhalational anesthesia technique may be used. If it is not available, then the patient can be maintained on total intravenous anesthesia (TIVA) using continuous infusion of propofol and fentanyl. Infusion or top-up of muscle relaxants is generally not needed, and patients can be maintained on positive pressure ventilation with TIVA.

Crystalloids can be used as maintenance fluids. As the procedure is not associated with blood loss, fluids should be administered judiciously. Temperature should be monitored, and warming blankets should be used as these patients are at a higher risk of hypothermia due to their frailty, cold environment of the gamma knife suite, and loss of thermoregulation under general anesthesia. Adequate padding of all pressure points should be done to prevent pressure sores due to long duration of the procedure. Also, care should be taken while transporting these patients from one place to another as they have fragile bones which are prone to fractures.

33.15.3 Extubation and Recovery

At the end of the procedure, most patients are extubated on table after adequately reversing the neuromuscular block. Antiemetics should be administered prior to tracheal extubation. The patients are monitored for 3–4 h after the procedure in the recovery room and discharged the same day [33–37].

33.16 What Are the Complications Associated with Gamma Knife Treatment?

The complication associated with gamma knife radiosurgery [38] may be due to the following:

Remote location: As the procedure involves moving the patient to various sites for imaging and procedure, many problems can be encountered which include machine and equipment failure, need for emergent airway management, nonavailability of assistance when needed, and difficult access for resuscitation. One should be prepared with anticipation and management of these problems.

Head frame: Prolonged application and lying down in supine position might cause undue pressure beneath the shoulders and can lead to pressure sores, so proper padding needs to be done for ensuring patient's comfort and safety. Also, since assistance might not always be available, one should be familiar with and able to use the necessary equipment for removal and adjustment of the head frame in case of emergency.

Anaphylaxis: It can happen due to contrast or drugs in susceptible patients. Such patients should be given H1 and H2 receptor blockers prophylactically, and availability of all necessary drugs and equipment for management of anaphylaxis should be ensured.

Prolonged duration of procedure: The procedure may sometimes last 4–6 h. All measures should be taken to ensure patient's comfort especially if the procedure is undertaken under local anesthesia or MAC. Constant communication and monitoring of the patient are vital in such a scenario. The anesthetic goals during general anesthesia include maintenance of fluid balance and prevention of hypothermia and hypoglycemia. The patient should be catheterized beforehand if such a long duration is anticipated.

Radiation exposure: It can lead to early and late complications which include.

early nausea, vomiting, headache, loss of hair (when the lesion is very superficial), and decreased seizure threshold. These complications are very rare as the radiation dose delivered to the normal brain is minimal.

Late—Vasogenic edema and radiation necrosis leading to focal neurological deficits or cranial nerve palsies.

The patients are therefore preemptively treated with steroids and antiemetics. Steroids are generally continued for 3–6 weeks for the prevention of brain edema and seizures in susceptible patients. Bevacizumab (anti-VEGF monoclonal antibodies) has also been tried in patients with vasogenic edema recalcitrant to the routine measures.

References

1. Alkabban FM, Ferguson T. Breast cancer. In: StatPearls. Treasure Island (FL): StatPearls Publishing; 2020.
2. Largillier R, Ferrero JM, Doyen J, Barriere J, Namer M, Mari V, Courdi A, Hannoun-Levi JM, Ettore F, Birtwisle-Peyrottes I, Balu-Maestro C. Prognostic factors in 1038 women with metastatic breast cancer. Ann Oncol. 2008;19(12):2012–9.
3. Chang J, Clark GM, Allred DC, Mohsin S, Chamness G, Elledge RM. Survival of patients with metastatic breast carcinoma: importance of prognostic markers of the primary tumor. Cancer. 2003;97(3):545–53.
4. Huang JF, Shen J, Li X, Rengan R, Silvestris N, Wang M, Derosa L, Zheng X, Belli A, Zhang XL, Li YM. Incidence of patients with bone metastases at diagnosis of solid tumors in adults: a large population-based study. Annals of translational medicine. 2020;8(7):482.
5. Xiao W, Zheng S, Liu P, Zou Y, Xie X, Yu P, Tang H, Xie X. Risk factors and survival outcomes in patients with breast cancer and lung metastasis: a population-based study. Cancer Med. 2018;7(3):922–30.
6. Tsukada Y, Fouad A, Pickren JW, Lane WW. Central nervous system metastasis from breast carcinoma autopsy study. Cancer. 1983;52(12):2349–54.
7. Barnholtz-Sloan JS, Sloan AE, Davis FG, Vigneau FD, Lai P, Sawaya RE. Incidence proportions of brain metastases in patients diagnosed (1973 to 2001) in the metropolitan Detroit cancer surveillance system. J Clin Oncol. 2004;22(14):2865–72.
8. Rostami R, Mittal S, Rostami P, Tavassoli F, Jabbari B. Brain metastasis in breast cancer: a comprehensive literature review. J Neuro-Oncol. 2016;127(3):407–14.
9. Kennecke H, Yerushalmi R, Woods R, Cheang MC, Voduc D, Speers CH, Nielsen TO, Gelmon K. Metastatic behavior of breast cancer subtypes. J Clin Oncol. 2010;28(20):3271–7.
10. Dawood S, Lei X, Litton JK, Buchholz TA, Hortobagyi GN, Gonzalez-Angulo AM. Incidence of brain metastases as a first site of recurrence among women with triple receptor–negative breast cancer. Cancer. 2012;118(19):4652–9.

11. Lin NU, Claus E, Sohl J, Razzak AR, Arnaout A, Winer EP. Sites of distant recurrence and clinical outcomes in patients with metastatic triple-negative breast cancer: high incidence of central nervous system metastases. Cancer. 2008;113(10):2638–45.
12. Albiges L, Andre F, Balleyguier C, Gomez-Abuin G, Chompret A, Delaloge S. Spectrum of breast cancer metastasis in BRCA1 mutation carriers: highly increased incidence of brain metastases. Ann Oncol. 2005;16(11):1846–7.
13. Song Y, Barry WT, Seah DS, Tung NM, Garber JE, Lin NU. Patterns of recurrence and metastasis in BRCA1/BRCA2-associated breast cancers. Cancer. 2020;126(2):271–80.
14. Evans AJ, James JJ, Cornford EJ, Chan SY, Burrell HC, Pinder SE, Gutteridge E, Robertson JF, Hornbuckle J, Cheung KL. Brain metastases from breast cancer: identification of a high-risk group. Clin Oncol. 2004;16(5):345–9.
15. Slimane K, Andre F, Delaloge S, Dunant A, Perez A, Grenier J, Massard C, Spielmann M. Risk factors for brain relapse in patients with metastatic breast cancer. Ann Oncol. 2004;15(11):1640–4.
16. Pestalozzi BC, Zahrieh D, Price KN, Holmberg SB, Lindtner J, Collins J, Crivellari D, Fey MF, Murray E, Pagani O, Simoncini E. Identifying breast cancer patients at risk for central nervous system (CNS) metastases in trials of the international breast cancer study group (IBCSG). Ann Oncol. 2006;17(6):935–44.
17. Ryberg M, Nielsen D, Osterlind K, Andersen PK, Skovsgaard T, Dombernowsky P. Predictors of central nervous system metastasis in patients with metastatic breast cancer. A competing risk analysis of 579 patients treated with epirubicin-based chemotherapy. Breast Cancer Res Treat. 2005;91(3):217–25.
18. Vogelbaum MA, Brown PD, Messersmith H, Brastianos PK, Burri S, Cahill D, Dunn IF, et al. Treatment for brain metastases: ASCO-SNO-ASTRO guideline; 2022. p. 331–57.
19. Bailleux C, Eberst L, Bachelot T. Treatment strategies for breast cancer brain metastases. Br J Cancer. 2021;124(1):142–55.
20. Dawood S, Broglio K, Esteva FJ, Ibrahim NK, Kau SW, Islam R, Aldape KD, Yu TK, Hortobagyi GN, Gonzalez-Angulo AM. Defining prognosis for women with breast cancer and CNS metastases by HER2 status. Ann Oncol. 2008;19(7):1242–8.
21. Melisko ME, Moore DH, Sneed PK, De Franco J, Rugo HS. Brain metastases in breast cancer: clinical and pathologic characteristics associated with improvements in survival. J Neuro-Oncol. 2008;88(3):359–65.
22. Stemmler HJ, Kahlert S, Siekiera W, Untch M, Heinrich B, Heinemann V. Characteristics of patients with brain metastases receiving trastuzumab for HER2 overexpressing metastatic breast cancer. Breast. 2006;15(2):219–25.
23. Eichler AF, Kuter I, Ryan P, Schapira L, Younger J, Henson JW. Survival in patients with brain metastases from breast cancer: the importance of HER-2 status. Cancer: interdisciplinary international journal of the American cancer. Society. 2008;112(11):2359–67.
24. Dawood S, Broglio K, Esteva FJ, Yang W, Kau SW, Islam R, Albarracin C, Yu TK, Green M, Hortobagyi GN, Gonzalez-Angulo AM. Survival among women with triple receptor-negative breast cancer and brain metastases. Ann Oncol. 2009;20(4):621–7.
25. Nam BH, Kim SY, Han HS, Kwon Y, Lee KS, Kim TH, Ro J. Breast cancer subtypes and survival in patients with brain metastases. Breast Cancer Res. 2008;10(1):1–8.
26. Schwartz M. Stereotactic radiosurgery: comparing different technologies. CMAJ. 1998;158(5):625–8.
27. Shaw E, Scott C, Souhami L, Dinapoli R, Kline R, Loeffler J, Farnan N. Single dose radiosurgical treatment of recurrent previously irradiated primary brain tumors and brain metastases: final report of RTOG protocol 90-05. Int J Radiat Oncol Biol Phys. 2000;47(2):291–8.
28. Berg RJ, Maheshwari K, Thapa S. Anesthetic considerations for gamma knife stereotactic radiosurgery in patients with intracranial lesions. Contemp Neurosurg. 2011;33(6):1–3.
29. Dagal A, Lam AM. Anesthesia for stereotactic radiosurgery and intraoperative magnetic resonance imaging. In: Ruskin KJ, Rosenbaum SH, Rampil IJ, editors. Fundamentals of Neuroanesthesia: a physiologic approach to clinical practice. Oxford, UK: Oxford University Press; 2013. p. 185–200.
30. Ghisi D, Fanelli A, Tosi M, Nuzzi M, Fanelli G. Monitored anesthesia care. Minerva Anestesiol. 2005;71(9):533–8.
31. Fahy CJ, Okumura M. Sedation for paediatric stereotactic radiosurgery: the dexmedetomidine experience. Anaesth Intensive Care. 2004;32(6):809–11.
32. Harris EA. Sedation and anesthesia options for pediatric patients in the radiation oncology suite. Int J Pediatr. 2010;2010:870921.
33. Edler A. Special anesthetic considerations for stereotactic radiosurgery in children. J Clin Anesth. 2007;19(8):616–8.
34. Bauman GS, Brett CM, Ciricillo SF, Larson DA, Sneed P, Stalpers LJ, Edwards M, Wara WM. Anesthesia for pediatric stereotactic radiosurgery. Anesthesiology. 1998;89(1):255–7.
35. Bone ME, Bristow A. Total intravenous anaesthesia in stereotactic surgery--one year's clinical experience. Eur J Anaesthesiol. 1991;8(1):47–54.
36. Sessler DI. Mild perioperative hypothermia. N Engl J Med. 1997;336(24):1730–7.
37. Stokes MA, Soriano SG, Tarbell NJ, Loeffler JS, Alexander E 3rd, Black PM, Rockoff MA. Anesthesia for stereotactic radiosurgery in children. J Neurosurg Anesthesiol. 1995;7(2):100–8.
38. Vachhrajani S, Fawaz C, Mathieu D, Menard C, Cusimano MD, Gentili F, Hodaie M, Kenny B, Kulkarni AV, Laperriere N, Schwartz M. Complications of gamma knife surgery: an early report from 2 Canadian centers. J Neurosurg. 2008;109(Supplement):2–7.

34 Case of Carcinoma Urinary Bladder for Proton Radiation Therapy

Rudranil Nandi and Srimanta Kumar Haldar

34.1 How Is the Cancer Burden in the World?

19 million new cases of carcinoma urinary bladder are diagnosed worldwide every year. It is estimated that one out of five may develop the disease before 75 years of age. The lowest incidence is 1 in 10 in South-Central Asia and Middle Africa and 1 in 2.5 in Australia and New Zealand. Presently, nearly 44 million such patients diagnosed within the last 5 years are alive [1].

34.2 What Is the Incidence of Urinary Bladder Cancer?

As per the GLOBOCAN 2020 database, urinary bladder carcinoma is the cause of approximately 3.0% (573,278 cases) of all recently diagnosed cancer and 2.1% (212,536 cases) of all cancer deaths worldwide. In India, it accounts for 1.6% of all newly diagnosed cancer and 1.3% of cancer deaths [1].

R. Nandi (✉) · S. K. Haldar
Department of Oncoanaesthesia, Tata Medical Center, Kolkata, West Bengal, India

34.3 Who Are more Affected with Urinary Bladder Cancer?

Urinary bladder carcinoma is more prevalent in the male population, with a ratio of 3:1, and is particularly common among the aged. The median age at the time of diagnosis varies from 69 years in men to 71 years in women. Nearly 90% of those affected are older than 55 years, with a mean age of 73 years at diagnosis. Men face a lifetime risk of one in 26, whereas women have a lower lifetime risk of one in 88. Whites are impacted about twice as often as Blacks or Hispanics, though Black patients are more likely to receive a diagnosis at an advanced stage. Over time, there has been a decrease in the incidence of the disease, leading to a decline in bladder cancer-related mortality for women, while the mortality rate remains steady for men. Bladder cancer is associated with various risk factors, although a significant number of patients are diagnosed without clear exposures [2].

34.4 What Are the Risk Factors of Bladder Cancer?

Recognized risk factors encompass male gender, advanced age, White ethnicity, contact with specific chemicals, use of certain drugs like cyclophosphamide, pelvic radiation, persistent bladder

N. Gupta et al. (eds.), *Problem Based Learning Discussions in Onco-Anesthesia and Onco-Critical Care*, https://doi.org/10.1007/978-981-99-6339-3_34

infection or irritation, previous history of bladder cancer in self or family, and smoking cigarette. Additionally, research suggests potential links with diabetes mellitus, obesity, and human papillomavirus. Prolonged use of pioglitazone independently associates with a slightly heightened risk of bladder cancer. A modest increase in risk may also be associated with the consumption of substantial amounts of processed red meat. Cigarette smoking stands out as the predominant contributor of elevated incidence of carcinoma bladder in Western countries. Moreover, intensity of smoking may correlate with the severity of bladder carcinoma. Heavy smokers are more prone to muscle-invasive and high-grade tumors. Occupational exposures in various industries, involving paint components (polyaromatic hydrocarbons), diesel exhausts, carcinogens associated with fire like benzene, and aromatic amines in the metal, auto, paper, hairdressing, and rubber industry, contribute to approximately 20% of new bladder cancer cases [3].

34.5 How Does Bladder Cancer Patients Present?

The primary indicator of bladder cancer commonly observed is painless hematuria, where blood in the urine is present. About 1.3% of individuals with asymptomatic microscopic hematuria (three or more RBCs/hpf), without an apparent benign cause, may have bladder cancer. Gross hematuria, or visible blood in the urine, is linked to a higher likelihood of malignancy, estimated at 20%. Irritative voiding symptoms often accompany bladder cancer, including urinary frequency, urgency, nocturia, and dysuria. If the tumor is situated near the bladder neck or urethra, obstructive symptoms like decreased or intermittent urine stream, incomplete voiding, or straining may be present. In cases of advanced disease, symptoms related to metastatic involvement may manifest in affected individuals [4].

34.6 What Are the Common Sites of Metastasis of Bladder Cancer?

Bladder cancer commonly metastasizes to various sites, including the lymph nodes, bones, lungs, liver, and peritoneum. Physical examination findings are typically inconspicuous in these, particularly in the absence of advanced or metastatic disease. However, in cases where the disease has progressed, physical examination may reveal palpable masses in the kidneys or bladder. This suggests that noticeable clinical signs often occur in advanced stages of bladder cancer or when metastasis has occurred [5].

34.7 What Are Different Types of Bladder Cancer and their Prognosis?

Bladder cancer is a diverse disease with varied clinical outcomes, and the predominant histologic type is urothelial cancer (UC) which is also referred to as transitional cell cancer. UC may originate from upper urinary tract, such as renal pelvis or ureter, but more commonly arises in the urinary bladder. The spectrum of bladder cancer includes slow-growing non-muscle-invasive bladder cancer (NMIBC) with a protracted presentation, to muscle-invasive bladder cancer (MIBC) that invade the detrusor muscle which are aggressive. MIBC often needs radical treatments like surgery, chemotherapy, and radiation. Patients with bladder cancer exhibit diverse life expectancies due to the presence of competing comorbidities.

The three primary concerns for cancer patients—survival, care experience, and future quality of life—apply to bladder cancer as well. MIBCs have an increased risk of spreading to lymph nodes and other organs. NMIBCs include carcinoma in situ (CIS), papillary tumors that are noninvasive, and papillary tumors that invade lamina propria. NMIBCs account for 70% of newly diagnosed bladder cancer and frequently require endoscopic assessments and resections [6].

34.8 What Is the Prognosis of Different Types of Bladder Cancer?

Non-muscle-invasive bladder cancers (NMIBCs) can be treated with curative intent, and patients with NMIBC have an approximately 90% 5-year overall survival (OS) rate. However, there is a progression risk, with 15–20% of NMIBCs advancing to muscle-invasive bladder cancer (MIBC). CIS and high-grade papillary tumors are more likely to progress to MIBC. The 5-year overall survival in patients having MIBC is in the range of 60–70% [7].

34.9 What Are the Various Management Options for Bladder Cancer?

Despite significant advancements in treating other cancer types, systemic therapy for bladder cancer had seen little change for over 30 years. However, in the past decade, an improved understanding of bladder s pathogenesis, combined with a growing interest in clinical drug development, has led to a rapid expansion of available treatment options. Bladder cancer management now involves five standard treatment types, the selection of which depends on the specific stage and type of the disease (Fig. 34.1). These are the following:

(a) Surgery.
(b) Radiation therapy.
(c) Chemotherapy.
(d) Immunotherapy.
(e) Targeted therapy [8].

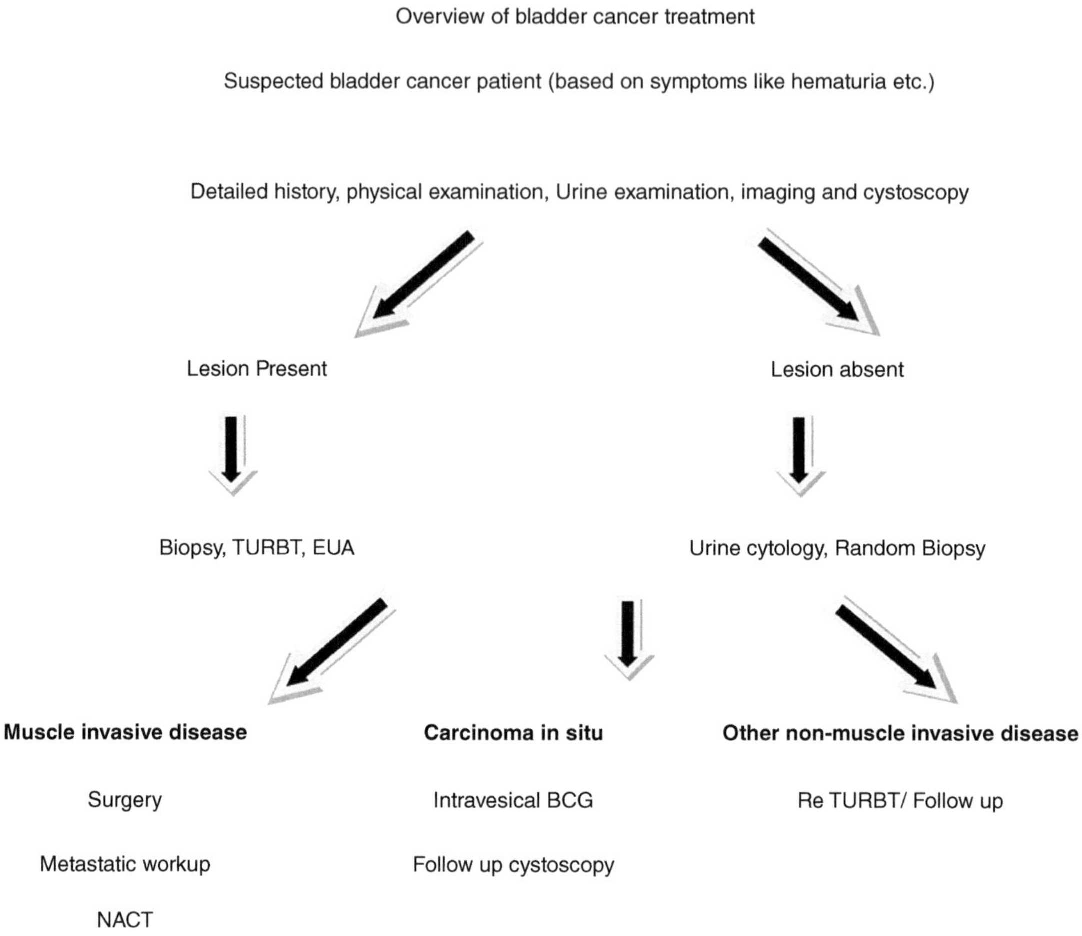

Fig. 34.1 Algorithm for the management of bladder cancer. (CT, computed tomography; TURBT, transurethral resection of bladder tumor) [9]. (*Reprinted from Sharma S, Ksheersagar P, Sharma P. Diagnosis and treatment of bladder cancer.* Am Fam Physician. *2009;80* [7]*:721*)

34.10 What Is Proton Radiation Therapy (PBT)?

High-energy protons have distinctive physical characteristics that allow for precise targeting and deposition of energy at desired sites, with minimal impact on healthy tissues. In contrast to photons used in conventional radiotherapy, which deposit their maximum energy upon entering tissue, protons travel in straight lines and deliver most energy when their path ends, known as the Bragg peak. This property of protons spares adjacent healthy tissue from the highest radiation effects.

The ability to precisely target deep-lying tissue and the central nervous system makes proton radiotherapy advantageous. It finds applications in the treatment of various conditions, including childhood brain tumors, retinoblastoma, prostate and bladder cancers, and hepatocellular carcinoma. Protons exhibit unique physical characteristics called Bragg peaks, and by overlaying several peaks, a region of uniform dose known as a spread-out Bragg peak (SOBP) can be tailored to the location and size of a tumor. Consequently, PBT delivers high-dose radiation to the target with minimal radiation-induced complications to nearby healthy tissue.

Recently, PBT has been found to be effective for bladder cancer, and this has led to an increased number of facilities worldwide [10].

34.11 What Are the Advantages of Proton Radiation Therapy?

(a) High-energy, precisely targeted proton beams can administer elevated doses of radiation to eliminate malignant cells, reducing recurrence rates in numerous cancer cases.
(b) Proton therapy is noninvasive and associated with fewer side effects.
(c) Patients undergoing proton therapy may exhibit increased tolerance for chemotherapy.
(d) Individuals undergoing treatment with proton therapy often experience a better quality of life.
(e) Proton therapy has demonstrated effectiveness in treating areas that have previously undergone radiotherapy [10].

34.12 What Are the Side Effects of PBT?

Side effects of PBT (Table 34.1) [11].

Table 34.1 Side effects of PBT

Short-term side effects
Nausea and vomiting
Fatigue
Alteration in taste
Diarrhea
Loss of hair
Headache
Blurring of vision
Mucositis
Radiation burns on the skin
Emotional upset due to repeated procedures
Long-term side effects
Claustrophobia
Regression in behavior
Hormonal dysfunction
Fertility impairment
Neurocognition problems
Changes in urinary bladder
Initiation of second tumor
Vascular problems like stroke and heart disease

34.13 What Are the Anesthetic Considerations in Patients Posted for Proton Radiation Therapy?

Anesthesia administration at proton therapy centers presents unique challenges due to factors such as the remote location, multiple treatment sessions (ranging from 10 to 30), and variable durations of individual sessions that may extend up to 90 min. Like conventional radiotherapy, immobilization devices like cradles and thermoplastic face masks are necessary. For young children and adults prone to claustrophobia or disorientation, deep sedation is often required for treatment.

The pre-procedural assessment should include a thorough medical history, location, position during treatment, and chemotherapy (previous or ongoing) along with their potential side effects. The preferred anesthetic technique for PBT is propofol-based total intravenous anesthesia (TIVA) without securing the airway. We need to provide supplemental oxygen through a face mask or nasal cannula and give antiemetics. Due to the prolonged sessions, extended length oxygen and suction tubing, as well as specialized anesthetic circuits, may be necessary for safe airway management. Additionally, extended length intravenous giving sets may be considered.

The extended treatment duration may result in a prolonged recovery. So an appropriately staffed and well-equipped recovery room is essential for patient safety [12, 13].

34.14 What Challenges an Anesthesiologist Face in an Outside Operating Room Environment?

The various challenges involved during treatment are the following:

(a) Anesthesia at a remote site with limited access to the patient involves staff members leaving the room during radiation delivery.

The patient is observed through video and monitoring screens.

(b) Loud ambient noise is present in the radiotherapy environment.
(c) The radiotherapy room is cold; therefore, it is advisable to increase the ambient temperature and use warming devices (applied outside the treatment field) as necessary.
(d) Radiation safety is crucial, necessitating protection and monitoring measures for staff members [14].

34.15 What Are the Patient-Related Concerns?

(a) A thorough pre-anesthetic evaluation is essential, considering both the local and systemic effects of the tumor, as patients may also be experiencing toxicities from concurrent chemo- and radiotherapy.
(b) Patients may experience delayed gastric emptying due to factors such as opioids, comorbidities, stress, and/or chemotherapy, increasing the risk of gastric content aspiration.
(c) Regular monitoring of laboratory values, including a full blood count and renal function, is crucial not only for safety reasons but also to assess the efficacy of treatment.
(d) There is a potential risk of upper respiratory tract infections (URTI) or sepsis during treatment.
(e) Careful consideration of the risk/benefit ratio is necessary when deciding whether to proceed or delay treatment.
(f) Inadequate nutrition may result from repeated episodes of nothing by mouth (NPO) for the procedure.
(g) Long-term venous access, such as a PICC or Hickman line under strict aseptic precautions, may be needed to avoid the need for daily.
(h) Patients may experience airway edema and swelling, and laryngospasm is a known complication in those with significant mucositis due to chemotherapy. Recurrent endotracheal intubation may increase the risk of subglottic stenosis [14].

34.16 What Positional Care Should Be Taken by Anesthesiologist During Proton Beam Radiotherapy in Other Tumors?

In modern radiotherapy, patients can be accurately positioned in the treatment room using automatic couches that offer 6° of freedom. This includes translation and rotations, allowing for precise and customized patient positioning during radiation therapy sessions.

Patients are sensitive to pressure injury since treatment tables are frequently firm and sessions last a prolonged period. The skin in the treatment area is especially vulnerable. The treatment of posterior fossa tumors may require the patient to be positioned in prone. Careful patient selection should be done for TIVA with an unprotected airway in prone position [15].

34.17 What Are the Implications of Tight-Fitting Immobilization Face Mask During Proton Therapy?

It may lead to airway compromise. The following issues might arise if face molds are used in case of head neck tumors:

(a) Impedes the patency of the airways.
(b) The location of any in place airway device.
(c) Impedes the chest movement during ventilation.
(d) In an emergency, delaying access to the airway.
(e) Result in pressure sores or skin damage.

The anesthesiologists should be involved in initial mask-molding process and anticipate weight gain around the neck that may occur due to administration of steroid during chemotherapy. This may lead to progressive tightening of the face masks, and the initial mask fitting should allow for extra room.

For patients who have undergone a craniotomy, considerations such as vocal cord paralysis and difficulty clearing oropharyngeal secretions should be carefully assessed before deciding to use the unprotected airway method.

While propofol has been widely utilized for procedural sedation and in intensive care settings, there is limited data on its safety for children undergoing daily prolonged procedures in an outpatient setting. Additionally, there is currently a lack of data on the safety and side effects associated with daily general inhalational anesthesia lasting up to 90 min over a 30-day period. As such, careful evaluation and monitoring are essential to ensure the safety and well-being of patients undergoing these procedures [16, 17].

34.18 Discuss the Pain and Palliative Care Management Strategies for Urinary Bladder Cancer Patient

The following key points and observations provide a comprehensive overview of the challenges and impact on the quality of life faced by patients diagnosed with bladder cancer, both non-muscle invasive (NMIBC) and muscle-invasive:

1. *Symptom burden:* Bladder cancer patients experience a considerable symptom burden, including blood in urine, urinary issues (frequency, urgency, incontinence, pain), gastrointestinal problems, fatigue, sleep disturbances, and impaired sexual function, particularly for those who have undergone radical procedures like cystectomy.
2. *Supportive care needs:* Patients have significant supportive care needs that extend beyond initial treatment. Emotional, cognitive, and sexual functioning is often impaired, emphasizing the need for comprehensive and ongoing support.
3. *Age-related differences:* Younger patients (<65 years old) report higher rates of financial difficulties, especially after radical cystectomy (RC). Mobility, usual activities, and pain are more commonly reported problems in this group.
4. *Comparisons with other cancers:* Bladder cancer patients experience more problems compared to patients with prostate and colorectal cancer, particularly in terms of mobility, usual activities, pain, sexual dysfunction, and financial toxicity.
5. *Treatment-specific impact:* The type of treatment, whether transurethral resection of bladder tumor (TURBT), radical cystectomy (RC), or radiotherapy (RT), has distinct impacts on various aspects of patients' lives. Sexual dysfunction is a significant concern, and patients undergoing RC may experience worse problems with body image, sexual intimacy, and enjoyment.
6. *Financial impact:* Younger patients receiving RC or TURBT report financial toxicity, with differences in employment disruption patterns between treatments. Lack of investment in supportive aspects of care and the necessity of multiple visits for BC management contribute to this financial burden.
7. *Quality of life differences:* Patients with NMIBC who receive adjuvant treatments have a better quality of life compared to those who undergo only endoscopic surgery. The lowest quality of life is reported for patients receiving RT for advanced BC.
8. *Sexual impact of radical treatments:* Radical treatments affect erection capability, ejaculation, and vaginal length. This may have sexual impact but pretreatment counselling and posttreatment support is often omitted.
9. *Female sexual issues:* Women's responses to questions about female sexual issues are lacking, indicating a need for further investigation into the impact of bladder cancer on women's sexual health [18].

34.19 What Are the Domains Where Bladder Cancer Patients Need Care?

Patients with bladder cancer need supportive care needs in following domains:

1. Communication with clinician.
2. Needs for daily living.
3. Information about health system.
4. Need for caregiver in family.
5. Psychosocial needs.
6. Physical and sexual needs.
7. Life expectancy and uncertainty discussion.
8. Coping impact of cancer treatment.
9. Financial crisis.
10. Impact on relationship with partner.
11. Life insurance [18].

References

1. Sung H, Ferlay J, Siegel RL, Laversanne M, Soerjomataram I, Jemal A, Bray F. Global cancer statistics 2020: GLOBOCAN estimates of incidence and mortality worldwide for 36 cancers in 185 countries. CA: Cancer J Clin. 2021;71(3):209–49. https://acsjournals.onlinelibrary.wiley.com/doi/10.3322/caac.21660.
2. Saginala K, Barsouk A, Aluru JS, Rawla P, Padala SA, Barsouk A. Epidemiology of bladder cancer. Med Sci. 2020;8(1):15.
3. Richters A, Aben KKH, Kiemeney LALM. The global burden of urinary bladder cancer: an update. World J Urol. 2020;38(8):1895–904.
4. Microhematuria: AUA/SUFU Guideline (2020)—American Urological Association 2023. https://www.auanet.org/guidelines-and-quality/guidelines/microhematuria.
5. Witjes JA, Bruins HM, Cathomas R, Compérat EM, Cowan NC, Gakis G, et al. European Association of Urology guidelines on muscle-invasive and metastatic bladder cancer: summary of the 2020 guidelines. Eur Urol. 2021;79(1):82–104.
6. Lenis AT, Lec PM, Chamie K, Mshs M. Bladder cancer: a review. JAMA. 2020;324(19):1980–91.
7. Grabe-Heyne K, Henne C, Mariappan P, Geiges G, Pöhlmann J, Pollock RF. Intermediate and high-risk non-muscle-invasive bladder cancer: an overview of epidemiology, burden, and unmet needs. Front Oncol. 2023 Jun;2(13):1170124.
8. Patel VG, Oh WK, Galsky MD. Treatment of muscle-invasive and advanced bladder cancer in 2020. CA: Cancer J Clin. 2020;70(5):404–23. https://doi.org/10.3322/caac.21631.
9. Diagnosis and Treatment of Bladder Cancer|AAFP. 2023. https://www.aafp.org/pubs/afp/issues/2009/1001/p717.html
10. Mohan R, Grosshans D. Proton therapy—present and future. Adv Drug Deliv Rev. 2017 Jan;15(109):26–44.
11. Dutz A, Agolli L, Baumann M, Troost EGC, Krause M, Hölscher T, et al. Early and late side effects, dosimetric parameters and quality of life after proton beam therapy and IMRT for prostate cancer: a matched-pair analysis. Acta Oncol. 2019;58(6):916–25.
12. Owusu-Agyemang P, Popovich SM, Zavala AM, Grosshans DR, Van Meter A, Williams UU, et al. A multi-institutional pilot survey of anesthesia practices during proton radiation therapy. Pract Radiat Oncol. 2016;6(3):155–9.
13. Owusu-Agyemang P, Grosshans D, Arunkumar R, Rebello E, Popovich S, Zavala A, et al. Non-invasive anesthesia for children undergoing proton radiation therapy. Radiother Oncol. 2014;111(1):30–4.
14. Wong T, Georgiadis PL, Urman RD, Tsai MH. Non-operating room anesthesia: patient selection and special considerations. Local Reg Anesth. 2020;13:1–9.
15. Devicienti S, Strigari L, D'Andrea M, Benassi M, Dimiccoli V, Portaluri M. Patient positioning in the proton radiotherapy era. J Exp Clin Cancer Res CR. 2010;29(1):47.
16. Adu-Poku O, Addison EK, Schandorf C, Hasford F, Inkoom S, Adom J, et al. Dosimetric effects of thermoplastic immobilizing devices on surface dose. Int J Med Phys Clin Eng Radiat Oncol. 2021;11(1):12–21.
17. Cappelli L, Poiset S, Greenberger B, Bar-Ad V. Thermoplastic mask-induced contact dermatitis: a case report. Cureus. 2022;14(4):e23815.
18. MacLennan SJ, MacLennan S. How do we meet the supportive care and information needs of those living with and beyond bladder cancer? Front Oncol. 2020;10:465.

Case of Ca Lung for EBUS and TBNA

35

Khushboo Pandey, Nishkarsh Gupta, and Anju Gupta

35.1 Discuss the Basic Principles of Bronchoscopy

Bronchoscopy refers to visualization of the airway with the help of a dedicated equipment working on the principle of optical fibers [1]. Its clinical application has been utilized for several diagnostic and therapeutic purposes. Further advancements in the technology have extended the field of interventional bronchoscopy by incorporation of physical properties of ultrasound waves. Such an equipment is known as endobronchial ultrasound (EBUS).

35.2 What Are the Equipment and Techniques Utilized for EBUS

35.2.1 Basic Description of EBUS

EBUS utilizes an inbuilt transducer with high-frequency ultrasound waves within the bronchoscope to visualize parabronchial and mediastinal structures [2]. Linear or radial EBUS are utilized nowadays in routine interventional pulmonary procedures. For diagnostic/therapeutic interventions, the transducer probe is negotiated through the working channel of the bronchoscope. Modern EBUS transducer probes are miniature in size, helping to overcome the poor penetration of ultrasound waves due to acoustic properties of air in lungs.

High-frequency EBUS transducer probes have good resolution, however, with a limited penetration due to shorter wavelength [3].

35.3 What Are Physiological Effects of Bronchoscopy?

The physiological cardiorespiratory perturbations imposed by flexible bronchoscopy have been well renowned [4]. The sympathetic stimulation due to activation of pressor response as a result of introduction of endoscope through the airway leads to moderate-severe cardiac manifestations in the form of tachypnea, desaturation, and worsening of pulmonary functions, especially in patients with limited cardiopulmonary reserve [5].

A decline in spirometric function such as FEV1, FVC, PEFR, and FEF 25–75 implies a possible bronchoconstriction due to insertion of scope [6].

Such manifestations are further profound in patients under rigid bronchoscopy due to the type of instrument and airway manipulation involved for visualization of airway.

K. Pandey · N. Gupta (✉) · A. Gupta
Onco-Anaesthesiology and Palliative Medicine, Dr. BRAIRCH, AIIMS, New Delhi, India

N. Gupta et al. (eds.), *Problem Based Learning Discussions in Onco-Anesthesia and Onco-Critical Care*, https://doi.org/10.1007/978-981-99-6339-3_35

35.4 What Are the Indications of EBUS?

Preliminary indications include the following [7]:

(a) Identification and localization of mediastinal structures adjacent to airway during interventional procedures
(b) Staging of hilar and mediastinal lymph nodes
(c) Biopsy of unknown solid structures in lung/pleura/mediastinum
(d) Sampling for suspected bronchopulmonary neoplasm [8]
(e) Diagnosis of infectious/inflammatory causes pertaining to thorax [9]
(f) Transbronchial needle aspiration (TBNA), conducted through therapeutic EBUS [10]

35.5 Discuss the Preoperative Evaluation and Optimization of Patients Posted for EBUS

Standard American Society of Anesthesiologists (ASA) guidelines are followed for preoperative evaluation [11], with special attention to airway assessment by the use of clinical as well as radiological parameters. Effect of previous anticancer treatments and comorbid conditions must be evaluated.

35.6 Discuss the Preparation and Safety Required for the Conduct of EBUS Procedure

Interventional pulmonary procedures are often conducted with a NORA facility; therefore, availability of equipment such as functional suctioning device, oxygen port, anesthesia drugs for induction, maintenance and reversal, monitoring devices and emergency drugs must be ensured. Nevertheless, anesthesia workstation must be appropriately functional. A difficult airway cart with all the airway devices must be always kept aside throughout the procedure. These procedures are dynamic and therefore mandate to ensure the availability of drugs and equipment for emergent clinical situations and cardiopulmonary resuscitation [12].

35.7 What Is the Anesthesia Technique Practiced for the Conduct of EBUS?

Such procedures are commonly performed under conscious sedation. Rarely, moderate to deep sedation or general anesthesia may be required in complex procedures. Delivery of anesthetic agent with total intravenous anesthesia (TIVA) technique is a recommended modality as open circuit during the procedure impedes the delivery of anesthetic agent. However, the incidence of complications has been found to be equivocal with both the techniques [13].

35.8 What All Modalities Are Available for Maintenance of Anesthesia?

Most of the procedures with EBUS are performed under conscious sedation, with topical anesthesia. Aerosolized lidocaine and/or spray-as-you-go technique can be used to facilitate bronchoscopy along with intravenous fentanyl and/or midazolam for conscious sedation. For induction and maintenance of general anesthesia with total intravenous anesthesia (TIVA), target-controlled infusion drug delivery system is a very useful modality. Propofol, ketamine, dexmedetomidine, and ketofol (1:1 mixture of ketamine and propofol) are commonly utilized drugs for intravenous anesthesia. Use of ketofol has been found to be equally effective as individual agents, incorporating beneficial properties of individual agents [14]. However, adverse effects of ketamine such as emergence delirium and increased secretions mandate close monitoring in the postoperative period. Inhalational-based anesthesia can be used for induction in children and short procedures with supplemental intravenous sedative-hypnotic drug boluses.

35.9 Discuss the Monitoring Techniques for the Procedure

Equipment for nonoperating room anesthesia (NORA) and monitoring devices must be ensured for availability and their proper functioning. Standard ASA monitoring with noninvasive blood pressure (NIBP), electrocardiograph (ECG), and pulse oximetry (SpO_2) is mandatory during the procedure. Additionally, the use of bispectral index (BIS) [15] end-tidal carbon dioxide (CO_2) monitoring and neuromuscular block monitoring in cases requiring general anesthesia is helpful for guiding the depth of anesthesia. Recently, transcutaneous probes for CO_2 monitoring [16] and electrical impedance tomography (EIT) [17] for monitoring of regional distribution of ventilation have been demonstrated to be helpful for the smooth conduct of such cases.

35.10 What All Oxygenation and Ventilation Strategies Can Be Utilized for EBUS?

Oxygenation and ventilation strategies are the most important aspect of the conduct of anesthesia during interventional pulmonary procedures.

A supraglottic airway device is the most commonly used airway conduit, to which a flexible catheter mount with a swivel adapter is attached and the EBUS bronchoscope is introduced through it. The self-sealing valve in the swivel adapter facilitates oxygenation and ventilation through one of the ports. These patients commonly present with compromised pulmonary functions; therefore the ability to tolerate relative hypoxia is limited. Anesthesiologists often find it challenging to maintain adequate oxygenation and ventilation during the conduct of interventional pulmonary procedures. The severity of clinical situation is further compounded by the presence of a difficult airway scenario. Several techniques have been utilized to maintain adequate oxygenation and ventilation, which include the following:

(a) Apneic oxygenation
(b) Spontaneous ventilation
(c) Controlled mechanical ventilation
(d) Jet ventilation
(e) High-frequency jet ventilation
(f) Noninvasive ventilation
(g) High-frequency nasal canula
(h) Continuous positive airway pressure

Apneic oxygenation is a cumbersome technique during the conduct of EBUS, as it involves intermittent oxygenation in between the procedure. Once the EBUS probe has been introduced, it is difficult to remove it and administer oxygen, thereafter reintroducing the EBUS scope after adequate saturation has been restored. Furthermore, repeated intubation utilized for oxygenation also predisposes for airway edema [18].

Spontaneous ventilation involves addition of topical anesthesia or airway-nerve blocks in order to facilitate bronchoscopy and prevent coughing/bucking or apneic spells. Ventilation can be assisted with the breathing circuit attached through side port of rigid bronchoscope or through the swivel connector of airway conduit [19].

Controlled mechanical ventilation is usually not required during the conduct of EBUS, as these are short procedures, well tolerated with conscious sedation and spontaneous ventilation.

Techniques of manual jet ventilation and high-frequency jet ventilation are feasible through RB, where the side port of RB is attached to a dedicated narrow bore jet-ventilating canula and the lumen of RB acts as an airway conduit [20].

Recently, utility of NIV, CPAP, and HFNC during interventional bronchoscopic procedures has been highlighted [21]. These modalities ensure paraoxygenation to maintain adequate oxygen saturation during the conduct of the procedure. It is especially beneficial for patients in critical care unit, undergoing bedside procedures. NIV mask in the form of nasal, oral, or helmet interface can be used to ventilate the patients during bronchoscopy while ensuring adequate gas exchange [22]. Additionally, CPAP face mask device can be utilized with variable FiO_2 in patients with acute respiratory failure defined as $PaO_2/FiO_2 < 300$ mmHg undergoing FOB.

Besides, HFNC is being utilized as an upcoming modality to prevent hypoxemic events during FOB [23]. The device can be used to maintain oxygenation throughout the procedure as a superior modality to conventional nasal canula [24].

35.11 What Are the Complications of EBUS Procedure?

Common complications encountered during the procedure include hypoxia, hypercapnia, and desaturation. Vigilant monitoring and management with oxygenation and ventilation are of paramount importance. Others include bleeding and airway edema, to be managed with electrocautery, topical anticoagulants, or vasoconstrictors or Fogarty catheter.

35.12 What Are the Contraindications of EBUS?

There are no specific contraindications of EBUS; those of fiberoptic bronchoscopy can be extrapolated to EBUS [25].

35.13 What Are the Limitations of EBUS?

1. Poor visualization and access for structures more than 2–3 cm beyond bronchial wall [26]
2. Operator dependent with a relatively long learning curve

35.14 Briefly Describe the Postoperative Care

Interventional pulmonary procedures are day care procedures; therefore, short-acting anesthetic agents are preferred, facilitating early discharge. Adequate recovery is as important as induction and maintenance of anesthesia. Intraoperative analgesia provided to combat laryngeal nociception with intravenous paracetamol usually suffices for the postoperative period as well. Role of steroids is controversial for airway edema; nevertheless, the latter is minimal in such EBUS interventions; therefore the use of steroids should be done as an individualized approach. Appropriate reversal of neuromuscular blockade along with supplementation of 100% oxygen until resumption of spontaneous breaths following withdrawal of bronchoscope is highly recommended. The incidence of reintubation in the postoperative care unit (PACU) has been reported to be up to 5–10% [27]; therefore, appropriate equipment should be readily available along with ASA standard monitors. Steam nebulization and bronchodilators are encouraged.

References

1. Cicenia J, Avasarala SK, Gildea TR. Navigational bronchoscopy: a guide through history, current use, and developing technology. J Thorac Dis. 2020;12(6):3263–71. https://doi.org/10.21037/jtd-2019-ndt-11.
2. Kuijvenhoven JC, Livi V, Morandi L, Cancellieri A, Annema JT, Trisolini R. The expanding role of endobronchial ultrasound in patients with centrally located intrapulmonary tumors. Lung Cancer. 2019;134:194–201. https://doi.org/10.1016/j.lungcan.2019.06.006. Epub 2019 Jun 24. PMID: 31319981.
3. Belanger AR, Akulian JA. An update on the role of advanced diagnostic bronchoscopy in the evaluation and staging of lung cancer. Ther Adv Respir Dis. 2017;11(5):211–21. https://doi.org/10.1177/1753465817695981. Epub 2017 Mar 8. PMID: 28470104; PMCID: PMC5933547.
4. Mohan A, Ansari A, Uniyal A, Upadhyay AD, Guleria R. Acute changes in physiological cardiopulmonary parameters during and after flexible fibreoptic bronchoscopy. Lung India. 2016;33:111–2.
5. Lundgren R, Haggmark S, Reiz S. Hemodynamic effects of flexible fiberoptic bronchoscopy performed under topical anesthesia. Chest. 1982;82:295–9.
6. Peacock AJ, Mitchell RB, Godfrey R. Effect of fiberoptic bronchoscopy on pulmonary function. Thorax. 1990;45:38–41.
7. Zou JY, Zhao WH, Chen JL, Du XK, Hu XW, Ye ZY. [The role of EBUS-TBNA in the systematic evaluation of lymph node staging and resectability analysis in non-small cell lung cancer].

Zhonghua Zhong Liu Za Zhi. 2019;41(10):792–795. Chinese. PMID: 31648504. https://doi.org/10.3760/cma.j.issn.0253-3766.2019.10.013.
8. Liam CK, Lee P, Yu CJ, Bai C, Yasufuku K. The diagnosis of lung cancer in the era of interventional pulmonology. Int J Tuberc Lung Dis. 2021;25(1):6–15. https://doi.org/10.5588/ijtld.20.0588. PMID: 33384039.
9. Tertemiz KC, Alpaydin AO, Karacam V. The role of endobronchial ultrasonography for mediastinal lymphadenopathy in cases with extrathoracic malignancy. Surg Endosc. 2017;31(7):2829–36. https://doi.org/10.1007/s00464-016-5293-z. Epub 2016 Oct 21. PMID: 27770251.
10. Santos LM, Figueiredo VR, Demarzo SE, Palomino ALM, Jacomelli M. The role of endobronchial ultrasound-guided transbronchial needle aspiration in isolated intrathoracic lymphadenopathy in non-neoplastic patients: a common dilemma in clinical practice. J Bras Pneumol. 2020;46(2):e20180183. https://doi.org/10.36416/1806-3756/e20180183. Epub 2020 May 11. PMID: 32402011; PMCID: PMC7462701.
11. Youn AM, Ko YK, Kim YH. Anesthesia and sedation outside of the operating room. Korean J Anesthesiol. 2015;68:323–31.
12. Wong T, Georgiadis PL, Urman RD, Tsai MH. Non-operating room anesthesia: patient selection and special considerations. Local Reg Anesth. 2020;13:1–9. Published 2020 Jan 8. https://doi.org/10.2147/LRA.S181458.
13. Bergbower EAS, Hong C, Gibbons M, Sachdeva A, Rock P, Anders MG. A retrospective analysis of respiratory complications under general anesthesia during EBUS-TBNA. J Community Hosp Intern Med Perspect. 2022;12(1):19–27. Published 2022 Jan 31. https://doi.org/10.55729/2000-9666.1003.
14. Ferguson I, Bell A, Treston G, New L, Ding M, Holdgate A. Propofol or Ketofol for procedural sedation and analgesia in emergency medicine—The POKER study: a randomised double-blind clinical trial. Ann Emerg Med. 2016;1:1–9.
15. Fadaizadeh L, Hoseyni MS, Shajareh E, Heydari G, Ardehali SH. Use of bispectrral index score for interventional bronchoscopy procedures. Tanaffos. 2015;14:246–51.
16. Ishiwata T, Tsushima K, Fujie M, Suzuki K, Hirota K, Abe M, et al. End-tidal capnographic monitoring to detect apnea episodes during flexible bronchoscopy under sedation. BMC Pulm Med. 2017;17:7.
17. Bialka S, Copik M, Rybczyk K, Owczarek A, Jedrusik E, Czyzewski D, et al. Assessment of changes of regional distribution in the lung tissue depending on the driving pressure applied during high frequency jet ventilation. BMC Anaesthesiol. 2018;31:101.
18. De Lima A, Kheir F, Majid A, Pawlowski J. Anaesthesia for interventional pulmonology procedures: a review of advanced diagnostic and therapeutic bronchoscopy. Can J Anaesth. 2018;65:1160.
19. Chadha M, Kulshrestha M, Biyani A. Anaesthesia for bronchoscopy. Indian J Anaesth. 2015;59:565–73.
20. Batra H, Yarmus L. Indications and complications of rigid bronchoscopy. Expert Rev Respir Med. 2018;12:509–20.
21. Pelaia C, Bruni A, Garofalo E, Rovida S, Arrighi E, Cammarota G, et al. Oxygenation strategies during flexible bronchoscopy: a review of the literature. Respir Res. 2021;22:253.
22. Sircar M, Onkar KJ, Chabbra GS, Bhattacharya S. Noninvasive ventilation-assisted bronchoscopy in high-risk hypoxemic patients. Indian J Crit Care Med. 2019;23:363–7.
23. D'Cruz RF, Hart N, Kaltsakas G. High-flow therapy: physiological effects and clinical applications. Breathe. 2020;4:1–10.
24. Su CL, Chiang LL, Tam KW, Chen TT, Hu MC. High-flow nasal canula for reducing hypoxemic events in patients undergoing bronchoscopy: a systematic review and meta-analysis of randomized trials. PLoS One. 2021;16:e0260716.
25. Muthu V, Sehgal IS, Dhooria S, et al. Endobronchial ultrasound-guided transbronchial needle aspiration: techniques and challenges. J Cytol. 2019;36(1):65–70. https://doi.org/10.4103/JOC.JOC_171_18.
26. Nogawa H, Matsumoto Y, Tanaka M, Tsuchida T. Diagnostic usefulness of bronchoscopy for peripheral pulmonary lesions in patients with idiopathic pulmonary fibrosis. J Thorac Dis. 2021;13(11):6304–13. https://doi.org/10.21037/jtd-21-1067. PMID: 34992810; PMCID: PMC8662480.
27. Conacher ID. Anaesthesia and tracheobronchial stenting for central airway obstruction in adults. Br J Anaesth. 2003;90(3):367–74. https://doi.org/10.1093/bja/aeg053.

Anesthesia and Cancer Recurrence 36

A. R. Karthik and Sushma Bhatnagar

36.1 Case Scenario

A 59-year-old postmenopausal lady is diagnosed with a T2N0M0 carcinoma breast and is planned for a simple mastectomy with sentinel lymph node biopsy. She undergoes the surgery under opioid and inhalational agent-based general anesthesia. Her postoperative period was uneventful. The receptor status of the excised specimen is found to be positive for estrogen and progesterone receptors and negative for HER2. The prognostic genetic marker recurrence score is 15 suggesting <1% benefit with chemotherapy to prevent a 10-year distant recurrence. She is advised by the oncologist to be started on letrozole and be on follow-up. After about a year, having read an article, she is anxious if the anesthesia she had received would be a risk factor for cancer recurrence or metastasis. How will you approach this patient? (Answer at the end.)

36.2 What Are the Common Survival Metrics Measured in Cancer Patients?

Standardized cancer-related endpoints are required for objective analysis of effect of anesthesia on cancer progression [1].

Overall survival rate (OS): The percentage of people in a study or treatment group who are still alive for a certain period of time after they were diagnosed with or started treatment for cancer. The cause of death is not specified, and it could be related or unrelated to cancer.

Five-year survival rate: It is the overall survival rate at 5 years of diagnosis or commencement of treatment.

Cancer-specific survival rate: The percentage of people in a study or treatment group who have not died from cancer in a specified period of time. Patients who died from causes other than cancer are not counted in this measurement.

Remission: It is the temporary or permanent absence of cancer.

Disease-free survival rate (DFS) or recurrence-free survival (RFS): The percentage of people in complete remission after completion of treatment. It can be further subclassified as biochemical recurrence-free survival (BRFS) or clinical recurrence-free survival (CRFS) based on the metric used to define recurrence/relapse.

Progression-free survival rate (PFS): The percentage of people who did not have new tumor growth or metastasis. The disease may have responded partially or completely to treatment. This includes patients who have stable cancer which does not grow or spread.

A. R. Karthik · S. Bhatnagar (✉)
Department of Onco-Anesthesiology and Palliative Medicine, Dr. BRA IRCH, AIIMS, New Delhi, India

N. Gupta et al. (eds.), *Problem Based Learning Discussions in Onco-Anesthesia and Onco-Critical Care*, https://doi.org/10.1007/978-981-99-6339-3_36

36.3 Briefly Summarize the Immunological Viewpoint of Cancer Recurrence

The patient's innate and adaptive immunity are implicated as the principal line of defense against tumor progression and metastasis. Three phases of the cancer immunoediting process have been postulated—elimination, equilibrium, and escape. In the elimination phase, the immune system detects and kills a developing tumor before it presents clinically. Some tumor cells survive the elimination phase, and the immune system prevents tumor cell outgrowth keeping them in a state of functional dormancy attaining the equilibrium phase. Rarely tumor cells escape the host's immune response and proliferate to become evident clinically. This is termed as the escape phase. Inflammation is a physiologic response to tissue stress situations like infection or tissue damage. Acute inflammation proceeds to the development of adaptive immunity. Chronic inflammation causes genotoxicity, cell proliferation, angiogenesis, and tissue invasion. If left uncontrolled, this can lead to tumor progression. The natural killer (NK) cells derived from lymphocytes play a major role in the recognition and lysis of cancer cells. The CD4+ Th1 cells and CD8+ cytotoxic T lymphocytes also play a role in protection against cancer. Various cytokines like interleukin-2, interleukin-10, interleukin-12, interferons, and tumor necrosis factor-α (TNF-α) protect against tumorigenesis. On the other hand, cytokines like vascular endothelial growth factor (VEGF) and transforming growth factor-β (TGF-β) produced by tumor cells play a role in escape from host immunity [2, 3]. Various other cytokines and immunological mechanisms have been implicated in tumor recurrence.

36.4 How Do the Commonly Used Anesthetic Agents Affect the Immune System?

Regional anesthesia has an opioid-sparing effect and reduces surgery-induced neuroendocrine stress response. It preserves NK cell response and increases antitumorigenic cytokines and inflammatory markers like C-reactive protein (CRP). Local anesthetics inhibit mesenchymal stem cell proliferation and epidermal growth factor receptor (EGFR) pathway. Lignocaine also exerts demethylating properties in vitro like chemotherapeutic agents.

Opioids cause immunosuppression, VEGF-dependent angiogenesis, epidermal growth factor pathway activation, mitogen-activated protein kinase (MAPK) pathway signaling, increased prostaglandin E-2 (PGE-2) production, neuroepithelial cell transforming gene-1 (NET-1) upregulation, nitric oxide (NO) synthesis, and reduced leukocyte transendothelial migration. The degree of immunosuppression of opioids shows considerable variation among themselves with morphine and fentanyl being more immunosuppressive.

Propofol shows antitumorigenic effect in animal studies by inhibition of cyclooxygenase (COX), reduction of hypoxia inducible factor-1α (HIF-1α), enhancing NK cell-mediated killing, and reduction of cancer cell invasiveness.

In vitro studies have demonstrated volatile anesthetic agents to be tumorigenic by increasing insulin like growth factors (IGFs) and HIF-1α. Some evidence has been conflicting with these findings showing that sevoflurane reduced cancer cell motility and invasion by reducing various matrix metalloproteinases. The results of in vitro studies involving inhalational agents have been heterogenous [2].

36.5 Based on Available Evidence, How Are the Anesthetic Agents and Anesthetic Techniques Implicated in Cancer Recurrence?

A meta-analysis of 1 randomized control trial (RCT) and 9 retrospective studies involving a total of 7866 patients with non-small cell lung cancer and breast and esophageal cancers concluded that usage of propofol-based total intravenous anesthesia (TIVA) is associated with better overall survival and disease-free survival [4]. In a meta-analysis of 20 RCTs with 2201 breast cancer patients, propofol-based intravenous anesthesia preserved anti-cancer immunity in comparison to inhalational anesthetics and offered better 2-year recurrence-free survival rates. But long-term outcomes were difficult to be measured given the small sample size [5]. In a systematic review of eight studies in patients undergoing various cancer surgeries, four of which reported overall mortality, it was seen that propofol-based TIVA had favorable survival rates compared to inhalational anesthesia. The quality of evidence was graded low [6]. Another large systematic review and meta-analysis of over 21,000 patients undergoing various cancer surgeries in 12 studies showed that TIVA was associated with slightly lower overall mortality but not with recurrence rates [7].

In a meta-analysis of ten studies in prostate cancer patients undergoing open radical prostatectomy, it was found that there was no reduction in biochemical recurrence-free survival (BRFS) based on anesthesia type. However, overall survival improved if regional anesthesia/analgesia was incorporated into the anesthetic regimen either alone or along with general anesthesia [8]. A systematic review of 15 studies in patients undergoing breast cancer surgery identified that paravertebral block use was associated with reduced inflammation and better immune response when compared with general opioid-based anesthesia, yet there was no influence on tumor recurrence or cancer-related survival [9]. A meta-analysis of 6 RCTs with 3139 patients undergoing various cancer resection surgeries reiterated that adjunctive use of regional anesthesia was not associated with reduced cancer recurrence [10].

A review of 4 studies in 746 patients undergoing major abdominal cancer surgery and surgeries for prostate cancer or colon cancer concluded that the evidence for regional anesthesia to prevent tumor recurrence was inadequate. However, the quality of evidence was graded low for all outcomes [11]. A meta-analysis of 14 studies, many of them in colon cancer, suggested that epidural anesthesia/analgesia was associated with better overall survival but not with recurrence-free survival [12]. Similar results were seen in another meta-analysis of 18 studies involving various cancers [13]. A meta-analysis of 9708 patients in 10 retrospective observational studies involving various cancers compared two groups: one received sole general anesthesia and the other received sole regional anesthesia for cancer surgery. The authors found no significant difference in the overall survival rate, cancer-related mortality, and time to cancer recurrence between the two groups. Since the evidence was of low quality, they could not make any recommendations [14]. On similar lines, a systematic review of six studies involving gastroesophageal cancer surgeries found that there was no convincing evidence to support or refute the usage of epidural anesthesia/analgesia to reduce cancer recurrence [15]. On the contrary, a meta-analysis of 21 studies, majority of them in colorectal cancer, concluded that neuraxial anesthesia with or without general anesthesia had better OS and reduced risk of cancer progression [16]. A meta-analysis of 37 studies, 3 of which were RCTs and 34 observational studies, was done on various late-stage cancers. Data from the RCTs suggested that regional anesthesia was not associated with better overall and disease-free survival, but data from retrospective cohort studies showed an association of regional anesthesia with better overall and disease-free survival rates [17].

A systematic review of 24 studies in patients with breast cancer including preclinical and clinical studies concluded that the contributory evidence for opioid usage (both in the perioperative period and in the chronic pain setting) in cancer recurrence is controversial [18]. A systematic review of 13 studies in patients undergoing colorectal surgery presented that no conclusive evidence was available to recommend against opioid usage in the perioperative period to reduce the risk of tumor recurrence [19].

36.6 Apart from Immunomodulation, How Does Perioperative Anesthesia Care Affect Long-term Oncological Outcomes?

Multimodal prehabilitation measures are required for improving the functional capacity of the cancer patient awaiting cancer surgery. Baseline functional capacity will most likely be reduced due to the disease process per se and neoadjuvant cancer-directed therapy. Prehabilitation will improve the baseline functional capacity and prepare the patient in a better way to tackle and get past the surgical stress period. This will also prepare the patient for early postoperative recovery and quicker return to intended oncologic treatment (RIOT). Timely completion of cancer-directed therapy before and after surgery is essential for preventing cancer recurrence. Hence proper planning of the perioperative journey plays a vital role in preventing cancer recurrence.

Appropriate mode of anesthesia during the intraoperative period is essential to provide an ideal surgical field conducive for major resection and reconstruction. For example, prevention of obturator jerk in urinary bladder carcinoma involving the lateral wall during transurethral resection is essential for adequate tumor clearance and prevention of complications like bladder perforation [20]. Keeping the brain lax during craniotomy is essential for adequate resection of brain tumors. Adequate lung isolation is required for resection of lung tumors.

Enhanced recovery after surgery (ERAS) care pathways should be incorporated in the perioperative period to enable early postoperative recovery and regaining of functional capacity.

36.7 Given the Equivocal Evidence for Anesthesia and Cancer Recurrence, What Should the Perioperative Plan of Action Be?

Our understanding of the effect of various anesthetic agents and techniques with respect to tumorigenesis and tumor prevention is primitive. The complex interplay of various factors in the perioperative period is yet to be elucidated to clarity. Certain interventions like reducing perioperative blood product transfusion in colon cancer patients have convincing evidence. But the evidence for majority of other interventions is equivocal. However, it is the anesthesiologist's responsibility to sail the patient through the storm of surgery with comfort and safety. It is established that surgery is both a physiologically and psychologically stressful situations. Anesthesia reduces the accompanying pain and stress response. Until confirmatory clinical evidence evolves, it is not prudent to deny or favor any particular agent or technique. The perioperative care plan should be personalized to that particular patient and disease process rather than based on preclinical evidence. It is also essential to generate high-quality evidence through well-powered prospective randomized trials with long-term follow-up, since early evidence suggests that anesthesia can be one of the various multifactorial determinants of cancer recurrence.

36.8 How Will you Approach the Patient Given in the Case Scenario?

The evidence for opioid and inhalational agent-based general anesthesia causing breast cancer recurrence is of low quality and inconsistent in clinical studies. The probability of recurrence cannot be reliably established solely based on the anesthetic technique used. Her other oncologic parameters point to a low risk of recurrence. Thus, she can be reassured and counselled to allay her anxiety. She should be encouraged to be on hormonal therapy and follow-up regularly.

References

1. Buggy DJ, Freeman J, Johnson MZ, Leslie K, Riedel B, Sessler DI, et al. Systematic review and consensus definitions for standardised endpoints in perioperative medicine: postoperative cancer outcomes. Br J Anaesth. 2018;121(1):38–44.
2. Sekandarzad MW, van Zundert AAJ, Lirk PB, Doornebal CW, Hollmann MW. Perioperative anesthesia care and tumor progression. Anesth Analg. 2017;124(5):1697–708.
3. Schreiber RD, Old LJ, Smyth MJ. Cancer immunoediting: integrating immunity's roles in cancer suppression and promotion. Science. 2011;331(6024):1565–70.

4. Yap A, Lopez-Olivo MA, Dubowitz J, Hiller J, Riedel B, the Global Onco-Anesthesia Research Collaboration Group, et al. Anesthetic technique and cancer outcomes: a meta-analysis of total intravenous versus volatile anesthesia. Can J Anesth Can Anesth. 2019;66(5):546–61.
5. Pang QY, Duan LP, Jiang Y, Liu HL. Comparison of outcomes after breast cancer surgery between inhalational and propofol-based intravenous anaesthesia: a systematic review and meta-analysis. J Pain Res. 2021;14:2165–77.
6. Soltanizadeh S, Degett TH, Gögenur I. Outcomes of cancer surgery after inhalational and intravenous anesthesia: a systematic review. J Clin Anesth. 2017;42:19–25.
7. Jin Z, Li R, Liu J, Lin J. Long-term prognosis after cancer surgery with inhalational anesthesia and total intravenous anesthesia: a systematic review and meta-analysis. Int J Physiol Pathophysiol Pharmacol. 2019;11(3):83–94.
8. Lee BM, Singh Ghotra V, Karam JA, Hernandez M, Pratt G, Cata JP. Regional anesthesia/analgesia and the risk of cancer recurrence and mortality after prostatectomy: a meta-analysis. Pain Manag. 2015;5(5):387–95.
9. Pérez-González O, Cuéllar-Guzmán LF, Soliz J, Cata JP. Impact of regional anesthesia on recurrence, metastasis, and immune response in breast cancer surgery: a systematic review of the literature. Reg Anesth Pain Med. 2017;42(6):751–6.
10. Lee ZX, Ng KT, Ang E, Wang CY, Binti Shariffuddin II. Effect of perioperative regional anesthesia on cancer recurrence: a meta-analysis of randomized controlled trials. Int J Surg. 2020;82:192–9.
11. Cakmakkaya OS, Kolodzie K, Apfel CC, Pace NL. Anaesthetic techniques for risk of malignant tumour recurrence. Cochrane Database Syst Rev. 2014;(11):CD008877.
12. Chen WK, Miao CH. The effect of anesthetic technique on survival in human cancers: a meta-analysis of retrospective and prospective studies. PLoS One. 2013;8(2):e56540.
13. Sun Y, Li T, Gan TJ. The effects of perioperative regional anesthesia and analgesia on cancer recurrence and survival after oncology surgery: a systematic review and meta-analysis. Reg Anesth Pain Med. 2015;40(5):589–98.
14. Ang E, Ng KT, Lee ZX, Ti LK, Chaw SH, Wang CY. Effect of regional anaesthesia only versus general anaesthesia on cancer recurrence rate: a systematic review and meta-analysis with trial sequential analysis. J Clin Anesth. 2020;67:110023.
15. Pérez-González O, Cuéllar-Guzmán LF, Navarrete-Pacheco M, Ortiz-Martínez JJ, Williams WH, Cata JP. Impact of regional anesthesia on gastroesophageal cancer surgery outcomes: a systematic review of the literature. Anesth Analg. 2018;127(3):753–8.
16. Weng M, Chen W, Hou W, Li L, Ding M, Miao C. The effect of neuraxial anesthesia on cancer recurrence and survival after cancer surgery: an updated meta-analysis. Oncotarget. 2016;7(12):15262–73.
17. Zhang YL, Pei LJ, Sun C, Zhao MY, Che L, Huang YG. Regional anesthesia and cancer recurrence in patients with late-stage cancer: a systematic review and meta-analysis. Chin Med J. 2021;134(20):2403–11.
18. Lucia M, Luca T, Federica DP, Cecilia G, Chiara M, Laura DM, et al. Opioids and breast cancer recurrence: a systematic review. Cancers (Basel). 2021;13(21):5499.
19. Diaz-Cambronero O, Mazzinari G, Cata JP. Perioperative opioids and colorectal cancer recurrence: a systematic review of the literature. Pain Manag. 2018;8(5):353–61.
20. Krishan A, Bruce A, Khashaba S, Abouelela M, Ehsanullah SA. Safety and efficacy of transurethral resection of bladder tumor comparing spinal anesthesia with spinal anesthesia with an obturator nerve block: a systematic review and meta-analysis. J Endourol. 2021;35(3):249–58.

Correction to: Paediatric Case of Mediastinal Mass for USG-/CT-Guided Biopsy

Sachidanand Jee Bharti and Wasimul Hoda

Correction to:
Chapter 22 in: N. Gupta et al. (eds.), *Problem Based Learning Discussions in Onco-Anesthesia and Onco-Critical Care*, https://doi.org/10.1007/978-981-99-6339-3_22

The (first name and last name) of [Wasimul Hoda] was unfortunately published with an error. The initially published version has now been corrected.

The updated version of this chapter can be found at https://doi.org/10.1007/978-981-99-6339-3_22

N. Gupta et al. (eds.), *Problem Based Learning Discussions in Onco-Anesthesia and Onco-Critical Care*, https://doi.org/10.1007/978-981-99-6339-3_37

GPSR Compliance

The European Union's (EU) General Product Safety Regulation (GPSR) is a set of rules that requires consumer products to be safe and our obligations to ensure this.

If you have any concerns about our products, you can contact us on ProductSafety@springernature.com

In case Publisher is established outside the EU, the EU authorized representative is:

Springer Nature Customer Service Center GmbH
Europaplatz 3
69115 Heidelberg, Germany

Batch number: 10731393

Printed by Printforce, the Netherlands